MRI
IN MEDICINE

The Nottingham Conference

MRI
IN MEDICINE
The Nottingham Conference

Edited by
Sir Peter Mansfield, FRS
The University of Nottingham, Nottingham, England

CHAPMAN & HALL

New York • Albany • Bonn • Boston • Cincinnati • Detroit • London • Madrid • Melbourne
Mexico City • Pacific Grove • Paris • San Francisco • Singapore • Tokyo • Toronto • Washington

Library of Congress Cataloging-in-Publication Data

MRI in medicine: the Nottingham conference / edited by Peter Mansfield
          p.   cm.
    Based on the 1st Nottingham Symposium on Magnetic Resonance in Medicine, held April 1994.
    Includes bibliographical references and index.
    ISBN 0-412-07391-9 (alk. paper)
    1. Magnetic resonance imaging--Congresses. I. Mansfield, P. II. Nottingham Symposium on Magnetic Resonance in Medicine (1sr: 1994)
    [DNLM: 1. Magnetic Resonance Imaging--congresses. WN 185 M9388 1995]
    RC78.7.N83M757 1995
    616.07'548--dc20
    DNLM/DLC
    for Library of Congress   95-31244
                                                                                                              CIP

Contents

SECTION II: MRI TECHNIQUES AND APPLICATIONS

Abstracts

SECTION III: METHODS AND APPLICATIONS IN MAGNETIC RESONANCE SPECTROSCOPY

Abstracts

SECTION IV: POSTER PRESENTATIONS

Preface

Since the independent invention of NMR imaging and subsequent publication in 1973 by two groups, one in the UK and one in the United States, the technique renamed magnetic resonance imaging (MRI) has revolutionized clinical diagnostic imaging to the point where it is currently the method of choice for the diagnosis of a range of pathologies, especially in the head and pelvis, in many clinical centers throughout the world. Of course, MRI has much more to offer, especially when combined with spectroscopy, which has also developed over the years and is now widely referred to as magnetic resonance spectroscopy (MRS).

The work described in this volume is based on a two-and-a-half day symposium entitled "The 1st Nottingham Symposium on Magnetic Resonance in Medicine," which took place in April 1994. The original intention of this meeting was to mark the establishment of two new magnetic resonance centers on the University of Nottingham campus, one in the Medical School and one in the Department of Physics, where the original pioneering work in MRI was conceived and implemented. But the meeting was also very successful in bringing together, at a focal point, many of the world's experts to present and discuss their current research work in MRI and MRS. The meeting was organized with plenary sessions followed by three parallel sessions, each of which was started with thematic seminars in three major topics, namely clinical MRI, MRI techniques and applications, and applications of MRS. The seminars were followed by contributed papers in the thematic topics.

Particular subtopics within the clinical MRI session included neuroimaging of the brain, cardiac imaging, and obstetric imaging. A complete list of subtopics is listed in the table of contents. In the MRI techniques and applications sessions, strong emphasis was placed on ultra-high-speed imaging and hyperfast imaging. Many contributions in high-speed imaging included neurofunctional imaging of the brain and, in particular, studies of signal changes within localized cortical regions in response to external stimuli and task activation.

In the MRS session considerable time was devoted to the study of dynamic metabolic pathways and processes. Muscle metabolism was also discussed as was MRS in cancer.

The structure of the program was such that there was sufficient time for some discussion following all the papers. All speakers and presenters of contributed papers and posters were invited to hand in manuscripts at the meeting. Most of the speakers produced a paper that is reproduced in this volume. Each paper is backed by numerous references provided by the authors for future reading.

I express my appreciation to all authors of the articles who kindly accepted our invitation to send in their contributions. I also take this opportunity to thank warmly Professor Axel Haase and the publishers for their enthusiastic response to the idea of publishing the Proceedings of the 1st Nottingham Symposium.

What became abundantly clear during the proceedings was that the general topics of MRI and MRS are still very much in a dynamic state with many exciting applications and new developments on the horizon.

For those of us privileged to participate in the meeting, few will have emerged without a sense of excitement and a greatly heightened appreciation of both the problems and challenges for the future. It is the aim of this volume to convey this sense of excitement and challenge to the reader.

MRI IN MEDICINE

The Nottingham Conference

After-dinner speech: Nottingham NMR recollections

E. R. Andrew

University of Florida, Gainesville, FL 32611, USA

The author notes a concentration of recent NMR-related anniversaries, including the 200th anniversary of the birth of George Green (1793) in Nottingham, the 150th anniversary of the birth of Boltzmann (1844), the 50th anniversary of the discovery of EPR by Zavoisky (1944), the 50th anniversary of the discovery of NMR (1945–1946). He describes how 30 years ago (1963) he introduced NMR to the Physics Department of Nottingham University, where he was joined by P. S. Allen, S. Clough, W. Derbyshire, and P. Mansfield, who over a 20-year period founded a highly successful school of NMR research. He emphasizes the need to explain NMR applications in a comprehensible manner to the general public and he looks forward to new future developments of NMR in medicine.

Keywords: NMR, MR imaging, magnetic resonance in medicine, encyclopedia of NMR, Nottingham, anniversaries.

It is a great pleasure to return to Nottingham where I spent 20 years of my earlier life and I am greatly moved to be the guest of honor this evening. It is perhaps a little like the Biblical return of the prodigal son who, you will remember, having squandered his inheritance in riotous living in a far-off country is welcomed home and the fatted calf is prepared for a welcome feast. Maybe nowadays it would have to be a not-fatted calf or at least a low-fat calf!

I do not know that I have been living particularly riotously in Florida, but we have certainly been living quite agreeably. I can testify that the sun shines brightly there most days, and as Dr. Balaban, Dr. Brady, Dr. Shulman, and others from more northerly states will be happy to be reminded, there is never any snow or ice in Florida, and I do have palm trees outside my Physics Office window, so you can see it is a real hardship for us to live over there! Furthermore, there is no retirement age, so I can spend all my days doing physics and, surprising as this may seem, there is not really much else I would rather be doing.

In case you should think that the University of Florida is just a glorified rest home without academic pretensions, I should mention that we recently put up a sufficiently good show to win, jointly with our colleagues at Florida State University, the competition

Address for correspondence: Department of Physics, 215 Williamson Hall, University of Florida, Gainesville, FL 32611, USA.

for $66 million from the National Science Foundation for the new U.S. National High Magnetic Field Laboratory, which is now built and is open for business. For high-resolution NMR we have a 600-MHz system and a 750-MHz system, a 900-MHz magnet (21 T) is at an advanced state of design, and a 1-GHz system is under consideration. Dr. Geoffrey Bodenhausen is coming from the University of Lausanne to be the laboratory's first NMR Director. So you may like to think of the University of Florida as a potential venue for your next sabbatical leave or to offer us a colloquium or seminar particularly in January or February.

Peter Mansfield said to me that since I am now rather venerable I might be a good person to say something about the early days of NMR in Nottingham. Actually, this seems to be a time when there is a current emphasis on history in our subject. We should note though what the great Scottish scholar Thomas Carlyle said, "History is a distillation of rumour"; his contemporary Bishop William Stubbs was more forthright when he said, "History is a pack of lies"; and as you know Henry Ford was even more succinct in the witness box saying, "History is bunk" [1]. Notwithstanding these warnings, last July in Nottingham, we celebrated the 200th anniversary of an outstanding local mathematical physicist George Green. He was responsible for Green's Theorem in electromagnetism and Green's functions in wide scientific use from quantum electrodynamics to aircraft design. Indeed, our Chairman, Sir Peter Mansfield, in his first major article [2] on magnetic resonance imaging (MRI) made use of Green's functions. George Green did most of his famous work while he was a miller in Nottingham [3], almost entirely self-taught (he only went to school for just over a year), and he did it before going to Cambridge University at the late age of 40. He never married but, nevertheless, had seven children. After graduation, as he was technically a bachelor, he was elected a Fellow of Gonville and Caius College at Cambridge University. Green's large windmill is in working order again and you can visit it while you are here in Nottingham. You can buy a bag of flour ground there and you can bring away a souvenir mug with Green's Theorem engraved on the exterior. During the celebrations last year, a floor tile in Westminster Abbey was dedicated to him, alongside those to Newton, Faraday, Kelvin, and Maxwell, the ultimate accolade.

More recently, we have been celebrating another major physicist with NMR connections, whose 150th birthday fell on 20 February 1994. This was Boltzmann. Boltzmann was Austrian but for a time was Professor of Mathematical Physics at Leipzig in Germany. Heisenberg later occupied this chair, and Felix Bloch, codiscoverer of NMR, obtained his doctorate there with Heisenberg. Felix had a fund of stories about Boltzmann and Heisenberg; he was born shortly before Boltzmann's death in 1906. In NMR we should all venerate Boltzmann who helps us to understand why our NMR signals are rather weak but are, nevertheless, measurable. A colleague of mine in the University of Florida, Yasu Takano, is making NMR measurements on metals down to microkelvin temperatures. Boltzmann is Yasu's friend, at least metaphorically, giving him enormously strong NMR signals.

This year we celebrate the 50th anniversary of the discovery of electron paramagnetic resonance (EPR) by Zavoisky in Kazan, Russia, in 1944 [4]. It is really quite extraordinarily remarkable that he was doing this work there at the height of the Second World War. The next AMPERE Congress will be held in Kazan in late August 1994 as a 50th anniversary celebration meeting.

Next, in 1995–1996, we celebrate the 50th anniversary of the discovery of NMR by Purcell, Torrey, and Pound and by Bloch, Hansen, and Packard [5, 6]. ISMAR (the International Society of Magnetic Resonance) is organizing this celebration at its conference in Sydney in July 1995. There is no special connection with Sydney, but it is a nice place to go and there is a strong concentration of NMR, MRI, and MRS in the New South Wales area.

The 50th anniversary of NMR is being given a great send-off with the planned publication in 1995 of the new *Encyclopedia of NMR* by Wiley. There will be about 600 entries written by some 400 experts. The world community of NMR is not enormous and as Ted Becker, one of the editors, pointed out to me, the effect has been that NMR work all around the world has temporarily come to a standstill for several months while everyone is furiously writing their sections of the encyclopedia to meet their deadlines.

Last year, 1993, we celebrated in the Physics Department at Nottingham University the 30th anniversary of doing NMR. My predecessor here as Professor of Physics and Head of Department was Professor L. F. Bates, an authority on classical magnetism. In the department there were groups working on electron paramagnetic resonance, acoustic paramagnetic resonance, and ferromagnetic resonance, and Professor Kenneth Stevens headed a group on related theory, but there was no nuclear magnetic resonance, a gap we proceeded to fill. When I came in 1963, I was very fortunate to find a nice new large physics building, money for new equipment, and for four new academic appointments in my field. Viewed from the stringencies of 1994 such a situation can only be regarded as quite remarkable. These four appointments were filled with very able NMR practitioners who have in different ways made their mark on the subject.

The first appointment was Stan Clough who came with me from the University of Wales. He became a Professor of Physics at Nottingham and was later Head of Department. He is a foremost authority on tunneling in NMR. Then we appointed Peter Allen who studied molecular dynamics at low temperatures by NMR until he emigrated to Canada in 1982. He is now at the University of Alberta where he is Professor of Applied Sciences in Medicine and is chairman of the department. Next came Bill Derbyshire who pioneered the NMR measurement of water in muscle, meat, and foodstuffs and now works with Rank Hovis MacDougall, as well as being a Professor of Food Science in Nottingham University. Finally, to complete our NMR Gang of Four (or Five including myself) was Peter Mansfield and his has been a great success story.

I first met Peter when he was a research student with Jack Powles at Queen Mary College, London and Jack asked me to be Peter's Ph.D. external examiner. I was very impressed and I invited him to join us here in 1964; so this is Peter's 30th year in Nottingham. Following on from the discovery of the solid echo with Jack, Peter's first work here was to develop multiple-pulse NMR in solids. The much sharpened responses from solids led him to suggest NMR diffraction with a field gradient to give spatial information. His first article on this topic [7], which included a one-dimensional NMR image, appeared in 1973, the same year as Paul Lauterbur's first paper on NMR imaging in *Nature* [8]. Since that first article, Peter has stayed at the forefront of NMR imaging ever since, introducing selective excitation, devising the fastest imaging methods using EPI, developing NMR microscopy, and overcoming the eddy current problem with active shielding. He has successfully patented his inventions to the benefit of the university and the British Exchequer. He has received many honors for his contributions, especially election to the Royal Society and his knighthood last year, and we are all very proud of him.

Our Gang of Five NMR practitioners held together for almost 20 years and I take great pride in the school of NMR research which developed from our separate but collective activities.

As we are meeting as a Conference on Magnetic Resonance in Medicine, it may be of interest to mention that the very first international conference on NMR imaging was held here in Nottingham in April 1976, 18 years ago [9]. Besides the Nottingham contingent, we had Paul Lauterbur from Stonybrook, Richard Ernst from Zurich, Hugh Clow from EMI, Jim Hutchison from Aberdeen, two colleagues from Holland, in fact, representation from almost all the groups then working, a total of about 25 people. The Society of Magnetic Resonance in Medicine attracts 100 times that number to its annual meetings, a measure of the growth of the subject.

There is no doubt that medical MRI has brought NMR to the notice and practical experience of the general public just like X-rays and ultrasound. We now have an educational responsibility to explain to the man in the street in an elementary way how it works. I was much intrigued by the recent approach of the Minister for Science, Mr. William Waldegrave, which I found most refreshing. British high-energy physicists wanted tens of millions of pounds to look for the Higgs boson. This could have come straight out of the comedy series "Yes, Minister," popular across the Atlantic, too. The Minister wanted to know what the Higgs boson was and why it was desirable to find it. He is not a scientist, but he has a first class honors degree in Greats at Oxford, so he is a classic example of the intelligent layman. Not being very satisfied with the answers, he issued a challenge at the Institute of Physics congress. He offered a bottle of champagne for the best answer in comprehensible terms as to what is a Higgs boson and why look for it, on a single sheet of paper. It attracted many entries and the five best, all given bottles of champagne, were printed in *Physics*

World [10] and make very good reading. It might be of interest to offer a bottle of champagne for the best explanation in terms comprehensible to the ordinary reader on one sheet of paper of, let us say, "Interventional MRI." After all, it will be an expensive business and will use public money.

For those of you visiting Nottingham for the first time, for what else besides the university and Magnetic Resonance is Nottingham famous? My mother worked in Nottingham as a photographer some 80 years ago and she used to say Nottingham was famous for four things: Robin Hood, lace, bicycles, and pretty girls. At that time (1907), she was probably one of them. But we can add to this list: D.H. Lawrence; Jesse Boot and Boots the Chemists; William Booth, the founder of the Salvation Army; Torville and Dean, the international skaters; dare I mention Players cigarettes whose contribution to excise duty is said to pay for about one-third of the cost of the National Health Service [11]; Lord Byron; Nottingham Forest football team, and one could go on.

Of all of these, Robin Hood reigns supreme and fits my historical theme. The sceptics should know (and I quote from the official brochure of the City of Nottingham [12]) that reference has been found to him in historical records back to A.D. 1230, where he is described as a fugitive from the law; he is said to have lived from 1160 to 1247. You can visit Edwinstowe Church, where Robin married Maid Marian. The Major Oak Tree, estimated at around 1400 years old, where Robin and his Merrie Men congregated, still stands nearby. You can see Little John's grave at Hathersage and Will Scarlett's in Blidworth and Friar Tuck's Well at Fountaindale. There is still a Sheriff of Nottingham, elected annually. What more proof do you need? You should visit Robin Hood's statue just outside the Castle wall in the city center and pay your respects.

As T. S. Eliot said, "Time present and time past are both present in time future" [1]. So let me end with a glimpse into the future opening up for Magnetic Resonance in Medicine. We may for example contemplate the following scenario. The famous neurosurgeon is awakened by telephone at 2 A.M. and is told of the necessity of an emergency operation. He is told that the patient has been readied in the double-doughnut interventional MRI magnet. So he jumps out of bed to his bedside on-line MRI workstation. He inserts his robotically controlled nonmagnetic miniscalpel through the keyhole prepared in the patient's cranium. He watches on his real-time 3D MRI display as he deftly weaves his scalpel around arteries and nerves until he reaches the lesion, which he cuts neatly away and makes good. Having retrieved his scalpel, he leaves his resident back in the hospital to stitch up the small entry hole, while 10 miles away he returns to bed and to sleep. Maybe in the 21st century, not so far off, this will, in fact, happen.

So, finally, let me congratulate Sir Peter on initiating this splendid series of symposia which will give us all an excellent excuse to return to Nottingham from time to time and learn about the latest advances in Magnetic Resonance in Medicine.

REFERENCES

1. *The Oxford Dictionary of Quotations,* 2nd ed. pp. 126, 197, 209, and 517. London: Oxford University Press, pages 126, 197, 209, 517 (1956).
2. Mansfield P, Grannell PK (1975) *Phys Rev B* **12**: 3618.
3. Cannell DM (1993) *George Green, Mathematician and Physicist* 1793–1841. London: Athlone Press.
4. Zavoisky EK, Altshuler SA, Kozyrev BM (1944) *Zhur Ekspt Theor Fiz* **10**: 121 (*in Russian*); see also Zavoisky, E (1965) J Phys USSR **9**: 211 and and Zavoisky, E (1946) J Phys USSR **10,** 170 and 197 (*in English*).
5. Purcell EM, Torrey HC, Pound RV (1946) *Phys Rev* **69**: 37.
6. Bloch F, Hansen WW, Packard ME (1946) *Phys Rev* **69**: 127.
7. Mansfield P, Grannell PK (1973) *J Phys C* **6**: L422.
8. Lauterbur P (1973) *Nature* **262**: 190.
9. Andrew ER (1985) *Proc Roy Soc Lond B* **225**: 399.
10. Higgs boson (1993) *Physics World,* September, page 26.
11. Bryson E (1974) *Portrait of Nottingham.* p. 23. London: Robert Hale.
12. *Robin Hood* (1993) City of Nottingham Publicity and Information Office.

The significance of MRI in myelin disorders

J. Valk[1*] and M.S. van der Knaap[2]

Departments of [1]Diagnostic Radiology and [2]Department of Child Neurology Free University Hospital, Amsterdam, The Netherlands

Systematic analysis of white matter changes on magnetic resonance (MR) images has increased the diagnostic quality of MR interpretation. For that purpose, structural elements were defined, relevant to the distinction of disease groups. Per disease group histograms were obtained of the frequency of involvement of these structural elements. On the reverse, this database could be used as the basis of an expert system. Loaded with the data of a new case, the program comes up with a differential diagnosis and probability percentage with confidence intervals per diagnostic item. The program has helped in identifying MR patterns in rare disorders.

Keywords: white matter disorders, myelin disorders, MRI of myelin disorders, pattern recognition.

PATTERN RECOGNITION

Histologically distinction is possible between a selective white matter disorders and selective myelin disorders. This distinction cannot be made in most cases by magnetic resonance imaging (MRI). We will, therefore, use white matter disorders (WMD) as a heading, including myelin disorders.

MRI has high sensitivity in visualizing WMD. To improve the specificity, we developed a systemic approach to the MR analysis of WMD [1]. Structural elements were defined relevant to distinguishing between entities. A scorings list was prepared and each of 43 items was scored per patient. The obtained data were collected in a database, which made it subsequently possible to obtain histograms of the frequency of involvement of structured elements per disease group (Fig. 1). Additional characteristics, such as calcification, cyst formation, necrosis, and hemorrhage were also scored. The program could now be used as an expert system. When data of a new case were imported in the program, the computer came up with a diagnostic suggestion, a probability percentage, and confidence intervals. All cases in the database (1483) were verified histologically or by laboratory investigations.

* Address for correspondence: Department of Diagnostic Radiology, Free University Hospital, P.O. Box 7057, 1007 MB Amsterdam, The Netherlands.

CLASSIFICATION

To use a pattern recognition program one obviously needs a practical classification of the concerned WMD. We proposed such a classification in previous work [1, 2].

WMD can be subdivided into acquired and hereditary disorders. The hereditary disorders can, in our opinion, best be classified by the cellular substructure, the organelle, in which the deficient enzyme is normally present. Accordingly, we distinguish lysosomal, peroxisomal, mitochondrial, and cytoplasmic disorders, disorders with a nuclear enzyme defect, and disorders of unknown etiology.

In the category of organic acid and amino acid metabolism disorders, the locations of the defect are not uniform and are not always known. This group is, therefore, treated as a separate entity.

The acquired disorders are clustered as inflammatory–infectious, toxic–metabolic, hypoxic–ischemic, and traumatic WMD. This classification serves its purpose for the pattern-recognition program and leaves enough space to integrate new findings.

LYSOMAL STORAGE DISORDERS

In lysosomal storage disorders, specific catabolic enzymes are absent and this causes the accumulation of metabolites. Four major categories of lysosomal storage disorders can be distinguished: the sphingolipido-

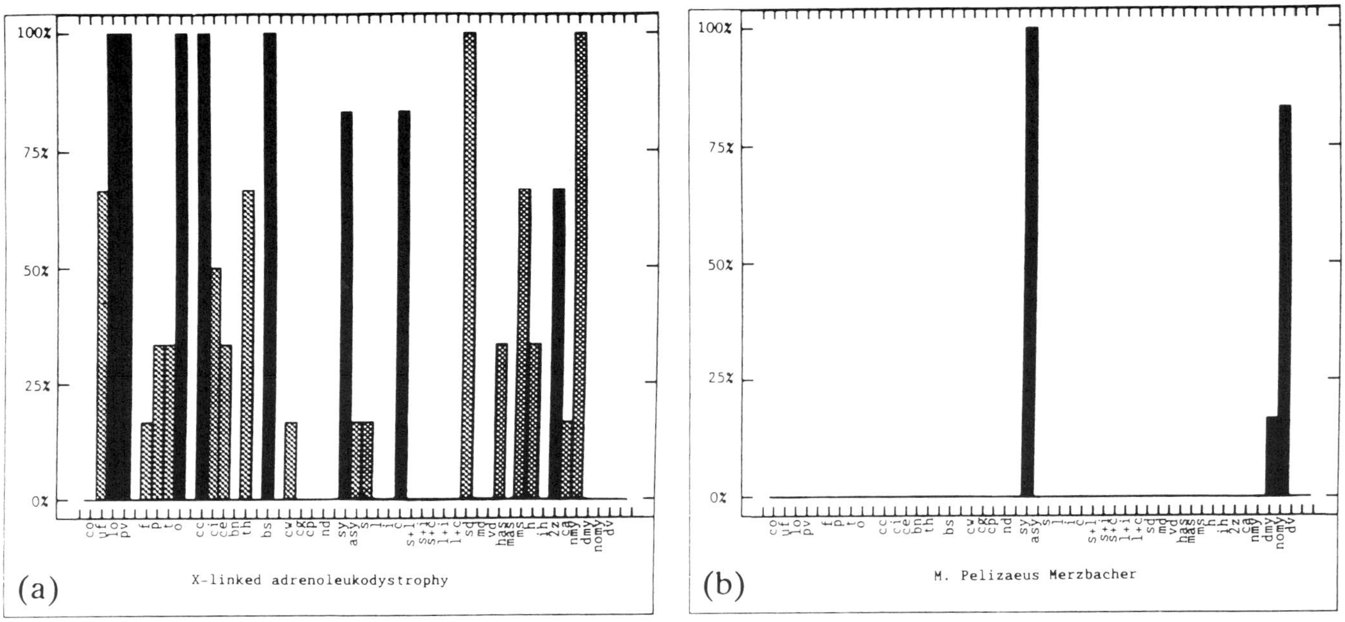

Fig. 1. Computer histograms of the frequency of involvement of structural elements in X-linked adrenoleukodystrophy and Pelizaeus–Merzbacher's disease.

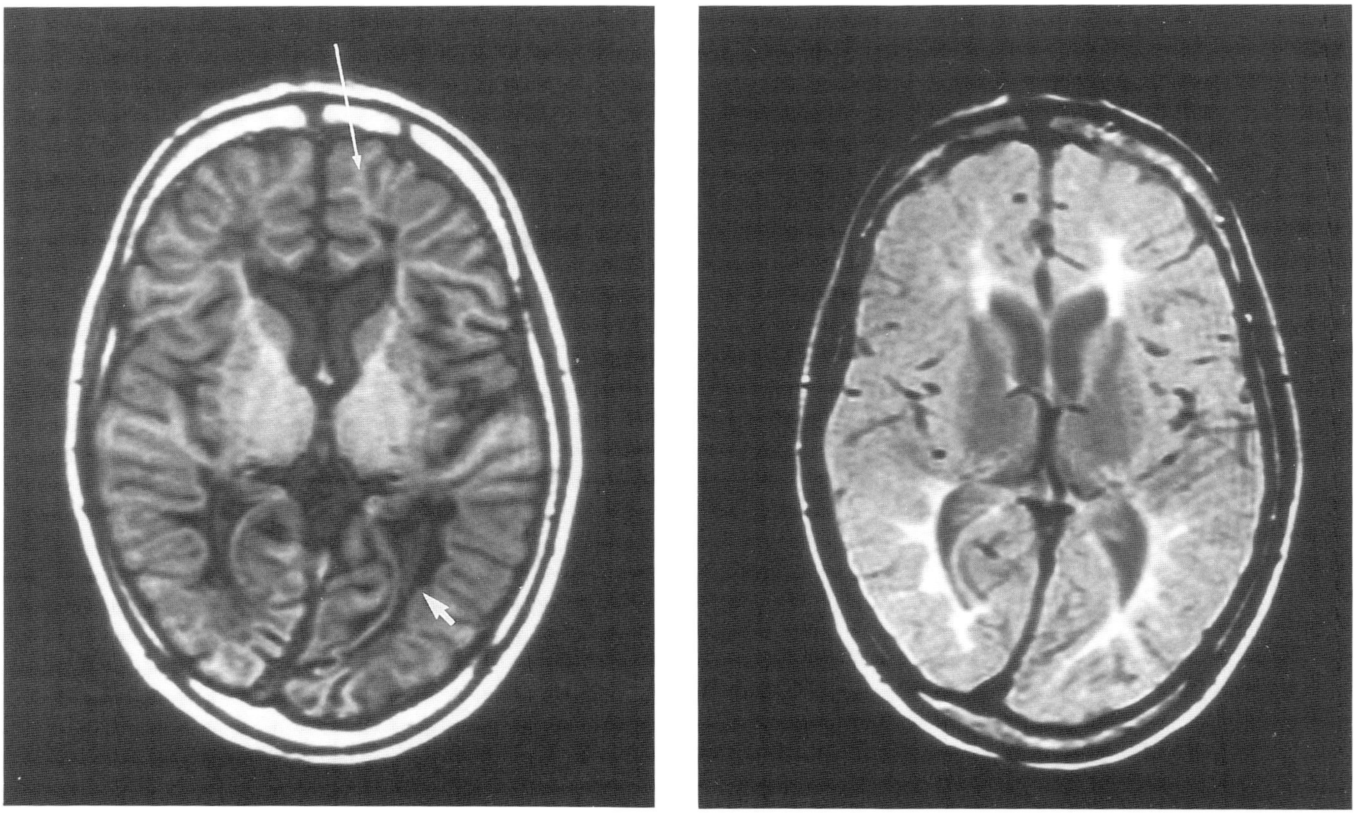

Fig. 2. Transverse T_1-weighted (a) and T_2-weighted (b) images in a patient with metachromatic leukodystrophy. Periventricular area with high signal intensity on the T_2-weighted image. The arcuate fibers are spared in the beginning [arrow in (a)].

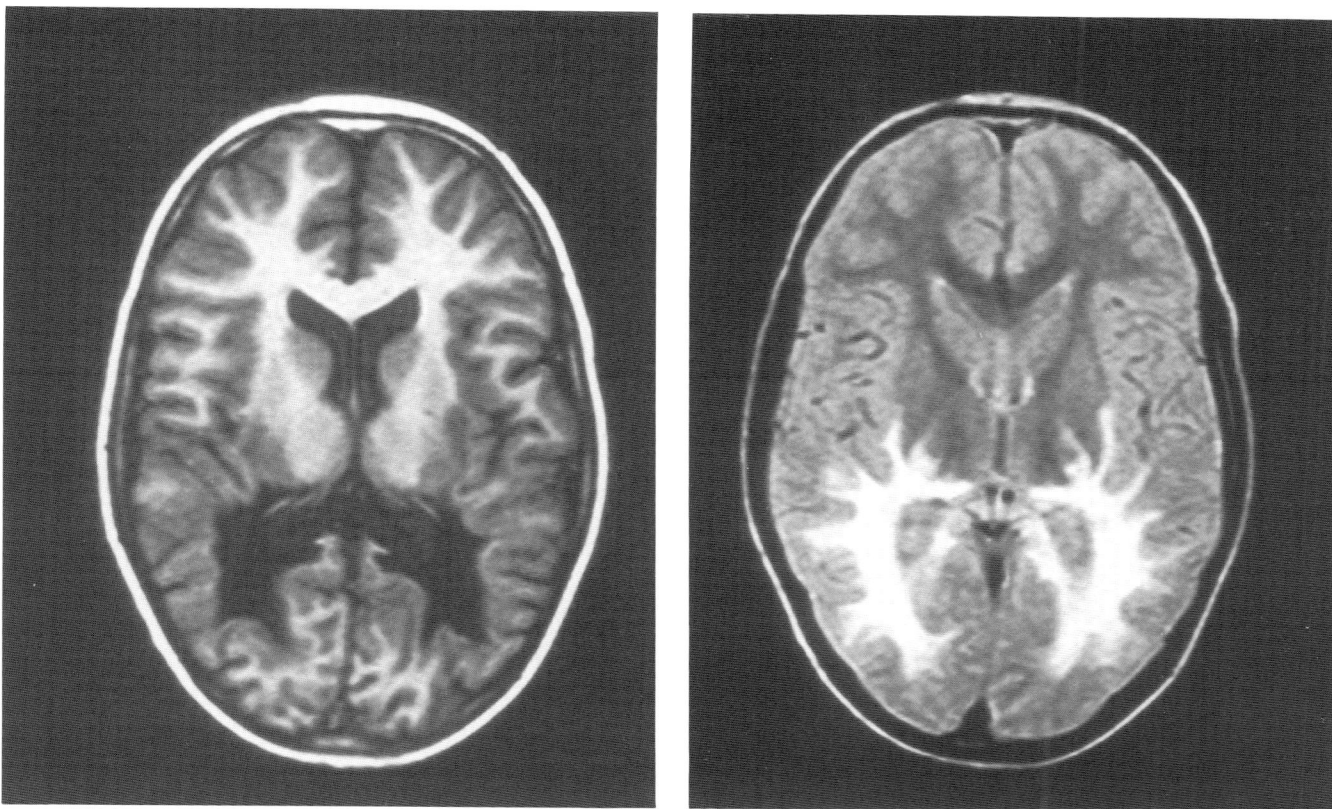

Fig. 3. Transverse T_1-weighted (a) and T_2-weighted (b) images in a patient with X-linked adrenoleukodystrophy. Typical bilateral occipital involvement, symmetrical, confluent, with dorsoventral gradient.

ses, the glycoproteinoses, the mucolipidoses, and the mucopolysacharidoses. A fifth category comprises various storage disorders involving glycogen, cystine, and long-chain fatty acid esters.

Among the sphingolipdoses, the MRI characteristics of two forms of leukodystrophy were described during the early phase of MRI development: metachromatic leukodystrophy and globoid cell leukodystrophy (Krabbe's disease) (Fig. 2) [2]. The MRI patterns of these disorders are now well established: symmetrical, confluent, periventricular lesions, spreading centrifugally, sparing the U-fibers [2, 3].

Gradually, more information is becoming available about the other lysosomal storage disorders. There have been reports on other sphingolipidoses, such as Fabry's disease and GM_2 gangliosidoses [4, 5], on some of the glycoproteinoses, such as fucosidosis and mannosidosis [6], and on the mucopolysaccharidoses, for example, Hunter's disease and Hurler's disease [7]. In five patients with Hurler's disease, cystic areas were described in the centrum semiovale, peritrigonal white matter, corpus callosum, and pericallosal region, corresponding to histological findings [8].

PEROXISOMAL DISORDERS

Over 40 enzymes have been identified within peroxisomes. Peroxisomes catalyze the oxidation of very-long-chain fatty acids; in most peroxisomal disorders, the failure to do so is prominent.

A number of MR patterns have emerged, of which some can be considered either pathognomonic for a specific disorder, as in X-linked adrenoleukodystrophy, or highly characteristic for a group of disorders, as in adrenomyeloneuropathy and Refsum's disease. The various patterns of peroxisomal disorders have been analyzed [9], and three can be distinguished: first, neuronal migration disturbances in combination with hypomyelination, dysmyelination, or demyelination; second, symmetrical demyelination of the posterior limb of the internal capsule, cerebellar white matter and brainstem tracts, and a variable involvement of cerebral hemispheres (Fig. 3); and third, symmetrical demyelination, exhibiting two zones, starting in the occipital area and spreading outward and forward with involvement of brainstem tracts [10].

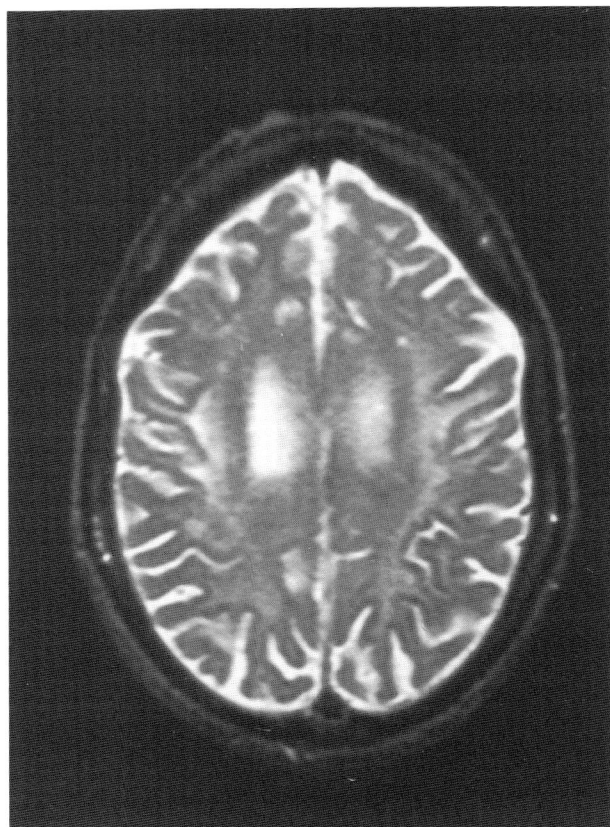

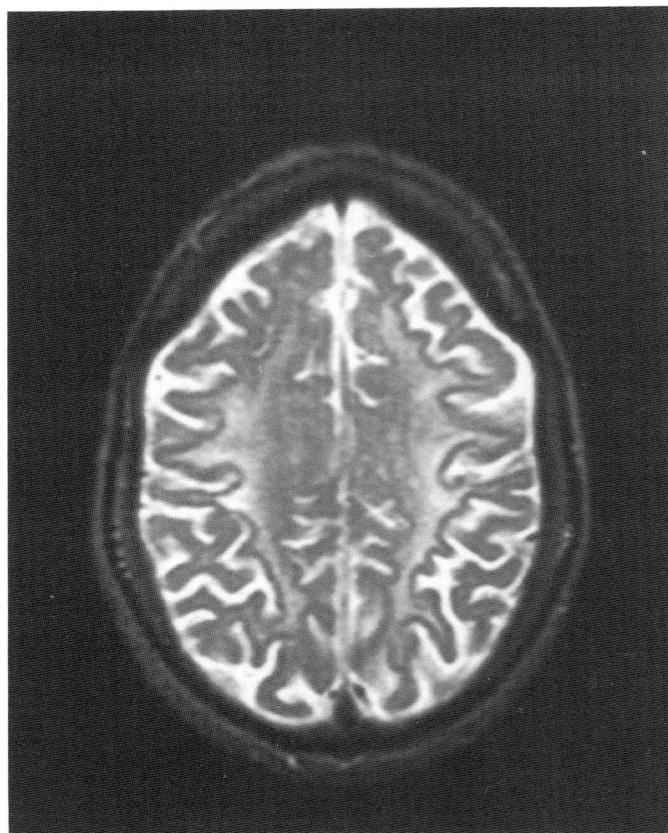

Fig. 4. Two T_2-weighted transverse images in patient with a mitochondrial disorder, Kearns–Sayre syndrome, showing the typical involvement of the arcuate fibers.

With a few exceptions of very rare disorders, MRI of most of the known peroxisomal disorders involving the brain has now been presented.

MITOCHONDRIAL DISORDERS

There is a wide variety of mitochondrial disorders, with considerable overlap [11]. Several encephalopathic forms can be distinguished clinically: mitochondrial encephalopathy, lactic acidosis, and strokelike episodes (MELAS); myoclonic epilepsy and ragged-red fibers (MERRF); the Kearns–Sayre syndrome (KSS) with a progressive ophthalmoplegia, retinal degeneration, cardiac defects, and encephalopathic signs; and Leigh's syndrome, a subacute necrotizing encephalopathy.

The MRI pattern of MELAS is not typical. Infarctlike lesions with an atypical distribution occurring at a young age suggests MELAS. Also, extensive cortical laminar necrosis has been described, bordered by gliotic tissue [12]. In MERRF, the MRI pattern is indistinct. A vacuolating myelinopathy may be seen in the central and cerebellar white matter, as well as the cerebellar peduncles, together with degeneration of the dentate nucleus. In KSS, extensive calcifications are reported using computer tomography (CT) and severe involvement of the white matter using MRI (Fig. 4). Leigh's syndrome is not caused by the failure of a single enzyme but may result from many mitochondrial defects. The lesions are located in the basal ganglia, brainstem tectum and tegmentum, periaqueductal gray matter, substantia nigra, thalamus, dentate nucleus, and spinal cord [13]. There is a remarkable resemblance to the distribution of lesions in Wernicke's encephalopathy, with the exception of the mammilary bodies, which are not involved in Leigh's syndrome.

DISORDERS OF ORGANIC ACID AND AMINO ACID METABOLISM

Disorders of organic acid and amino acid metabolism form a heterogeneous group. Many of the enzymes

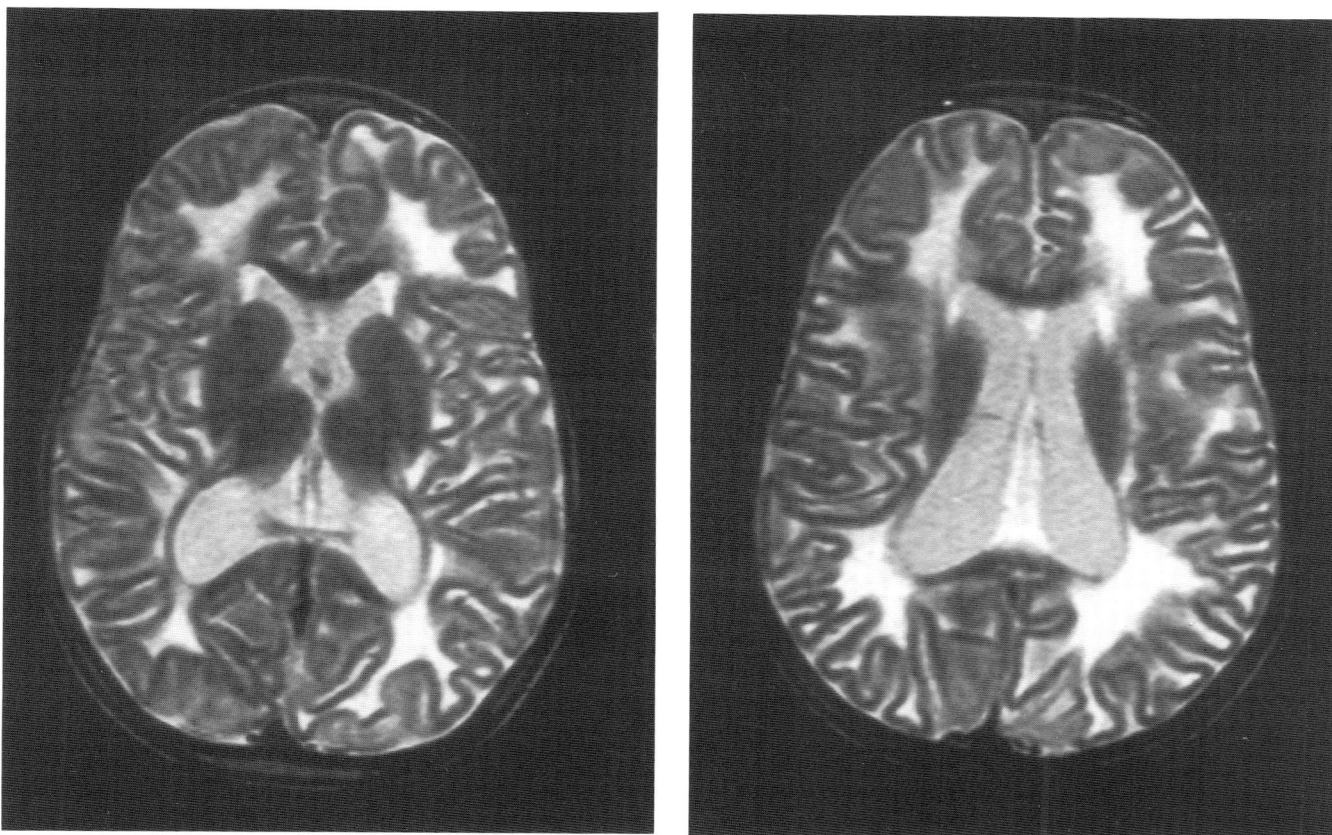

Fig. 5. Two T_2-weighted transverse images showing the typical image of white matter swelling caused by either vacuolating myelinopathy, swelling of astrocytes or increased intercellular water. These images can be seen in Canavan's disease, and in a number of other disorders.

involved are located in the cytoplasm, but a number of enzymes are mitochondrial or peroxisomal, and the location of others is unknown. Therefore, certain organic acidurias may occur in peroxisomal or mitochondrial dysfunction.

Many new characteristic MRI patterns have been reported in this group of disorders, undoubtedly related to the nature and location of the enzymatic defect and the consequences of the resulting biochemical derangement. First, there is a group with prevalent lesions in the arcuate fibers, which are confluent and generalized or patchy and irregular. This pattern can be with or without cerebellar involvement. Second, there is a group of disorders with preferential involvement of the basal ganglia, in particular the caudate nucleus and the putamen, and combined with WMD. Third, there is a group with periventricular white matter lesions. Fourth, there are disorders with WMD and calcifications. Finally, there is an unusual pattern with two kinds of edema having a typical pattern of spread. The manifestations described may be accompanied by other abnormalities, such as pericerebral fluid

collections, arachnoid cysts, cerebellar hypoplasia, and corpus callosum agenesis. We will mention some examples briefly.

In some cases, there is a tendency for primary involvement of the most recently formed myelin, i.e., the subcortical arcuate fibers. This, for example, is seen in Canavan's disease, L-2-hydroxyglutaric aciduria, and other conditions that share a vacuolating myelinopathy histologically (Fig. 5). In Canavan's disease, the involvement of the arcuate fibers is symmetrical and homogeneous. The spread of the disease is in most cases centripetal. However, two cases have been reported with a more central beginning of the disease [14]. In L-2-hydroxyglutaric aciduria, the arcuate fiber involvement is irregular, leading to a rather specific pattern that should suggest the possibility of this type of disorder (Fig. 6).

In another group of organic and amino acidopathies, the deficiency of mitochondrial proteins affects the energy metabolism of the cells. The basal ganglia, in particular the caudate nucleus and the putamen, are extremely susceptible to such effects. This has been

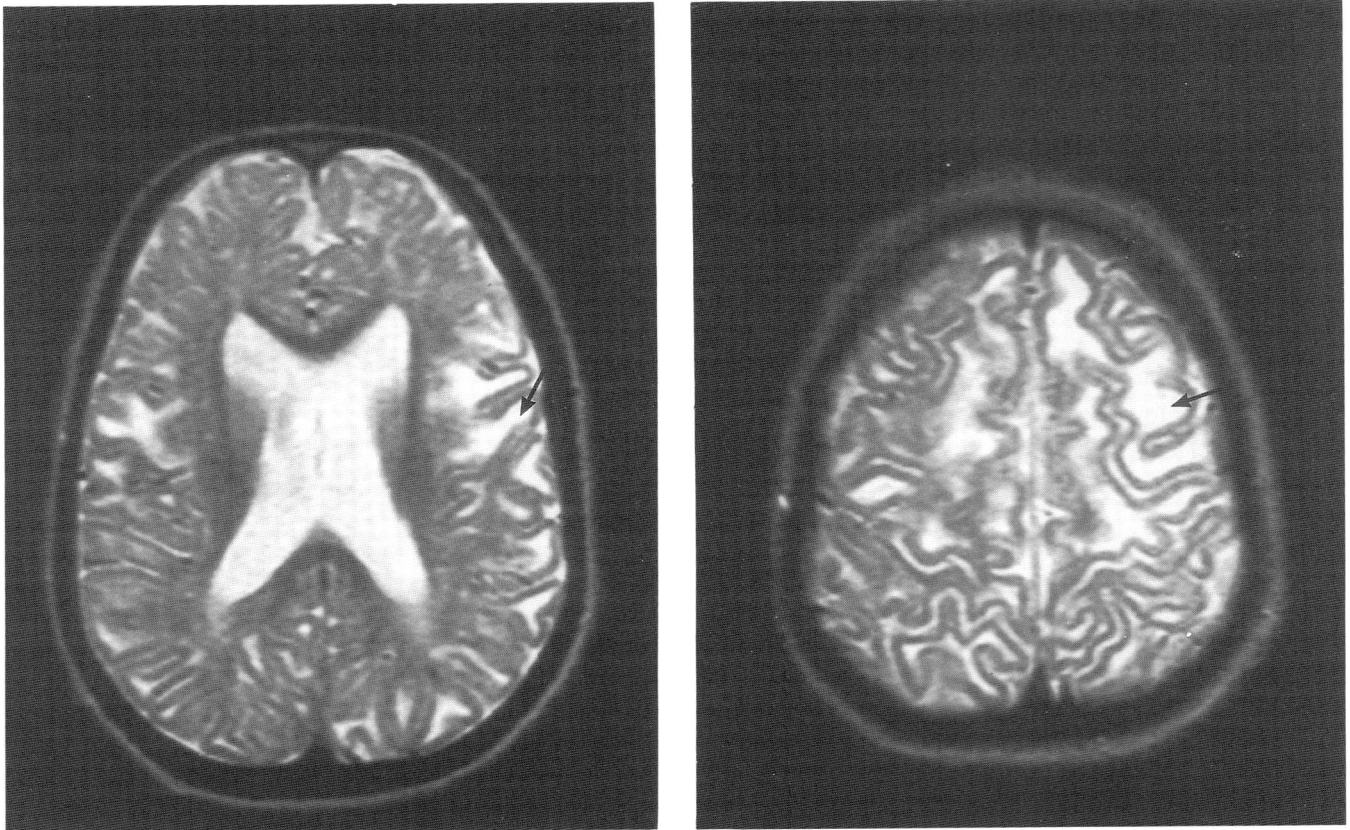

Fig. 6. Pattern recognition helped in finding highly characteristics patterns for rare disorders. In these two T_2-weighted transverse images irregular white matter swelling direct subcortical is seen. Together with a number of other features the images are diagnostic of L-2OH-glutaric acidemia.

reported in glutaric aciduria type I, together with the presence of bilateral arachnoid cysts and frontotemporal atrophy [15]. Involvement of basal nuclei is also seen in methylmalonic acidemia [16].

In other cases, the lesions are located in the periventricular region. Phenylketonuria is a good example. A number of reports have been published on the long-term effects of phenylketonuria in patients in whom the dietary restrictions were not fully implemented [17, 18–20]. The MRI changes in the white matter were located mainly in the periventricular frontal and occipital white matter. There was no close relationship between the severity of the MRI signal changes and the clinical condition. In a variant of phenylketonuria, dihydropteridine reductase deficiency, extensive bilateral calcifications have been reported [21] in addition to severe periventricular white matter changes.

Maple syrup urine disease shows very specific CT and MRI patterns, initially with generalized, diffuse edema, in combination with localized, more severe edema involving the deep cerebellar white matter, the dorsal part of the brainstem, the cerebral peduncles,

and the dorsal limb of the internal capsule. This edema disappears during the second month of life [22], leaving atrophy behind. In other amino and organic acidopathies, prevalent atrophy has been described, for example, in nonketotic hyperglycinemia [23].

The examples given here demonstrate sufficiently that in the organic and amino acidopathies, various patterns can develop. A further subdivision of this category in relation to the specific biochemical action that results from the enzymatic defect would probably lead to more homogeneous subgroups with fitting MRI.

MISCELLANEOUS

In both Pelizaeus–Merzbacher disease, a disorder of proteolipid protein synthesis, and Alexander's disease, presumably primarily a disorder of astrocytes, the recognition of the MRI pattern can prompt diagnosis *in vivo* [24–28]. MRI reflects beautifully the histological findings in these diseases (Fig. 7).

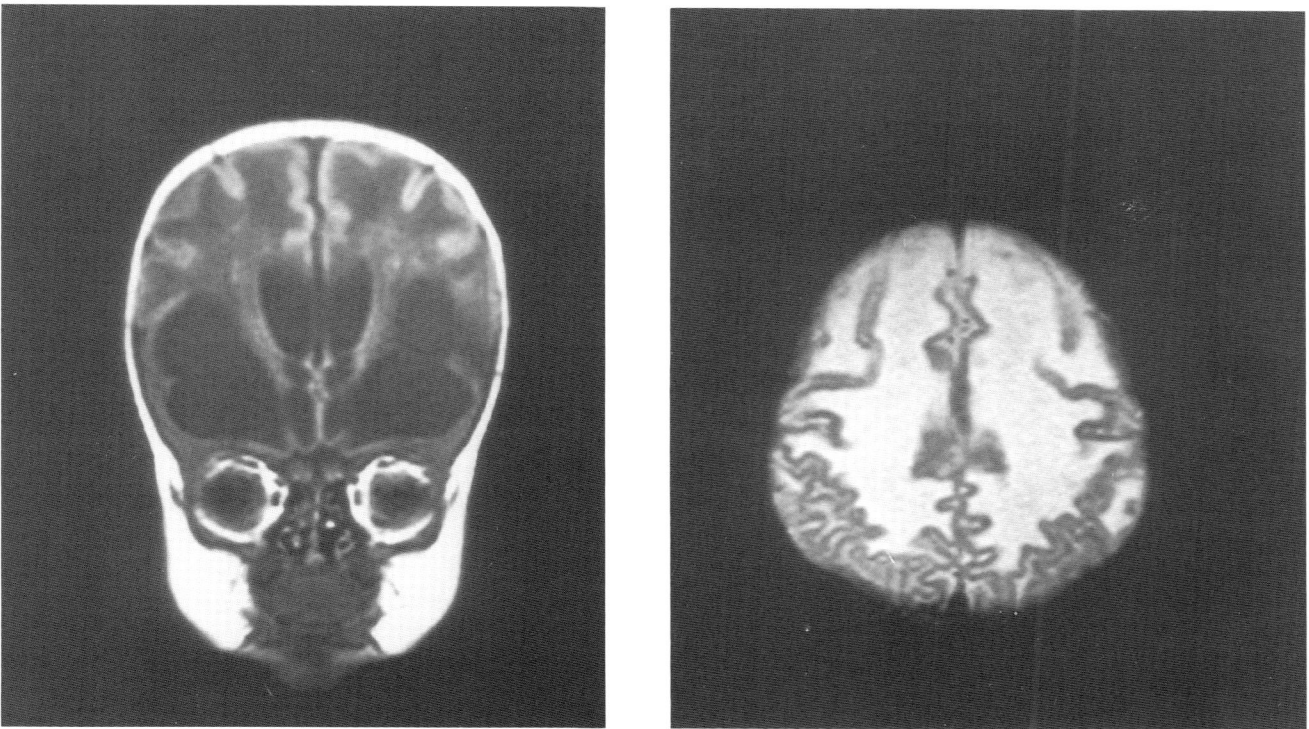

Fig. 7. T_1-weighted coronal (a) and T_2-weighted transverse (b) images in patient with Alexander's disease. The swelling of the white matter is caused by swollen astrocytes. There is a ventrodorsal gradient; in the frontal and temporal regions the lesions become easily cystic.

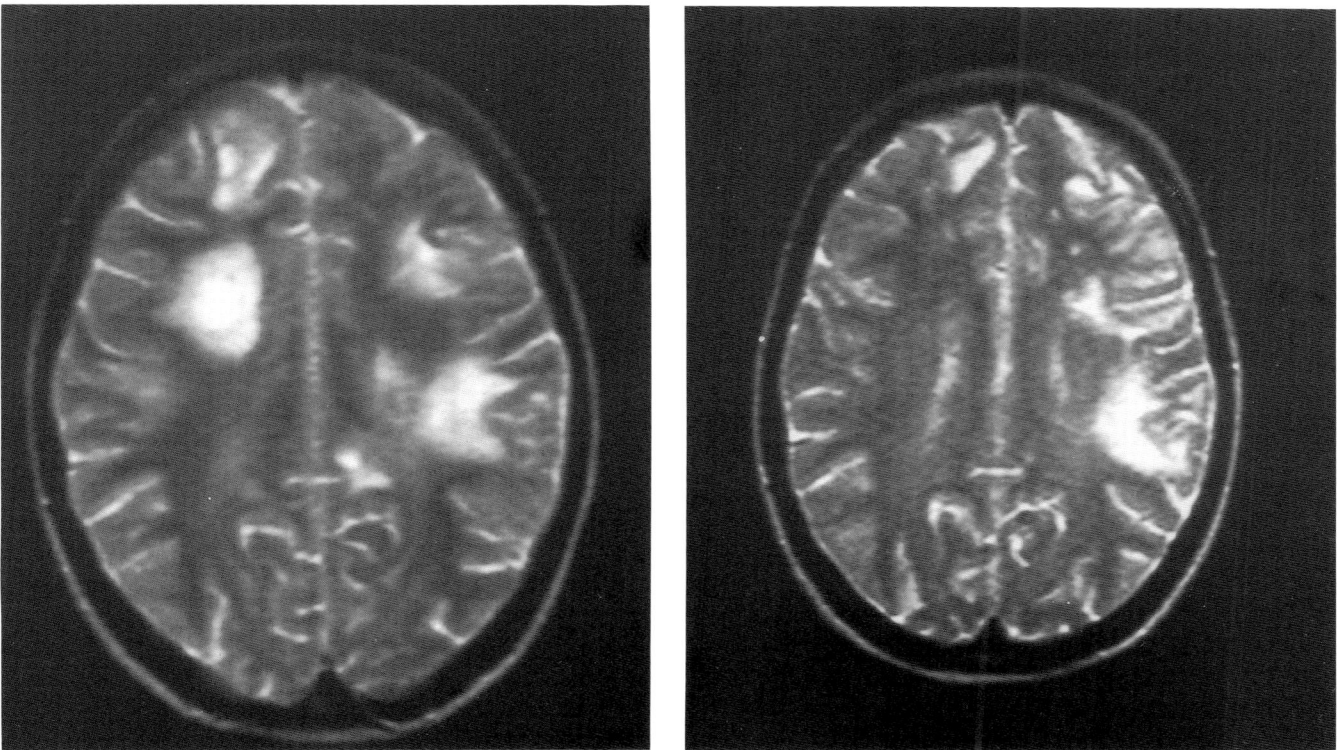

Fig. 8. Two T_2-weighted transverse images in two different patients with acute disseminated encephalitis. Large, irregular, asymmetric, confluent lesions, of which some may enhance.

In a number of myelin disorders, MRI expression of the underlying white matter swelling is striking. We have seen this generalized or focal expansion of the white matter in Canavan's disease, L-2-hydroxyglutaric aciduria, pyruvate carboxylase deficiency, congenital muscular dystrophy, and toxic heroin encephalopathy. In all these cases there is swelling of the white matter, but the image pattern differs from that of vasogenic or cytotoxic edema. In vasogenic edema the typical digitation of the edema is seen, often in combination with the underlying cause of this type of edema. Cytotoxic edema is intracellular, caused by anoxia or intoxication of the cell, and involves both gray and white matter; it causes loss of distinction between the two and has a moderate mass effect. Vacuolating leukoencephalopathy causes a mild swelling of the white matter, expanding the arcuate fibers and leading to a typical image of the stretched cortical lining. The swelling seen in Alexander's disease is due to astrocytic swelling with identical MR features.

Recently, the value of neuroimaging in metabolic disease affecting the central nervous system has been summarized in an editorial [29]. We agree with Naidu and Moser that continued interaction between clinicians, neuroradiologists, and neuroscientists leads to improved understanding and delineation of various disorders and their phenotypes. This, in turn, should lead to earlier recognition and more effective therapeutic intervention and genetic counseling.

ACQUIRED WHITE MATTER DISORDERS

Noninfectious–inflammatory disorders

Among the noninfectious–inflammatory disorders, multiple sclerosis (MS) in its various forms has rightfully obtained most attention, thanks to the diagnostic role of MRI, but also to the emerging role of gadolinium-DTPA (Gd-DTPA)-enhanced MRI to monitor the effects of treatment in MS [30, 31]. MRI may show dissemination in time and space of lesions and contribute to the diagnosis of laboratory-supported definite MS. Its role is then comparable to that of other laboratory tests. Gd-DTPA-enhanced MRI, however, is a better monitor of subclinical activity of lesions than any other noninvasive test. The confidence of the diagnosis of MS using MRI and the correlation with clinical symptoms have long been considered to be rather poor. Recently, however, it appears that the diagnosis of MS can be made with more confidence using MRI if specific conditions are met [32–37]. Attention has been drawn to cases of MS in young children and adolescents, by no means a rare occur-

rence [38–40]. Confirmation also has been obtained about quite a number of other diseases mimicking MS lesions on MRI, such as acute disseminated encephalomyelitis (Fig. 8), neurosarcoidosis, all types of vasculitis, tropical spastic paraparesis, Lyme disease, amyloid angiopathy, and chronic demyelinating polyneuropathy [41–47]. The question of the true extent of MS plaques and the quality of the apparently noninvolved white matter has been addressed recently with diffusion imaging. It is too early to establish the role of this technique, but it certainly shows that MRI will continue to provide us with new information at the molecular level [48–51]. Magnetization transfer imaging may be a new indirect way to look at the biochemistry of membranes and remyelination, but this method still has to prove its clinical relevance. Magnetic resonance spectroscopy (MRS) is coming of age and has already contributed to the understanding of the composition of newly formed and older MS lesions. In the newer lesions, surprisingly, both free fatty acids and lactate have been reported. Further analysis of this phenomenon can be expected in the near future [52, 53].

Infectious disorders

Infectious disorders involving mainly or only the white matter are exceptional. Two examples are cytomegalovirus (CMV) infection and AIDS encephalopathy. Encephalopathy in patients with AIDS has been described by many authors, as have superimposed infections and tumors [54–57]. The pattern of CMV and AIDS encephalopathy are nearly identical on MRI. Both show a periventricular diffuse, mild demyelination, not involving the U-fibers. Proton MRS may show abnormalities, in particular of *N*-acetyl aspartate, in the brain of AIDS patients with normal imaging studies [58].

Hypoxic–ischemic lesions

In post-hypoxic–ischemic lesions, periventricular white matter lesions occur in both very young infants and older people. In infants and children, MRI has proved to be the imaging modality of choice for follow-up of post-hypoxic–ischemic damage. There is a good correlation between the severity of the abnormalities and the extent of the CNS lesions. Selective white matter and neuronal damage have also been identified in other areas [59–64]. In older people, uncertainty about the significance of the periventricular white matter lesions remains, in particular in view of the many asymptomatic cases. Histologically, these lesions represent widened Virchow–Robin spaces, white matter pallor, demyelination, gliosis, or lacunar infarctions [65–68].

Toxic–metabolic encephalopathies

A much neglected area in neuroimaging is the toxic–metabolic encephalopathies. The most commonly reported are the alcohol-related syndromes, in particular Wernicke's encephalopathy, central pontine and extrapontine myelinolysis [69–72], and fetal alcohol syndrome. The Marchiafava–Bignami syndrome is well known but rare in most countries.

Wilson's disease, one of the endogeneous forms of toxic–metabolic encephalopathy, has been shown to have more or less extensive white matter involvement. Focal abnormalities are found in the lenticular, thalamic, and caudate nuclei, as well as in the brainstem and, the cerebellar and cerebral white matter in a variable pattern. No correlation has been found between the severity of the clinical condition and the MRI findings [73].

Changes in both gray and white matter have been reported in hepatocerebral syndromes, probably as a result of hyperammonemia and the release of excitatory amino acids. MRS has shown the abnormal metabolic findings [74–76].

In many other conditions, the existing knowledge about WMD in, for example, posttraumatic, postradiotherapeutic, and postcytostatic findings has been confirmed [77, 78].

CONCLUSION

MRI has proven its value in the diagnosis of WMD. If an imaging modality is required in the workup of a patient suspected of having WMD, then MRI should be the first choice. A systematic analysis, as suggested in our pattern recognition program, will help to improve the diagnostic quality and contribution of MR.

ACKNOWLEDGMENT

We thank Anita Dompeling for secretarial assistance in preparing the manuscript.

REFERENCES

1. Van der Knaap MS, Valk J, de Neeling N, Nauta JJP (1991) Pattern recognition in magnetic resonance imaging of white matter disorders in children and young adults. *Neuroradiology* **33**: 478–493.
2. Valk J, van der Knaap MS (1989) *Magnetic Resonance of Myelin, Myelination and Myelin Disorders*. Berlin: Springer-Verlag.
3. Demaerel Ph, Wilms G, Verdru P, Carton H, Baert AL (1990) MR findings in globoid cell leucodystrophy. *Neuroradiology* **32**: 520–522.
4. Morgan SH, Rudge P, Smith SJM, Bronstein AM, Kendall BE, Holly E, Young EP, Crawford M D'A, Bannister R (1990) The neurological complications of Anderson–Fabry disease: investigation of symptomatic and presymptomatic patients. *Quart J Med* **75**: 491–504.
5. Brismar J, Brismar G, Coates R, Gascon G, Ozand P (1990) Increased density of the thalamus on CT scans in patients with GM$_2$ gangliosidosis. *AJNR* **11**: 125–130.
6. Dietemann JL, Filippi de la Palavesa MM, Tranchant C, Kastler B (1990) MR findings in mannosidosis. *Neuroradiology* **32**: 485–487.
7. Shimoda-Matsubayashi S, Kuru Y, Sumie H, Ito T, Hattori N, Okuma Y, Mizuno Y (1990) MRI findings in the mild type of mucopolysaccharidosis II (Hunter's syndrome). *Neuroradiology* **32**: 328–330.
8. Afifi AK, Sata Y, Waziri MH, Bell WE (1990) Computed tomography and magnetic resonance imaging of the brain in Hurler's disease. *J Child Neurol* **5**: 235–241.
9. Van der Knaap MS, Valk J (1991) The MR spectrum of perioxisomal disorders. *Neuroradiology* **33**: 30–37.
10. Van der Knaap MS, Valk J (1989) MR of aderenoleukodystrophy: histopathologic correlations. *AJNR* **10**: S12–S14.
11. Sandhu PS, Dillon WP (1991) MR demonstration of leukoencephalopathy associated with mitochondral encephalomyopathy: case report. *AJNR* **12**: 375–379.
12. Fujii T, Okuno T, Ito M, Mothoh K, Hamazaki S, Okada S, Kusaka H, Mikawa H (1990) CT, MRI, and autopsy findings in brain of a patient with MELAS. *Pediatr Neurol* **6**: 253–256.
13. Yamagata T, Yano S, Okabe I, Miyao M, Momoi MY, Yanagisawa M, Hirata H, Komatsu K (1990) Ultrasonography and magnetic resonance imaging in Leigh disease. *Pediatr Neurol* **6**: 326–329.
14. Brismar J, Brismar G, Gascon G, Ozand P (1990) Canavan disease: CT and MR imaging of the brain. *AJNR* **11**: 805–810.
15. Hald JK, Nakstad PH, Skjeldal OH, Stromme P (1991) Bilateral arachnoid cysts of the temporal fossa in four children with glutaric aciduria type I. *AJNR* **12**: 407–409.
16. Andreula CF, Blasi de R, Carella A (1991) CT and MR studies of methylmalonic acidemia. *AJNR* **12**: 410–412.
17. Thompson AJ, Smith I, Brenton D, Youl BD, Rylance G, Davidson DC, Kendall B, Lees AJ (1990) Neurological deterioration in young adults with phenylketonuria. *Lancet* **336**: 602–605.
18. Shaw DWW, Weinberger E, Maravilla KR (1990) Cranial MR in phenylketonuria. *J Comput Assist Tomogr* **14**: 458–460.
19. Pearsen KD, Gean-Marton AD, Levy HI, Davis KR (1990) Phenylketonuria: MR imaging of the brain with clinical correlation. *Radiology* **177**: 437–440.
20. Shaw DWW, Maravilla KR, Weinberger E, Garretson J, Trahms CM, Scott CR (1991) MR imaging of phenylketonuria. *AJNR* **12**: 403–406.
21. Sugita R, Takahashi S, Ishii K, Matsumoto K, Ishibashi T, Sakamoto, Narisawa K (1990) Brain CT and MR findings

in hyperphenylalaninemia due to dihypdropeteridine reductase deficiency (variant of phenylketonuria). *J Comput Assist Tomogr* **14**: 669–703.

22. Brismar J, Aqeel A, Brismar G, Coates R, Gascon G, Ozand P (1990) Maple syrup urine disease: findings on CT and MR scans of the brain in 10 infants. *AJNR* **11**: 1219–1228.

23. Press GA, Barshop BA, Haas RH, Nyhan WL, Glass RF, Hesselink JR (1989) Abnormalities of the brain in nonkeotic hyperglycinemia: MR manifestations. *AJNR* **10**: 315–321.

24. Van der Knaap MS, Valk J (1989) The reflection of histology in MR imaging of Pelizaeus–Merzbacher disease. *AJNR* **10**: 99–103.

25. Silverstein AM, Hirsh DK, Trobe JD, Gebarski SS (1990) MR imaging of the brain in five members of a family with Pelizaeus–Merzbacher disease. *AJNR* **11**: 495–499.

26. Bobele GB, Garnica A, Bradley Schaefer G, Leonard JC, Wilson D, Marks WA, Leech RW, Brumback RA (1990) Neuroimaging findings in Alexander's disease. *J Child Neurol* **5**: 253–258.

27. Hess DC, Fischer AQ, Yaghmai F, Figueroa R, Akamatsu Y (1990) Comparative neuroimaging with pathologic correlates in Alexander's disease. *J Child Neurol* **5**: 248–252.

28. Shah M, Ross JS (1990) Infantile Alexander disease: MR appearance of a biopsy-proved case. *AJNR* **11**: 1105–1106.

29. Naidu SB, Moser HW (1991) Value of neuroimaging in metabolic diseases affecting the CNS. *AJNR* **12**: 413–416.

30. Sharief MK, Phil M, Thompson EJ (1991) The predictive value of intrathecal immunoglobulin synthesis and magnetic resonance imaging in acute isolated syndromes for subsequent development of multiple sclerosis. *Ann Neurol* **29**: 147–151.

31. Harris JO, Frank JA, Patronas N, McFarlin DE, McFarland HF (1991) Serial gadolinium-enhanced magnetic resonance imaging scans in patients with early, relapsing–remitting multiple sclerosis: Implications for clinical trials and natural history. *Ann Neurol* **29**: 548–555.

32. Zerrin Yetkin F, Haughton VM, Anne Papke R, Fischer ME, Rao SM (1991) Multiple sclerosis: Specificity of MR for diagnosis. *Radiology* **178**: 447–451.

33. Truyen L, Gheuens J, Van de Vyver FL, Parizel PM, Peersman GV, Martin JJ (1990) Improved correlation of magnetic resonance imaging (MRI) with clinical status in multiple sclerosis (MS) by use of an extensive standardized imaging-protocol. *J Neurol Sci* **96**: 173–182.

34. Quint DJ (1991) Multiple sclerosis and imaging of the corpus callosum. *Radiology* **180**: 15–17.

35. Gean-Martin AD, Gilbert Vezina L, Marton KI, Stimac GK, Peyster RG, Taveras JM, Davis KR (1991) Abnormal corpus callosum: a sensitive and specific indicator of multiple sclerosis. *Radiology* **180**: 215–221.

36. Paty DW, McFarlin DE, McDonald WI (1991) Magnetic resonance imaging and laboratory aids in the diagnosis of multiple sclerosis. *Ann Neurol* **29**: 3–5.

37. Lynch SG, Rose JW, Smoker W, Petajan JH (1990) MRI in familial multiple sclerosis. *Neurology* **40**: 900–903.

38. Millner MM, Ebner F, Justich E, Urban C (1990) Multiple sclerosis in childhood: contribution of serial MRI to earlier diagnosis. *Dev Med Child Neurol* **32**: 769–777.

39. Osborn AG, Harnsberger HR, Smoker WRK, Boyer RS (1990) Multiple sclerosis in adolescents. *AJNR* **11**: 489–494.

40. Ebner F, Millner MM, Justich E (1990) Multiple sclerosis in children: value of serial MR studies to monitor patients. *AJNR* **11**: 1023–1027.

41. Shermann JL, Stern BJ (1990) Sarcoidosis of the CNS: comparisons of unenhanced and enhanced MR images. *AJNR* **11**: 915–923.

42. Zuheir AL, Kawi M, Bohlega S, Banna M (1991) MRI findings in Neuro-Behçet's disease. *Neurology* **41**: 405–408.

43. Rafto SE, Milton WJ, Galetta SL, Grossman RI (1990) Biopsy-confirmed CNS Lyme disease: MR appearance at 1.5 T. *AJNR* **11**: 482–484.

44. Loes DJ, Biller J, Yuh WTC, Hart MN, Godersky JC, Adams Jr HP, Keefauver SP, Tranel D (1990) Leukoencephalopathy in cerebral amyloid angiopathy: MR imaging in four case. *AJNR* **11**: 485–488.

45. Hawke SHB, Hallinan JM, McLeod JG (1990) Cranial magnetic resonance imaging in chronic demyelinating polyneuropathy. *J Neurol Neurosurg Psychiatry* **53**: 794–796.

46. Williams DW, Elster AD, Kramer SI (1990) Neurosarcoidosis: gadolinium-enhanced MR imaging. *J Comput Assist Tomogr* **14**: 704–707.

47. Fernandez RE, Rothberg M, Ferencz G, Wujack D (1990) Lyme disease of the CNS: MR imaging findings in 14 cases. *AJNR* **11**: 479–481.

48. Doran M, Bydder GM (1990) Magnetic resonance perfusion and diffusion imaging. *Neuroradiology* **32**: 392–398.

49. Doran M, Hajnal JV, Van Bruggen N, King MD, Young IR, Bydder GM (1990) Normal and abnormal white matter tracts shown by MR imaging using directional diffusion weighted sequences. *J Comput Assist Tomogr* **14**: 865–873.

50. Hajnal JV, Doran M, Hall AS, Collins AG, Oatridge A, Pennock JM, Young IR, Bydder GM (1991) MR imaging of anisotropically restricted diffusion of water in the nervous system: technical, anatomic, and pathologic considerations. *J Comput Assist Tomogr* **15**: 1–18.

51. Sakuma H, Nomura Y, Takeda K, Tagami T, Nakagawa T, Tamagawa Y, Ishii Y, Tsukamoto T (1991) Adult and neonatal human brain: diffusional anisotropy and myelination with diffusion-weighted MR imaging. *Radiology* **180**: 229–233.

52. Miller DH, Austin SJ, Connelly A, Youl BD, Gadian DG, McDonald WI (1991) Proton magnetic resonance spectroscopy of an acute and chronic lesion in multiple sclerosis. *Lancet* **5**: 58–59.

53. Sappey-Marinier D (1990) High-resolution NMR spectroscopy of cerebral white matter in multiple sclerosis. *Magn Reson Med* **15**: 229–239.

54. Chrysikopoulos HS, Press GA, Grafe MR, Hesselink JR, Wiley CA (1990) Encephalitis caused by human immunodeficiency virus: CT and MR imaging manifestations

with clinical and pathologic correlation. *Radiology* **175**: 185–191.

55. Grafe MR, Press GA, Berthoty DP, Hesselink JR, Wiley CA (1990) Abnormalities of the brain in AIDS patients: correlation of postmortem MR findings with neuropathology. *AJNR* **11**: 905–911.

56. Kieburtz KD, Ketonen L, Zettelmaier AE, Kido D, Caine ED, Simon JH (1990) Magnetic resonance imaging findings in HIV cognitive impairment. *Arch Neurol* **47**: 643–645.

57. Tien RD, Chu PK, Hesselink JR, Duberg A, Wley C (1991) Intracranial cryptococcosis in immunocompromised patients: CT and MR findings in 29 cases. *AJNR* **12**: 283–289.

58. Menon DK, Baudouin CJ, Tomlinson D, Hoyle C (1990) Proton MR spectroscopy and imaging of the brain in AIDS: evidence of neuronal loss in regions that appear normal with imaging. *J Comput Assist Tomogr* **14**: 882–885.

59. Barkovich AJ, Truwit CL (1990) Brain damage from perinatal asphyxia: Correlation of MR findings with gestational age. *AJNR* **11**: 1087–1096.

60. Valk J, van der Knaap MS, Grauw de T, Taets v Amerongen AHM (1991) The role of imaging modalities in the diagnosis of posthypoxic–ischemic and hemorrhagic conditions of infants (part I or two). *Klin Neuroradiol* **1**: 72–79.

61. Byrne P, Welch R, Johnson MA, Darrah J, Piper M (1990) Serial magnetic resonance imaging in neonatal hypoxic–ischemic encephalopathy. *J Pediatr* **117**: 694–700.

62. Konishi Y, Kuriyama M, Hayakawa K, Konishi K, Yasujima M, Fujii Y, Sudo M (1990) Periventricular hyperintensity detected by magnetic resonance imaging in infancy. *Pediatr Neurol* **6**: 229–232.

63. Feldman HM, Scher MS, Kemp SS (1990) Neurodevelopmental outcome of children with evidence of periventricular leukomalacia on late MRI. *Pediatr Neurol* **6**: 296–302.

64. Dietrich RB, Vining EP, Taira RK, Hall TR, Philipart M (1990) Myelin disorders of childhood: correlation of MR findings and severity of neurological impairment. *J Comput Assist Tomogr* **14**: 693–698.

65. Leifer D, Buonanno PS, Richardson EP Jr (1990) Clinicopathologic correlations of cranial magnetic resonance imaging of periventricular white matter. *Neurology* **40**: 911–918.

66. Yamaguchi H, Fukuyama H, Harada K, Yamaguchi S, Moyoshi T, Doi T, Kumura J, Iwasaki Y, Asato R, Yonekura Y (1990) White matter hyperintensities may correspond to areas of increased blood volume: correlative MR and PET observations. *J Comput Assist Tomogr* **14**: 905–908.

67. Bradley WG, Whitemore AR, Watanabe AS, Davis SJ, Teresi LM, Homyak M (1991) Association of deep white matter infarction with chronic communicating hydrocephalus: implications regarding the possible origin of normal-pressure hydrocephalus. *AJNR* **12**: 31–39.

68. Hachinski V (1991) Binswanger's disease: neither Binswanger's nor a disease. *J Neurol Sci* **103**: 1.

69. Gallucci M, Bozzao A, Splendiani A, Masciocchi C, Passariello R (1990) Wernicke encephalopathy: MR findings in five patients. *AJNR* **11**: 887–892.

70. Victor M (1990) MR in the diagnosis of Wernicke–Korsakoff syndrome. *AJNR* **11**: 895–896.

71. Donnal JF, Ralph Heinz E, Burger PC (1990) MR of reversible thalamic lesions in Wernicke syndrome. *AJNR* **11**: 893–894.

72. Koci TM, Chiang F, Chow P, Wang A, Chiu LC, Itabshi H, Mehringer CM (1990) Thalamic extrapontine lesions in central pontine myelinolysis. *AJNR* **11**: 1229–1233.

73. Prayer L, Wimberger D, Kramer J, Grimm G, Oder W, Imhof H (1990) Cranial MRI in Wilson's disease. *Neuroradiology* **32**: 211–214.

74. Chamuleau RAFM, Bosman DK (1991) What the clinician can learn from MR glutamine/glutamate assays. *NMR Biomed* **4**: 103–108.

75. Ross BD (1991) Biochemical considerations in 1H spectroscopy. Glutamate and glutamine; myo-inositol and related metabolites. *NMR Biomed* **4**: 59–63.

76. Kreis R, Farrow N, Ross BD (1991) Localized 1H NMR spectroscopy in patients with chronic hepatic encephalopathy. Analysis of changes in cerebral glutamine, choline and inositols. *NMR Biomed* **4**: 109–116.

77. Valk PE, Dillon WP (1991) Radiation injury of the brain. *AJNR* **12**: 45–62.

78. Wilson DA, Nitschke R, Bowman ME, Chaffin MJ, Sexauer CL, Prince JR (1991) Transient white matter changes on MR images in children undergoing chemotherapy for acute lymphocytic leukemia: correlation with neuropsychologic deficiencies. *Radiology* **180**: 205–209.

MRI correlates of disease course and activity in multiple sclerosis

Lance D. Blumhardt,[1]* Silas Barbosa,[2] Neil Roberts[2], Dibendu Betal[2] and Christophe Gratin[2]

[1]University of Nottingham, Nottingham, NG7 2UH UK
[2]University of Liverpool, Liverpool, UK

We have carried out a comparative cross-sectional study of patients with relapsing and remitting MS (multiple sclerosis) (RRMS) ($n = 9$), primary progressive MS (PPMS) ($n = 7$), and secondary progressive MS (SPMS) ($n = 10$) using image analysis techniques to determine the number and volume of Gd-DTPA-enhancing lesions. RRMS patients had more lesions than either PPMS or SPMS (ns), and the mean volume of the lesions ($p = 0.006$) and the total volume of enhancing lesions ($p < 0.03$) were significantly larger in patients with RRMS compared with PPMS. The prevalence of blood-brain barrier (BBB) breakdown appears to be similar in PPMS and SPMS, with the higher rate in RRMS suggesting a suppressive effect of disease duration (and/or age). Similarly, the volume of the lesion load overall was negatively correlated with disease duration (ρ -0.56, $p < 0.003$). Differences between PPMS and RRMS/SPMS patients in the volume of the enhancing lesions may reflect differences in the ability of these patients to suppress the immune-mediated damage to axons which may follow episodic BBB breakdown and which is not visualized on conventional magnetic resonance imaging.

Keywords: multiple sclerosis, MRI, image analysis, lesion volume

INTRODUCTION

Magnetic resonance imaging (MRI) evidence of disease activity in multiple sclerosis (MS) is increasingly used as an outcome measure in treatment trials [1], and gadolinium (Gd-DTPA) enhancement to assess the integrity of the blood brain barrier (BBB) markedly improves sensitivity. The majority of studies of new lesion development have been carried out in patients with relapsing and remitting MS (RRMS) and there are little quantitative data currently available on the levels of disease activity associated with different disease courses. Previous studies have relied on lesion counts and/or arbitrary scales of lesion size or confluence for semiquantitative assessment [2–5]. In order to determine the effectiveness of potential treatments, it is essential to measure MR abnormalities accurately and, if possible, to correlate these with measures of disability and clinical outcome.

We report here the results from a cross-sectional study of the prevalence of Gd-DTPA-enhancing lesions and their volume as estimated by image analysis techniques in different groups of MS patients. A report on a serial study in these patients is in preparation.

METHODS

Patient material

We studied 26 informed and consenting patients from a MS research clinic (L.D.B.) with RRMS ($n = 9$), primary progressive MS (PPMS) ($n = 7$), and secondary progressive MS (SPMS) ($n = 10$). For the RRMS, PPMS, and SPMS patients, respectively, the mean ages were 33 (26–42), 48 (41–56), and 43 (32–56), the mean symptom durations were 52 ± 27.3 months, 72 ± 25.2 months, and 112 ± 88.5 months, the mean Kurtzke Expanded Disability Status Scores (EDSS) scores [6] were 3.6 (1.5–6), 3.6 (1.5–6), and 4.3 (2–6), and the

* Address for correspondence: Division of Clinical Neurology, Faculty of Medicine, University Hospital, Queens Medical Centre, Nottingham NG7 2UH, UK.

mean ambulation index [8] scores 2.0 (0-3), 2.5 (2-4) and 2.4 (1-4).

All patients satisfied the Washington committee criteria [7] for definite MS. The patients with PPMS had all presented with an isolated progressive myelopathy and had never experienced relapses or remissions. They all had oligoclonal bands in the cerebrospinal fluid (CSF) and paraclinical evidence (abnormal visual evoked potentials or brain MRI) of "clinically silent" lesions remote from the spinal cord. The SPMS cases were all in a phase of spinal progression with documented evidence of an earlier phase of relapses and remissions. The patients with PPMS and SPMS were matched for age and disability and the duration of their progressive phase.

MRI protocol

All patients were investigated using a 1.5-Tesla SIGNA (General Electric, Milwaukee, Wisconsin, USA) whole-body MR imaging system. The manufacturer's head coil was used to transmit and receive the radiofrequency (RF) pulses. On a true mid-line sagittal image, generated by prior localization in the axial and coronal scanning planes, a line was drawn through the top of sphenoid sinus and the superior surface of the cerebellum. This line denoted the center of the middle slice of a series of 31 dual-echo, spin-echo [TR 2000 ms; TE 30 and 80 ms; 1 NEX; acquisition matrix 128×128; slice thickness 4 mm; field of view (FOV) 24 cm] contiguous axio-oblique slices. Gadolinium dimeglumine (Gd-DTPA) (Magnevist, Schering AG) was administered intravenously in a dose of 0.2 mmol kg^{-1}. Within 5 min of the injection, the acquisition of 31 contiguous T_1-weighted spin-echo images (TR 600 ms; TE 30 ms; 1 NEX; acquisition matrix 128×128; slice thickness 4 mm; FOV 24 cm) was commenced using the same axio-oblique scanning plane. There were no significant side effects of Gd-DTPA.

Image preprocessing and quantification of MRI parameters

MR images were transferred to a SUN 3/160 (SUN Microsystems, California, USA) hosted CONTEXTVISION (Struers AB) image analysis system. Also available on a SUN SPARC 2 computer connected to the network was ANALYZE software (Mayo Foundation, Milwaukee, USA), comprising facilities for sizing and oblique section reformatting of the images.

Individual lesion thresholding was achieved using a purpose developed routine from CONTEXTVISION. A small region containing the lesion transect to be segmented was selected and isolated from the rest of the image. This was thresholded and the result stored.

The process was repeated for successive lesion transects on successive images until all the lesions were segmented. The volume of the lesion load was obtained automatically as the product of the total number of pixels on the binary images containing the segmented lesions and the voxel volume.

Statistics

Differences between patient groups were assessed with Student's t-test or the Mann–Witney test where appropriate to the normality of the data (Wilks test). Confidence intervals were set at the 95% level and all significance values quoted are two-tailed. For correlation analyses, we used the nonparametric Spearman's rank test.

RESULTS

MRI analysis

Numbers of lesions

The majority of the patients (24/26, 92%) had one or more enhancing lesions on their first scan. All patients with RRMS had enhancing lesions, compared with 6/7 (86%) of the PPMS and 9/10 (90%) of the SPMS patients.

A total of 230 enhancing areas were identified in the 24 patients (average 10 lesions per patient, range 0–43). One hundred eighty-seven (81%) of these (average 8.1 per patient, range 1–38) were greater than five pixels in area. All statistical analyses were restricted to lesions with a diameter of more than five pixels.

The highest number of enhancing lesions occurred in RRMS patients and the lowest in PPMS patients; there were 104 abnormalities in the RRMS group, 56 in the SPMS group, and 27 in the PPMS patients. The number of enhancing lesions *per patient* were in the ranges 2–37, 0–7, and 0–14 with means of 11.6 ± 12.35, 3.9 ± 2.37, and 6.2 ± 4.32, for the RRMS, PPMS, and SPMS groups, respectively. The intergroup variances were high, particularly for the RRMS and SPMS patients, and the differences between these group means were not significant.

Volumes of enhancing lesions and lesion load

For the RRMS and SPMS patients, there was a wide interpatient variation in the total lesion volumes: the mean volumes per patient were 2.585 ± 4.037 cc and 0.961 ± 1.552 cc, respectively. By contrast, the lesion load in the PPMS patients was significantly smaller (0.237 ± 0.132 cc; $p = 0.03$) with much less interpatient variation.

The mean volumes of individual lesions also showed marked intergroup differences. The largest lesions were in the RRMS group and the smallest in the PPMS groups (0.219 ± 0.471 cc and 0.056 ± 0.040 cc, respectively; $p = 0.006$). The average lesion volume in the SPMS patients (0.167 ± 0.314 cc) was similar to that of the RRMS patients.

An analysis of the distribution of lesion volumes showed that the RRMS and SPMS had similar bimodal distributions with main peaks at 0.033 cc and above 0.314 cc (see Fig. 1). The PPMS patients had a skewed unimodal distribution with a dominant peak at 0.033 cc and no lesions larger than 0.165 cc.

Clinical correlations

There were no significant correlations between MRI lesion volumes and disability measures. The volume of enhancing tissue for all patients was negatively corre-

lated with symptom duration (ρ −0.56, CI −0.78 to −0.23, $p = 0.003$) and age (ρ −0.45, CI −0.72 to −0.08, $p = 0.02$).

DISCUSSION

Previous studies have concluded that enhancing lesions (and, therefore, BBB disruption) occur much less frequently in PPMS than either RRMS or SPMS [2, 3]. A recent study reported enhancing lesions in 62% of the scans of SPMS patients compared to 37% for RRMS and 14% for PPMS [3]. In one serial study [2], only 50% of patients with PPMS had new lesions and only 5% of these enhanced. In contrast, we have found enhancing lesions in most patients (i.e., 100% for RRMS, 90% for SPMS, and 86% for PPMS patients). These discrepancies may be due in part to the higher field strength of our system and the greater accuracy of the image analysis techniques and perhaps to the small numbers of patients in each study.

Large differences in the numbers of enhancing lesions per patient have been reported in the above different clinical groups. Kappos and co-workers [4] noted only 0.3 lesions per patient in "primary chronic progressive" disease compared with 10.8 and 3.7 lesions per patient in "relapsing progressive" and "secondary chronic progressive" disease, respectively. In the present study, the younger RRMS patients had much higher counts than either of the progressive groups, perhaps suggesting a suppressive effect of disease duration (or age) on events at the BBB.

Previous studies have reported differences between PPMS and SPMS for arbitrary scores of "lesion size" and "total lesion load." On T_2-weighted images, SPMS cases had larger and more confluent lesions than those with PPMS, and it was concluded that SPMS patients had a significantly higher lesion load [9, 10]. High Gd-DTPA scores and high variance have been found in SPMS and RRMS, and low scores and low variance in the PPMS cases [5]. Further, in a serial study, whereas the majority of new lesions enhanced in SPMS, only a minority did so in PPMS [2].

In support of previous studies [2, 5], we have found marked differences in the volume of enhancing tissue, with small lesions and low lesion load in patients with PPMS, and larger lesions and higher lesion load in patients with RRMS and SPMS. The RRMS patients had more lesions at almost all volumes and the PPMS the least. Both the SPMS and RRMS groups had an additional "subpopulation" of larger lesions resulting in a quasibimodal distribution. By contrast, the PPMS patients were characterized by a less variable population of mainly small lesions.

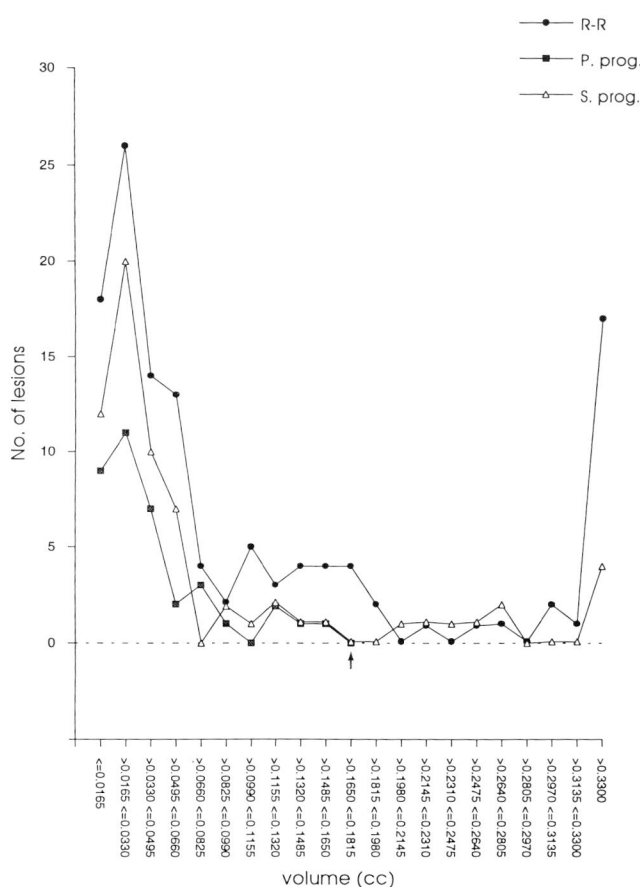

Fig. 1. Relationship between number and volume of lesions by disease course. Note that no lesions in the PPMS group exceeded 0.165 cc (arrow). Note that lower limit of 0.017 cc includes lesions of five pixels or less. R-R = RRMS; P. prog. = PPMS; S. prog. = SPMS.

We found no relationship between the volume of the enhancing lesion load and disability measures. However, we did find negative correlations between the volume of enhancing tissue and both disease duration and age. This is in conflict with other studies using arbitrary Gd-DTPA scores where authors concluded that the fall in relapse rate was not related to a reduced amount of activity [5]. Instead, our data would suggest that there is a reduction in both the number of BBB breakdowns and the extent of the inflammatory response with disease duration and/or age.

Our observations that the smallest volumes of Gd-PTA enhancement occur in the patients with the worst prognosis for disability (i.e., PPMS) and that the inflammatory response correlates negatively with disease duration would suggest that the volume of enhancing tissue reflects, at least in part, the patient's ability to suppress the immune-mediated attack on the myelin, although not the unvisualized axonal damage that is presumably responsible for the irreversible neurological deficits.

ACKNOWLEDGMENTS

We gratefully acknowledge support from the Cancer and Polio Research Fund Ltd. and the Marilyn Houlton Trust for Motor Neuron disease.

REFERENCES

1. Paty DW, Li DKB, the UBC MS/MRI Study Group (1993) *Neurology* **43**: 662.
2. Thompson AJ, Kermode AG, Wicks D, MacManus DG, Kendall BE, Kingsley DPE, McDonald WI (1991) *Ann Neurol* **29**: 53.
3. Wiebe S, Lee DH, Karlik SJ, Hopkins M, Vandervoort MK, Wong CJ, Hewitt L, Rice GPA, Ebers GC, Noseworthy JH (1992) *Ann Neurol* **32**: 643.
4. Kappos L, Stadt D, Rohrbach E, Keil W (1988) *Neurology* **38** (Suppl 1): 255.
5. Thorpe JW, Kingsley DPE, Macmanus DG, McDonald WI, Miller DH (1993) *Proc Annual Meeting Soc. Mag. Res. Med.* **12**: 1454.
6. Kurtzke JF (1983) *Neurology* **33**: 1444.
7. Poser CM, Paty DW, Scheinberg L, McDonald WI, Davis FA, Ebers GC, Johnson KP, Sibley WA, Silberberg DH, Tourtellotte WW (1983) *Ann. Neurol.* **13**: 227.
8. Hauser SL, Dawson DM, Lehrich JR, Beale MF, Kevy SV, Propper RD, Mills RD, Weiner HL (1983) *New Engl J Med* **308**: 173.
9. Thompson AJ, Kermode AG, MacManus DG, Kendall BE, Kingsley DPE, Moselely IF, McDonald WI (1990) *Br Med J* **300**: 631.
10. Thompson AJ, Kermode AG, MacManus DG, Kingsley DPE, Kendall BE, Moseley IF, McDonald WI (1989) *Lancet* **i**: 1322.

Clinical magnetic resonance imaging study
of focal cerebral ischemia

A. L. Krivoshapkin,* G. P. Streltsova and M. G. Jacobson

Research Institute of Traumatology and International Tomography Centre, Novosibirsk, Russia

Of the 47 patients with focal cerebral ischemia (FCI), 26 patients had completed stroke, 5 suffered from severe head injury, and 16 patients had anterior circulation aneurysms. Twenty-one stroke patients underwent bypass surgery and all traumatic patients underwent cerebral revascularization by omental graft. Aneurysm patients were surgically treated by neck clipping. In seven of them, aneurysm were occluded by nonferromagnetic (NFM) Ni-Ti alloy clips. In each case, comparative magnetic resonance imaging (MRI), computerized tomography (CT), and angiography (AG) findings were evaluated both before and after operation. MRI was much more sensitive than CT for detecting the ischemic tissue in all groups of patients. The difference in infarct area appreciated by MRI and CT in stroke patients turned out to be determined by the time between the onset of ictus and examination. MRI was particularly valuable for following up patients with FCI after cerebral revascularization by bypass surgery and omental graft. MRI was capable of replacing both postoperative AG and CT in patients operated on with NFM clips.

Keywords: MRI, CT, cerebral revascularization nonferromagnetic clip.

There is increasing interest in imaging the patients with ischemic cerebrovascular disease today because new therapies are emerging [1]. By and large, both computerized tomography (CT) and magnetic resonance imaging (MRI) have demonstrated anatomic correlates in stroke patients, but MRI has proven to be more sensitive to tissue changes than any other imaging modality [2].

The aim of the present study was to evaluate the advantages of MRI over CT for detecting focal cerebral ischemia (FCI) in patients with different cerebrovascular diseases.

CLINICAL MATERIALS AND METHODS

These series included 47 patients with FCI: 26 patients had completed stroke, 5 suffered from severe head injury, and 16 patients had anterior circulation aneu-

rysms. Twenty-one stroke patients underwent bypass surgery [3]. All traumatic patients were operated on by means of microsurgical omentum transplantation for cerebral revascularization [4]. Aneurysm patients were surgically treated by neck clipping. In seven of them, aneurysm were successfully occluded by nonferromagnetic (NFM) Ni-Ti alloy clips that have been especially developed at our institute. In each case, clinical course, MRI, CT, and angiography (AG) findings were evaluated.

The MR images were performed on a 0.28-T MR imaging system manufactured by Bruker Inc., Germany. All CT scans were performed on a Tomoscan CX/S system manufactured by Philips, Holland.

RESULTS

Our study showed that there was a significant degree of tissue specificity obtainable from the MRI parameters so the image provided easy identification of both small or mild cerebral infarcts. There were no bone artifacts with which to contend. It was particularly valuable for detecting infarctions in the basal ganglia. These lesions were seen by MRI but not by CT. The infarct volume detected by MRI had much greater

* Address for correspondence: Department of Neurosurgery, Institute of Traumatology, 17 Frunze Street, 630091 Novosibirsk, Russia.

extent than that appreciated by CT. The difference in infarct area evaluated by MRI and CT in stroke patients was determined by the time between the onset of ictus and examination. For 6 months after stroke, it was 60 + 8%. Six months later, this index was 3.5 times less. If the difference of the infarct volume detected by MRI and CT was more than 30% the patients appeared to have benefited from bypass surgery as demonstrated clinically as well as with postoperative TCD (transcranial Doppler) and MRI. On the other hand, patients with lesser difference showed insignificant or no postoperative improvement of neurological deficits.

In traumatic patients, MRI was capable of clearly demonstrating the reduction of ischemic area after the operation, intracranial microsurgical omentum transplantation.

In aneurysm patients, MRI was particularly excellent in detecting the true size of the aneurysm. The multiplanar tissue specificity obtainable from the MRI parameters so the capabilities of MRI were an advantage over CT as well as its ability to visualize vascular structures without a contrast agent. Postoperative MRI scans in patients operated on with NFM clips were quite useful to appreciate the thrombosis of clipped aneurysm and the evidence of any cerebral ischemia.

ILLUSTRATIVE CASE REPORTS

Case 1

A 26-year-old right-handed man was taken to the clinic on January 16, 1993, 11 months after severe head injury. Examination showed both sever hemiparesis of his right extremities and aphasia. CT and MRI revealed vast ischemic lesion in the left frontal lobe. The patient showed significant improvement after intracranial microsurgical omentum transplantation. Postoperative MRI demonstrated the diminution of the ischemic area by 30% (Fig. 1).

Case 2

A 56-year-old right-handed man suffered a spontaneous subarachnoid hemorrage on March 23, 1992, manifested by an intense headache, memory disturbance, and moderate stiff neck. Contrast enhancement CT (CECT) examination demonstrated a round area of hyperdensity in the suprasellar cistern on the right side due to the anterior communicating artery (ACA) aneurysm. Cerebral angiography revealed the large ACA aneurysm with a wide neck. Frontal and axial MRI showed the "signal void" region due to the patent lumen of the ACA aneurysm. The patient underwent occlusion of the aneurysm by means of neck clipping with a NFM clip. Postoperative CECT

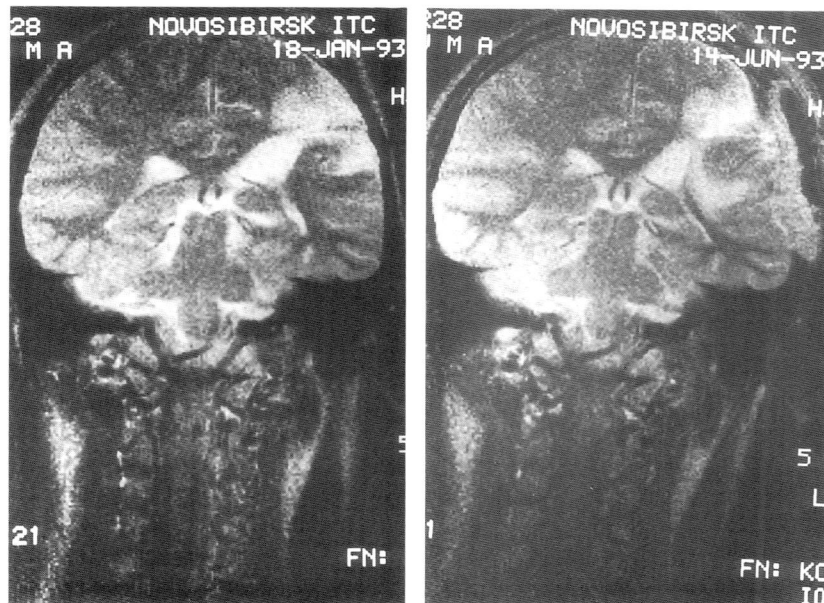

Fig. 1. Frontal MRI (T_2-weighted images) showing hypersignal in the left frontal lobe due to severe head injury before operation (on the left) and after surgery (on the right). The ischemic area after microsurgical omentum transplantation is smaller by 30%.

showed that the suprasellar region could be seen faintly because of metallic artifacts due to the intracranial vascular clip. At the same time, MRI clearly demonstrated complete aneurysm occlusion (Fig. 2).

DISCUSSION

Both CT scan and MRI are valuable techniques for imaging the patients with ischemic cerebrovascular disease [1]. Although cerebral angiography still remains the definitive study, in some cases representing the "gold standard" for vascular evaluation, the advent of CT has greatly changed the role of AG in the investigation and follow-up of patients with subarachnoid hemorrhage [5]. MRI is the imaging modality of choice in the late stages of subarachnoid and parenchimal hemorrhages and the also ideal method in detecting the presence and analyzing large aneurysms [6]. Based on the "flow void" without any contrast agent, intracranial aneurysms could only be recognized by MRI. Our comparative MRI and CT study showed that MRI appeared to be superior to CT in the detection and diagnosis of a number of cerebrovascular diseases. CT is not as sensitive as MRI on focal cerebral ischemia due to the limitation of contrast resolution, the presence of bone or NFM metal artifacts, and poorer visualization of infarcted tissue [7]. So the specificity of CT scanning alone in the diagnosis of cerebrovascular pathology with small ischemic lesions has been questioned. Our study demonstrated that the diminution of the ischemic lesion after cerebral revascularization was first and foremost the result of the reduction of the area with slightly prolonged relaxation times in MRI which could not be recognized by CT and likely to be an ischemic penumbra [8–10]. MRI turned out to be especially valuable for following up patients with FCI after cerebral revascularization by such procedures as bypass surgery and microsurgical omentum transplantation. Therefore, we believe that MRI is capable providing a substrate for understanding the pathophysiology of focal cerebral ischemia in addition to the anatomical correlates and improving the outcomes of both medical and surgical treatment of patients with cerebrovascular diseases. CT presently is the best method in evaluating the postoperative aneurysm patients [11] so long as MRI is contraindicated in the follow-up of patients who underwent surgery for intracranial aneurysms due to the presence of ferromagnetic vascular clips. In our series, MRI was capable of replacing both postoperative AG and CT in patients operated on with weak paramagnetic clips. No artifacts of NFM Ni-Ti alloy clips and no clip motion during postoperative MRI were observed.

Thus, in many respects, MRI can be a significant step beyond CT for imaging the patients with ischemic cerebrovascular disease. These results indicate that MRI is the modality of choice to examine patients with FCI and follow them up after cerebrovascular operations.

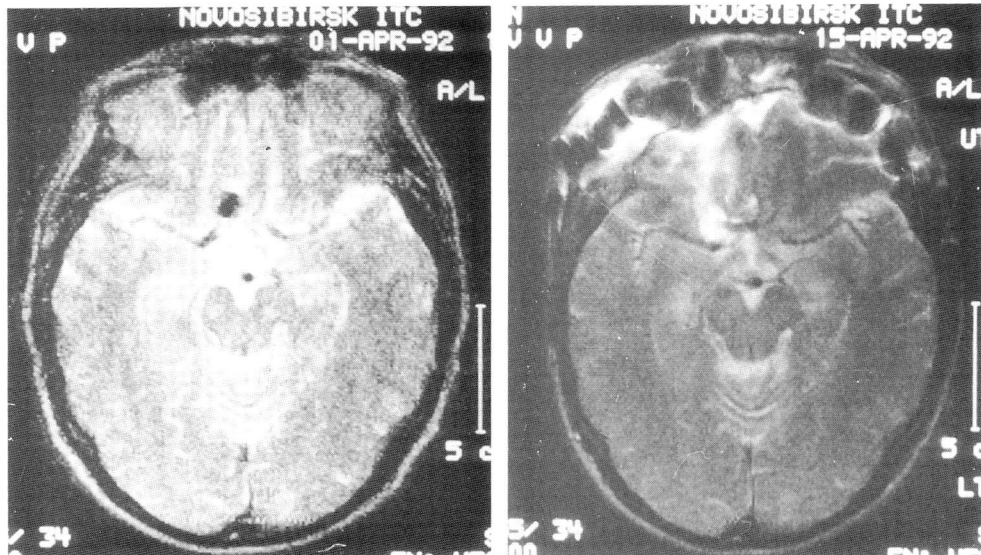

Fig. 2. Axial MRI (T_2-weighted images) showing the large ACA aneurysm (on the left). The complete thrombosis within the lumen of the ACA aneurysm as well as the presence of the right frontal ischemic area following aneurysm neck occlusion by means of the NFM clip (on the right).

ACKNOWLEDGMENTS

We thank Dr. Samuil S. Rubinovich for constant interest and Mrs. Irina A. Bahtina for invaluable technical assistance.

REFERENCES

1. Latchaw RE (1991) Imaging the patients with ischemic cerebrovascular disease. *Stroke Clin Updates* **2**: 13–16.
2. Latchaw RE (1990) NMR imaging of the human brain—insights into neurological diseases. In *NMR: Principles and Application to Biomedical Research* Pettegrew J, ed) pp. 550–585. New York: Springer-Verlag.
3. Yasargil MG, Yonekawa Y (1977) Results of microsurgical extra-intracranial arterial bypass in the treatment of cerebral ischemia. *Neurosurgery* **21**: 22–24.
4. Miyamoto S, Kikuchi H, Karasawa J et al. (1990) Cerebral revascularization by omental graft for moyamoya disease. In *The Omentum: Research and Clinical Application* (Goldsmith HS, ed) pp. 159–164. New York: Springer-Verlag.
5. TerBrugge KG, Rao KCVG, Lee SH (1983) Cerebral vascular anomalies. In Cranial Computed Tomography. (Lee SH, Rao KCVG, eds), pp. 547–583. New York: McGraw-Hill Book Co.
6. Huk WJ (1990) Vascular malformations. Aneurysms. In *MRI of Central Nervous System Diseases* (Huk WJ, Gademann G, Friedmann G, eds) pp. 332–334. New York: Springer-Verlag.
7. Bradley WG, Waluch V, Yadley RA, Wicoff RR (1984) Comparison of CT and MR in 400 patients with suspected diseases of the brain and cervical spinal cord. *Radiology* **152**: 695–702.
8. Astrup J, Siesjo BK (1981) Thresholds in cerebral ischemia—the ischemic penumbra. *Stroke* **12**: 723–725.
9. Samson V, Baron JC, Bousser MG, Rey A, Derlon JM, David P, Comoy J (1985) Effect of extra-intracranial arterial bypass on cerebral blood flow and oxygen metabolism in humans. *Stroke* **16**: 609–616.
10. Samson V, Baron JC, Bousser MG, Rey A, Roux FX, Derlon JM, Comoy J, David P, Comar D (1985) Consequences hemodynamigues et metaboliques regionales de l'anastomose temporo-sylvienne etude de quinze patiente par tomographie par emissionale positrons. *Neurochirurgie* **31**: 31–36.
11. Stark DD, Bradley WG (1988) Intracranial aneurysm. In Magnetic Resonance Imaging (Stark DD, Bradley WG, eds) pp. 476–482. St. Louis, MO: The C.V. Mosby Company.

3D TOF MRA: role in evaluation of intracranial aneurysms following embolization with platinum coils

D. J. Wilcock,[1]* T. Jaspan[2] and S. Evans[2]

[1]Sub-department of Academic Radiology and [2]Department of Radiology, University Hospital, Nottingham NG7 2UH, UK

Several patients with intracranial aneurysms at our hospital have recently been treated with embolization of the aneurysm itself with detachable platinum coils. This has been done as part of a multicenter trial of GDC platinum coils. We report our experience in the follow-up of these patients with magnetic resonance (MR) after the embolization procedure. We present several illustrative cases and discuss the information that can be gained from the spin-echo images, the magnetic resonance angiography (MRA) source data, and the maximum intensity projection (MIP) reconstructions. We also examine the relative merits and limitations of MR in this role including thrombus formation, susceptibility artifact, and estimation of size and morphology of the aneurysms. We discuss the role of MRA in the planning of the embolization procedure.

Keywords: magnetic resonance imaging, angiography, aneurysms, embolization.

CASE REPORTS

Patient 1

A 42-year-old woman presented with recurrent left-hemisphere infarcts. Digital subtraction angiogram (DSA) demonstrated a large elongated saccular aneurysm of the extracranial internal carotid artery (Fig. 1a). The neck of this aneurysm was wide. Due to the high cervical position of the lesion, the patient was referred for endovascular treatment of the aneurysm.

Two platinum coils were placed within the fundus of the aneurysm. At the end of the procedure, the aneurysm was largely occluded, but a significant neck to the lesion remained into which one loop of the platinum coil projected. An incomplete embolization was achieved as a nondetachable coil system was used and placement of a further coil would have potentially jeopardized the parent vessel. The GDC coil system was not available at the time of the procedure; however, the coil material was identical to that used for the

GDC system. The internal carotid artery remained patent at the end of the procedure.

Magnetic resonance (MR) imaging was performed for assessment 20 months later. On both the MRA source data (Fig. 1b) and the maximum intensity projection (MIP) reconstructions (Fig. 1c), the neck of the aneurysm is seen to remain patent, but the distal two-thirds of the lumen had been occluded. In addition, flow in the carotid artery distal to the aneurysm was visualized. Circle of Willis magnetic resonance angiography (MRA) demonstrated the intracranial vessels to be normal.

Patient 2

This 45-year-old man presented with a subarachnoid hemorrhage from a large left middle cerebral artery aneurysm. He underwent three separate embolization procedures over the next year.

After the first embolization, spin-echo (SE) axial T_2-weighted scans showed the left middle cerebral aneurysm with a complex signal intensity pattern (Fig. 2a) with a peripheral low signal related to mural calcification, lamellated hyperintensity in keeping with subacute thrombi, and a central area of mixed but essentially low signal which could be related to the platinum GDC coil ball or a flow void.

* Address for correspondence: Sub-department of Academic Radiology, University Hospital, Nottingham NG7 2UH, UK.

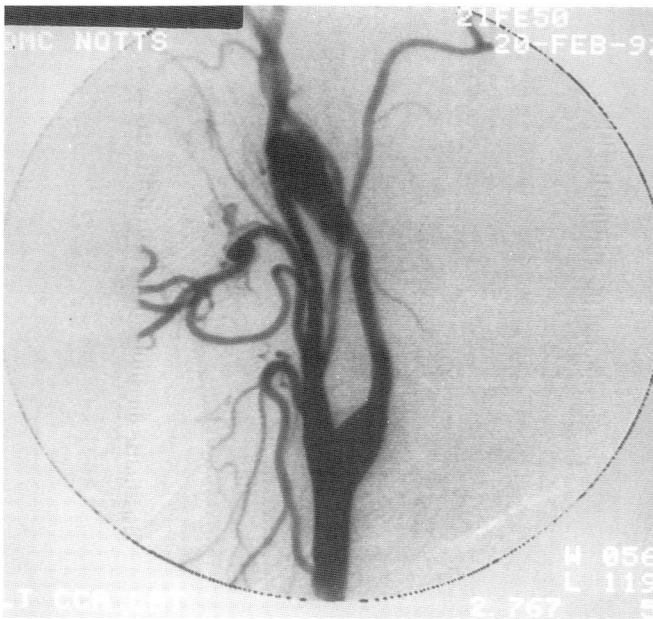

(a)

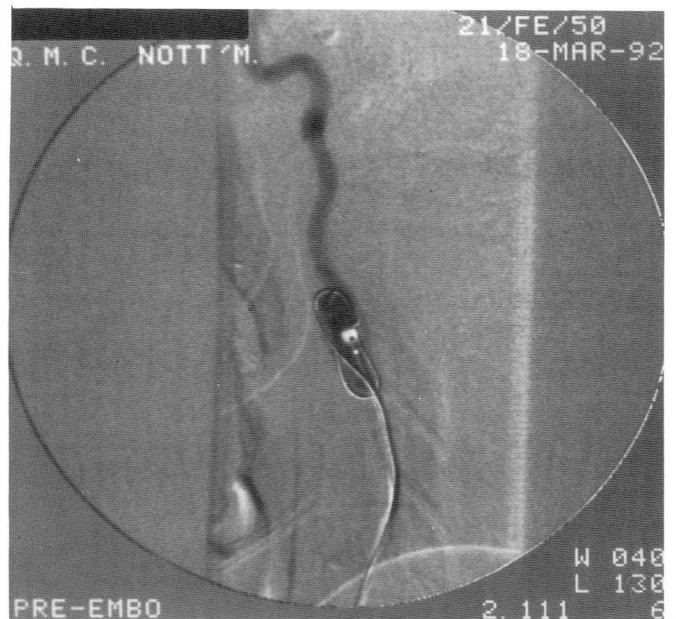

(b)

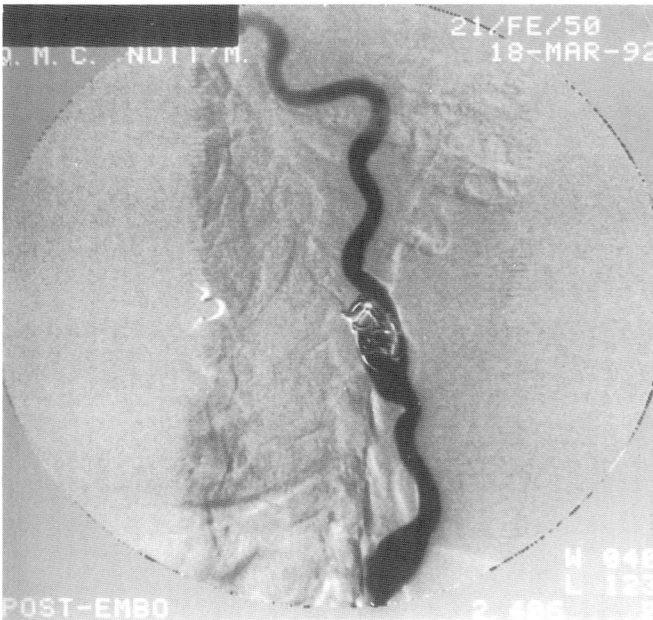

(c)

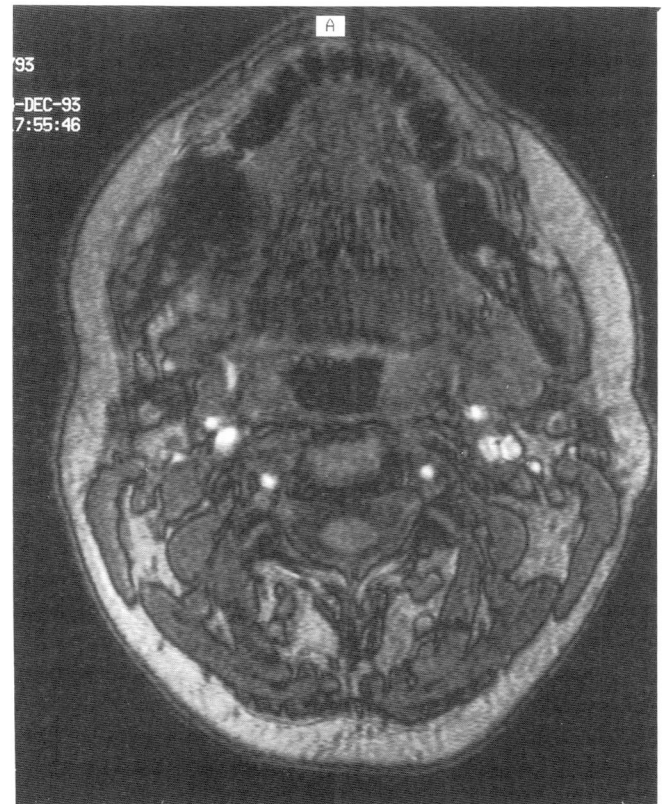

(d)

Fig. 1. A 42-year-old woman who presented with recurrent left hemisphere infarcts (Patient 1). (a) DSA demonstrates the large elongated saccular aneurysm of the extracranial internal carotid artery. (b) DSA during embolization of the aneurysm with GDC coils. (c) DSA at the end of the procedure showing occlusion of the majority of the aneurysm and patency of the distal internal carotid artery. (d) MRA source data demonstrating flow in the neck of the aneurysm.

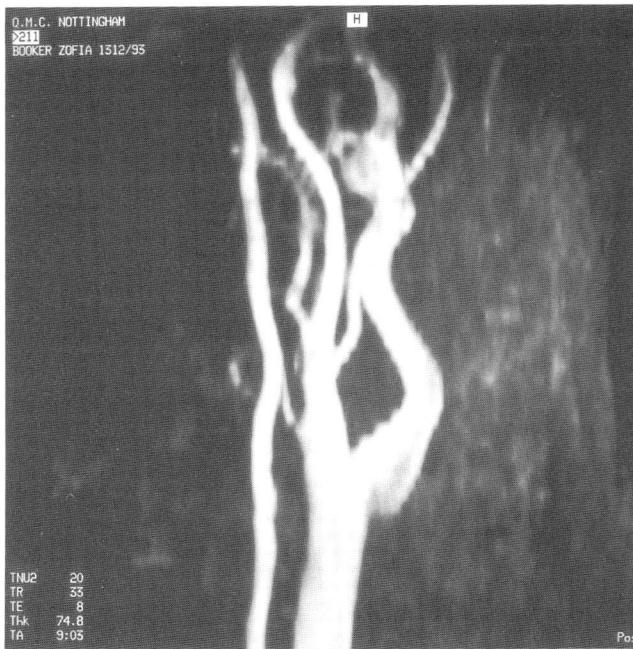

(e)

Fig. 1. (e) MIPed reconstruction shows the neck of the aneurysm to be patent but the distal two-thirds of the lumen had been occluded. Also, flow in the carotid artery distal to the aneurysm is visualized.

MRA acquired at the same time showed flow within the residual pouch and patency of the distal vessels, although the signal was attenuated (compared to the right) due to slow flow and saturation effects.

After the second embolization, SE images demonstrated more thrombi in the aneurysm, but the aneurysm has continued to enlarge.

The third embolization further occluded the aneurysm; however, a small residual pouch was deliberately left, as M2 vessels emanated from it. There was good concordance between the MRA and conventional X-ray angiogram; however, difficulty in separating thrombi from flow in large aneurysms with MIPed MRA images was experienced in this case (Fig. 2b). High signal from methemoglobin on gradient recalled echo (GE) images is incorporated into the reconstructed MIPed images. Phase contrast angiography would be very useful in distinguishing the subacute thrombi from flow in large aneurysms.

Patient 3

This 52-year-old woman presented with a subarachnoid hemorrhage. Conventional angiography at the time demonstrated a large aneurysm at the origin of

(a)

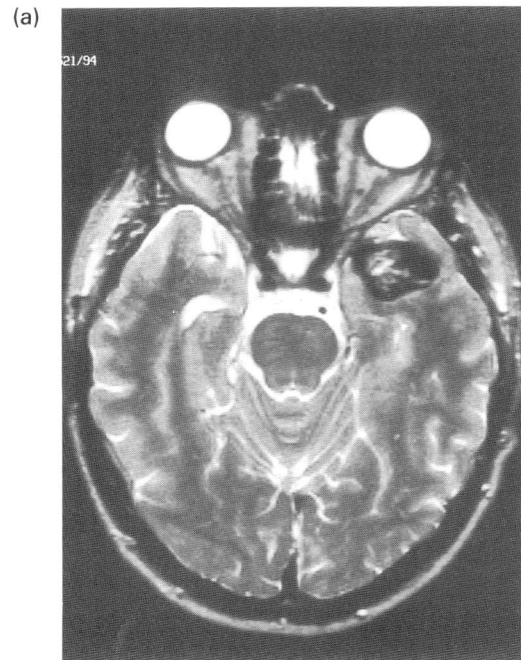

(b)

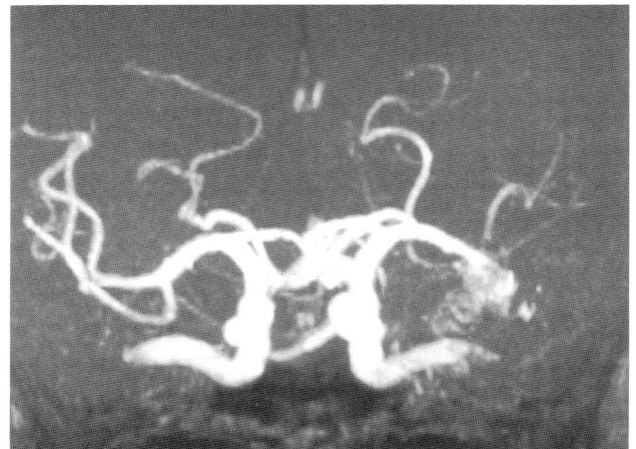

Fig. 2. A 45-year-old man who presented with a subarachnoid hemorrhage from a large left middle cerebral artery aneurysm. He underwent three separate embolization procedures over the next year (Patient 2). (a) Following embolization, axial T_2-weighted scans showed the left middle cerebral aneurysm with a complex signal intensity pattern with peripheral low signal related to mural calcification, hyperintensity in keeping with subacute thrombi and centrally low signal which could be related to the platinum GDC coil balls or might represent a flow void. (b) MRA after the third and final embolization. Difficulty in separating thrombi from flow in large aneurysms was experienced in this case. High signal from met hemoglobin on gradient-echo images is incorporated into the reconstructed MIPped images.

(a)

(b)

(c)

(d)

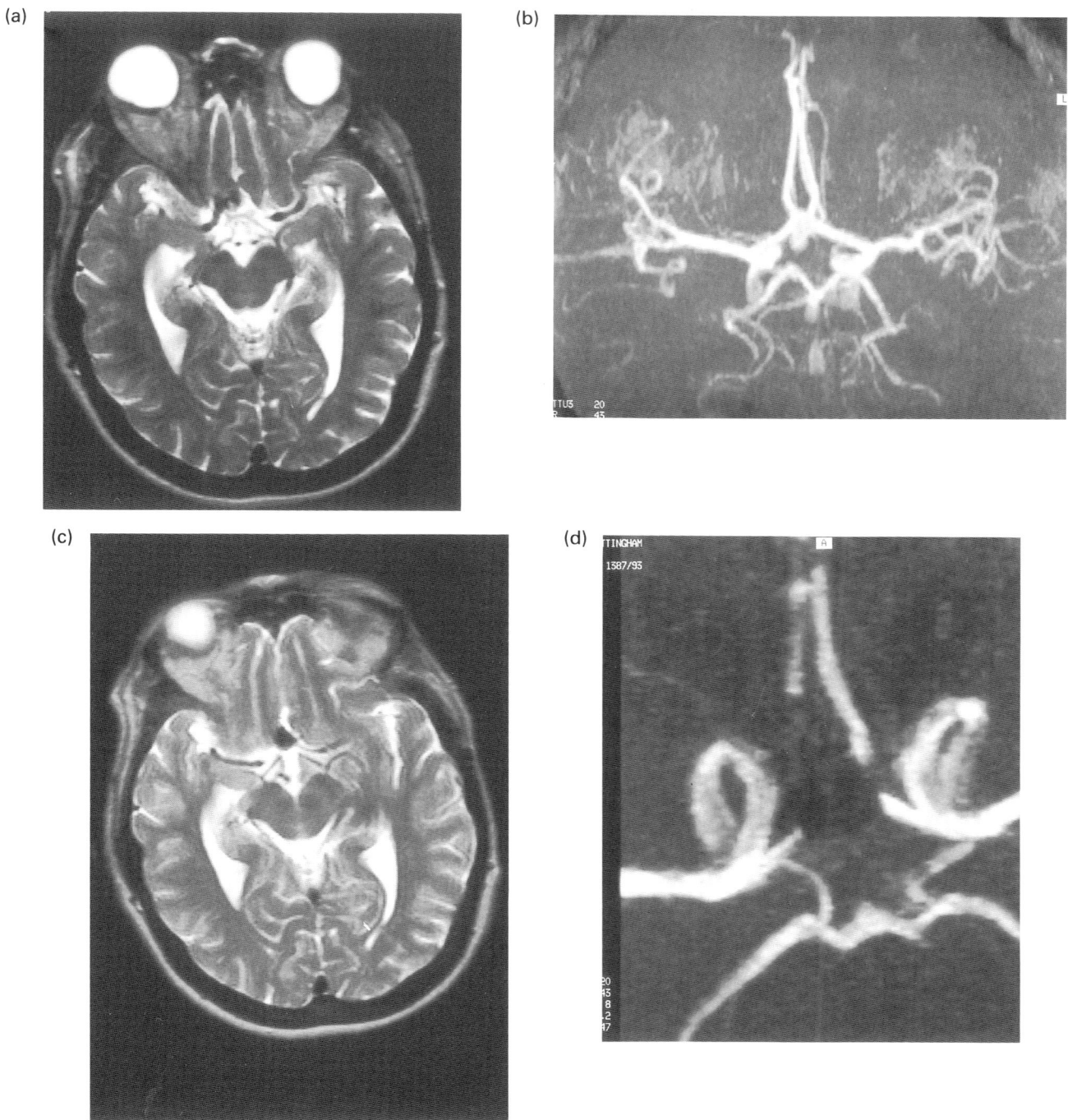

Fig. 3. A 52-year-old woman with a large aneurysm at the origin of the left anterior cerebral artery (Patient 3). (a) Prior to embolization, spin-echo images demonstrate the aneurysm which contains some thrombi (high signal). (b) Prior to embolization, MRA MIPed images demonstrate the aneurysm to contain flowing blood. (c) Postembolization, spin-echo images demonstrate dense loss of signal from the aneurysm (susceptibility effect). (d) Postembolization MRA shows nonvisualization of the parent vessels due to the susceptibility effect of the coils.

(a)

(b)

(c)

(d)

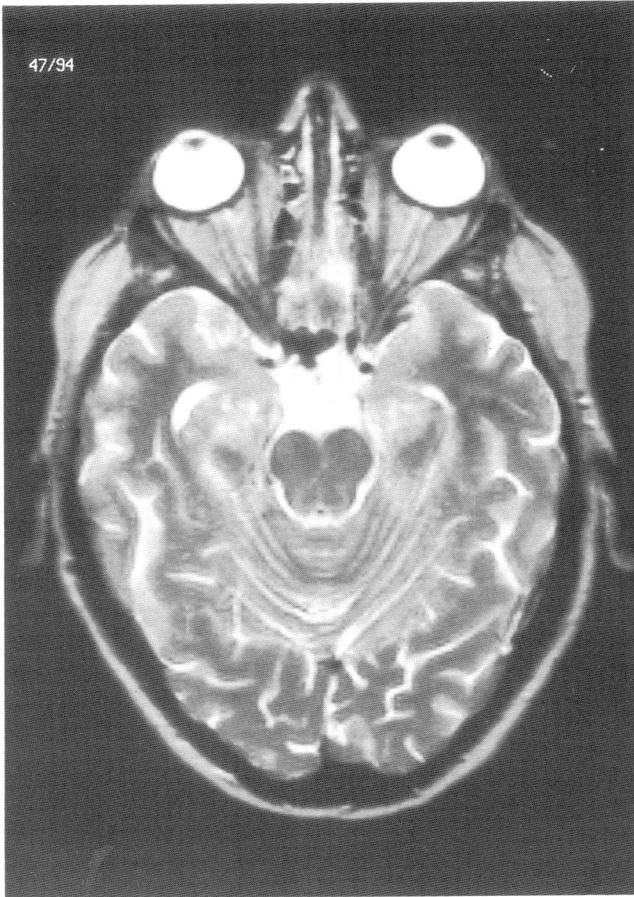

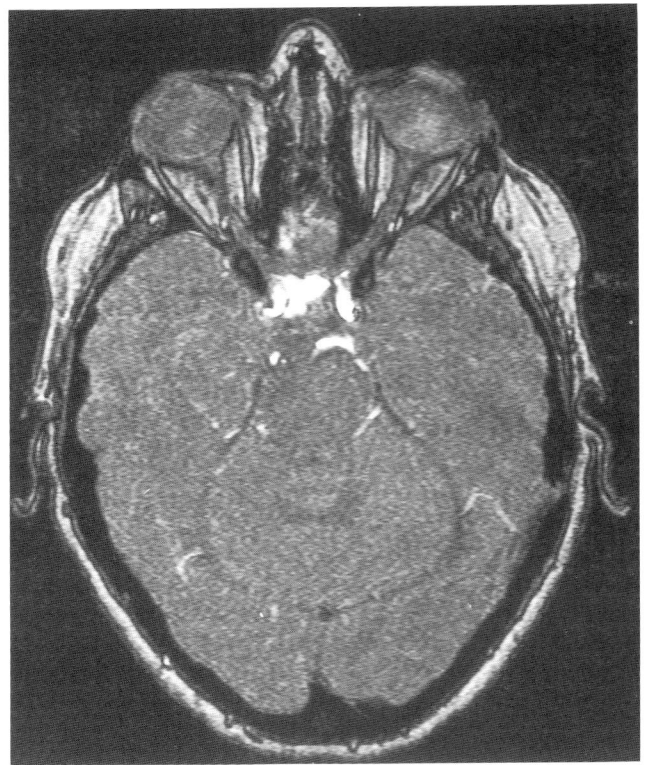

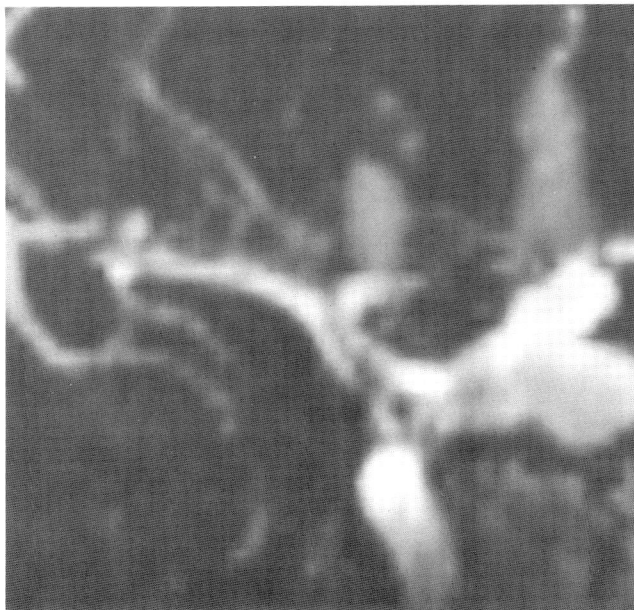

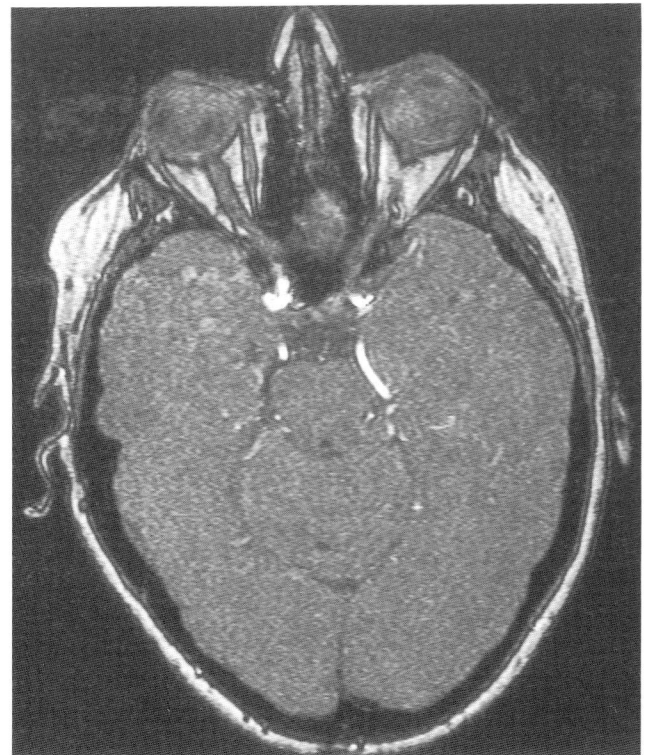

Fig. 4. A 50-year-old woman with a large aneurysm at the origin of the right ophthalmic artery (Patient 4). (a) Spin-echo images demonstrate the aneurysm. (b) Prior to embolization, MRA source images demonstrate the aneurysm to contain flowing blood. (c) Prior to embolization, MRA MIPed images demonstrate a bilobed aneurysm with hematoma superiorly. (d) Postembolization, MRA source images show no flow in the aneurysm. (Continued on page 332.)

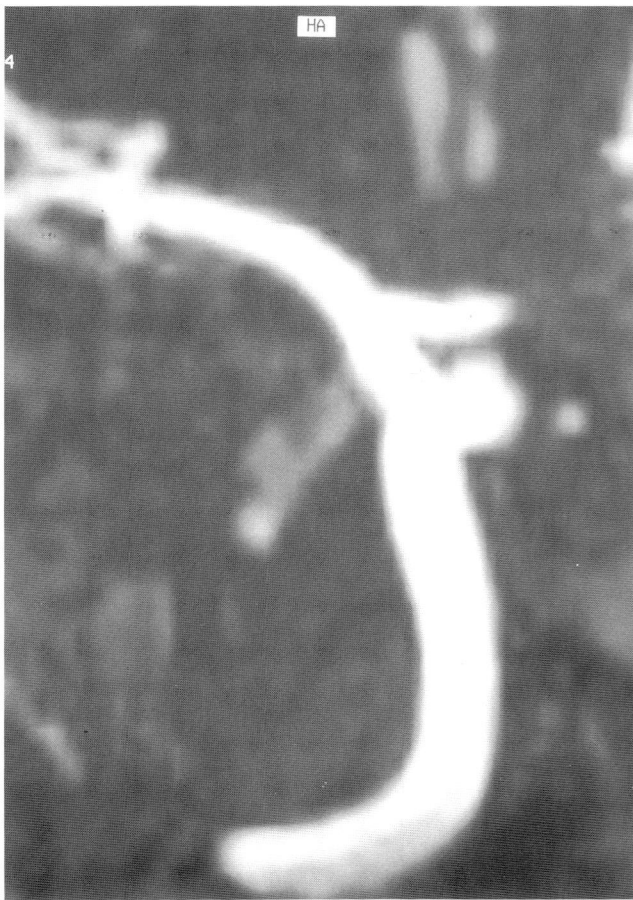

(e)

Fig. 4. (e) Postembolization, flow in a small residual pouch is seen on MRA MIPed images, but the aneurysm is largely occluded.

the left anterior cerebral artery. This was subsequently wrapped at surgery.

Eight months later, the aneurysm was assessed with MR. The spin-echo images demonstrated the aca aneurysm to contain some high-signal thrombi (Fig. 3a). The MRA sequence demonstrated flow within the aneurysm (Fig. 3b). These images allowed assessment of size and morphology, enabling an appropriate choice of coils and approach.

On the same day, embolization was undertaken using three GDC coils with almost complete obliteration of the aneurysmal sac. Two days later, assessment by MRA showed a low signal in the aneurysm on both T_1 and T_2 spin-echo sequences (Fig. 3c). This could possibly have represented a flow void, but the dense loss of signal indicates a susceptibility artifact from the platinum coils. The postembolization MRA (Fig. 3d) demonstrated loss of signal in the region of the

aneurysm and the parent vessel due to the susceptibility artifact from the platinum coil mass, but the distal aca was visualized and the proximal segment was presumed to be patent.

Patient 4

A 50-year-old woman presented with a subarachnoid hemorrhage. Conventional angiography demonstrated a large aneurysm at the origin of the right ophthalmic artery. Two weeks later, MRA was performed to assess the aneurysm. MRA source data confirmed flow within the lumen (Fig. 4b). The reconstructed images demonstrated a bilobed aneurysm with hematoma superiorly (Fig. 4c). Four days later, embolization with six GDC coils caused almost complete obliteration of the aneurysm.

Flow in a small residual pouch is seen on both the MRA source data (Fig. 4d) and the MIPed reconstructions (Fig. 4e), but the aneurysm remained largely occluded. Measurements of the aneurysmal size were made from the MIPed images.

Patient 5

This 54-year-old woman had a giant basilar artery tip aneurysm, and bilateral middle cerebral artery aneurysms demonstrated on conventional arteriography.

She was treated with embolization in which tungsten spiral microcoils and platinum coils were inserted into the basilar tip aneurysm. Later, computer tomography (CT) showed densely packed coils, producing a severe radial artifact and was not useful. The spin-echo coronal sequence clearly demonstrated a large aneurysm burrowing into the brainstem (Fig. 5a). Spin-echo images also demonstrated extensive changes in the surrounding diencephalic structures and posterior internal capsule on the left side, probably representing a combination of edema and ischemia.

MR angiography demonstrated a persistent residual pouch and gave some evidence of the internal flow dynamics (Fig. 5b). It also demonstrated the bilateral moderate-sized middle cerebral artery aneurysm.

Phase ghosting was helpful in this case, as it established pulsatility of the aneurysm (Fig. 5c).

This incompletely embolized aneurysm continued to grow and subsequently ruptured with the death of the patient.

DISCUSSION

The use of three-dimensional time-of-flight (3D TOF) MR angiography in the evaluation of intracranial

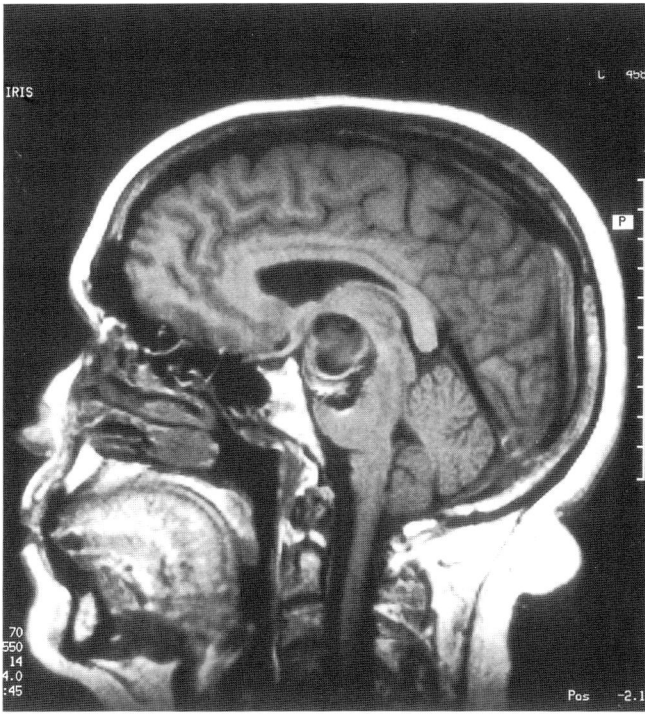

(a)

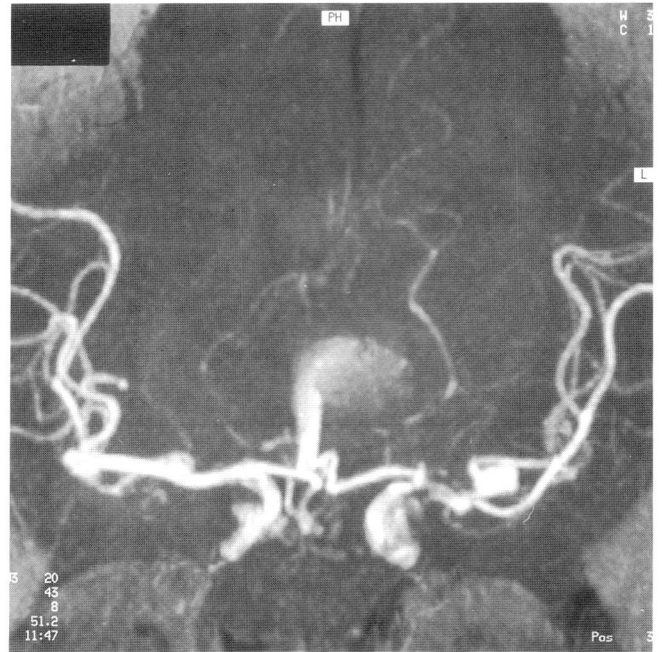

(b)

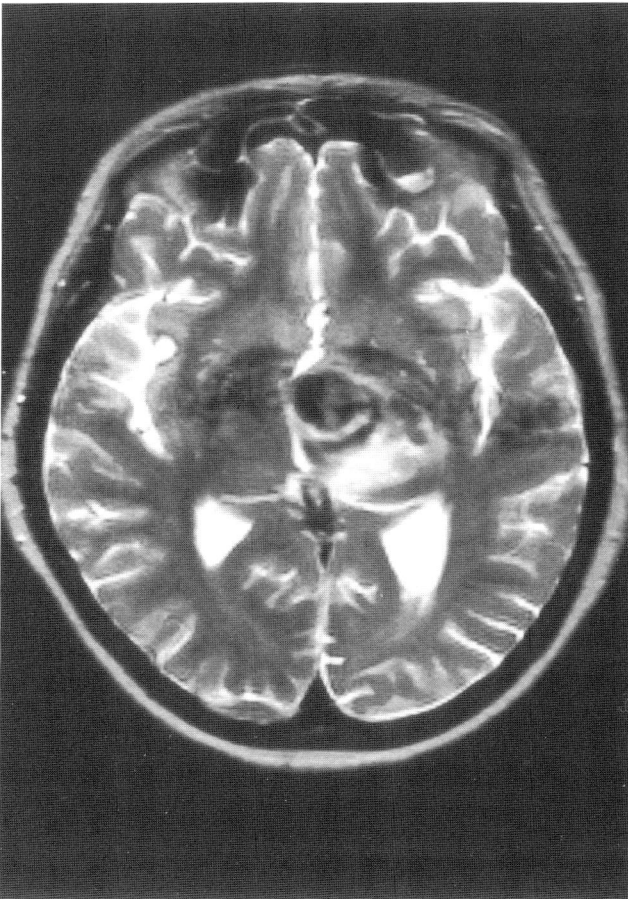

(c)

Fig. 5. A 54-year-old woman with a giant basilar artery tip aneurysm and bilateral middle cerebral artery aneurysms (Patient 5). (a) Spin-echo coronal sequences demonstrate a large aneurysm burrowing into the brainstem. (b) Phase ghosting establishes pulsatility of the aneurysm. (c) MRA MIPed demonstrates a persistent residual pouch and shows the internal flow dynamics.

aneurysms treated by endovascular balloon occlusion has been previously reported [1]. To our knowledge, this is the first report of MRA of platinum microcoils in cerebral aneurysms. All patients were imaged using a Siemen's 1.5-T Magnetom scanner. The MR angiography sequence used has the following parameters: TR = 43, TE = 8, flip angle = 20, field of view = 200, slice thickness = 52 mm, matrix = 256 × 512 oversampled, number of acquisitions = 1, acquisition time = 11 min 47 s).

The platinum coils produce an area of signal loss on SE images which could be mistaken for a flow void. Signal loss due to susceptibility artifacts from platinum coils is qualitatively different from a flow void from which it can be distinguished (patient 3). However, the susceptibility artifact is also small, as predicted by *in vitro* and *in vivo* experimental studies [2].

The 3D MRA TOF sequence is sensitive to paramagnetic substances and these will appear as bright objects in the MIP reconstructions. Therefore, a subacute thrombus produces high-signal simulating flow on TOF images. This problem has been previously described [3]. Phase contrast techniques would be useful to overcome the T_1 shortening effect of methaemoglobin on MIPed images and demonstrate more clearly residual slow flow in large aneurysms.

Platinum emboli in the cerebral hemispheres as a complication of this procedure has been reported in a recent communication to the FDA. We reviewed all the spin-echo images for evidence of platinum emboli, but none was detected.

CONCLUSION

MRA is a quick outpatient, serial noninvasive monitoring technique in the evaluation of cerebral aneurysms which have been embolized with platinum coils. MRA has the advantages of not requiring a general anesthetic, no radiation burden, and increased comfort, which is important in those patients who need repeated examinations. Platinum coils did not cause a clinically significant susceptibility problem.

MRA also has an important role in the planning of the embolization procedure. External and internal dimensions of aneurysms may be demonstrated and this helps in the selection of coil size and selecting the approach to the aneurysm.

Problems with MRA include limited spatial resolution, degradation due to motion artifact, high-signal subacute thrombi simulating flow on GR images, and slow flow leading to saturation effects and reduced signal.

REFERENCES

1. Tsuruda JS, Sevick RJ, Halbach VV (1992) Three-dimensional time-of-flight MR angiography in the evaluation of intracranial aneurysms treated by endovascular balloon occlusion. *Am J Nucl Reson* **13**(4): 1129–1136.
2. Marshall MW, Teitelbaum GP, Kim HS, Marshall MW, Teitelbaum GP, Kim HS, Deveikis J (1991) Ferromagnetism and magnetic resonance artefacts of platinum embolization microcoils. *Cardiovasc Intervent Radiol* **14**(3): 163–166.
3. Strother CM, Eldevik P, Kikuchi Y, Graves V, Partington C, Merlis A (1989) Thrombus formation and structure and the evolution of mass effect in intracranial aneurysms treated by balloon embolization: emphasis on MR findings. *Am J Nucl Reson* **10**(4): 787.

Dynamic T_1 studies of gadolinium uptake in brain tumors using LL-EPI

A. Freeman,[1] P. Gowland,[1] D. Jellineck,[2] D. Wilcock,[3] J. Firth,[2]
B. Worthington,[3] P. Mansfield[1]*, and G. Ratcliffe[4]

*Magnetic Resonance Centre, Department of Physics and Departments of [2]Neurosurgery
and [3]Academic Radiology University of Nottingham NG7 2RD, UK
[4]Squibb Diagnostics, Hounslow, Middlesex, TW3 3JA, UK*

Using ultrafast T_1 mapping (LL-EPI), the uptake from a bolus injection of Gd-DO3A (ProHance) into the sagittal sinus and a brain tumor has been monitored. The measurement of absolute T_1 removes the possible error in uptake curves created from T_1-weighted sequences caused by changes in T_2^* and simplifies the calculation of ProHance concentration. The LL-EPI sequence has an acquisition time of 1.2 s and is repeated every 4 s to obtain uptake curves with a high temporal and spatial resolution. Optimization of the LL-EPI sequence has been performed to obtain a precision of 5% over the T_1 range 0.3–1.2 s.

Keywords: fast T_1 mapping, LL-EPI, dynamic Gd uptake.

INTRODUCTION

Dynamic imaging using contrast agents such as gadolinium chelates can potentially improve the specificity of magnetic resonance imaging (MRI). We have previously demonstrated the use of dynamic uptake studies of Gd-DTPA to assess brain tumors using T_1-weighted inversion recovery echo-planar imaging (IR-EPI) [1]. It was possible to correlate calculated vascularity and permeability indices with histologically determined tumor grade and the surgeon's assessment of vascularity by modeling the transfer of contrast agent into the capillaries and across the blood-brain barrier. However, the change in signal intensity with contrast agent concentration is due to changes in both T_1 and T_2 relaxation rates, so imaging sequences that are sensitive to both these relaxation times limit the accuracy of the techniques. This article describes the application and optimization of a rapid direct T_1 measurement sequence which overcomes these problems.

Models of contrast agent uptake in tumors require a knowledge of the arterial concentration (input function) as well as the tumor concentration of the agent. This is because of the individual variation in both the rate of mixing of contrast agent in the blood and rate of removal of the contrast agent by the kidneys. A bolus injection of contrast agent takes about 20 s to distribute into the blood stream and so a temporal resolution of a few seconds is required to adequately monitor the input function. A similar temporal resolution is required for the tumor to monitor the vascular phase, which could have a time constant almost as rapid as the input function. A simple and noninvasive method of measuring the input function to the tumor is to use a vessel visible in the same plane as the tumor; to achieve this high spatial resolution in a T_1 map is required.

METHOD

Sequence optimization

The Look–Locher sequence, which uses a single spin inversion followed by multiple low-angle readout pulses can be used in combination with EPI [2] to generate high-resolution T_1 maps in a few seconds with a repeatability of 5% [3]. To use this sequence in rapid studies of contrast agent uptake it is necessary to

---

* Address correspondence to Sir Peter Mansfield, Magnetic Resonance Centre, University of Nottingham, University Park, Nottingham NG7 2RD, UK.

(i) decrease the T_1 map acquisition period to maintain adequate temporal resolution and (ii) minimize the gradient duty cycle to prevent overheating of gradient amplifiers. Monte Carlo simulations were used to minimize the number of pulses and select the optimum pulse spacing to maintain the reproducibility of T_1 measurements over the T_1 range 1.4–0.3 s found in the blood stream before and after a standard 0.1 mmol kg^{-1} dose of Gd-DO3A (Gadoteridol, Pro-Hance, Squibb Diagnostics). A reproducibility of 5% relative standard deviation (SD) in T_1 was deemed adequate for the uptake models, where

$$\text{Relative standard deviation of } T_1 = \frac{\text{SD (fitted } T_1)}{\text{simulated } T_1} \%.$$

The experiment was simulated by repeatedly fitting T_1 to calculated data with the addition of Gaussian noise. The standard deviation of T_1 was compared with different sequence parameters and an optimum sought. A signal-to-noise ratio (S/N) of 40 : 1 was used, which is the expected S/N of a standard 90° EPI scan using the head coil. Linear pulse spacing only was investigated. The simulation (Fig. 1) shows that a sequence with $N = 6$ (number of readout pulses), readout pulse angle = 45°, $t_i = 0.01$ s (time from the inversion pulse to first readout) and $t_a = 0.2$ s (separation time between remaining readout pulses) had a 5% relative standard deviation of T_1 over the T_1 range of 0.3–1.2 s and an acquisition time of 1.2 s. Further simulations showed that an otherwise identical sequence with

$N = 8$ had the desired reproducibility over a T_1 range of 0.3–1.5 s; however, six samples were used for this pilot study to ensure reliability of the gradients.

Patient scanning

LL-EPI was used on a dedicated 0.5-T EPI scanner to generate T_1 maps in 1.2 s, comprising 128 × 128 pixel arrays with a voxel size of 2.5 × 2.5 × 10 mm^3. The sequence was initially repeated every 4 s for 30 min after a bolus injection of ProHance to provide a time uptake curve with a high temporal resolution.

Image analysis

Two regions of interest were chosen from the T_1 maps: one over the sagittal sinus and the other over the tumor chosen from the enhanced area at the peak of the uptake curve. These regions were followed through the complete time course to produce a T_1 uptake curve. The relative contrast agent concentration is known to be proportional to changes in longitudinal relaxation rate, so the concentration C was simply calculated using

$$C = \frac{1}{k}\left(\frac{1}{T_{1m}} - \frac{1}{T_{1i}}\right)$$

where k is the relaxivity (mM^{-1} s^{-1}) of Gd ProHance in the tissue, T_{1m} is the T_1 measured from the region of

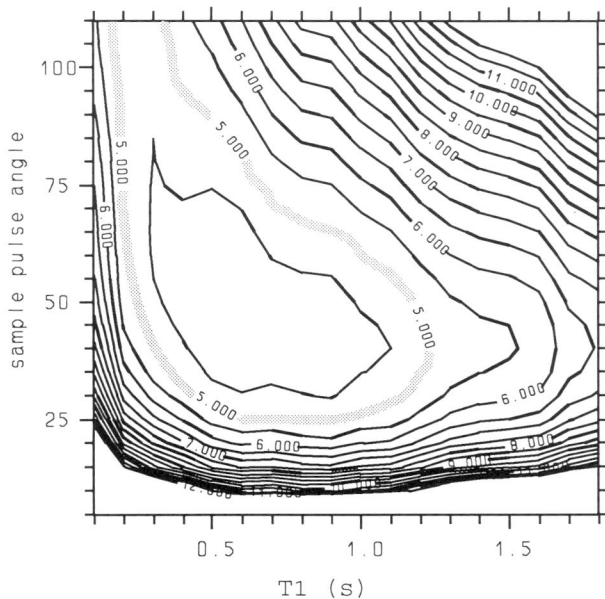

Fig. 1. Contour map of relative standard deviation of T_1 for sample pulse angle against T_1. This was produced for the LL-EPI sequence with $N = 6$, $t_i = 0.01$ s, $t_a = 0.2$ s, S/N = 40 : 1. The 5% contour is highlighted.

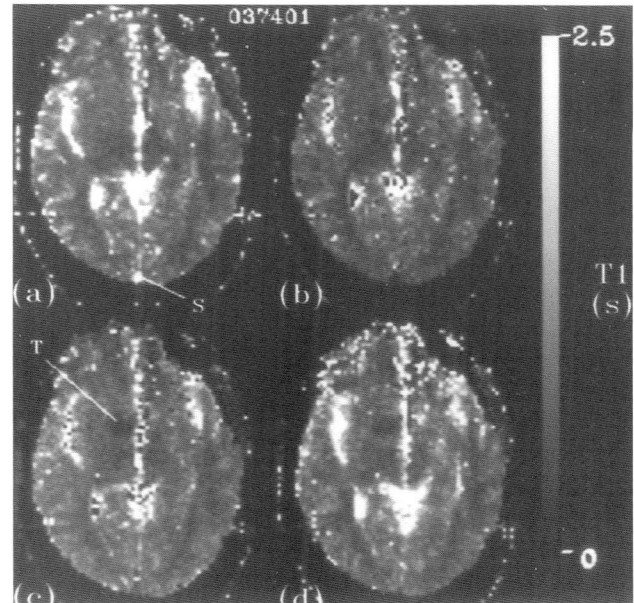

Fig. 2. Four LL-EPI T_1 maps using parameters $N = 6$, $t_i = 0.02$, $t_a = 0.2$, pulse angle = 45°; (a) before injection of contrast agent and at (b) 50 s, (c) 450 s and (d) 1200 s following contrast agent injection. S = sagittal sinus; T = tumor.

interest and T_{1i} is the T_1 before the ProHance injection of the same region of interest.

RESULTS

Four typical T_1 maps from a patient with a lymphoma are shown in Fig. 2. The change in T_1 in the sagittal sinus is visible in image (b) followed by the slower ProHance uptake into the tumor in image (c). The final image (d) shows a very gradual washout of ProHance from this particular lymphoma.

A graph of relative Gd ProHance concentration for the complete time course is given in Fig. 3 which shows an initial rapid uptake into the tumor and slower later phase. This curve will be modeled to provide quantitative vascularity and permeability indices using techniques described in Ref. 1.

DISCUSSION

Although the LL-EPI sequence measures absolute T_1 and is insensitive to T_2^*, in all cases it has been assumed that T_1 and T_2^* do not change significantly over the LL-EPI acquisition period of 1.2 s. However, in the initial uptake phase, T_1 and T_2^* will be changing rapidly. But simulations show that even for the most rapid changes in T_1 and T_2^* observed in the sagittal sinus, the fitted T_1 lies within the actual range of T_1 occurring during acquisition and is weighted toward the T_1 at the time of the inversion pulse; therefore, this is not a significant problem.

CONCLUSION

Simulations have shown that using LL-EPI it is possible to measure T_1 with sufficient reproducibility and low enough gradient duty cycle over the T_1 range 0.3–1.2 s to be able to monitor the change in Gd ProHance concentration by direct T_1 measurements. It is envisaged that this range will be increased by nonlinear sampling. These measurements will improve the accuracy of the fitted model parameters (blood volume, perfusion rate, and blood-brain barrier permeability) and should provide a robust assessment of tumor stage and response to treatment.

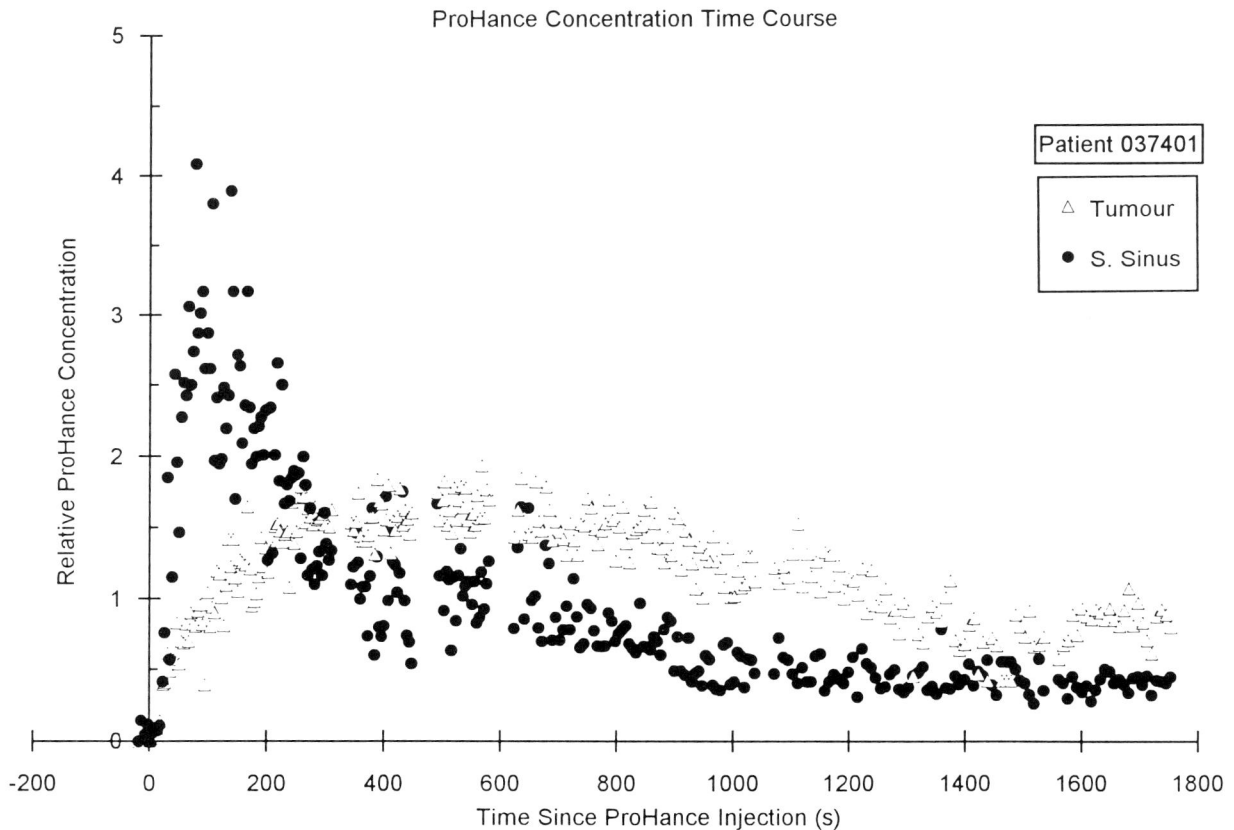

Fig. 3. Time course of relative Gd ProHance concentration for the tumor and sagittal sinus.

ACKNOWLEDGMENT

This work is supported by Squibb Diagnostics. The EPI program is funded by the MRC.

REFERENCES

1. Gowland P, Mansfield P, Bullock P, Stehling M, Worthington B, Firth J (1992) Dynamic studies of gadolinium uptake in brain tumors using inversion-recovery echo-planar imaging. *Magn Reson Med* **26:** 241–258.

2. Howseman A, Stehling M, Chapman B, Coxon R, Turner R, Ordidge R, Cawley M, Glover P, Mansfield P, Coupland R (1988) Improvements in snap-shot nuclear magnetic resonance imaging. *Br J Radiol* **61:** 822–828.

3. Gowland P, Mansfield P (1993) Accurate measurement of T_1 in vivo in less than 3 seconds using echo-planar imaging. *Magn Reson Med* **30:** 351–354.

Quantitative analysis of Gd-DTPA enhanced dynamic MR images by simplex minimization

D. L. Buckley,[1]* R. W. Kerslake,[2] S. J. Blackband[1] and A. Horsman[1]

[1]Centre for MR Investigations, Hull Royal Infirmary, Hull HU3 2JK UK
[2]Magnetic Resonance Centre, University Hospital, Nottingham NG7 2RD, UK

The introduction of fast clinical imaging techniques enables the dynamic sampling of contrast agent kinetics. The quantity of data generated by such techniques demands the application of automated analysis tools to provide objective assessments of contrast washin/washout characteristics across an entire image. Using a simple compartmental model, the washin/washout characteristics may be defined in terms of a biexponential function. Curve fitting to this nonlinear function may be approached using a nonlinear least squares technique. We demonstrate an alternative technique, simplex minimization, to be more robust in a comparative study using Monte Carlo simulation. The application of the technique is illustrated by pixel-by-pixel analysis of dynamic data obtained from a patient with primary carcinoma of the breast.

Keywords: dynamic MRI, simplex minimization, nonlinear least squares, breast neoplasm.

INTRODUCTION

Dynamic imaging before, during, and after injection of dimeglumine gadopentetate (Gd-DTPA) appears useful in many clinical magnetic resonance (MR) examinations [1–3]. Rapid contrast kinetics may be observed both with a high spatial and temporal resolution using fast gradient-echo imaging sequences. However, assessment of these data sets is hampered by the lower signal-to-noise ratio (S/N) implicit in a faster imaging sequence and by the large number of images that must be assessed. Qualitative analysis typically involves choosing clearly enhancing regions and then visually assessing these areas using a cine-loop viewer. This method is both subjective and time-consuming without providing the clinician with data across the entire image. Quantitative techniques that provide complete image-wide pixel-by-pixel information are likely to prove more sensitive and will also avoid user subjectivity. Contrast kinetics may be modeled mathematically in terms of a few simple parameters [1, 2]. Curve fitting

to the dynamic image data provides estimates of these parameters. Thus, a theoretical model for the behavior of contrast agent on a pixel-by-pixel basis may be constructed.

Compartmental models are often described in terms of a number of exponential functions [1, 2, 4]. Curve fitting to a multiple exponential function requires the use of a nonlinear curve-fitting routine. The standard technique, nonlinear least squares (NLLS), has been used previously to fit multiexponential functions not only in the quantitative analysis of Gd-DTPA enhancement profiles [1, 2, 4, 5] but also in the analysis of multicompartment NMR relaxation decays [6]. Although NLLS provides a useful tool in the modeling of a large range of nonlinear systems, its effectiveness in the fitting of multiple-exponential functions has been questioned [7]. In particular, the accuracy of convergence appears to be sensitive to the initial choice of parameter estimates. In the following report, we compare the performance of NLLS by the method of Marquardt [8] with a more generalized minimization technique, simplex minimization [9], in the fitting of a biexponential function. The application of the simplex method is then demonstrated in the analysis of contrast enhancement of a breast tumor.

---

* Address for correspondence: Centre for MR Investigations, Hull Royal Infirmary, Anlaby Road, Hull HU3 2JZ, UK.

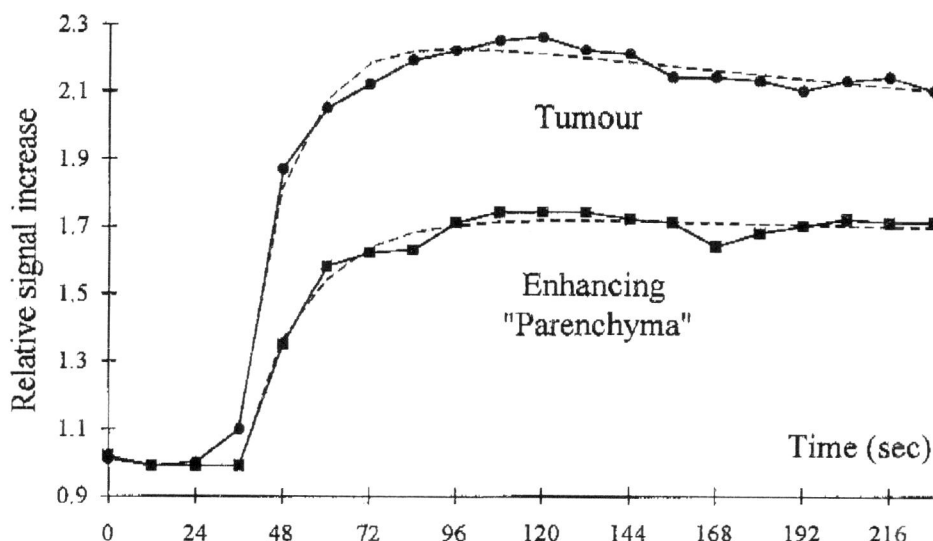

Fig. 1. Distribution of error in the estimate of parameter $a[4]$ [see Eq. (1)] using data with a S/N of 20 : 1. Graphs show percentage error along the x axes and frequency along the y axes. Upper graphs calculated using simplex minimization; lower graphs using NLLS by the method of Marquardt. Variation of initial parameter estimate about correct value (a) 5%, (b) 15%, and (c) 25%.

METHODS

Curve fitting

The model chosen for curve fitting is a general form of a biexponential function that may be used to model contrast kinetics:

$$S = \frac{a[1] \exp(-a[2]t) - a[3] \exp(-a[4]t)}{a[4] - a[2]} \quad (1)$$

where $a[1]$–$a[4]$ represent the separable parameters and t is the independent variable. Values for S were generated using Monte Carlo simulation. One thousand curves, each of 1000 data points, were generated using known parameter values. To these data was added pseudorandom noise with a Gaussian distribution. The width of the noise distribution could be predetermined and had a coefficient of variation (CV) between 5% and 15%. In order to compare the performance of the techniques in relation to the initial parameter estimate, the choice of estimate was also varied using a pseudorandom distribution. The width of this Gaussian distribution, centered on the correct parameter value, was varied between 5% and 45% (CV). Hence, each curve was submitted to the two curve-fitting routines given a pseudorandom initial estimate of each parameter. The distribution of error in the final calculation of each parameter was then plotted at each noise level and initial estimate variation. A convergence failure was defined as any convergence occurring outside the 99.9% confidence limit of

a specific error distribution at each noise level. This distribution was obtained using the simplex method and an initial estimate CV of 5%. Thus, the relative failure rate could be calculated for each technique at each noise level and initial estimate CV.

Imaging

Imaging of a patient with primary carcinoma of the breast was carried out on a 1.5-T Signa MR system (IGE Medical Systems, WI, USA) using a dedicated phased-array breast coil. The study was approved by the local ethics committee and the patient gave written, informed consent. Using a fast SPGR sequence (TR/TE 11.2/4.2 ms, flip 30°, NEX = 2), 100 images may be obtained in a little under 5 min. Thus, 25 images at 4 slice locations were collected with a temporal resolution of 11.6 s. Into an antecubital fossa vein 0.1 mmol kg^{-1} body weight of Gd-DTPA was injected immediately prior to image set 4. Data were then transferred to a SUN workstation where curve fitting was undertaken using software developed at the Centre.

RESULTS

The relative failure rates of each technique at noise levels of 10% and 15% are presented in Table 1.

Parameter images calculated from the dynamic study clearly highlighted areas of Gd-DTPA enhancement

Table 1. Relative percentage failure rates (see text for definition) for curve fitting by simplex minimization and NLLS by the method of Marquardt.

Method	Noise (CV)	Initial estimate variation (CV)								
		5%	10%	15%	20%	25%	30%	35%	40%	45%
Simplex	10%	0.1	0.1	0.1	0.1	0.1	0.1	0.2	0.4	0.3
	15%	0.1	0.1	0.1	0.1	0.1	0.1	0.2	0.6	0.3
NLLS	10%	0.1	0.1	0.1	0.1	0.1	0.4	0.9	1.2	2.2
	15%	0.1	0.1	0.1	0.1	0.1	0.4	0.9	1.1	2.2

not restricted to the lesion. The parameters were not distributed homogeneously throughout the lesion. Washin was seen to be more rapid at the tumor margins, although the maximal enhancement was greatest within the tumor boundary. The extent of enhancement observed in the parameter images exceeded that demonstrated in a fat-suppressed postcontrast, T_1-weighted image.

DISCUSSION

Simplex minimization provides a more robust method of fitting data to a biexponential function than NLLS by the method Marquardt. The error distribution is defined partially by the distribution of initial parameter estimates. This sensitivity to initial estimates makes Marquardt's method inappropriate for the analysis of routinely acquired dynamic MR data. The initial estimates must be obtained from the image data when a priori information is not available and, as such, are influenced by propagation of the error governed by the image S/N. Even if a priori information is available regarding contrast kinetics within the tumor, it may not be applicable to the data obtained from other regions of the image.

One of the fundamental reasons for this sensitivity relates to an approximation used in the NLLS method [7], which holds for multiple exponential functions only in a very small region close to the minimum of the parameter space. Erratic behavior results when initial estimates take the search procedure far from the global minimum. As the simplex technique makes no such assumptions [9], convergence is predominantly noise governed. This has implications for the multiexponential analysis of NMR relaxation decays. If accurate automated fitting is to be achieved using image data and NLLS, then very good initial estimates are required. Typically, both the quality and quantity of the data are limited. Although simplex minimization will still suffer from poor quality data, producing results of a low precision, the accuracy of the results will not be affected by the choice of initial estimate.

We have used simplex minimization to quantify contrast agent kinetics in the breast in terms of a simple compartmental model. The technique is robust and fully automated. Synthetic images represent parameters calculated by the curve-fitting highlight areas of enhancement and demonstrate the heterogeneous distribution of contrast characteristics within tumors.

ACKNOWLEDGMENTS

This work was funded by the Yorkshire Cancer Research Campaign. The phased-array breast coil was supplied by IGE Medical Systems as part of an ongoing research agreement.

REFERENCES

1. Larsson HBW, Stubgaard M, Frederiksen JL, Jensen M, Henriksen O, Paulson OB (1990) Quantitation of blood-brain barrier defect by magnetic resonance imaging and gadolinium-DTPA in patients with multiple sclerosis and brain tumours. *Magn Reson Med* **16**: 117–131.
2. Tofts PS, Kermode AG (1991) Measurement of the blood-brain barrier permeability and leakage space using dynamic MR imaging. 1. Fundamental concepts. *Magn Reson Med* **17**: 357–367.
3. Flickinger FW, Allison JD, Sherry RM, Wright JC (1993) Differentiation of benign from malignant breast masses by time-intensity evaluation of contrast enhanced MRI. *Magn Reson Imaging* **11**: 617–620.

4. Brix G, Semmler W, Port R, Schad LR, Layer G, Lorenz WJ (1991) Pharmacokinetic parameters in CNS Gd-DTPA enhanced MR imaging. *J Comput Assist Tomogr* **15**: 621–628.

5. Müller-Schimpfle M, Brix G, Layer G, Schlag P, Engenhart R, Frohmuller S, Heß T, Zuna I, Semmler W, van Kaick G (1993) Recurrent rectal cancer: Diagnosis with dynamic MR imaging. *Radiology* **189**: 881–889.

6. Clayden NJ, Hesler BD (1992) Multiexponential analysis of relaxation decays. *J Magn Reson* **98**: 271–282.

7. Gans P (1992) *Data Fitting in the Chemical Sciences by the Method of Least Squares.* Chichester: John Wiley and Sons.

8. Bevington PR (1969) *Data Reduction and Error Analysis for the Physical Sciences.* New York: McGraw-Hill.

9. Nelder JA, Mead R (1965) A simplex method for function minimisation. *Computer J* **7**: 308–313.

Evaluation of myocardial function and perfusion in ischemic heart disease

Charles B. Higgins,* Maythem Saeed, Michael Wendland, Michael Bourne, Johannes Steffans, and Hajime Sakuma

Department of Radiology, University of California, San Francisco, CA 94143, USA

Ischemic heart disease is the most frequently encountered cardiac disease. Magnetic resonance imaging (MRI) can be used to investigate several facets of this disease. A number of studies over the past several years have shown the capability of cine MRI for quantifying regional myocardial function and for identifying abnormalities of regional myocardial wall thickening in the basal or vasodilated states due to ischemia. Contrast-enhanced inversion recovery fast gradient echo and echo-planar imaging have been applied for monitoring the first passage of contrast media through the myocardium. This technique has depicted regional perfusion deficits in the basal state or in the vasodilated states induced by vasodilators. Recent studies have also disclosed the feasibility of using MR techniques for displaying the morphology of the major coronary arteries and for measuring blood flow velocity in the coronary arteries and coronary bypass grafts. Thus, MRI has the capability for evaluation of morphology and flow in the coronary arteries and for assessment of function and perfusion of the myocardium.

Keywords: cine MRI, ischemic heart disease, myocardial function, myocardial perfusion.

Ischemic heart disease is the most frequent cause of morbidity and mortality in advanced industrialized societies. Consequently, the importance of any noninvasive cardiac imaging techniques is defined by its effectiveness for the evaluation of ischemic heart disease. Noninvasive techniques are usually applied to detect the presence of regional myocardial ischemia by demonstrating either regional myocardial dysfunction or regional myocardial perfusion deficits in the basal or vasodilated states. Several studies in recent years have shown the capability of magnetic resonance imaging (MRI) for demonstrating regional myocardial ischemia either indirectly as regional contractile dysfunction or directly as a regional perfusion deficit. This article will examine progress in the application of MRI for the evaluation of regional myocardial function and perfusion in ischemic heart disease.

* Address for correspondence: Radiology Department, Box 0628, University of California, San Francisco, CA 94143, USA.

EVALUATION OF REGIONAL MYOCARDIAL FUNCTION BY MRI

Cine GRE and multiphasic spin-echo imaging have been used to measure wall thickening and wall motion during the cardiac cycle in order to obtain information about cardiac function in patients with ischemic heart disease [1–4] (Fig. 1). MR imaging has provided reproducible quantification of the normal extent of wall thickening during systole in the various regions of the left ventricle (LV) [5]. A decrease in wall thickening has been observed at sites of prior myocardial infarction [5] and the identification of regional myocardial dysfunction in ischemic heart disease by cine GRE imaging has correlated well with the same observations made by contrast ventriculography [1, 6, 7]. Using uptake of ^{99}Tc-methoxyisobutyl-isonitrile (MIBI) on single-proton emission tomography (SPECT) as reference for residual viability at sites of myocardial ischemic injury, Sechtem and coworkers [8, 9] found that regional end diastolic wall thickness of less than 6

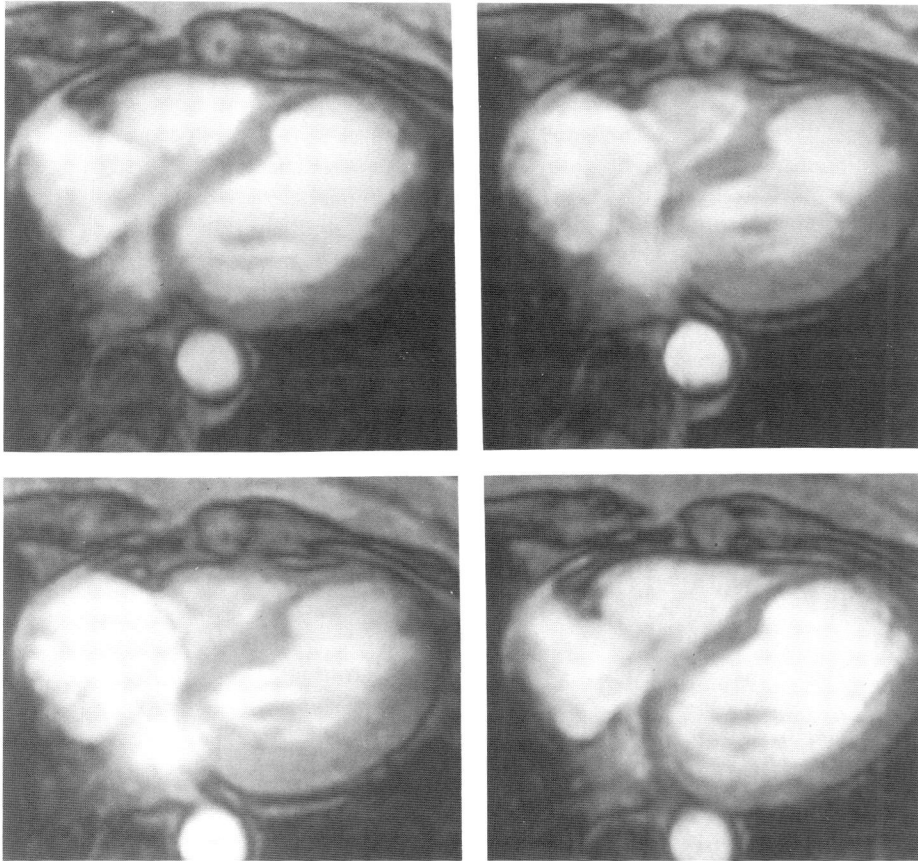

Fig. 1. Cine MRI of a patient with an anteroseptal myocardial infarction. Images are shown for early (upper left), mid (upper right), and late (lower left) systole and diastole (lower right). There is severe wall thinning and lack of systolic wall thickening in the anteroseptal region, consistent with prior transmural myocardial infarction.

mm and systolic wall thickening of less than 1 mm on cine MRI are indications of nonviable transmural infarctions.

Comparative studies between uptake of ^{18}F-fluorodeoxyglucose (FDG) in positron emission tomography (PET) and cine MR imaging have generally concluded that preserved wall thickness and systolic wall thickening provide reliable evidence that regions with moderate reduction in blood flow and FDG activity represent viable myocardium [10]. On the other hand, absence of systolic wall thickening can be caused by either hibernating or nonviable myocardium [11]. The discordance of metabolic activity as shown by moderate or normal uptake of FDG and absent wall thickening seem to be indicative of hibernating myocardium. Severely reduced or absent FDG uptake associated with significant wall thinning and no systolic wall thickening indicate nonviable myocardium [10].

Another method for measuring wall thickening, wall motion, and wall deformation has been achieved by myocardial tagging using spatial presaturation of the myocardium [12, 13]. This method provides precise tracing of the normal and abnormal "in-plane" rotation and "through-plane" displacement of the ventricle. Therefore, measurements of wall motion and wall thickening can be corrected for in-plane and through-plane movement and can supply precise information about these parameters in ischemic heart disease. The myocardial tagging method has been shown to be a unique method for assessing the abnormal motion of the peri-infarction zone of the myocardium [14]. Kramer and coworkers [14] found that left ventricular dilatation and eccentric hypertrophy during remodeling are associated with persistent differences in segmental function between adjacent and remote noninfarcted myocardium, which may reflect increased wall stress in the adjacent regions.

Cine GRE imaging provides accurate and highly reproducible measurements of left ventricular volumes, ejection fraction, and myocardial mass [15]. Such images, when encompassing the entire heart, provide a three-dimensional data set at multiple phases of the cardiac cycle, including end diastole and end systole. Consequently, the measurements of volumes and mass are not dependent on assumption of geometrical models, as is required for such measurements obtained by echocardiography and X-ray ventriculography. Because of asymmetry of the ventricle caused by regional infarction and the remodeling of the left ventricle, formulas for calculating volumes and mass based on geometrical models have questionable validity, whereas MR imaging has been accurate for measuring LV mass in the abnormally shaped ventricle after transmural infarction [16].

In addition to studies performed at rest, cine GRE imaging has been performed during pharmacological stress testing imposed by the administration of dipyridamole [17–19] or dobutamine [20–22]. In patients with known coronary artery disease but normal LV function at rest, cine GRE imaging has been performed in order to visualize wall motion or wall thickening abnormalities in the potentially ischemic myocardium induced by the use of pharmacological agents which either increase myocardial oxygen requirement or induce disparity of blood flow or both. Baer et al. [19] found that dipyridamole-induced wall motion abnormalities shown by cine MR imaging correlated closely with results of myocardial stress scintigraphy. The sensitivity of dipyridamole MRI for the localization of hemodynamically significant stenoses of major coronary arteries was 84%, whereas the specificity reached 89% when compared to coronary arteriography as the gold standard. Pennell et al. [20] used dobutamine for inducing pharmacological stress during MR imaging. They found a 91% sensitivity and 100% specificity for detection of significant coronary artery disease and no significant differences were noted between MRI and thallium in the detection or localization of coronary arterial stenoses. Baer et al. [21] compared dobutamine cine GRE with MIBI–SPECT and found good correlation for the detection of ischemic segments. These studies have characterized noninfarcted jeopardized myocardium as having normal systolic wall thickening in the basal state, but during dobutamine stress, wall thickening is reduced in the jeopardized segment of the left ventricle.

Likewise, van Rugge et al. [22] showed in 30 symptomatic patients an 81% sensitivity and a 100% specificity for predicting significant stenoses shown by coronary arteriography. Therefore, cine MR imaging during pharmacological stress serves as a new method for detection and localization of hemodynamically significant coronary arterial stenoses.

Evaluation of regional myocardial perfusion by MRI

The development of fast imaging techniques enables the monitoring of the first-pass kinetics of distribution of MR contrast agents for the purpose of estimating regional myocardial perfusion (Figs. 2–5). Several studies in animals [23–29] and in patients [28–32] have employed either fast gradient echo sequences or echo-planar imaging in order to monitor regional myocardial blood flow.

Atkinson et al. [23] used fast gradient echo sequences to study myocardial perfusion in isolated rat hearts with ligated coronary arteries. In this study a preparatory inversion recovery pulse was used for accentuating T_1-enhancing effects. After an injection of a gadolinium-DTPA bolus, a marked difference in contrast enhancement between perfused and nonperfused segments of the heart during the first pass of the contrast agent was observed. Another study assessed the first passage of MR contrast media using fast GRE sequences with preparation pulse to accentuate T_1-weighting (inversion recovery fast GRE) and magnetic susceptibility effect (driven equilibrium fast GRE). With these sequences the ischemic region has been depicted as a low signal intensity region using Gd-DTPA, and as a high signal intensity region using Dy-DTPA-BMA during the first pass of these agents [24].

In order to enhance the difference between normal and hypoperfused myocardium, the vasodilator dipyridamole has been used in several studies [25, 26]. Miller et al. [25] studied the effect of dipyridamole stress in dogs with coronary artery stenosis. This study found a close correlation between myocardial blood flow and signal intensity after gadolinium administration. Delineation between hypoperfused and normal myocardium was improved after dipyridamole. The normal myocardium showed a 78% increase in signal intensity, whereas the hypoperfused area increased by only 49% after dipyridamole. Schaefer et al. [26] found that the sensitivity of MR imaging to detect hypoperfused myocardium increased from 48% before the administration of dipyridamole to 75% after application of the drug. Whereas Miller et al. [25] used a multislice T_1-weighted spin-echo technique to obtain postcontrast images, Schaefer et al. [26] used T_1-weighted gradient-recalled sequences.

More recently, a first pass of gadolinium-based contrast media administered after dipyridamole stress and monitored using inversion recovery fast GRE has demonstrated potentially ischemic areas not identified in the basal state. In a canine model of nonocclusive stenosis used in our laboratory, dynamic contrast-enhanced MRI in the basal state has shown no perfusion defect, but after infusion of dypridamole, this

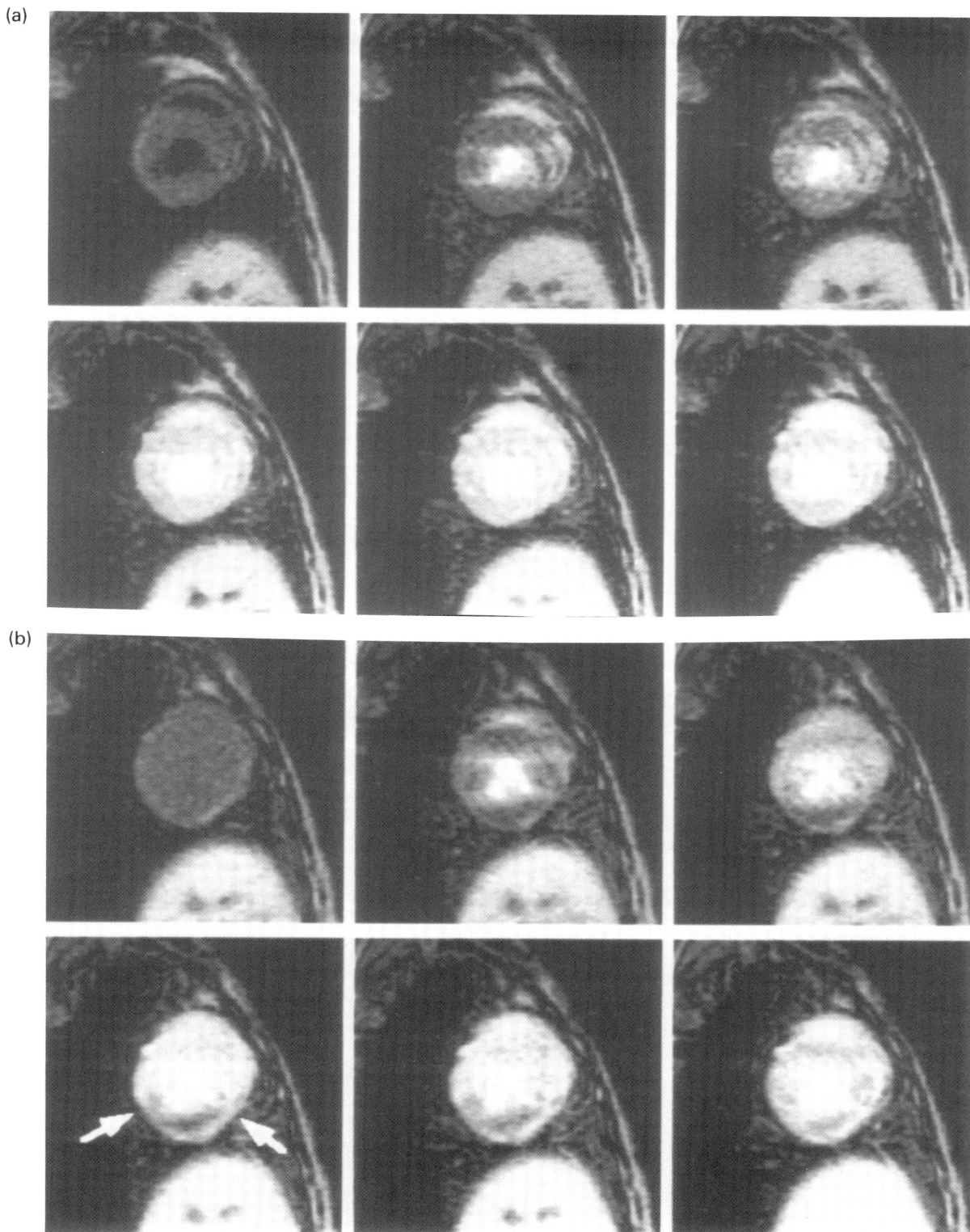

Fig. 2. Series of inversion recovery prepared fast gradient echo images in the basal state [top (a)] and in the vasodilated state [bottom (b)] induced by dipyridamole infusion in a dog with a nonocclusive stenosis of the left circumflex coronary artery. In each instance, images are shown before contrast media and during the first pass of contrast media through the heart. Images are acquired at 1–2-s intervals. In the basal state the perfusion defect is not evident. In the vasodilated state the perfusion defect (arrows) is demarcated due to initial exclusion of the gadolinium chelate during the first pass of contrast media.

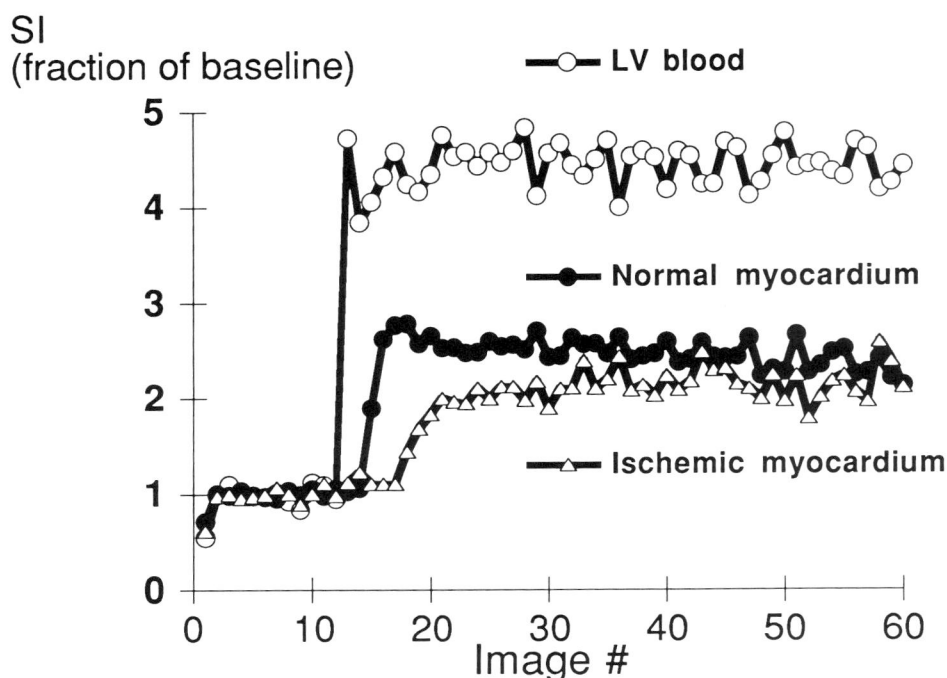

Fig. 3. Signal intensity versus time curves during the first pass of a gadolinium chelate through the heart of a dog with acute coronary occlusion. Signal intensity was measured on inversion recovery fast gradient echo images acquired at 1–2-s intervals. For a short interval there is greater enhancement of normal compared to ischemic myocardium. After the 30th image, demarcation between the two regions is not possible.

sequence displays a perfusion defect during the first pass of gadolinium chelates through the heart (Fig. 2). The dynamic study uses inversion recovery fast gradient echo sequences and 0.03–0.05 mmol kg^{-1} of the contrast medium.

Echo-planar imaging has also been applied to monitor the first pass of gadolinium DTPA-BMA (gadodiamide) injection in hearts of normal rats and rats with coronary occlusion [29]. Inversion recovery echo-planar imaging combined with a low dose of gadolinium DTPA-BMA showed a 63% increase in signal intensity after the administration of the contrast agent in normal myocardium, whereas the ischemic zone showed only slight enhancement. Gradient-recalled echo-planar imaging combined with a higher dose of gadolinium DTPA-BMA caused marked signal loss in normal myocardium due to the magnetic susceptibility effect of high concentrations of this agent, whereas the signal of the ischemic zone remained nearly unchanged [29]. Both approaches allowed clear differentiation between ischemic and normally perfused myocardium.

The effectiveness of contrast-enhanced first-pass MR perfusion imaging not only for detection but also for quantification of myocardial ischemia was evaluated in dogs by Wilke et al. [33]. Fast gradient echo

sequences were used to follow the first pass of Gd-DTPA in dogs with varying grades of stenosis of the left anterior descending coronary artery. Imaging performed before and after application of dipyridamole showed that MR perfusion imaging can define different levels of myocardial perfusion. By comparing absolute myocardial blood flow with signal intensity versus time curves obtained from MR images it was found that the inverse mean transit time of the MR contrast agent yielded a linear correlation with absolute blood flow in the myocardium. These results suggest that quantification of myocardial blood flow may be feasible using first-pass MR perfusion imaging.

MR perfusion imaging has been used to study normal volunteers [23, 30, 32] and patients with coronary artery disease, with [28] and without [30, 32] pharmacological stress. In normal volunteers, fast GRE imaging has been used to follow a bolus of contrast agent through the cardiac chambers and the myocardium providing temporal information about the transit of the contrast agent. In patients with ischemic heart disease, the first transit of a gadolinium contrast medium monitored with inversion recovery fast GRE demonstrated transient perfusion deficits (Fig. 4) and a difference in the intensity versus time curve for ischemic compared to normal regions.

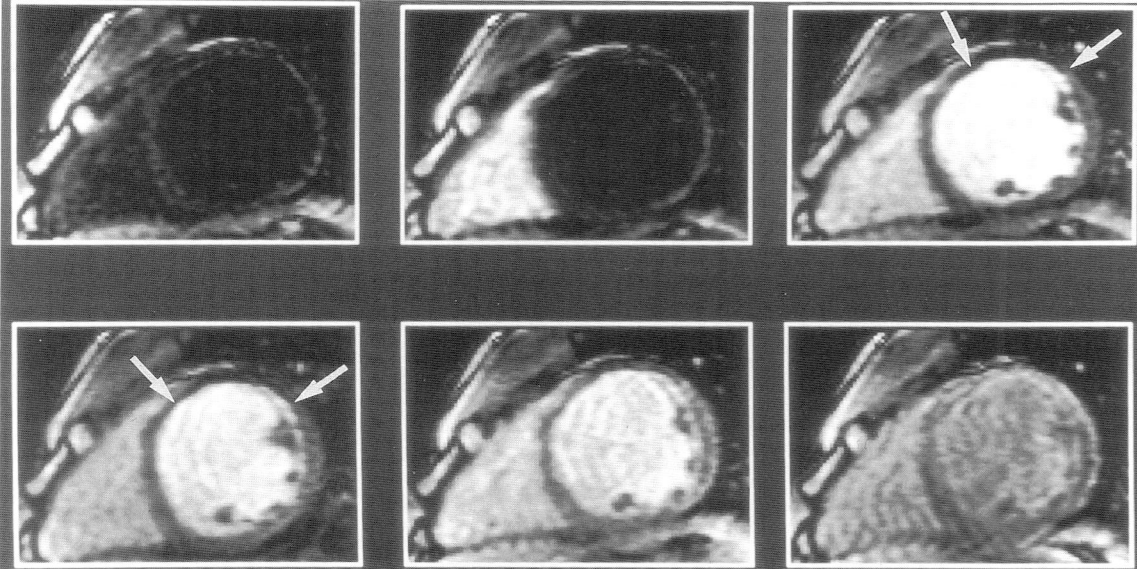

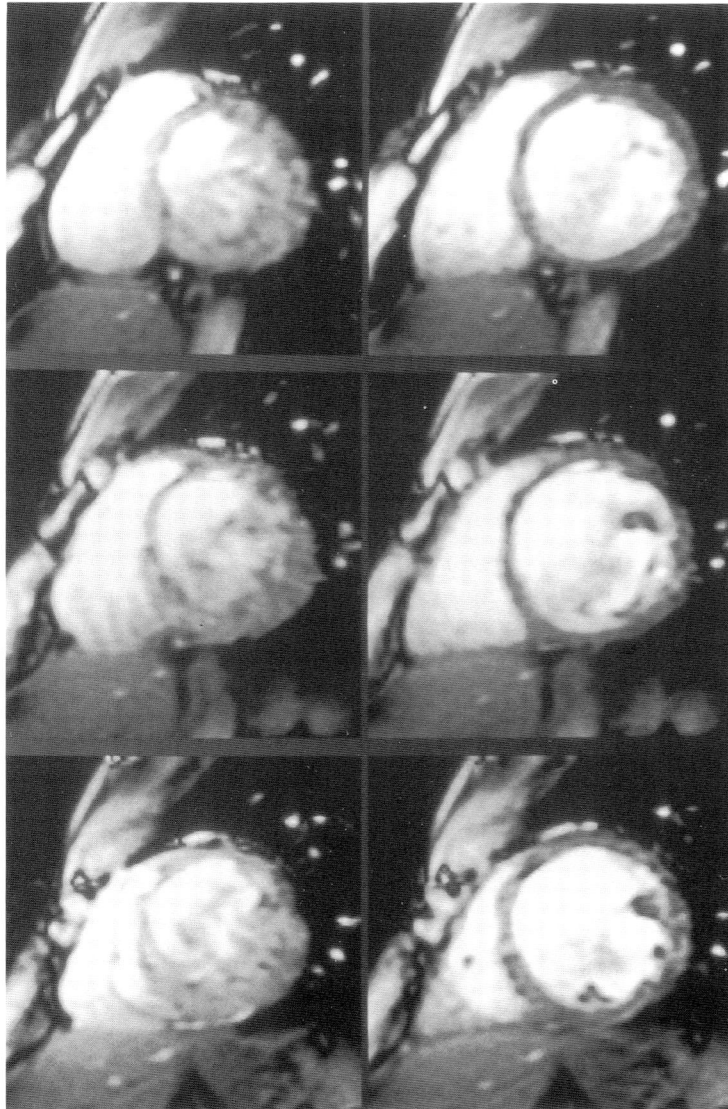

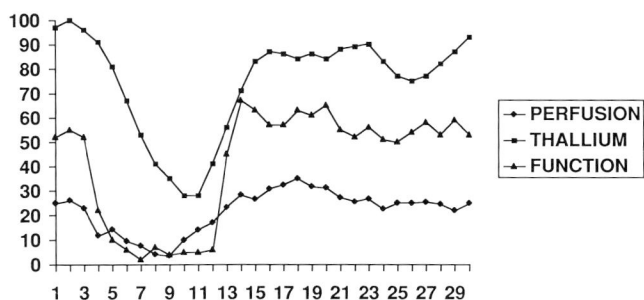

Fig. 5. Comparison of thallium perfusion with MR perfusion as shown by dynamic contrast-enhanced MRI and regional wall thickening as shown by breath hold cine MRI in a patient with a fixed thallium defect of the inferior segment of the left ventricle. The values for each of 30 segments (horizontal axis) are shown. The segments showing wall thickening and MR perfusion abnormalities correlate spatially with the thallium perfusion defect.

Studies performed by Wilke et al. [28] and Manning et al. [30] have shown that first-pass contrast-enhanced myocardial perfusion imaging can detect areas of hypoperfused myocardium in patients with coronary artery disease. In each of these studies, differences in the signal intensity versus time curves between the normally perfused segments and the segments supplied by stenotic arteries were observed after the bolus administration of Gd-DTPA. Wilke et al. [28] observed a delay in signal increase of the hypoperfused myocardium compared to normal myocardium, and these areas correlated well with abnormal areas shown by technetium scintigraphy. Manning et al. [30] were able to identify abnormal myocardium as areas of reduced peak signal intensity and diminished upslope of the intensity versus time curve.

Preliminary results by Schaefer et al. [31] suggested that pharmacological stress induced by dipyridamole injection could enhance detection of hypoperfused myocardium by MR perfusion imaging. Although they did not compare predipyridamole and postdipyridamole images, they demonstrated a difference in

signal intensity between normal and hypoperfused myocardium.

We have recently combined functional and perfusion imaging of patients with ischemic heart disease during the same MR study (Figs. 4 and 5). In a group of patients with perfusion deficits previously demonstrated by thallium scintigraphy, breath hold cine MRI has been used to display the extent of the deficit in wall thickening, whereas inversion recovery prepared fast gradient echo imaging during the first pass of gadodiamide injection (Omniscan, Nycomed, Oslo, Norway) has been used to demonstrate the perfusion deficit. Concordance has been shown between the thallium deficit and the functional and perfusion deficits as defined by MRI (Figs. 4 and 5).

REFERENCES

1. Sechtem U, Sommerhoff BA, Markiewicz W, White RD, Cheitlin MD, Higgins CB (1987) Regional left ventricular wall thickening by MRI: evaluation in normal subjects and patients with global and regional dysfunction. *Am J Cardiol* **59:** 145–151.
2. Fisher MR, von Schulthess GK, Higgins CB (1985) Multiphasic cardiac magnetic resonance imaging: normal left ventricular wall thickening. *Am J Radiol* **145:** 27–40.
3. Pflugfelder PW, Sechtem UP, White RD, Higgins CB (1988) Quantification of regional myocardial function by rapid (cine, magnetic resonance imaging. *Am J Radiol* **150:** 523–530.
4. Semelka RC, Tomei E, Wagner S, Mayo MD et al (1990) Interstudy reproducibility of dimensional and functional measurements between cine magnetic resonance studies in the morphological abnormal left ventricle. *Am Heart J* **119:** 1367–1373.
5. Peschock RM, Rokey R, Malloy GM, McNamee P et al. (1989) Assessment of myocardial systolic wall thickening using nuclear magnetic resonance imaging. *J Am Coll Cardiol* **14:** 653–659.
6. McDonald KM, Parrish T, Wennberg P et al. (1992) Rapid accurate and simultaneous noninvasive assessment of right and left ventricular mass with nuclear magnetic resonance imaging using the snapshot gradient method. *J Am Coll Cardiol* **19:** 1601–1607.
7. Underwood S, Rees RSO, Savage PE et al. (1986) Assessment of regional left ventricular function by magnetic resonance. *Br Heart J* **56:** 334–339.
8. Baer FM, Smolarz K, Jungehuelsing M, Beckwilm J, Theissen P et al. (1992) Chronic myocardial infarction: assessment of morphology, function and perfusion by gradient-echo magnetic resonance imaging and ^{99m}Tc-methoxyisbutyl-isonitrile-SPECT. *Am Heart J* **123:** 636–645.
9. Sechtem U, Voth E, Schneider C, Theissen P, et al. (1993) Assessment of residual viability in patients with myocar-

Fig. 4. Perfusion [top (a)] and functional [bottom (b)] scans in a patient with a fixed thallium defect in the anteroseptal region of the left ventricle. The dynamic contrast enhanced (inversion recovery prepared fast gradient echo) sequence shows a perfusion defect (arrows) in the anteroseptal and anterior region of the left ventricle. The function study consists of breath hold cine MRI at basal, mid, and apical levels. Images are shown at each level in late systole and late diastole. There is absence of systolic wall thickening in the anteroseptal and anterior wall of the left ventricle.

dial infarction using magnetic resonance imaging. *Int J Cardiac Imaging* **9**: 931–40.

10. Perrone-Filardi P, Bacharach S, Dilsizisan B, Maurea S, Frank JA, Bonow RO (1992) Regional left ventricular thickening. Relation to regional uptake of ^{18}F-fluordeoxyglucose and ^{201}Tl in patients with chronic coronary artery disease and left ventricular dysfunction. *Circulation* **86**: 1125–1137.

11. Perrone-Filardi P, Bacharach S, Dilsizian V, Maurea S, Marin-Neto JA et al. (1992) Metabolic evidence of viable myocardium in regions with reduced wall thickness and absent wall thickening in patients with chronic ischemic left ventricular dysfunction. *J Am Coll Cardiol* **20**: 161–168.

12. Zerhouni EA, Parish DM, Rogers WJ et al. (1988) Human heart: tagging with MR imaging—a method for noninvasive assessment of myocardial motion. *Radiology* **169**: 59–63.

13. Clark NR, Reichek N, Bergey P, Hoffman EA et al (1991) Circumferential myocardial shortening in the abnormal human left ventricle. Assessment by magnetic resonance imaging using spatial modulation of magnetization. *Circulation* **84**: 67–74.

14. Kramer CM, Lima JA, Reichek N, Ferrari VA et al. (1993) Regional differences in function within noninfarcted myocardium during left ventricular remodeling. *Circulation* **88**: 1279–1288.

15. Wagner S, Auffermann W, Buser P, Semelka RC, Higgins CB (1991) Functional description of the left ventricle in patients with volume overload, pressure overload, and myocardial disease using cine magnetic resonance imaging. *Am J Cardiac Imaging* **5**: 87–97.

16. Shapiro EP, Rogers WJ, Beyar R, Soulen RL et al. (1989) Determination of left ventricular mass by magnetic resonance imaging in hearts deformed by acute infarction. *Circulation* **79**: 706–711.

17. Pennell DJ, Underwood SR, Longmore DB (1990) Detection of coronary artery disease using MR imaging with dipyridamole. *J Comput Assist Tomogr* **14**: 2167–2170.

18. Baer FM, Smolarz K, Jungehulsing M et al. (1992) Feasibility of high-dose dipyridamole-magnetic resonance imaging for the detection of coronary artery disease and comparison with coronary angiography. *Am J Cardiol* **69**: 51–56.

19. Baer FM, Smolarz K, Theissen P, Voth E, Schichta H, Sechtem U (1993) Identification of hemodynamically significant coronary artery stenoses by dipyridamole-magnetic resonance imaging and ^{99m}Tc-methoxyisobutyl-isonitrile-SPECT. *Int J Card Imag* **9**: 133–145.

20. Pennell DJ, Underwood SR, Manzara CC, Swanton RH, Walker JM, Ell PJ, Longmore DB (1992) Magnetic resonance imaging during dobutamine stress in coronary artery disease. *Am J Cardiol* **70**: 34–40.

21. Baer FM, Voth P, Theissen P, Schichta H, Sechtem U (1993) Dobutamine–MRI in comparison to simultaneously assess ^{99m}Tc–MIBI–SPECT for the localization of hemodynamically significant artery stenoses (Ab-

stract). In *Book of Abstracts: Society of Magnetic Resonance in Medicine 1993.* p. 224. Berkeley, CA: Society of Magnetic Resonance in Medicine.

22. van Rugge FP, van der Wall EE, de Roos A, Bruschke AV (1993) Dobutamine stress magnetic resonance imaging for detection of coronary artery disease. *J Am Coll Cardiol* **22**: 431–439.

23. Atkinson JA, Burstein D, Edelman RR (1990) First pass cardiac perfusion: evaluation with ultrafast MR imaging. *Radiology* **174**: 757–762.

24. Saeed M, Wendland MF, Sakuma H, Chew W. Laurerma K et al. (1993) Detection of myocardial ischemia using first pass contrast-enhanced inversion recovery and driven equilibrium fast GRE imaging. (Abstract). In: *Book of Abstracts: Society of Magnetic Resonance in Medicine, 1993.* p. 536. Berkeley, CA: Society of Magnetic Resonance in Medicine.

25. Miller DD, Holmvang G, Gill JB et al. (1989) MRI detection of myocardial perfusion changes by gadolinium-DTPA infusion during dipyridamole hyperemia. *Magn Reson Med* **10**: 246–255.

26. Schaefer S, Lange R, Gutekunst D, Parkley RW, Willerson JT, Peshock RM (1991) Contrast-enhanced magnetic resonance imaging of hypoperfused myocardium. *Invest Radiol* **26**: 551–556.

27. Schmiedl U, Ogan MD, Paajanen H et al. (1987) Albumin labeled with Gd-DTPA as an intravascular, blood-pool enhancing agent for MR imaging: biodistribution and imaging studies. *Radiology* **162**: 205–210.

28. Wilke N, Engels G, Koroneos A, Feistel H et al. (1992) First pass myocardial perfusion imaging with ultrafast gadolinium-enhanced MR imaging at rest and during dipyridamole administration. (Abstract). *Radiology* **185**: 33.

29. Wendland MF, Saeed M, Masui T, Derugin N, Moseley ME, Higgins CB (1993) Echoplanar MR imaging of normal and ischemic myocardium with gadodiamide injection. *Radiology* **186**: 535–542.

30. Manning WJ, Atkinson DJ, Grossman W, Paulin S, Edelman RR (1991) First-pass nuclear magnetic resonance imaging studies using gadolinium-DTPA in patients with coronary artery disease. *J Am Coll Cardiol* **18**: 959–965.

31. Schaefer S, Van Tyen R, Saloner D (1992) Evaluation of myocardial perfusion abnormalities with gadolinium-enhanced snapshot MR imaging in humans. *Radiology* **185**: 795–801.

32. van Rugge FP, Boreel JJ, van der Waal EE et al. (1991) Cardiac first pass and myocardial perfusion in normal subjects assessed by subsecond Gd-DTPA enhanced MR imaging. *J Comput Assist Tomogr* **15**: 989–995.

33. Wilke N, Simm C, Zhang J, Ellermann J et al. (1993) Contrast enhanced first pass myocardial perfusion imaging: correlation between myocardial blood flow in dogs at rest and during hyperemia. *Magn Reson Med* **29**: 485–497.

Functional evaluation in congenital and acquired heart disease

D. B. Longmore,[1] D. M. Firmin,[2] J. Keegan,[2] G. Z. Yang,[2] P. Gatehouse[2] and S. R. Underwood[2]

[1]Brompton MR Enterprises
[2]Royal Brompton Hospital, 92 Fulham Road, London SW3 6HR, UK

INTRODUCTION

Approximately half of the readers of this article will die of cardiovascular disease—a further quarter will die of cancer and 12% of lung disease. At present, vast intellectual and financial resources have been and are being applied to magnetic resonance (MR) studies, ignoring these three vital areas. All but a handful of the world's 9000 MR machines are not available to cardiologists, oncologists, and lung specialists and they are used to study less than 3.5% of all disease. Approximately three in every thousand live births manifest one of the commoner congenital heart diseases, pulmonary artery stenosis, atrial septal defect, patent ductus arteriosis, and the more complicated tetralogy of Fallot although there are many other complicated forms of congenital disease. However, acquired cardiovascular disease consisting of blockage of arteries to vital organs with plaques of atheroma is responsible for most mortality and morbidity.

MR, the most powerful diagnostic instrument yet conceived, is needed and should be urgently applied in two main areas: to study the population with existing congenital and acquired heart disease and for population screening to enable an understanding of the natural history of the disease, secondary prevention, and to monitor the efficacy of preventive measures.

IMAGING STRATEGY

In order to achieve these goals, additional magnetic resonance techniques are required which are not necessary for brain, joint, or spine imaging. These include cardiac gating, velocity mapping using the field even echo rephasing (FEER) [1] technique associated with rapid imaging [2–4] and a method of producing relevant images in the correct planes. A transverse (transaxial image of the chest) is used to measure the angle of the heart to the left. A scan in this plane produces a vertical long axis (VLA) image through the left atrium and the left ventricle. From this, the downward angle of the heart is measured, and a double oblique image from below is produced to provide a horizontal long axis (HLA) showing the five functional chambers of the heart and the coronary arteries in cross section (Fig. 1). The HLA image shows the right atrium, the right ventricle, the left atrium, the left ventricle, and the left ventricular outflow tract as well as the tricuspid and mitral valves and the right and left coronary arteries. Also from the HLA image, planes can be selected perpendicular to the HLA to produce the so-called short axis (SA) image (Fig. 2).

Functional evaluation using MR in patients with existing disease provides a safer, cost-effective method of achieving a more comprehensive diagnosis and monitoring the efficacy of therapeutic measures. Its wide range of capabilities enables anatomical and functional information about the cardiovascular system to be obtained at one sitting, without the need to invade the patient with catheters or the use of contrast agents [5]. The diagnostic power and, from the patient's point of view, the simplicity of an MR examination means that, for the first time, population screening for presymptomatic cardiovascular disease is a reality. Furthermore, the application of secondary preventive measures can be tested by using repeated MR studies. While the heart and circulation are being studied it is only a small step to include screening for breast cancer [6, 7] and, with the new ultra short TE sequences, to study the lung.

FUNCTIONAL ASSESSMENT OF CONGENITAL HEART DISEASE

There are three discreet areas in the assessment and management of congenital heart disease. All best studied by MR [8, 9].

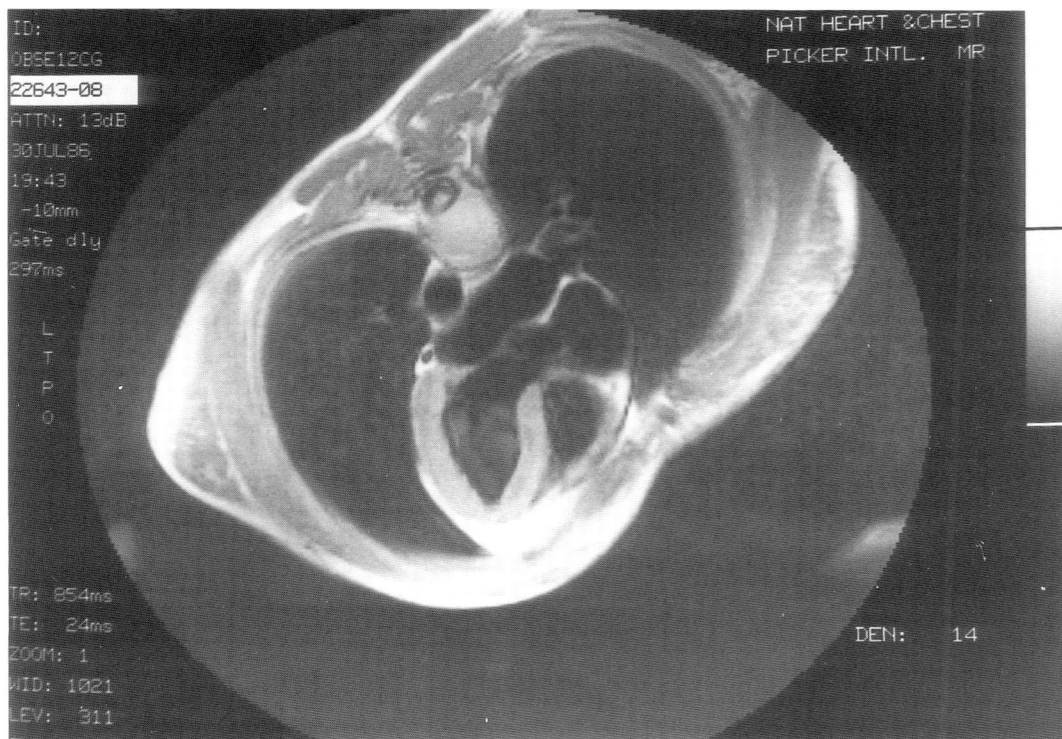

Fig. 1. A double oblique horizontal long axis image of a normal heart acquired at the beginning of systole showing the right atrium. The tricuspid valve, the right coronary artery, the left atrium, the mitral valve, the left coronary artery, the left ventricle, and the left ventricular outflow tract.

The neonate and infants, later in life when the less-catastrophic abnormalities begin to manifest themselves and to follow up the results of surgical intervention [10, 11].

THE FUNCTIONAL ASSESSMENT OF NEONATES AND INFANTS

The small size of an infant and its inability to lie still, combined with the complexity of many congenital abnormalities, necessitates a rapid imaging technique. Only two rapid techniques are currently available, echo planar (EP) with velocity mapping [12] and turbo-FLASH [13, 14] with velocity mapping. The former gives a better ultimate signal-to-noise (S/N) ratio and can freeze movement within the less than the 50-ms acquisition time needed to obtain a velocity-encoded image, whereas the FLASH technique requires acquisition for over 200 ms (there is no stage in the cardiac cycle of an infant when the heart is relatively still for 200 ms) of the same part of the cardiac cycle for 16 or more heart beats. At all stages throughout life the filling and contraction of the heart varies from beat to beat. This variability is never more marked than in the neonate with congenital disease. However, velocity mapping can be used successfully [15] with either technique to find a jet, measure its velocity, and, from the velocity measurement, calculate the gradient and, therefore, the severity of the lesion using a modified Bernoulli equation [16]. Velocity mapping combined with good anatomical imaging commonly yields more information than can be obtained from a cardiac catheter angiogram. The combination of an ultrasound scan and an MR examination are now always sufficient to make an accurate and complete diagnosis and both to indicate whether surgery is necessary and to guide the surgeon. This combination of techniques give an insight into the compensatory mechanisms which can allow an infant with gross abnormalities to survive to childhood when operative intervention is easier and safer. Most MR assessment of congenital heart disease has been undertaken in children who have survived infancy with or, in less serious cases, without palliative surgery. MR is frequently the only technique that can make a correct and complete diagnosis, yielding information about the lesions and their functional significance. It is the only available technique for the repeated long-term follow-up of children postoperatively [17–19]. It is

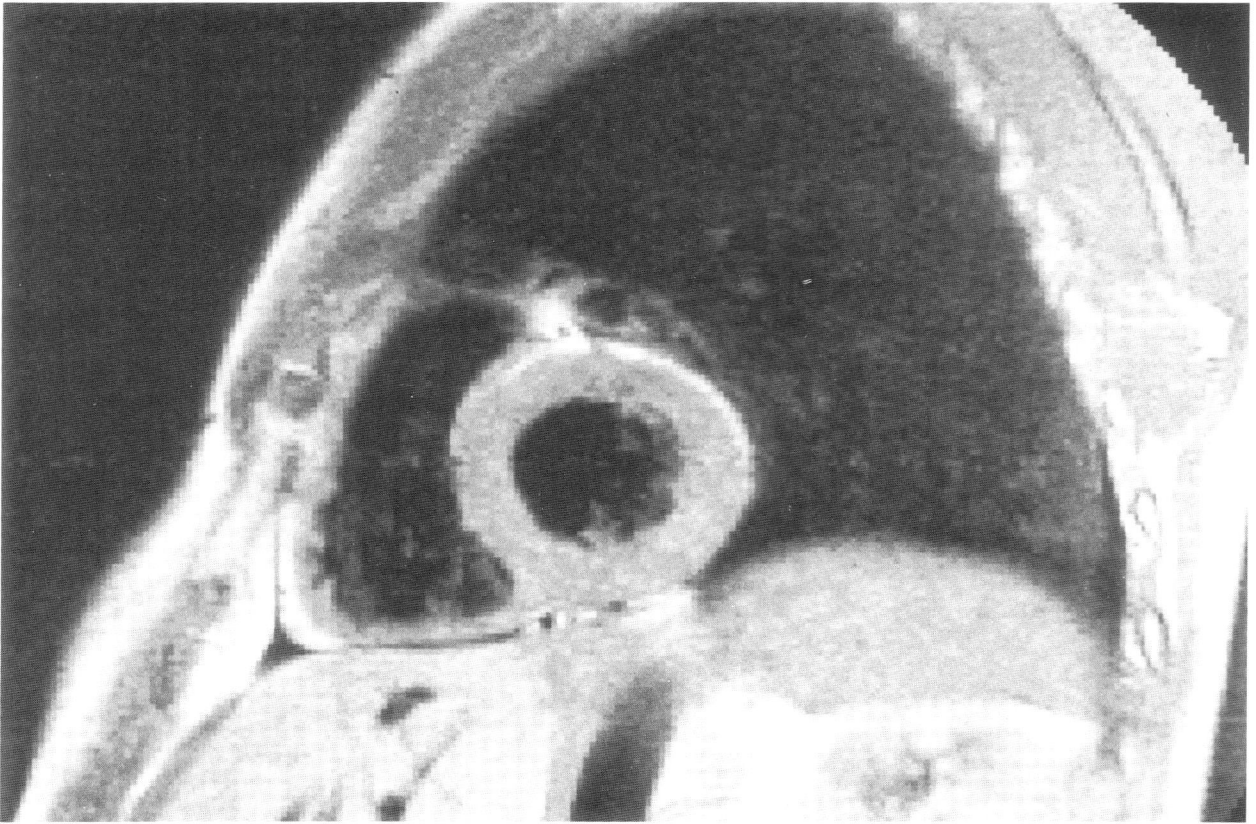

Fig. 2. A double oblique short axis view of a normal heart looking from the apex toward the base taken from an MR cine timed at end diastole. The right ventricle wrapped round the doughnut-shaped left ventricle is seen against the chest wall. A coronary artery is seen on the upper surface of the left ventricle; a coronary artery and a coronary sinus are seen on the diaphragmatic surface. The section, 4 mm thick, is taken near the base of the heart above the level of the papillary muscles, and the chordae tendinae are seen in the cavity of the ventricle.

vital in postoperative cases to undertake a full functional assessment including velocity mapping because calcified obstructions are not visualized on anatomical studies and can only be demonstrated by blood velocity mapping. MR is uniquely able to detect the afferent and efferent vessels to an artereovenus malformation, helping the surgeon to plan an operation. In multiple AV malformations (Klippel, Tralawney syndrome), the measurement of the total blood flow through the AV malformations can predict the impending onset of high-output heart failure [20].

FUNCTIONAL ASSESSMENT OF ACQUIRED HEART DISEASE

Functional assessment of valve disease

Valve disease may be acquired or present as a late manifestation of congenital heart disease. A small proportion of the population are born with a bicuspid aortic valve which will frequently function normally until the patient is in their early forties, by which time calcification causing stenosis and regurgitation results from the abnormal vibrations and stresses on the two cusps [21]. MR can be used to measure the jet velocity, to calculate the gradient [22], and to measure the regurgitant fraction. This can be done directly using velocity mapping or by comparing the ratio of the stroke volumes of the right and left ventricles which in the normal is unity [23, 24]. Narrowing of the pulmonary valve [25] is the commonest congenital deformity of the heart, but it too may not prove to be significant until adult life when the gradients can be measured. The mitral and aortic valves are damaged by disease notably rheumatic fever, which at the present time is uncommon in the western world but still commonly causes valve disease in developing countries. The stenosis and regurgitation due to rheumatic fever can be visualized as areas of signal loss on gradient echo images [26, 27] but are best measured directly using velocity mapping with very short echo times [28] because multivalve disease invalidates comparison of stroke volumes from the two sides of the heart.

Functional assessment of traumatic cardiovascular disease

The commonest traumatic cardiovascular lesion due to road traffic and other accidents is a partial tear of the aorta, causing a dissecting aneurism. These can be detected with a computer tomography (CT) scan or an anatomical MR [29] image which usually reveals the site of injury. However, by its very nature, the dissection travels down the length of the aorta and sometimes backward toward the origin of the coronary arteries. Before any repair can be attempted it is essential to determine where the blood is flowing and which branches to vital organs arise from the true lumen and which from the false lumen. Tears and penetrating injuries such as stab wounds to the heart can be seen on MR images, and blood can be demonstrated flowing in and out of false aneurisms.

Functional assessment of inflamatory lesions

Heart muscle can be affected directly by viral illnesses such as the ME virus, glandular fever, or by inflamatory/allergic processes such as rheumatic fever. Alcohol, drugs, and other toxic materials can also cause generalized dysfunction of the myocardium. Cine MR imaging supplemented with measurements of global ventricular function, as described below, are usually adequate to study these conditions.

Functional assessment of neoplastic disease in the cardiovascular system

Primary tumors of the heart muscle are uncommon but are readily seen on MR scans. Tumors in the atria can float through the artrioventricular valves during artrial systole and be blown back into the atria during ventricular systole, causing valve dysfunction which can be measured. (Anatomical images do not distinguish between intracardiac blood clot and tumor; however the FEER velocity mapping technique reveals the presence of clot.) Tumors in the right atrium which do not have an obvious connection to the atrial wall are frequently extensions of tumors in other parts of the vascular system that have grown into the atrium. Their hemodynamic significance can be determined by velocity mapping. More frequently, the heart is invaded by a local tumor such as a lung cancer with hilar glandular involvement. In these cases, cardiac function can be impaired either by stiffening of the wall or reduction of chamber size by the mass of tumor tissue or directly by tumor replacing contractile elements of the heart. The heart is frequently the site of benign fibrous tumors that can be checked for malignant change by repeated studies.

Degenerative heart disease

Most cardiovascular deaths are due to various forms of degenerative heart disease, of which the commonest are atherosclerotic disease and hypertension. MR can be used to distinguish between ventricular function which is abnormal because of a reduced blood supply, constriction of the heart by scar tissue around it, and dysfunction due to damage of the heart itself, usually as a result of an inadequate blood supply due to coronary artery disease [30]. Ventricular function can be studied globally or regionally.

Global ventricular function

Global ventricular function can be measured using MR both in the resting state and with pharmacological stress to mimic exercise. Volume measurements can be obtained either by summating the areas of multislice covering the ventricles in systole or diastole or area length calculations of VLA and HLA systolic and diastolic images. Subtraction of the systolic volume from the diastolic volume provides an accurate measure of the stroke volume which can be compared with the residual volume to give an ejection fraction. The use of pharmacological stress can reveal abnormalities of global function either by changes of ejection fraction or by changes in velocity and acceleration of blood in the aorta [31, 32]. In the normal heart, increasing doses of a pharmacological stress agent such as dobutamine cause an increase in aortic blood flow, velocity, and acceleration. But in the abnormal heart, increasing the dose produces increased performance up to a limit of pharmacological stress at which the "fall-off" starts to give an indication of the extent of the myocardial damage followed by decreasing velocity and acceleration.

Regional ventricular function

Global ventricular function can be at the lower limits of normal or slightly impaired yet regions of the ventricle may be contracting suboptimally, not contracting or even moving paradoxically (bulging during systole, further disadvantaging ventricular function).

Multislice VLA, HLA, or most usefully, SA views of the heart can be used to assess regional thickening and movement of the heart wall during contraction. The addition of pharmacological stress highlights areas that fail to contract normally and can indicate which coronary artery is failing to provide an adequate blood supply to the affected region.

The inner surface of the heart muscle is under maximum stress during cardiac contraction and is furthest away from the blood supply that enters the heart from its outer surface. The first sign that the heart is becoming injured is its failure to "actively relax" to enable filling at the beginning of diastole to be followed later in the disease process by a failure of contraction. Velocity mapping of the inner surface of the heart in the direction of the long axis of the heart provides a sensitive measure of the elasticity and capability of the heart to fill actively and of failure to contract [33].

Measurements such as global and regional ventricular function demonstrate the effect rather than the cause of reduced ventricular function, which is most commonly due to a diminished blood supply due to atheromatous disease partially blocking the coronary arteries.

ATHEROMATOUS DISEASE, CORONARY ARTERY DISEASE, AND POPULATION SCREENING

Atheromatous disease is progressive and from demographic studies and animal experimentation is known to be reversible in its early presymptomatic stages.* You the reader, hopefully a normal subject, require answers to three fundamental questions about atheromatous disease: Have I got it? Are the atheromatous plaques of a type which can ulcerate and cause sudden death? Can MR monitor the efficacy of preventive and therapeutic measures? An MR machine capable of functional imaging and velocity mapping is capable of answering all these questions.

Have I got it? Coronary artery disease appears not to coexist with a normal compliant arterial system. Therefore, measurements of aortic compliance or its reciprocal, the velocity along the aorta of the onset of the arterial pulsewave, can be used to determine whether the subject is normal or an arteriopath. Aortic compliance can be determined directly by measuring the volume of the arch of the aorta at peak systole

---

* Atheromatous disease was unknown in central Europe after World War I. Postmortem studies at the London Hospital from 1908 to 1940 showed a steady increase in coronary artery disease. Casualties in the Siege of Lenigrad in World War II showed no arterial disease, likewise there was no atheromatous disease in the concentration camps, whereas young soldiers killed in the Korean and Vietnam wars showed massive diffuse disease. Experimental atheroma in laboratory animals regresses with starvation. Atheromatous disease does not coexist with wasting diseases. It also varies not only from time to time but from place to place with wide variations in its incidence in apparently genetically similar populations in different countries.

when it is most dilated and at the end of diastole when its elastic recoil reduces it to its smallest volume [34, 35]. An alternative is to measure the onset of the arterial pulsewave in the ascending aorta and at the end of the arch of the aorta during peak systolic flow. In a normal subject under the age of 55, the pulsewave takes an average of 32 ms to traverse the arch, whereas if the transit time of the leading edge of the pulsewave takes less than 12 ms, diffuse arterial disease is present. This simple screening test divides subjects into three clearly defined populations—athletes who have remained fit, those in the normal range, and those with arterial disease.

Are the atheromatous plaques of a type that can ulcerate and cause sudden death? If the patient is shown to be an arteriopath by the screening tests outlined above, arterial plaques in the larger vessels can be found on spin-echo images of the vessel walls. The presence of the plaque can be confirmed and artifacts excluded by detecting acceleration upstream of the obstruction, increased velocity across it, and deceleration downstream of it. Water and fat images of the plaque are then acquired by using Dixon's selective reading of fat and water or Hinks selective exitation of fat and water. A subtraction image shows the percentage of lipid present. Plaques may have a lipid content of 0% to 28%. A plaque with a high lipid content is at risk of rupture and ulceration, which will be followed by an acute thrombosis on its surface and the potential for sudden death [36]. A very low lipid content implies a fibrous scar which, though narrowing the vessel, is not immediately life-threatening. At the present stage of development, MR studies of coronary arteries is based on a single breath hold to acquire 16 turbo-FLASH images. The resolution using this technique is not yet adequate to visualize atheromatous plaques in the coronary arteries and to do chemical shift imaging in them [37]. Furthermore, fat suppression techniques are needed in order to produce accurate images of the coronary arteries and velocity measurements in them, avoiding phase changes due to the presence of fat. The techniques are, however, adequate for determination of the hemodynamic significance of coronary plaques. The way ahead for coronary imaging depends on the development of velocity-encoded echo-planar and spiral imaging, both of which are proven techniques and should yield sufficient resolution to enable analysis of coronary plaques. At present, the inference has to be made that the lipid content of plaques in the coronary arteries is similar to that in plaques elsewhere in the circulation as is usually the case.

Can MR monitor the efficacy of preventive and therapeutic measures? Simple preventive measures including strict diet and exercise have been shown to cause regression of atheromatous plaques, and in subjects with very high cholesterol and other lipid levels, lipid-lowering agents may be necessary. The advantage of MR is that the studies can be repeated regularly to monitor the progress of preventive measures.

THE FUTURE

More versatile magnetic resonance machines capable of echo-planar imaging and spiral velocity mapping will become available. These machines will use a new generation of open access magnets in which ultrasound and laser intervention will be done using direct MR vision. Ultrasound surgery with MR vision has the advantage that the ultrasound energy can be applied at a low level to confirm that it is focused on the area of interest and then at a higher therapeutic energy. The massive intellectual pool of knowledge will be switched from neuroradiology to cardiology, oncology, and to the lung.

CONCLUSIONS

Functional evaluation of the cardiovascular system using rapid imaging (spiral echo planar), chemical shift, and velocity mapping is capable of making the diagnosis in congenital and acquired cardiovascular disease which, between them, cause the largest number of deaths of any disease in the western world and massive morbidity and suffering. Furthermore, for the first time in the history of medicine, there is the opportunity to apply preventive measures to eradicate the epidemic of preventable arterial disease. There needs to be a change of emphasis and a switching of resources to apply to the most common diseases rather than to those which are most easily studied. There also needs to be proper training in cardiovascular MR, not so much for imagers as for cardiologists and experts in vascular disease.

REFERENCES

1. Bryant DJ, Payne JA, Firmin DN, Longmore DB (1984) Measurement of flow with NMR imaging using a gradient pulse and phase difference technique. *J Comput Assist Tomogr* **8**: 588–593.
2. Mansfield P (1977) Multi-planar image formation using NMR spin echoes. *J Phys C* **10**: L55–L58.
3. Mansfield P, Pykett IL (1978) Biological and medical imaging by NMR. *J Magn Reson* **29**: 355–373.
4. Rzedzian RR, Pykett IL (1987) Instant images of the human heart using a new, whole-body MR imaging system. *Am J Roentgenol* **149**: 245–250.
5. Mohiaddin RH, Longmore DB (1993) Functional aspects of cardiovascular magnetic resonance imaging. Techniques and application. *Circulation* **88**: 264–281.
6. Porter BA, Smith JP (1993) Breast cancer MR detection and staging. *Magn Res*
7. Kaiser WA (1992) MRM promises earlier breast cancer diagnosis. *Diagn Imaging* **9**: 88–93.
8. Boxer RA, Singh S, LaCorte MA, Goldman M, Stein HL (1986) Cardiac magnetic resonance imaging in children with congenital heart disease. *J Pediatr* **109**: 460–464.
9. Wolff F, Barutho J, Wecker D, Brechenmacher C, Chambron J (1986) Apport de l'imagerie par resonance magnetique dans les cardiopathies congenitales. *Arch Mal Coeur* **79**: 1563–1568.
10. Rees RSO, Firmin DN, Mohiaddin RH, Underwood SR, Longmore DB (1989) Application of flow measurements by magnetic resonance velocity mapping to congenital heart disease. *Am J Cardiol* **64**: 953–956.
11. Rees RSO, Somerville J, Warnes C, Underwood SR, Firmin DN, Klipstein RH, Longmore DB (1988) Comparison of magnetic resonance imaging with echocardiography and radionuclide angiography in assessing cardiac function and anatomy following Mustard's operation for transposition of the great arteries. *Am J Cardiac* **61**: 1316–1322.
12. Firmin DN, Gatehouse PD, Longmore DB (1992) Comparison of snapshot quantitative flow imaging techniques (Abstract). *Magn Reson Med* **11**: 2915.
13. Haase A, Frahm J, Matthaei D, Hanicke W, Merboldt KD (1986) FLASH imaging: rapid NMR imaging using low flip angle pulses. *J Magn Reson* **67**: 258–266.
14. Frahm J, Haase A, Matthaei D (1986) Rapid NMR imaging of dynamic processes using the FLASH technique. *Magn Reson Med* **3**: 321–327.
15. Rees RSO, Firmin DN, Mohiaddin RH, Underwood SR, Longmore DB (1986) Application of flow measurements by magnetic resonance velocity mapping to congenital heart disease. *Am J Cardiol* **64**: 953–956.
16. Kilner PJ, Firmin DN, Rees RSO, Martinez J, Pennell DJ, Mohiaddin RH, Underwood SR, Longmore DB (1991) Valve and great vessel stenosis: assessment with magnetic resonance jet velocity mapping. *Radiology* **178**: 229–235.
17. Rees RSO, Somerville J, Underwood SR, Wright J, Firmin DN, Klipstein RH, Longmore DB (1987) Magnetic resonance imaging of pulmonary arteries and their systemic connections in pulmonary atresia: comparison with angiographic and surgical findings. *Br Heart J* **58**: 621–626.
18. Rees RSO, Somerville J, Warnes C, Underwood SR, Firmin DN, Klipstein RH, Longmore DB (1988) Comparison of magnetic resonance imaging with echocardiography and radionuclide angiography in assessing cardiac function and anatomy following Mustard's operation

for transposition of the great arteries. *Am J Cardiol* **61:** 1316–1322.

19. Sampson C, Martinez J, Rees S, Somerville J, Underwood R, Longmore DB (1990) Evaluation of Fontan's operation by magnetic resonance imaging. *Am J Cardiol* **65:** 819–821.

20. Huber M, Longmore DB, Firmin DN, Assheuer J, Bewermeyer H, Heiss WD (1989) MR tomography flow measurement in cerebral arteriovenous angioma. *Digitale Bilddiagnostik* **9:** 1–4.

21. Kilner PJ, Manzara CC, Mohiaddin RH, Pennell DJ, St John Sutton MG, Firmin DN, Underwood SR, Longmore DB (1993) Magnetic resonance jet velocity mapping in mitral and aortic valve stenosis. *Circulation* **87:** 1239–1248.

22. Mohiaddin RH, Longmore DB (1993) Functional aspects of cardiovascular magnetic resonance imaging. Techniques and application. *Circulation* **88:** 264–281.

23. Longmore DB, Klipstein RH, Underwood SR, Firmin DN, Hounsfield GH, Watanabe M, Bland C, Fox KM, Poole-Wilson PA, Rees RSO, Denison DN, McNeilly AM, Burman ED (1985) Dimensional accuracy of magnetic resonance in studies of the heart. *Lancet* **i:** 1360–1362.

24. Watanabe M, Hosoda Y, Longmore DB (1986) Left and right ventricular dimensions and functions measured by ECG-gated NMR cardiac imaging. *J Cardiogr* **16:** 343–352.

25. Rees RSO, Somerville J, Underwood SR, Wright J, Firmin DN, Klipstein RH, Longmore DB (1987) Magnetic resonance imaging of pulmonary arteries and their systemic connections in pulmonary atresia: comparison with angiographic and surgical findings. *Br Heart J* **58:** 621–626.

26. Evans AJ, Blinder RA, Herfkens RJ et al. (1988) Effects of turbulence on signal intensity in gradient echo sequences. *Invest Radiol* **23:** 512–518.

27. Mohiaddin RH, Pennell DJ (1992) Magnetic resonance assessment of stenosis and regurgitation of the cardiac valves and great vessels. In: *Percutaneous Balloon Valvuloplasty* (Chang TO, ed), pp. 185–213. New York: Igaku-Shoin Medical Publishers.

28. Kilner PJ, Firmin DB, Rees RSO, Martinez JE, Pennell DJ, Mohiaddin RH, Underwood SR, Longmore DB (1990) Magnetic resonance jet velocity mapping for assessment of valve and great vessel stenosis. *Radiology* **178:** 229–235.

29. Goldman AP, Kotler MN, Scanlon MH, Ostrum B, Parameswaran R, Parry WR (1986) The complementary role of magnetic resonance imaging. Doppler echocardiography and computed tomography in the diagnosis of dissecting thoracic aneurysms. *Am Heart J* **111:** 970–981.

30. Mohiaddin RH, Wann SL, Underwood SR, Firmin DN, Rees RSO, Longmore DB (1990) Vena caval flow: assessment with cine MR velocity mapping. *Radiology* **177:** 537–541.

31. Pennell DJ, Underwood SR, Ell PJ, Swanton RH, Walker JM, Longmore DB (1990) Dipyridamole magnetic resonance imaging: a comparison with thallium-201 emission tomography. *Br Heart J* **64:** 362–369.

32. Pennell DJ, Underwood SR, Manzara CC, Ell PJ, Swanton RH, Walker JM, Longmore DB (1992) Magnetic resonance imaging during dobutamine stress in coronary artery disease. *Am J Cardiol* **70:** 34–40.

33. Karwatowski SP, Mohiaddin R, Yang GZ, Firmin DN, St John Sutton M, Underwood SR, Longmore DB (1994) Assessment of regional left ventricular long-axis motion with MR velocity mapping in healthy subjects. *J Magn Reson Imaging* **4**(2).

34. Mohiaddin RH, Underwood SR, Bogren HG, Firmin DN, Klipstein RH, Rees RSO, Longmore DB (1989) Regional aortic compliance studied by magnetic resonance imaging: the effects of age, training and coronary artery disease. *Br Heart J* **62:** 90–96.

35. Mohiaddin RH, Schoser K, Amanuma M, Burman ED, Longmore DB (1990) MR imaging of age-related dimensional changes of thoracic aorta. *J Comput Assist Tomogr* **14:** 748–752.

36. Mohiaddin RH, Sampson C, Firmin DN, Longmore DB (1991) Magnetic resonance morphological, chemical shift and flow imaging in peripheral vascular disease. *Eur J Vasc Surg* **5:** 383–396.

37. Edelman RR, Manning W, Burstein D, Paulin S (1991) Coronary arteries; breath-hold MR angiography. *Radiology* **181:** 641–643.

Magnetic resonance velocity vector mapping in aortic aneurysms

R.H. Mohiaddin,* H.G. Bogren, G.Z. Yang, P.J. Kilner and D.N. Firmin

Royal Brompton Hospital, National Heart and Lung Institute, London SW3 6NP UK

We used magnetic resonance imaging with cine velocity vector mapping to study blood flow patterns in the thoracic aorta of patients with aortic aneurysms. Spin-echo images of the thoracic aorta were acquired in orthogonal and oblique planes. Cine phase-shift velocity maps were then acquired in selected aortic planes, with velocity encoded in two orthogonal directions. The two-directional velocity data were processed to generate flow vector maps depicting flow distribution in the chosen plane. Diameter ratios between the aortic valves and aneurysmal ascending aortas were reduced, causing blood to enter as a relatively narrow stream with lateral vortical, recirculating flow. In atherosclerotic aneurysms, there was abnormal angulation between the left ventricular outflow tract and ascending aorta, causing the stream to attach to the anterior aortic wall, with recirculating flow posteriorly. In Marfan patients, the primary stream was central with vortices on either side. In patients with coarctation, the main stream attached to the posterior wall of the descending aorta, with recirculation anteriorly. Magnetic resonance imaging with cine velocity mapping allows comprehensive assessment of aortic anatomy and blood flow patterns. Sequential studies at early stages may provide new information about the natural history of aortic aneurysms.

Keywords: magnetic resonance imaging, blood flow, aortic aneurysm.

INTRODUCTION

Although the role of the hydraulic forces in the formation and propagation of aortic aneurysms has long been discussed, it is still poorly understood. These hydrodynamic forces are usually generated as a result of a stream of blood flowing through a narrowed area in a vessel of larger diameter and the stresses and consequent strains encountered, all capable of contributing in time toward weakness of the vascular wall [1]. We used magnetic resonance imaging (MRI) with multidirectional velocity mapping to study the relationship between aortic morphology and aortic flow patterns in patients with aortic aneurysms.

* Address for correspondence: Magnetic Resonance Unit, Royal Brompton Hospital, Sydney Street, London SW3 6NP, UK.

MATERIALS AND METHODS

Subjects

Sixteen patients with aortic aneurysms were studied. The etiology is as follows: atherosclerosis [2], Marfan's syndrome [3], and poststenotic dilatation due to coarctation [4]. Four patients had aortic valve regurgitation.

Magnetic resonance imaging

A Picker International machine operating at 0.5 T was used. Anatomical images of the thoracic aorta were acquired in orthogonal and oblique planes using spin-echo imaging (Fig. 1a). Cine phase-shift velocity mapping was then used to measure velocity in oblique sagittal or coronal planes through the aorta. During each acquisition, velocity was encoded twice, one in the direction of the read (vertical in the figure) and the other in the direction of the phase (horizontal in the figure) encoding gradients (Fig. 1b and c). This was done simultaneously by interleaving [3].

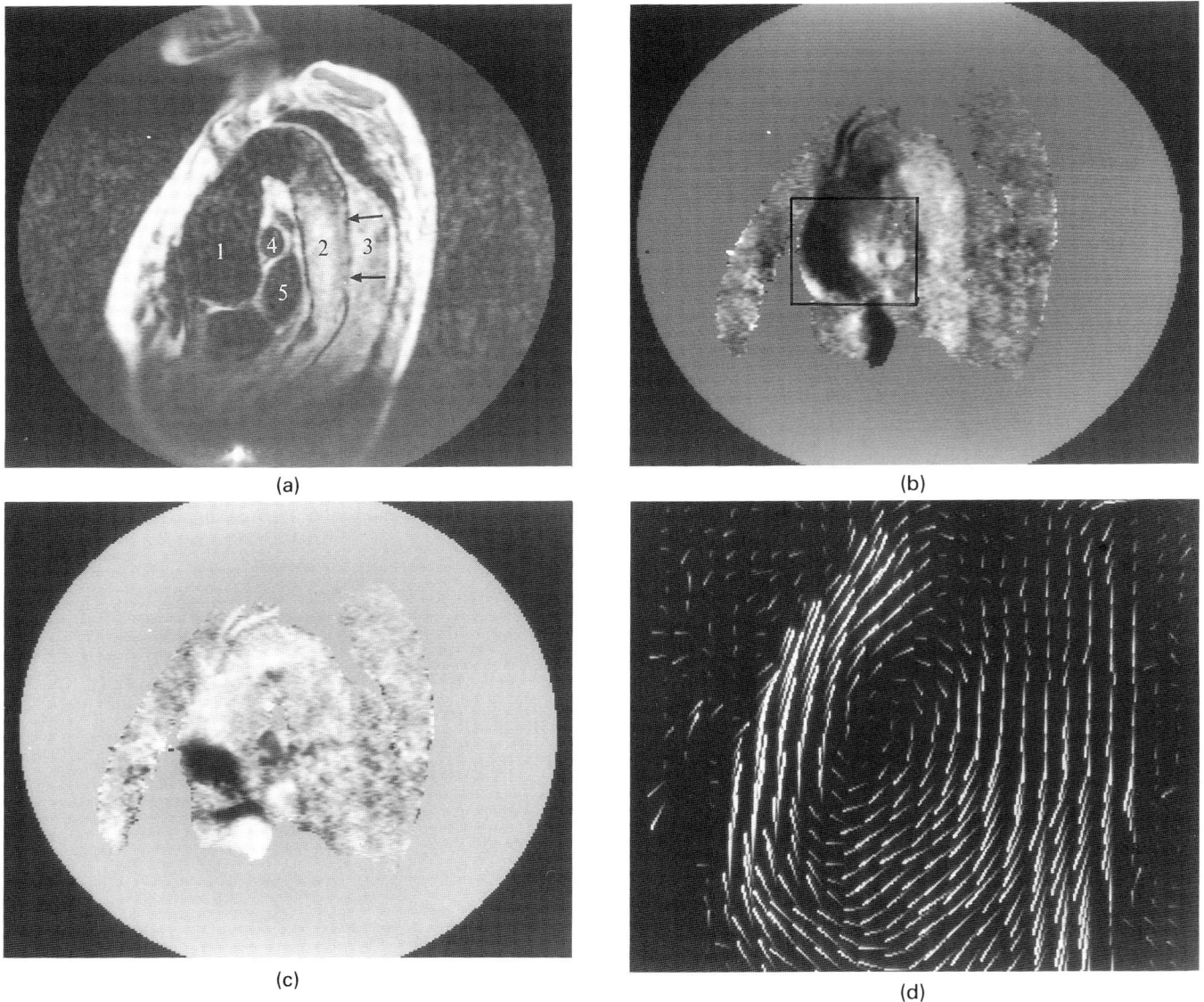

Fig. 1. A spin-echo image (a) in an oblique sagittal plane through the thoracic aorta of patient with dilated aorta and dissection involving the descending aorta, with systolic velocity maps encoded vertically (b) and horizontally (c). Vector maps in a corresponding plane to (a) acquired during early systole, demonstrating primary and secondary flow in a dilated aortic segment indicated by the rectangular area on (b). 1: ascending aorta, 2: true lumen, 3: false lumen, 4: right pulmonary artery, 5: left atrium, arrows: intimal flap.

Visualization of flow

Maps of orthogonal velocity components were processed into multiple computer-generated streaks (Fig. 1d) whose orientation, length, and movement corresponded to velocity vectors in the chosen plane [3, 5].

RESULTS

The thoracic aorta was grossly dilated in all patients. The diameter ratio between aortic valve annulus and the ascending aorta was greatly reduced, forcing the blood to enter the ascending aorta as a narrow jet during systole and creating vortices of secondary flow. These vortices migrate distally during the course of ventricular systole. The direction of the primary jets and the secondary vortices vary in the different groups. In atherosclerotic aneurysm, there is an abnormal angle between the left ventricular outflow tract and the ascending aorta directing the jet toward the anterior aortic wall and creating secondary vortices in posteriorly (Figs. 1 and 2a). In patients with Marfan's

(a)

(b)

(c)

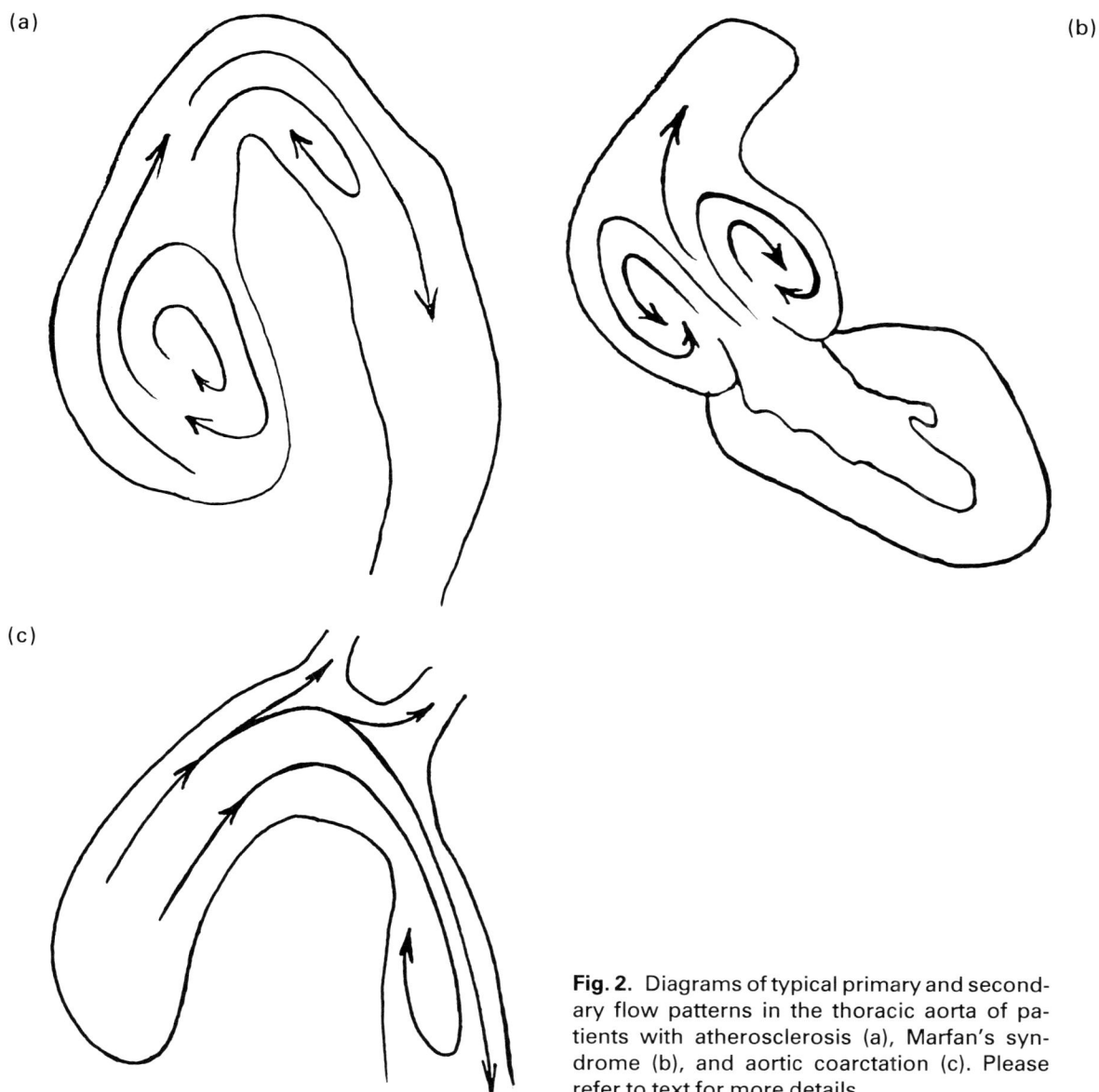

Fig. 2. Diagrams of typical primary and secondary flow patterns in the thoracic aorta of patients with atherosclerosis (a), Marfan's syndrome (b), and aortic coarctation (c). Please refer to text for more details.

syndrome, the primary jet is central with two vortices on either side (Fig. 2b). In patients with coarctation, the narrow jets is directed toward the posterior wall of the descending aorta causing local circulation anteriorly (Fig. 2c). There is a large retrograde in the thoracic aorta in patients with aortic valve regurgitation.

DISCUSSION

Blood flow must obey the principles of conservation of mass, momentum, and energy, but prediction of the actual movements of unsteady blood flow in compliant vessels of variable geometry is practically impossible. We have presented results demonstrating that noninvasive display of anatomy and visualization of multidirectional flow patterns in living vessels is feasible and that there appears to be clear differences between patterns of flow observed in these patients and those previously reported in normal subjects [6]. This study demonstrates clearly the influence of aortic morphology on the primary and secondary flow patterns in the thoracic aorta.

Patients with a dilated aorta showed an irregular

vortical flow pattern in the ascending aorta. The formation of these vortices may be related to the abnormal ratio between aortic valve diameter and aortic diameter. The preferential inflow of blood toward the anterior aortic wall, on the other hand, may be related to the abnormal angle between aortic valve and ascending aorta.

Several anatomical factors affect the character of flow in a vessel, for example, branch-to-trunk ratios less than 1 [7] and acute angles of branching [4], arterial tapering [8], and vessel distensibility [2, 9]. In cases of aortic coarctation without a significant obstruction, abnormal flow can be caused by these anatomical factors. In patients with significant aortic obstruction, blood flow is complex. By conservation of mass, total flow at every cross section of the vessel must be constant. When the area of the vessel is decreasing (stenosis), the average velocity must increase, which requires an acceleration and a pressure gradient in the direction of flow. If the area increases (poststenotic dilatation), the adverse pressure gradient may be large enough to cause the flow near the wall to change direction while the higher velocity fluid in the center of the tube continues in the same direction. This results in a region of recirculation in the outer region of an expanding tube, whereas the fluid in the center of the tube effectively separates from the tube walls. The conversion of the high kinetic energy of the swiftly moving stream into high potential energy of lateral pressure was postulated to be a factor in the development of poststenotic dilatation [1]. In addition, the lower velocity due to widening of the vessel, according to the Bernoulli equation, would itself increase lateral pressure and cause an even greater dilatation [1].

MR velocity mapping has unique potential for the acquisition of multidimensional and multidirectional velocity data [10]. Velocities in a pulsatile flow field are distributed in the four dimensions of space and time, and measurement of three components is more appropriate than two components to determine the local velocity vector. In this study, velocity measurements were confined to two directions in selected planes mainly because of the long acquisition time and the difficulty of handling and displaying the vector of three-dimensional velocity data. However, given current developments in rapid imaging, together with improvements in data storage, handling, and displaying of multidirectional velocity, these limitations may become less important [11, 12].

CONCLUSION

MRI with multidirectional velocity mapping is a powerful noninvasive tool which allows comprehensive assessment of aortic morphology and aortic flow patterns. Sequential studies of patients with aortic aneurysms at an early stage could provide new information about the natural history of this disease.

REFERENCES

1. Holman E (1955) The development of arterial aneurysms. *J Surg Gyn Obstr* **100**: 599–611.
2. Bogren HG, Mohiaddin RH, Klipstein RH, Firmin DN, Underwood SR, Rees RSO, Longmore DB (1989) The function of the aorta in ischemic heart disease: A magnetic resonance and angiographic study of aortic compliance and blood flow patterns. *Am Heart J* **118**: 234–247.
3. Mohiaddin RH, Yang GZ, Kilner PJ (1994) Visualization of flow by vector analysis of multidirectional cine magnetic resonance velocity mapping. *J Comput Assist Tomogr* **18**: 383–392.
4. Roach MR (1977) The effects of bifurcations and stenoses on arterial disease. In *Cardiovascular Flow Dynamics and Measurements* (Hwang NHC and Norman NA, eds) pp 489–539. Baltimore, MD: University Park Press.
5. Yang GZ, Burger P, Kilner PJ, Mohiaddin RH (1991) In vivo blood flow visualization with magnetic resonance imaging. *IEEE Proceedings of Visualization. San Diago, CA*, pp. 202–209.
6. Kilner PJ, Yang GZ, Mohiaddin RH, Firmin DN, Longmore DB (1993) Helical and retrograde secondary flow patterns in the aortic arch studied by three-directional magnetic resonance velocity mapping. *Circulation* **88**: 2235–2247.
7. Walburn FJ, Blick EF, Stein PD (1979) Effect of the branch-to-trunk area ratio on the transition to turbulent: Implications in the cardiovascular system. *Biorheology* **16**: 411–417.
8. Walburn FJ, Stein PD (1981) Effect of vessel tapering on the transition to turbulent flow: Implications in the cardiovascular system. *J Biomech Eng* **103**: 116–120.
9. Stein PD, Sabbah HN (1980) Hemorheology of turbulence. *Biorheology* **17**: 301–319.
10. Firmin DN, Gatehouse PD, Yang GZ, Kilner PJ, Longmore DB (1992) Rapid 7-dimensional imaging of pulsatile flow (Abstract). *Soc Magn Reson Med* **11**: 2915.
11. Gatehouse PD, Firmin DN, Hughes RL, Collins S, Longmore DB (1994) Real time blood flow imaging by spiral scan phase velocity mapping. *J Magn Res Med* **31**: 504–512.
12. Mohiaddin RH, Gatehouse PD, Firmin DN (1994) Exercise-related changes in aortic flow measured by magnetic resonance spiral echo-planar phase-shift velocity mapping *J Magn Reson Image* 1994 (in press).

Short-echo-time magnetic resonance phase-shift velocity mapping for assessment of heart valve and great vessel stenoses: three years' experience

Philip J. Kilner,* David N. Firmin, Raad H. Mohiaddin, Cynthia Sampson, and S. Richard Underwood

Magnetic Resonance Unit, Royal Brompton Hospital, London SW3 6NP UK

Shortening the echo times of magnetic resonance (MR) sequences used for phase-shift velocity mapping to 3.6 ms has extended use of the technique to measurement of velocities in turbulent, poststenotic jet flows. We used a 0.5-T MR machine and field even-echo rephasing (FEER) sequences with 3.6 ms echo times for jet velocity mapping. *In vitro* trials used continuous flow through a phantom with a 6-mm stenosis. Fifteen patients with mitral and/or aortic valve stenosis and 20 patients with repaired aortic coarctation were studied prospectively, with Doppler ultrasonic measurement of peak jet velocity performed independently on the same day. The clinical contribution of MR jet velocity mapping, used during a 3-year period in 306 patients with congenital and acquired disease of heart valves, great vessels, and conduits, was assessed retrospectively. The 3.6-ms sequence allowed accurate measurement of jet velocities up to 6 m s^{-1} *in vitro* ($r = 0.996$). Prospective studies in patients showed good agreement between MR and Doppler measurements of peak velocity: $n = 38$; range, 1.2–6.1 m s^{-1}; mean, 2.7 m s^{-1}; mean of differences (Doppler–MR), 0.22 m s^{-1}; standard deviation of differences, ± 0.38 m s^{-1} ($\pm 14\%$). MR jet velocity mapping proved particularly valuable for assessment and localization of stenoses at sites where ultrasonic access was limited. The technique represents a diagnostic advance which can obviate the need for catheterization in selected cases.

Keywords: MRI, velocity mapping, stenosis, hemodynamics, coarctation, valve disease.

INTRODUCTION

Magnetic resonance (MR) phase-shift velocity mapping has become established as a method for accurate measurement of nonturbulent intravascular flow [1–4]. However, loss of MR signal from regions of turbulent flow can preclude measurement of poststenotic jet velocities and limit the clinical usefulness of the technique. Shortening the echo time of MR sequences used to 3.6 ms effectively surmounts this problem. It allows recovery of signal from all but the most intensely turbulent regions of poststenotic blood flow and enables application of the technique to jet velocity measurement. We have previously published results of *in vitro* and clinical trials of short-echo-time MR jet velocity measurement [5, 6], and we have reported use of the technique in specific applications [7–9]. Other groups have also used and evaluated jet velocity mapping in patients with mitral and aortic valve stenosis [10–12].

The purpose of this article is to summarize our experience of MR jet velocity mapping, giving results of our principal *in vitro* and clinical validation studies and reviewing clinical applications of the technique, as we have used it, over a 3-year period.

METHODS

For all studies, a 0.5-T Picker MR 2055 machine was used, fitted with modified gradient coils allowing $G_{max} = 14$ mT m^{-1}, rise time = 400 μs, dB/dt (max) = 8.75 T s^{-1}. Surface chest receiver coils were used.

---

* Address for correspondence: Magnetic Resonance Unit, Royal Brompton Hospital, Sydney Street, London SW3 6NP, UK.

Field even-echo rephasing (FEER) sequences with 14, 6, and 3.6 ms echo times were used for phase shift velocity mapping [5, 6].

Details of imaging technique were adapted to specific studies. Electrocardiographic gating was used in all patients, usually to acquire 16 frames covering the systolic and/or diastolic flow periods. Velocity maps representing slices 6–10 mm thick with a 40-cm field of view were acquired in 2 × 128 phase-encoding steps.

Spin-echo and cine gradient-echo pilot acquisitions were used to locate jets, working toward accurate identification of the location and direction of the poststenotic jet. A TE 6 ms cine acquisition, without velocity encoding, was often used for identification of jet location because, for high-velocity jets, this showed localized signal loss around the jet core, effectively outlining the jet. Once visualized, the jet core could be cut through accurately, either longitudinally or transversely, by the final velocity mapping slice.

For mapping velocities in the plane of the jet, velocity was encoded in the read gradient direction, with the jet aligned in this direction (Fig. 1). For mapping of velocities through the plane of a slice transecting the jet, velocity was encoded in the slice select gradient direction, and the slice was located immediately downstream of the orifice in order to avoid the region of high acceleration on the upstream side.

Subtraction of reference from velocity-encoded phase images was performed using Picker software. The process was designed to subtract out all but velocity-related phase shifts.

Velocity of pixels on the resulting velocity maps was represented by a gray scale. Peak jet velocity was estimated from an average of at least four pixels in the central jet core region.

In vitro studies

In vitro studies used continuous flow through a phantom containing a 6-mm stenosis. Peak jet velocity measurements by MR and continuous-wave Doppler ultrasound were compared with jet velocities calculated from the flow rate and orifice area [5].

Patients

Fifteen patients with mitral and/or aortic valve stenosis (18 studies) and 20 patients with repaired aortic coarctation were studied prospectively, all of them having Doppler ultrasonic measurement of peak jet velocity performed independently on the same day.

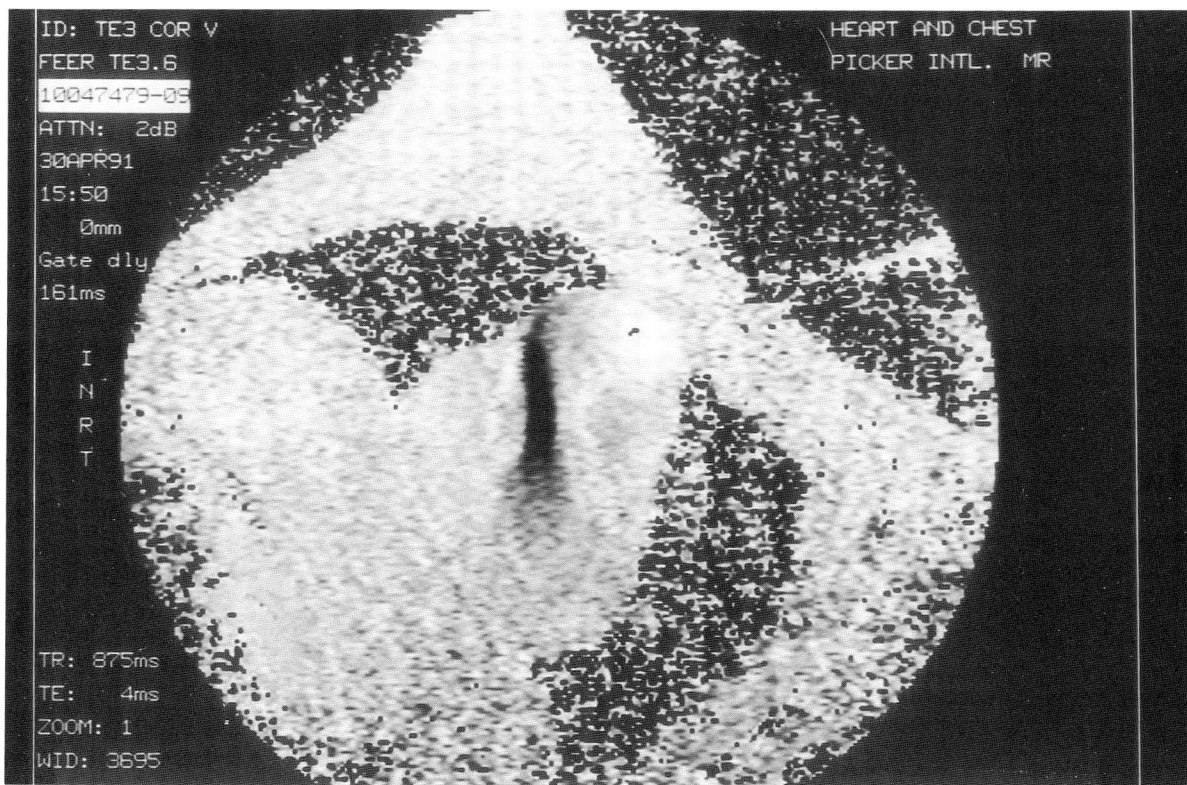

Fig. 1. Systolic velocity map frame, TE 3.6 ms, in a patient with aortic stenosis. The jet above the stenosed valve, with a peak velocity of 3.6 m s^{-1}, appears as a dark streak up the center of the image.

The use of MR jet velocity mapping in 306 patients aged 8–72 (mean age 32) in the 3-year period up to July 1993 was reviewed retrospectively. Diagnoses included repaired or native aortic coarctation (165), ventriculo-pulmonary conduit stenosis (67), valvar and subvalvar stenosis (39), pulmonary artery stenosis (18), and obstruction following Mustard and Fontan operations (31).

RESULTS

In vitro studies

Both the magnetic resonance TE 3.6 ms and the continuous-wave Doppler jet velocity measurements correlated well with the calculated mean jet velocities *in vitro* ($r = 0.996$ and $r = 0.997$, respectively). Full mapping of the jet, with accurate peak velocity measurement, was possible for jet velocities up to 6 m s^{-1} using the TE 3.6 ms sequence, as long as the slice was correctly located and as long as the slice thickness did not exceed the orifice diameter. An artifact, the "edge spike" artifact, was found to cause localized velocity overestimation in pixels bordering the jet at high jet velocities, or at lower velocities if sequences with longer echo times were used.

Prospective clinical studies

Prospective studies in patients with mitral or aortic stenosis or repaired aortic coarctation showed good agreement between MR and Doppler measurements of peak velocity: $n = 38$; range, 1.2–6.1 m s^{-1}; mean, 2.7 m s^{-1}; mean of differences (Doppler–MR), 0.22 m s^{-1}; standard deviation of differences, ± 0.38 m s^{-1} ($\pm 14\%$).

Retrospective review of clinical use

Over a 3-year period, 349 jet velocity map studies were attempted in 306 patients. In 273 (78%) of these, velocity map quality was sufficiently good for determination of the location of stenosis and for jet velocity measurement. Failures, which were apparent from degraded velocity map appearances, were attributed to patient movement, inaccurate slice location, or machine failure. There were no problems regarding anatomical access or alignment with flow, except in a few cases ($n = 6$) where the presence of metal within a few millimeters of the region of interest (e.g., the supporting ring of a Hancock valved conduit) precluded accurate jet velocity measurement.

The most important patient groups, in terms of patient numbers and clinical usefulness of velocity mapping, were adult patients with repaired aortic coarctation and adults with ventriculo-pulmonary conduits (inserted for Fallot's tetralogy, pulmonary atre-

sia, or transposition of the great arteries). In these patients, as in patients with pulmonary artery stenoses and obstructions following Mustard or Fontan operations, adequate visualization by ultrasound was rarely possible.

There were also a few patients ($n = 4$) referred with aortic and/or subaortic stenosis in whom adequate ultrasonic assessment had not been possible. In these, jet velocity mapping provided important additional information.

Regarding the orientation of velocity map planes, we chose to use slices aligned with the jet more often than slices transecting the jet (although in some cases, both were acquired). The former gave clear depiction of jet location in relation to upstream and downstream flows, whereas the latter gave information on jet cross-sectional area and orifice shape.

DISCUSSION

The *in vitro* trials and the prospective clinical studies showed that short-echo-time MR jet velocity mapping has sufficient accuracy and range to be useful in clinical assessment of stenoses of heart valves, great vessels, and conduits in adults. In the prospective studies and in general clinical use, the consistency of velocity map image quality was good.

Jet velocity mapping increases the diagnostic value of MR imaging as a second-line investigation after transthoracic echocardiography. The advantages of MR velocity mapping over continuous-wave Doppler are freedom of access to jets at any point and in any direction through the heart and great vessels, reliable depiction of the location of the jet, and ability to map through-plane as well as in-plane velocities. But the technique does not acquire data in real time and is (at present) unable to search across volumes interactively. Pilot acquisitions have to be used carefully to identify the location and direction of a jet. With experience, and as long as the patient remains still, this works very well, but it can be relatively time-consuming.

In terms of patient tolerance and noninvasiveness, the technique is more acceptable for repeated follow-up investigation than transesophageal echocardiography and gives better access to the great vessels and pulmonary arteries. In selected cases, use of the technique obviates the need for catheterization. We have found the very short echo time (3.6 ms) to be necessary for recovery of adequate signal from high-velocity jets and for minimization of artifacts. The "edge spike" artifact appears to be caused by phase shifts arising not from velocity but from sudden deceleration of blood at the lateral borders of a jet.

Velocity measurements from such regions should be avoided.

At present, the use of jet velocity mapping is limited by the lack of suitably equipped MR machines. This is regrettable, as the technique extends the usefulness of MR investigation in cardiology and has potential for further development.

REFERENCES

1. Moran PR (1982) A flow velocity zeugmatographic interlace for NMR imaging in humans. *Magn Reson Imaging* **1:** 197–203.
2. Nayler GL, Firmin DN, Longmore DB (1986) Blood flow imaging by cine magnetic resonance. *J Comput Assist Tomogr* **10:** 715–722.
3. Underwood SR, Firmin DN (1991) *Magnetic Resonance of the Cardiovascular System.* Oxford: Blackwell Scientific Publications.
4. Mostbeck GH, Caputo GR, Higgins CB (1992) MR measurement of blood flow in the cardiovascular system. *Am J Radiol* **159:** 453–461.
5. Kilner PJ, Firmin DN, Rees RSO, Martinez JE, Pennell DJ, Mohiaddin RH, Underwood SR, Longmore DB (1991) Valve and great vessel stenosis: Assessment with MR jet velocity mapping. *Radiology* **178:** 229–235.
6. Kilner PJ, Manzara CC, Mohiaddin RH, Pennell DJ, Sutton MStJ, Firmin DN, Underwood SR, Longmore DB (1993) Magnetic resonance jet velocity mapping in mitral and aortic valve stenosis. *Circulation* **87:** 1239–1248.
7. Martinez JE, Mohiaddin RH, Kilner PJ, Khaw K, Rees RSO, Somerville J, Longmore DB (1992) Obstruction in extracardiac ventriculopulmonary conduits: Value of magnetic resonance imaging with velocity mapping and Doppler echocardiography. *J Am Coll Cardiol* **20:** 338–344.
8. Mohiaddin RH, Kilner PJ, Rees RSO, Longmore DB (1993) Magnetic resonance volume flow and jet velocity mapping in aortic coarctation. *J Am Coll Cardiol* **22:** 1515–1521.
9. Sampson C, Kilner PJ, Hirsch R, Rees RSO, Somerville J, Underwood SR. (1994) Venoatrial pathways after Mustard operation for transposition of the great arteries: anatomic and functional imaging. *Radiology* **193:** (in press).
10. Sondergard L, Thomsen C, Stahlberg F, Gymoese E, Lindvig K, Hilderbrandt P, Henriksen O (1992) Mitral and aortic valvular flow: quantification with MR phase mapping: *J Magn Reson Imaging* **2:** 295–302.
11. Sondergard L, Stahlberg F, Thomsen C, Stensgard A, Lindvig K, Henriksen O (1993) Accuracy and precision of MR velocity mapping in measurement of stenotic cross sectional area, flow rate and pressure gradient. *J Magn Reson Imaging* **3**(2): 433–437.
12. Eichenberger AC, Jenni R, von Schultess GK (1993) Aortic valve pressure gradients in patients with aortic valve stenosis: quantification with velocity-encoded cine MR imaging. *Am J Radiol* **160:** 971–977.

Magnetic resonance imaging of coronary arteries and coronary stenosis

D.J. Pennell,* H.G. Bogren, J. Keegan, D.N. Firmin and S.R. Underwood

Magnetic Resonance Unit, Royal Brompton Hospital, London SW3 6NP, UK

Coronary artery imaging is an important investigation for the management of coronary artery disease. Alternative noninvasive imaging would be useful, but the small caliber and tortuosity of the coronary vessels and cardiac and respiratory motion create formidable imaging problems. We first studied 21 normal subjects and 5 with coronary artery disease established by X-ray contrast angiography, of whom 2 had undergone bypass grafting. Of these, 22 were imaged successfully. Identification of the artery was possible for the left main stem, left anterior descending, right coronary, and left circumflex arteries respectively in 95%, 91%, 95%, and 76%. The arterial diameter at the origin could be measured in 77%, 77%, 81%, and 63%. The mean $\pm$SD arterial diameter in each case (4.8 $\pm$ 0.8, 3.7 $\pm$ 0.5, 3.9 $\pm$ 0.9, and 2.9 $\pm$ 0.6 mm) was not significantly different from reference values (all p = ns). The mean length of artery visualized was 10.4 $\pm$ 5.2, 46.7 $\pm$ 22.8, 53.7 $\pm$ 27.9, and 26.3 $\pm$ 17.5 mm. In 12 normal males, the total coronary area was 30.9 $\pm$ 9.2 mm^2 and the ratio compared with body surface area was 16.4 $\pm$ 4.4 mm^2 m^{-2} (both p = ns compared with reference values). In seven patients, with X-ray contrast coronary angiography, the proximal arterial diameter measured by magnetic resonance was 3.9 $\pm$ 1.1 mm, and by X-ray contrast angiography 3.7 $\pm$ 1.0 mm (p = ns). We then studied 17 patients with angina. Imaging of just the relevant artery was performed and analysis was blinded to the X-ray angiography results. Stenosis was identified on the magnetic resonance (MR) images by localized reduction in vessel signal intensity. Stenosis location by MR was assessed by measurement of its distance from a reference vessel, with correlation to the X-ray findings. X-ray coronary angiography showed 23 stenoses of which 15 (65%) were correctly located by blind assessment of the MR images. Of the eight remaining stenoses, a further 5 (63%) were correctly located on the MR images after retrospective comparison (overall sensitivity 87%). There were three lesions thought to represent stenosis by MR, which on review of the X-ray angiogram proved to be a minor stenosis <50% (two cases) or a tortuous vessel (one case). Greater signal loss was seen in the more severe stenoses. The stenosis length by MRI was greater than by X-ray (8.4 versus 5.1 mm, p < 0.001). The overestimation of stenosis length may be due to turbulence.

Keywords: flow MRI, coronary angiography MRI, X-ray angiography.

INTRODUCTION

Imaging of the coronary arteries is important in the management of coronary artery disease, but X-ray contrast angiography requires arterial catheterisation and carries a small risk of death and other complications [1, 2]. At present, there is no satisfactory alternative. Although X-ray contrast coronary angiography provides little information on coronary flow or the vessel wall, it is an essential examination prior to revascularization by coronary bypass surgery or angioplasty.

Magnetic resonance (MR) angiography has progressed in recent years, challenging conventional angiography for the carotid [3] and renal [4] vessels and proving to be superior to the conventional technique for peripheral angiography [5]. However, magnetic resonance angiography of the coronary vessels has been hindered by a combination of formidable problems. These include their small caliber, cardiac motion, respiratory motion, tortuosity, and proximity to other tissues of high water density. None of these

* Address for correspondence: MR Unit, Royal Brompton Hospital, Sydney Street, London SW3 6NP, UK.

problems, however, is insurmountable, and images of the coronary arteries [6, 7] and coronary artery bypass grafts [8, 9] were first acquired using standard MR techniques several years ago, but the technique was unreliable and the resolution was limited because of the long imaging times. Technological advances have now made fast imaging possible, with single-image acquisition times as low as 10 ms using the echo-planar technique [10], 300 ms using the Fast Low Angle Shot (FLASH) technique [11], and the possibility of magnetic resonance fluoroscopy at 12.5 frames per second [12]. Recent studies suggest that such fast-imaging techniques alleviate the above problems [13, 14]. We report our experience of fast gradient-echo imaging of normal and stenosed coronary arteries [15].

METHODS

Magnetic resonance imaging was performed using a velocity-compensated gradient-echo sequence (TE 6.5 ms, TR 15.7 ms) and a segmented *k*-space technique, such that 8 phase-encoding steps were acquired in each cardiac cycle, with complete imaging over 16 cardiac cycles during breath-holding. The acquisition window for the eight phase-encoding steps was 126 ms, which was positioned in mid to late diastole. Fat signal suppression was employed, using frequency-selective preexcitation and dephasing prior to water excitation. Studies were performed using a 1.5-T system (Picker International Vista scanner, Cleveland Heights, OH, USA), with a 60-cm patient bore. The field of view used was 20 cm and the slice thickness 4 mm, giving an in-plane pixel size of 1.6 × 0.8 mm. A surface coil over the anterior chest was used. The duration of imaging was approximately 1 h.

RESULTS

The left main stem (95%), left anterior descending (91%), and right coronary arteries (95%) were identified in nearly all subjects, but the left circumflex artery was more difficult (76%). The majority of the missed arteries occurred early in our experience, but the left circumflex artery continued to pose problems. The mean diameter of the arteries measured by magnetic resonance was not significantly different from reference values from quantitative X-ray coronary angiography [16]. The length of the left main stem was 10.4 mm and varied from 3.6 to 20.2 mm, which is similar to the reference range [17]. The mean length of artery seen by longitudinal imaging was greatest for the

right coronary (53 mm) and left anterior descending arteries (46 mm), and least for the left circumflex artery (26 mm). The diagonal arteries were seen in five of the last nine subjects, after the use of the tilted transaxial imaging of the proximal left anterior descending artery, as described above. In 12 normal males, the total coronary area, defined as the sum of the areas of the proximal arteries [18], was 30.9 ± 9.2 mm^2 (range 19.4–57.2), and the total coronary area to body surface area ratio was 16.4 ± 4.4 mm^2 m^{-2} (range 10.9–27.9). Both were not significantly different from reference values [15, 17]. The interobserver variation for measurement of the diameter of the proximal arteries was 7% for the left main stem, 12% for the left anterior descending artery, 11% for the right coronary artery, and 18% for the left circumflex artery.

Comparison of magnetic resonance and X-ray contrast coronary angiography

The proximal arterial diameter measured by magnetic resonance was 3.9 ± 1.1 mm, and by X-ray contrast angiography 3.7 ± 1.0 mm (p = ns). The mean difference between the measurements was 0.2 ± 0.5 mm, and the coefficient of variation was 13.7%. Coronary artery disease was present in five of the seven patients with previous X-ray contrast angiography. The occluded left anterior descending artery was identified in all four patients and there was clear similarity between the magnetic resonance and conventional coronary images. The insertion of the bypass graft distal to the left anterior descending artery occlusion was identified, and comparison made with conventional angiography. In one patient, right coronary artery occlusion was identified, and vein grafts to the right coronary and left circumflex arteries visualized.

Coronary artery stenosis

We then studied 17 patients with angina. Imaging of just the relevant artery was performed and analysis was blinded to the X-ray angiography results. Stenosis was identified on the MR images by localised reduction in vessel signal intensity. Stenosis location by MR was assessed by measurement of its distance from a reference vessel, with correlation to the X-ray findings.

X-ray coronary angiography showed 23 stenoses, of which 15 (65%) were correctly located by blind assessment of the MR images. Of the eight remaining stenoses, a further five (63%) were correctly located on the MR images after retrospective comparison (overall sensitivity 87%). There were three lesions thought to represent stenosis by MR which on review of the X-ray angiogram proved to be a minor stenosis <50% (two cases) or a tortuous vessel (one case). Greater signal loss was seen in the more severe stenoses. The stenosis length by MRI was greater than by X-ray (8.4 versus 5.1 mm, $p < 0.001$). The overestimation of stenosis length may be due to turbulence.

DISCUSSION

Coronary artery imaging by magnetic resonance imaging is progressing rapidly. The problems of small vessel size and tortuosity have been tackled and the preliminary results are very encouraging. Faster imaging perhaps with spiral acquisitions may further reduce motion artefact in the images. In addition, the shorter readout times would allow multislice imaging within a single breath-hold which would also eliminate misregistration between different breath-hold images. Magnetization transfer may also assist in improving contrast in the images by reducing myocardial signal. Considerable further development is required before a clinical investigation can be envisaged, but the future promises to be very interesting.

REFERENCES

1. Kennedy JW, Baxley WA, Bunnel IL et al. (1982) Mortality related to cardiac catheterisation and angiography. *Cathet Cardiovasc Diagn* **8**: 323–340.
2. Davis K, Kennedy JW, Kemp HG, Judkins MP, Gosselin AJ, Killip T (1979) Complications of coronary arteriography from the collaborative study of coronary artery surgery (CASS). *Circulation* **59**: 1105–1112.
3. Fram EK, Heiserman JE (1993) Carotid and vertebral arteries. In *Magnetic Resonance Angiography, Concepts and Applications* (Potchen EJ, Haacke EM, Siebert JE, Gottschalk A, eds.) pp. 498–518. St. Louis, MO: C.V. Mosby.
4. Kent KC, Edelman RR, Kim DD, Steinman TI, Porter DH, Skillman JJ (1991) Magnetic resonance imaging: A reliable test for the evaluation of proximal atherosclerotic renal arterial stenosis. *J Vasc Surg* **13**: 311–318.
5. Owens RS, Carpenter JP, Baum RA, Perloff LJ, Cope C (1992) Magnetic resonance imaging of angiographically occult runoff vessels in peripheral arterial occlusive disease. *New Engl J Med* **326**: 1577–1581.
6. Underwood SR (1991) Imaging of acquired heart disease. In *Magnetic Resonance of the Cardiovascular System* (Underwood SR, Firmin DN, eds.) pp. 41–67. London: Blackwell.
7. Underwood SR (1988) Magnetic resonance imaging of the cardiovascular system. In *Perspectives in Cardiology, 1988* (Sobel BE, Julian DG, Hugenholtz PG, eds.) pp. 344–359. London: Current Medical Literature.
8. Underwood SR, Firmin DN, Klipstein RH, Rees RSO, Longmore DB (1987) Magnetic resonance velocity mapping: Clinical applications of a new technique. *Br Heart J* **57**: 404–412.
9. White RD, Caputo GR, Mark AS, Modin GW, Higgins CB (1987) Coronary artery bypass graft patency: Noninvasive evaluation with MR imaging. *Radiology* **164**: 681–686.
10. Stehling MJ, Howseman AM, Ordidge RJ et al. (1989) Whole body echo-planar MR imaging at 0.5 T. *Radiology* **170**: 257–263.
11. Frahm J, Merboldt KD, Bruhn H, Gyngell ML, Hänicke W, Chien D (1990) 0.3 second FLASH imaging of the human heart. *Magn Reson Med* **13**: 150–157.
12. Riederer SJ, Tasciyan T, Farzaneh F, Lee JN, Wright RC, Herkfens RJ (1988) MR fluoroscopy: Technical feasibility. *Magn Reson Med* **8**: 1–15.
13. Edelman RR, Manning WJ, Burstein D, Paulin S (1991). Coronary arteries: Breath-hold MR angiography. *Radiology* **181**: 641–643.
14. Manning WJ, Li W, Boyle NG, Edelman RR (1993) Fat-suppressed breath-hold magnetic resonance coronary angiography. *Circulation* **87**: 94–104.
15. Pennell DJ, Keegan J, Firmin DN, Gatehouse PD, Underwood SR, Longmore DB (1993) Magnetic resonance imaging of coronary arteries: Technique and preliminary results. *Br Heart J* **70**: 315–326.
16. Dodge JT, Brown BG, Bolson EL, Dodge HT (1992) Lumen diameter of normal coronary arteries. Influence of age, sex, anatomic variation, and left ventricular hypertrophy or dilatation. *Circulation* **86**: 232–346.
17. Abramson DI, Dobrin PB (1984) In *Blood Vessels and Lymphatics in Organ Systems* p. 320. Orlando, FL: Academic Press.
18. MacAlpin RN, Abbasi AS, Grollman JH, Eber L (1973) Human coronary artery size during life. A cinearteriographic study. *Radiology* **108**: 567–576.

Differential diagnostics of portal hypertension studied by MR imaging

G.P. Streltsova,[1]* G.A. Morgunov,[2] M.G. Jakobson,[1] A.V. Strygin[1] and I.I. Shterental[1]

[1]*International Tomography Center of Russian Academy of Sciences, Siberian Branch, Novosibirsk, Russia*
[2]*Medical Institute, Novosibirsk, Russia*

This study has examined the ability of magnetic resonance imaging (MRI) to reveal the features of intrahepatic and extrahepatic portal circulation in portal hypertension syndrome (PHS). A retrospective analysis of the abdominal MRI examinations of 96 patients was performed. The spin-echo imaging technique was used to obtain coronal, transaxial, and sagittal images for all patients. The main distinctive features of revealed extrahepatic PHS in nine patients were the thrombosed lumen of the portal vein, the widespread net of collateral vessels around the portal vein, and the widened hepatic artery. The smooth liver surface without evident disturbances of the architectonics of intrahepatic vasculature was depicted in all patients and the caudal lobe hypertrophy was observed in five patients. The widening of the azygos vein was displayed in six of nine patients and hemiazygos vein was delineated in one case. Typical morphologic features of liver cirrhosis and different degrees of the stenosis of the intrahepatic segment of the inferior vena cava (IVC) (10–30%) were found in 28 patients. More than 30% stenosis of the IVC was displayed in 7 of 18 patients (average 28%) with the preascitic liver cirrhosis and in all patients with ascites (average 47%). In two patients the Budd–Chiari syndrome was characterized by the reduced caliber or by the absence of hepatic veins, the comma-shaped intrahepatic collateral vessels, and the constriction of the intrahepatic IVC. The primary ascending thrombosis of the IVC (1 patient) and the occlusion or direct extensions of tumor (16 patients) were usually well seen on MR images.

Keywords: MRI, portal hypertension syndrome, portal vein thrombosis, liver cirrhosis.

INTRODUCTION

Portal hypertension syndrome (PHS) is characterized by a pressure gradient between the portal and systemic venous vessels. A distinguishing feature of the PHS is the existence of numerous causes of portal circulation blockade which leads to some variants of regional circulatory disturbances among which the liver cirrhosis predominates. The aim of our research was to estimate the opportunities of magnetic resonance imaging (MRI) in the differential diagnostics of various forms of portal circulation blockade in comparison with the complex X-ray instrumental examination to reveal the particular signs of MRI and to predict possible complications of the current disease.

* Address for correspondence: Diagnostic Department, International Tomography Center, Russian Academy of Sciences Siberian Branch, Institutskaya Street, 3A, Novosibirsk 630090, Russia.

MATERIALS AND METHODS

Magnetic resonance images of 98 patients were analyzed. Among the causes of PHS were confirmed liver cirrhosis ($n = 27$), thrombosis of the portal vein ($n = 9$), Budd–Chiari syndrome ($n = 2$), primary ascending thrombosis of the inferior vena cava (IVC) ($n = 1$), hyperkinetic version of PHS caused by multifocal liver hemangiomas ($n = 1$), and malignant tumors with stenosis or occlusion of the IVC ($n = 16$). The reference group included 42 patients who had no disturbances of portal system circulation. MRI was performed on a Bruker BMT-1100 iron-shielded resistive MR tomography system operated at 0.28 T field strengths corresponding to 12 MHz proton resonance frequency. According to diagnostic aims, the axial, coronal, and sagittal imaging planes were used. All images were produced using the spin-echo (SE), rapid acquisition with relaxation enhancement (RARE), and the 2DFT. The T_1-weighted multislice single echo (MSSE, TR

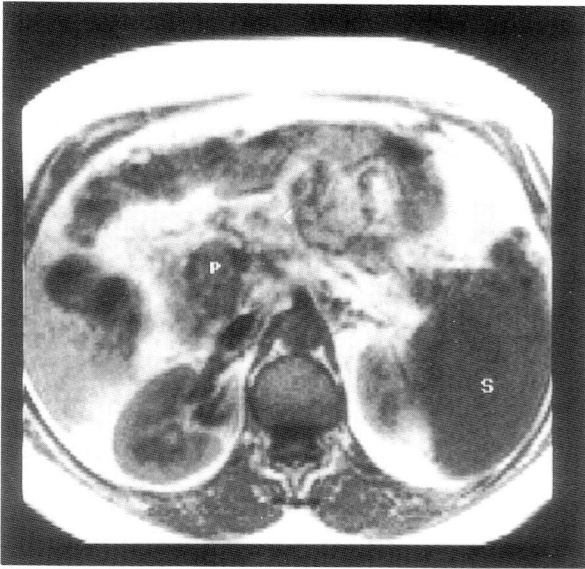

Fig. 1. Thrombosis of the portal vein. Numerous collateral vessels around the portal vein (*p*). SE 370/15/4.

370/TE 23 ms) and T_2-weighted multislice multiecho (MSME, TR 1200–1800/TE 120 ms) sequences were employed. The length of the IVC stenosis and the stenosis index were defined by 10 axial slices. The stenosis index was calculated in percent as a ratio of the cross-sectional area of the infrahepatic segment of IVC to the least cross section of the intrahepatic segment.

RESULTS AND DISCUSSION

MRI compared with angiography is remarkable with its unique ability to define the vasculature without intravenous contrast material. The ability to distinguish the lumen of vessel from its wall and from surrounding tissues is determined by the fundamental principle of MRI, i.e., by the fact that MR signal intensity decreases proportionally to the velocity of nuclei moving through the imaged volume. Therefore, the absence of signal takes place in the vessels with rapid laminar flows. As a result, the extrahepatic and intrahepatic vasculature is clearly delineated. Analyses of the MR images of the reference group has testified that the use of three orthogonal planes allows one to obtain clear images of the extrahepatic and intrahepatic vasculature providing the portal circulation. The IVC, the portal vein trunk, its main right and left branches, the drain hepatic veins, the splenic and superior mesenteric vessels, as well as the azygos vein were depicted in all patients, whereas the proximal segment of the common hepatic artery was delineated only in 40% patients in the axial plane [1]. The 15% and less physiological stenosis of IVC occurred in 25% of patients; however, two patients exhibited 19% and 23% stenosis. The azygos vein, 4–6 mm in diameter, was depicted in 80% patients. Among the main characteristic features of the images taken in patients with extrahepatic PHS was the absence of portal vein trunk (five patients). Sometimes it was possible to distinguish the thrombosed lumen of the portal vein (four patients) and the recanalization with the signal flow void (one patient). The combined thrombosis of the portal vein trunk and its right branch took place in one case. The combined thrombosis of the portal vein trunk and the splenic vein was observed in one patient as well. The availability of a numerous collateral vessels around the thrombosed portal vein was the second significant peculiarity of the extrahepatic portal hypertension. The increased compensatory flow of arterial blood and, as a consequence, the enlarged diameter of the hepatic artery allowed the delineation of this vessel in all patients, with the length of visible segment increased. The widened azygos vein was displayed in six of nine patients and the hemiazygos vein was delineated in one patient. We assumed that the widening of the azygos vein indicated the formation of collateral circulation of gastro-oesophageal type, which initiated varication of the esophagus followed by hemorrhage. This assumption has been confirmed, in a complex instrumental X-ray investigation, by visually enlarged contrasting azygos vein diameter as well as by increased pressure and the degree of blood oxygenation in the azygos vein as compared to the superior vein cava. A decrease in liver size was observed only in one case. Different degrees of caudate lobe hypertrophy were observed in five patients. A considerable increase in splenic dimensions was found in all cases; a new-grown lien was found in two of six patients who underwent surgical intervention (splenectomy). Thirty-six percent and 46% stenosis of the intrahepatic segment of IVC appeared in two cases. In the cases of liver cirrhosis, the features of MRI were different, depending on the stage of the disease. The morphological peculiarities of liver cirrhosis have been described in detail elsewhere [2–4]. The IVC stenosing (average 28%) was found in 7 of 18 patients with the preascitic stage of liver cirrhosis. Considerable widening of splenic artery and vein diameter and moderate widening of portal vein trunk, its right and left branches, as well as superior mesenteric and asygos vein were observed in all patients. The caliber of the drain hepatic veins was rather small, and sometimes the contours of veins were uneven. The delineation of the common hepatic artery was

(A)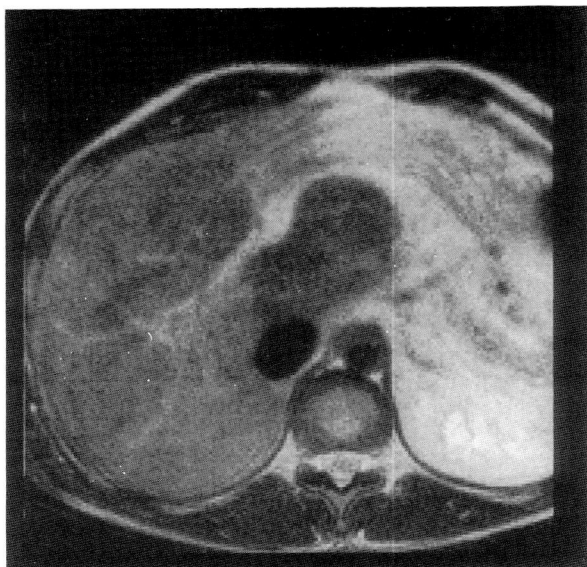

(B)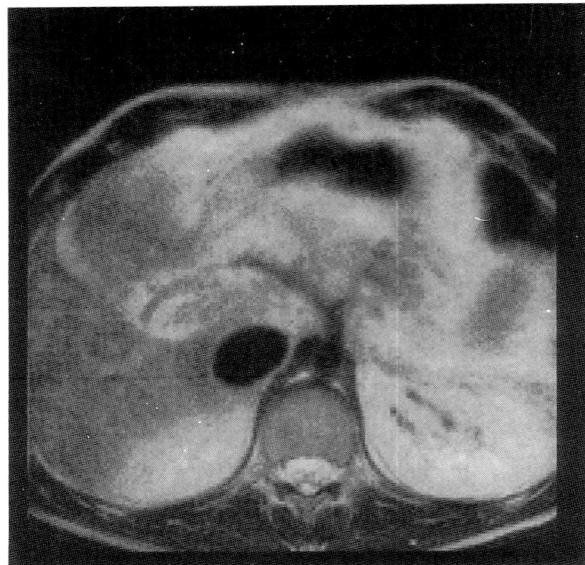

(C)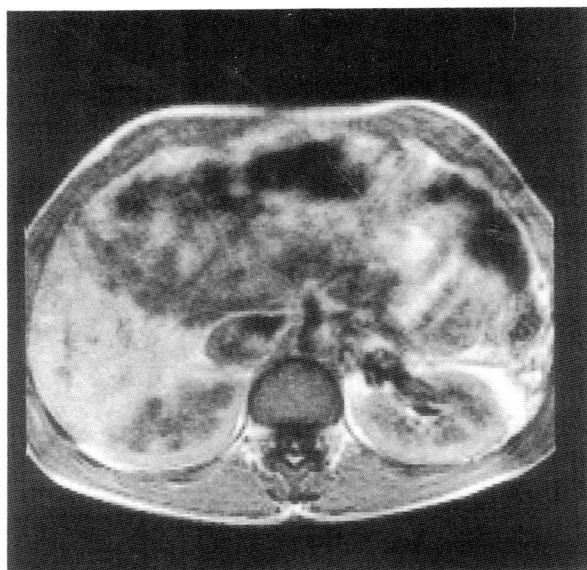

Fig. 2. Thrombosis of the portal vein and its main branches. (A) The flow void is absent in the portal veins. Hypertrophy of the caudal lobe. RARE 3000/21/2; (B) the widened hepatic artery; (C) The collateral vessels in front of the left kidney. The splenorenal shunt is patent. SE 370/15/4.

possible in 4 of 18 patients (22%). In the ascitic liver cirrhosis, considerable decrease in liver size was observed in eight patients, and only one patient exhibited the considerably increased liver size. The left lobe hypertrophy was found in one patient, but the caudate lobe hypertrophy took place in six (67%) patients. The splenomegaly was displayed in all cases. These were the largest dimensions of the lien in this category of patients. The end stage of ascitic liver cirrhosis was characterized by considerable disturbances of the architectonics of both the intrahepatic and extrahepatic vascular beds. The IVC stenosing took place in all patients, and the index stenosis varied within 28–70% (average 47%). In all cases, the portal vein diameter

was widened and the portovertebral angle was decreased. This process was not observed in patients with preascitic liver cirrhosis. The portal and drain hepatic veins were often narrowed and greatly deformed, so, as a rule, they were difficult to identify. The collateral vessels were often displayed near the splenic hilum. The common hepatic artery was seen only in three patients (33%).

The Budd–Chiari syndrome was characterized by reduction in caliber or absence of hepatic veins, comma-shaped intrahepatic collateral vessels, and constriction of the intrahepatic IVC. The hepatic veins obliteration was combined with the left portal vein thrombosis. In the other case, the ascendent IVC thrombosis was complicated by thrombosis of drain hepatic veins, superior mesenteric, and the portal veins. In both cases, MR findings were confirmed by angiography data.

CONCLUSION

The application of the intrahepatic and extrahepatic circulation method to the investigation of different forms of portal circulation blockade has shown the high informativity and prognostic value of MRI, which compares well with the complex instrumental X-ray investigation.

MRI appears to be an effective means for evaluating the blockade portal circulation level, for prognosing the development of portal hypertension complications (esophageal hemorrhage and ascitis), and for correct choice of the method of treatment.

The MRI must be carried out before the angiography and, in most cases, can replace the dangerous invasive investigation.

REFERENCES

1. Fisher M, Wall S, Hricak H, et al. (1985) Hepatic vascular anatomy on magnetic resonance imaging. *Am J Radiol* **144:** 739.
2. Itai Y, Ohnishi S, Ohtomo K et al. (1987) Regenerating nodules of liver cirrhosis: MR imaging. *Radiology* **165:** 419.
3. Itai Y, Ohtomo K, Kokubo T, et al. (1988) CT and MR imaging of postnecrotic liver scars. *J Comput Assist Tomogr* **12**(6): 971.
4. Weisslerder R, Stark DD (1989) *MRI Atlas of the Abdomen,* Koln: Deutscher Arzte-Verlag GmbH.
5. Okuda K, Takayasu K, Iwamoto S (1989) Angiography in the diagnosis of liver disease. *Semin Liver Dis* **9**(1): 50.
6. Whalen E (1990) Liver imaging—Current trends in MRI, CT, and US. Am J Radiol **155:** 1125.

New developments in MRI contrast enhancement

Robert C. Brasch

Contrast Media Laboratory, Department of Radiology, University of California, San Francisco, CA 94143-0628, USA

Ongoing developments in contrast media for magnetic resonance imaging (MRI) should lead to an improvement in sensitivity for the detection of disease, better definition of normal and pathologic anatomy, added functional information, and an expansion of diagnostic MRI applications. Currently available for clinical use are four low-molecular-weight gadolinium complexes which distribute in the extracellular fluid space and highlight defects in the blood-brain barrier. An estimated 20–45% of patients undergoing MRI examination receive one of these governmental-approved gadolinium complexes. In addition, contrast agents differing in purpose and primary magnetic effect, both paramagnetic proton relaxation and magnetic susceptibility agents, are being developed. These include agents for enhancing the blood pool, myocardium, liver, lymph nodes, tumors, and gastrointestinal lumen. Criteria for suitability of new contrast agents include diagnostic efficacy, safety, stability, pharmacology, and cost.

Keywords: contrast-enhanced MRI, tissue-specific contrast media, hepatic contrast media, oral contrast media, blood pool contrast media.

In general, the goal of magnetic resonance imaging (MRI) contrast enhancement is to add functional information to the generally remarkable morphologic information available from the unenhanced images. In some cases, anatomic information may also be improved. Contrast agents, specifically those of high-dose efficiency and those directed to specific tissues, may expand the role of MR into areas of medicine as yet relatively untouched by the MR revolution. Table 1, subject to frequent modification and not intended to be all-inclusive, may be helpful for identifying some of the many contrast agents now under development, their type of enhancement, and their primary distribution pattern. Ultimately to be governmental-approved and used widely, a candidate contrast agent must prove itself to be both efficacious and safe.

Address for Correspondence: Contrast Media Laboratory, Department of Radiology, University of California, San Francisco, 513 Parnassus Avenue, San Francisco, CA 94143-0628 USA.
* Portions of this manuscript have been previously published in a review article by the author: New directions in the development of MR imaging contrast media. *Radiology* **183**:1–11 (1992).

MEANS OF ALTERING MRI CONTRAST

Signal intensity on MR images is primarily determined by proton relaxation times (T_1 and T_2) and by proton density [1, 2]. The presence of a pharmaceutical can be imaged if it locally alters one or more of these variables. Perhaps the simplest strategy is to displace water, for example, by filling the gastrointestinal tract with a fluorocarbon emulsionlike perfluorooctylbromide (PFOB, Imagent™), recently approved in the United States, thereby decreasing proton density and intraluminal signal intensity. However, the majority of contrast agents are chosen for their ability to shorten primarily the T_1 or the T_2 times of tissues.

The ability of certain chemicals to decrease proton relaxation times depends on the creation of local magnetic fields that fluctuate with appropriate frequency components. The varying field experienced by nearby protons will depend not only the characteristics of the agent, including magnetic moment and electron spin relaxation time but also on the nature of their molecular interactions with protons, such as inner- and outer-sphere coordination and diffusional

Table 1. Classification of MR contrast agents.

	Extracellular	Intracellular or cell bound	Gastrointestinal
Positive enhancers	Low molecular weight Gd-DTPA Gd-DOTA Gd-HP-DO3A Gd-DTPA-BMA Gd-BOPTA Nitroxides Macromolecular/blood pool Albumin-(Gd-DTPA)$_x$ Dextran-(Gd-DTPA)$_x$ Polylysine-(Gd-DTPA)$_x$ PEG-Polylysine-(Gd-DTPA)$_x$ Paramagnetic liposomes	Hepatocyte directed Gd-BOPTA Gd-EOB-DTPA Mn-DPDP Fe-HBED Fe-EHPD Lymph node Polylysine-(Gd-DTPA)$_x$-dextran Adrenal gland Polylysine-(Gd-DTPA)$_x$-NH$_2$ RES directed Paramagnetic liposomes Tumor directed Metalloporphyrins Antibody-(Gd-DTPA)$_x$ Calcification directed Gd-DTPA-diphosponate	Water miscible Gd-DTPA Ferric ammonium citrate Water immiscible Vegetable oils Fats Sucrose polyester
Negative enhancers	Low molecular weight Dys-DTPA Dys-DTPA-BMA Macromolecular/blood pool MION PION USPIO Albumin-(Dys-DTPA)$_x$	Hepatocyte directed AG-USPIO MION-ASF RES directed SPIO, USPIO, MION, Superparamagnetic liposomes Lymph nodes USPIO MION-46 Antigen directed MION-immunoglobulin MION-Fab	Water miscible SPIO Barium sulfate suspensions Clays Water immiscible Gas-producing pellets PFOB

translation. Both T_1 and T_2 times are effected, but not necessarily to the same extent. For practical purposes it is useful to divide this consideration of relaxation agents into two subclasses: (1) paramagnetic, positive enhancers and (2) susceptibility effect, negative enhancers. To the physical chemist this separation is arbitrary because the principles defining the interactions of both subclasses with protons are the same, simply variations on a spectrum of interactions [2].

Positive enhancers

Certain metals, including Mn(II), Fe(III), and GD(III), and stable free radicals, such as nitroxides and melanin, contain unpaired electrons. The unpaired electrons cause these substances to be strongly paramagnetic, at least 1800 times stronger than the hydrogen

nucleus with a single unpaired proton. Gd(III) ions, the paramagnetic core of available gadolinium complexes, contain seven unpaired electrons, yielding very strong T_1 relaxation properties. On a molecular basis, the strong paramagnetism of these metal ions will disturb the relaxation of nearby water protons, causing both T_1 and T_2 relaxation times to decrease. Although both T_1 and T_2 times are affected, the T_1 shortening effect predominates on MRI at low concentrations of paramagnetic ions. Shortening of T_1 times in tissues, as observed following the intravenous administration of gadolinium complexes in the standard 0.1-mmol kg^{-1} dose, will produce an increase in signal intensity [3, 4]. This change in tissue relaxation will be best seen on T_1-weighted images. Somewhat paradoxically, at high concentrations, for instance in the concentrated urine of the bladder after administration of a gadolinium complex, the T_2 shortening effect of paramagnetic agents predominates over the T_1 shortening effect and signal intensity decreases.

Negative enhancers

Ferromagnetic substances consist of a crystalline array of many paramagnetic elements that when placed in an external magnetic field behave in synchrony. Superparamagnetic particles such as iron oxide particles, including both ferrites and magnetites, may be considered a subgroup of ferromagnetic substances which lack magnetic memory. One effect of such an array of strongly paramagnetic elements is to produce a localized disturbance in magnetic field homogeneity. The effect on proton relaxation depends on the compartmentalization and arrangement of the particles. Nearby protons will experience this field inhomogeneity, a so-called "outer sphere" or "susceptibility effect," causing rapid dephasing of spins and a resultant decrease in T_2 and T_2^*. The effects of superparamagnetic particles on T_1 relaxation are relatively minor compared to the T_2 effects; the particles cannot get close enough to free protons to produce a significant "inner-sphere" interaction. Predominant shortening of T_2 and T_2^* produces a loss of local signal intensity. This negative enhancement, essentially a localized blackening of the image, is seen best on T_2-weighted and gradient echo pulse sequences.

Superparamagnetic iron oxide particles are not the only formulations that produce a strong susceptibility effect. Certain metals such as dysprosium, having a large magnetic moment but little effect on T_1 relaxation, have been used in metal complexes to induce negative enhancement. For example, echo-planar T_2-weighted imaging was successfully applied to demonstrate a localized loss of perfusion in a stroke model after injection of dysprosium-DTPA-BMA, a low-osmolality susceptibility contrast agent [5]. In this study, the ischemic area was better shown with a negative contrast agent, dysprosium-DTPA-BMA, than with the corresponding positive enhancer, gadolinium-DTPA-BMA.

EXTRACELLULAR AGENTS

Low-molecular-weight contrast agents (<1000 daltons) designed to enhance the extracellular fluid spaces and blood-brain barrier defects can no longer be considered a "new direction" and will not be discussed here in detail. Governmental-approved gadolinium complexes now in clinical use include gadolinium-DTPA dimeglumine (Magnevist™, gado-pentatate dimeglumine, Schering AG, Berlin, Germany), Gd-DOTA meglumine (Dotaram™, Guerbet Laboratories, Aulnay-sous-Bois, France), Gd-HP-DO3A (Prohance™, Squibb Diagnostics, Princeton, NJ, USA), and Gd-DTPA-bismethylamide (Omniscan™, Nycomed AG, Oslo, Norway). As a class, these gadolinium complexes are highly effective contrast enhancers with favorable safety profiles.

BLOOD POOL AND CAPILLARY INTEGRITY MARKERS

Contrast enhancing agents are also being developed to specifically enhance the blood pool. Multiple applications have been envisioned and tested in preclinical feasibility studies including enhanced angiography, assessments of relative tissue blood volume, estimation of tissue perfusion, and detection of abnormal capillary permeability [6]. Several approaches seem feasible for the design of blood pool markers; the critical factor is molecular size. Both macromolecular paramagnetic formulations and superparamagnetic particles of sufficient molecular weight, generally $>50\,000$ daltons, after intravenous injection will escape only very slowly from the vascular compartment. Tissue enhancement levels will be near constant for minutes to hours. The apparent volume of distribution of macromolecular contrast agents (MMCMs), for example, albumin-(Gd-DTPA)$_{30}$ is approximately 0.05 L kg of tissue, like the blood volume. As blood pool markers, MMCMs have the potential to be applied for estimates of blood flow or perfusion, using the classical principles of dye dilution. Unfortunately, Gd-DTPA and other ECF contrast media have inherent disadvantages for estimates of blood volume and perfusion (except in the brain with an intact capillary barrier). Plasma concentration of Gd-DTPA declines by 70% within 5 min of administration [7]. On the first pass through the capillary bed, 50% or more of circulating Gd-DTPA diffuses from the blood into the extravascular compartment. Simultaneously, glomerular filtration contributes to a rapidly declining plasma concentration. MMCMs are designed to be too large for diffusion through normal capillaries and glomerular endothelium and, thus, to be more reliable blood pool markers.

In addition to blood volume and perfusion estimates, the prolonged intravascular retention of MMCMs permits imaging of multiple body regions without repeated dosing. Similarly, the requirement for critical timing of image acquisitions is canceled: Enhancement of normal tissues using MMCMs is virtually identical at 5 min and 50 min postadministration.

MMCMs have not yet been clinically tested, but several polymeric formulations have been studied in animals including albumin-$(Gd-DTPA)_{30}$, dextran-$(Gd-DTPA)_{15}$, polylysine-$(Gd-DTPA)_{60}$ [6], and gadolinium-labeled Starburst™ dendrimers [8]. Each of these polymers demonstrates extremely high T_1 relaxivity, from 40 to 1070 times higher than Gd-DTPA on a per mole basis [6, 8]. This high-dose efficiency is due to the multiplicity of gadolinium ions (as many as 170) attached to each polymeric molecule and to the slowing of molecular rotation of each paramagnetic subunit. The slower rotational correlation time of gadolinium complexes bound to macromolecules, compared to Gd-DTPA alone, more closely approximates the tumbling rate of water.

MRI blood pool contrast agents have been shown useful to define tissue ischemia and/or the adequacy of reperfusion procedures in multiple organs, notably the heart, lungs, kidneys, and brain [6, 9–12]. As might be anticipated when using an intravascular marker, acute vascular occlusion results in an absent or blunted enhancement of tissues distal to the occlusion, dependent on the presence and adequacy of collateral circulation. The contrast differences between ischemic and normally perfused regions remain constant for an extended period, eliminating problems created by the gradual wash-in of smaller ECF contrast agents into ischemic zones.

Just as low-molecular-weight contrast agents, like Gd-DTPA dimeglumine, are used to define abnormal capillary permeability in the CNS, macromolecular enhancers have proven useful to define abnormalities of capillary integrity in extra-CNS tissues. The capillary endothelium of normal tissues are relatively impervious to MMCMs. But following various tissue injuries, capillary integrity is destroyed and large molecules may diffuse into the interstitial space. This abnormal capillary permeability is a relatively early response to disease but is not highly specific, being observed in neoplasia [13], irreversible myocardial ischemia [10], inflammation, pulmonary edema [11], and response to chemotherapy [14]. On MR images enhanced with a MMCM this abnormal capillary leakiness is marked by a time-dependent increase in local signal intensity; circulating blood levels of contrast agent stay constant while the interstitium gradually accumulates more of the leaked macromolecules. From analysis of time–intensity curves it may be feasible to quantify and grade abnormalities in capillary integrity [15].

High-dose efficiency, prolonged tissue enhancement which eliminates the criticality of image timing, the ability to gauge tissue blood volume and perfusion, and the ability to evaluate changes in capillary integrity provide strong motivations to develop a clinically acceptable macromolecular contrast agent. Remaining challenges are to identify one or more well-tolerated formulations lacking immunologic reactivity. Ideally, a MMCM can be designed to provide near-constant intravascular concentrations for up to 1 h postadministration and yet be efficiently metabolized to permit complete elimination of the metal complex over a period of days.

THE HEART

The primary goal of cardiac MRI contrast enhancement has been to better define the status of myocardial perfusion. Nonenhanced MRI cannot discriminate ischemic myocardium, but noninfarcted myocardium, from healthy myocardium. The limitations imposed on the use of ECF contrast media for perfusion imaging, namely, rapidly changing plasma concentrations and rapid transcapillary diffusion, were detailed in the previous section. However, contrast differences between acutely infarcted and normal myocardium can be significantly improved using Gd-complexes, as shown by animal and clinical investigations. On delayed images, the infarcted myocardium has greater signal intensity (gradual washin of contrast agent) than normal myocardium (gradual washout).

With the availability of very rapid serial image acquisitions it may now be feasible to assess relative myocardial blood flow using even low-molecular-weight ECF contrast media. Acquisition times with echo-planar imaging are in the range of 30–50 ms and can be gated to a specific phase of the cardiac cycle. Monitoring of the first-pass kinetics, assuming that the contrast media molecules remain primarily in the intravascular compartment, provides a means to estimate regional myocardial perfusion. Using a standard echo-planar technique, the T_2^* effect is accentuated, especially at higher field strengths, favoring the use of a magnetic susceptibility contrast agent such as dysprosium-DTPA-BMA (Salutar, Sunnyvale, CA, USA) [16]. In animals with coronary artery occlusion, on immediate postcontrast images this contrast agent effectively erases the signal from normally perfused myocardium, leaving the region of ischemia as an easily defined zone of higher signal.

Kinetics of macromolecular blood pool contrast agents may also be monitored by rapid acquisition techniques to assess regional myocardial perfusion and offer advantages of high-dose efficiency and minimal transcapillary diffusion. The adequacy and timeliness of interventional techniques to restore perfusion to ischemic myocardial segments can also be assessed using MMCM. In experimental myocardial ischemia of less than 30 min followed by release of the coronary artery occlusion, MMCM (albumin-Gd-DTPA) enhancement of the myocardium immediately returns to normal levels. However, with coronary occlusion of 60 min or more followed by reperfusion, the enhancement of the involved region gradually increases over time, indicating abnormal capillary permeability, correlating closely with permanent damage shown by histopathology and MR spectroscopy [10]. A single administration of this blood pool agent is adequate to demonstrate the initial ischemic stage, the return of myocardial perfusion after release of the coronary artery occlusion, and the reperfusion-induced injury of capillary integrity.

Another agent tested for enhancement of the myocardium is manganese dipyridoxal diphosphonate (Mn-DPDP, Salutar, Sunnyvale, CA, USA) [17]. In a dose of 400 μmol kg^{-1} the signal of normal myocardium increased 125% for over 1 h compared to only a 16% increase in the ischemic zone of a rat coronary occlusion model.

LIVER AGENTS

The role of abdominal MRI can be expected to expand with the availability of effective contrast enhancement agents, especially when used in conjunction with faster acquisition times and artifact reduction techniques. Of critical importance is the recognition of focal hepatic lesions, particularly metastatic deposits. Even small ones must be detected accurately. Primary liver lesions also must be identified and accurately characterized, including neoplasms, cysts, focal nodular hyperplasia, and hemangiomas.

The competition is keen to develop clinically acceptable contrast agents for the liver. Although both negative and positive enhancers have been proposed, a function-based classification is more practical for consideration of the divergent approaches to liver enhancement. Certain agents are targeted to the hepatocytes, whereas others are designed for phagocytosis by the reticuloendothelial system (RES). These differences in cellular distribution within the liver may contribute to potential differences in tolerance and efficacy.

Hepatocyte-directed liver agents

Available gadolinium complexes distribute throughout the extracellular fluid compartments producing enhancement of the liver and, depending on vascularity, of liver tumors. There is no hepatocyte-specific uptake or biliary excretion of these ECF agents. When used with dynamic imaging sequences and bolus injection, liver-tumor contrast is increased in many cases during the initial 2–3 min [18]. Subsequently, liver-tumor contrast may be diminished by the slow diffusion of the contrast agent into the tumor.

Certain paramagnetic complexes, including both Fe(III) and Gd(III), have been shown to be taken up by hepatocytes and subsequently excreted in the bile. The mechanism for this hepatocyte uptake has been shown to be via a relatively nonspecific receptor known as the hepatocyte anion transporter. The physiological role of this receptor is thought to rid the body of noxious anionic substances, including bilirubin. Early tested Fe(III) complexes, including Fe-EHPD and Fe-HBED, were found to have preferential hepatobiliary excretion in rodents but significantly less potential for liver enhancement in patients based on human radiotracer kinetic data.

More recently introduced complexes with relatively high hepatobiliary excretions include Gd-(benzyloxy-proprionictetraacetate) (BOPTA) (Bracco, Milan, Italy) and Gd-ethoxybenzyl-DTPA (Gd-EOB-DTPA) (Schering A.G., Berlin, Germany) [19]. Both formulations are also partially excreted by the kidney, providing the potential to simultaneously evaluate renal and hepatocellular functions. Gd-EOB-DTPA demonstrates 10% protein binding, an LD$_{50}$ in mice of 10 mmol kg^{-1}, 66–75% hepatobiliary excretion in rodents, and more than 200% liver enhancement at a dose of 0.1 mmol kg^{-1} [19]. In addition to the obvious potential to improve sensitivity for parenchymal liver mases, the potential to evaluate biliary anatomy using these hepatobiliary agents offers a significant advantage over particulate liver contrast agents, which are not subject to biliary excretion.

Superparamagnetic iron oxide particles can be directed to specific receptor systems of the liver, and other tissues, by attachment of substrates specific for the receptor. For example, ultrasmall iron oxide particles coated with aisaloglycoprotein (ASG) can be directed to normal hepatocytes which have ASG receptors on their surface [21, 22]. The induced loss of signal intensity in liver parenchyma produces sharp contrast with metastases and hepatocellular cancers, tissues which do not contain ASG receptors. Reimer et al. noted that the relative effectiveness for reduction of liver signal intensity was superior using the ASG-coated small iron oxide particles, mean size 12 nm, than from the larger AMI-25 particles, 72 nm [22].

RES-DIRECTED LIVER AGENTS

Particulate substances and liposomes administered intravenously are cleared from the blood by cells of the reticuloendothelial system (RES), concentrated in the liver, spleen, and bone marrow. Kupffer cells represent only 2% of the liver volume, whereas hepatocytes compose 78% of the volume. Normal RES physiology has been used to target numerous contrast enhancing materials, including paramagnetic liposomes [23] and dextran-coated superparamagnetic iron oxide particles [24].

Superparamagnetic iron oxide (SPIO) particles, like paramagnetic chelates, consist of two components: the magnetic ingredient (iron oxide core) and a "coating" to make particles water soluble and biocompatible. The central iron oxide core is responsible for the magnetic properties, whereas the coating of particles determines biodistribution. Central iron oxide cores may be monocrystalline, termed MION for monocrystalline iron oxide nanoparticles, or polycrystalline, have different sizes, be composed of different types of iron oxides, and have widely varying T_2 relaxivities typically ranging from 5 to 200 (mM s)$^{-1}$. Because of their unique surface-bound hydrophilic coatings, pharmaceutical iron oxide formulations are not strictly ferrites or magnetites. Both ferrite ($Fe_2M_xO_4$, where M is a metal cation) and magnetite (Fe_3O_4) are water-insoluble crystals that are poorly suited for clinical use.

Various surface coatings of pharmaceutical iron oxides have been examined, including polysaccharides such as dextran, starch, and arabinogalactan. Once administered intravenously, these surface-bound molecules are capable of interaction with plasma and cell-bound proteins and are, along with the overall size, major determinants of biodistribution. For example, polygalacosylated agents are taken up by hepatocyte galactose-recognizing receptors, whereas polyglucosylated agents (dextran) are primarily taken up by phagocytic cells of the RES; surface-modified SPIO may be directed to specific receptor systems or antigenic sites.

Advantages of iron-oxide-based contrast media are their specificity for cells of the RES, their potent magnetic properties making them detectable at very low tissue concentrations, and their potential for *in vivo* degradation to innocuous metabolites. The iron ultimately is added to the normal body stores. Potential disadvantages of these agents are their colloidal properties, particularly for larger particles, the past observation of some adverse effects in clinical trials, and the technically challenging synthesis.

Coated iron oxide particles, formulated as AMI-25 (Advanced Magnetics, Cambridge, MA, USA) with a median particle diameter of 50 ± 29 nm, have been tested extensively in animal models and in clinical trials for liver–spleen enhancement. These superparamagnetic ferrites, producing a negative enhancement on T_2-weighted images, are rapidly cleared from the circulation by the RES with a half-life of 8 min. Extremely effective T_2-relaxation agents, clinically tested doses of superparamagnetic particles, have ranged from 10 to 50 µmol Fe kg^{-1}. Useful enhancement of the liver is achieved in less than 1 h and persists for more than 1 day; liver signal intensity returns to precontrast levels by 7 days. The size threshold for MRI detection of hepatic metastases is significantly reduced from approximately 10 mm without enhancement to 3 mm after contrast administration [24].

LYMPH NODE ENHANCEMENT

Targeting MRI contrast media to lymph nodes would be a boon to cancer staging. Currently, the MR identification of an abnormal node relies exclusively on demonstration of nodal enlargement. Unfortunately, unenhanced signal intensities of normal and metastatic nodes overlap considerably so that intensities alone cannot be used for differentiation. Ideally, a nodal metastasis would be identifiable using lymph-node-specific contrast enhancement by absent or focally abnormal enhancement, even in a normal-sized node.

Three strategies for delivery of contrast agents to lymph nodes seem possible; subcutaneous injection of particulates, picked up by the lymph vessels and deposited in the lymph nodes; endolymphatic administration; and intravenous injection of lymphotropic agents that circulate in the blood before extraction by lymph node macrophages. Although in an experimental setting, interstitial and intra-lymphatic administration routes are the most direct and certain approachs for agent delivery to lymph nodes, these routes are clinically less practical compared to intravenous administration.

Recently, feasibility has been shown for an IV administration route of certain ultrasmall superparamagnetic iron oxide (USPIO) formulations which significantly accumulate in lymph nodes [25, 26]. USPIO and, even smaller monocrystalline iron oxide nanopolymers (MIONs), can transmigrate through capillary walls by vesicular transport and through interendothelial junctions to gain access to the interstitial space. From the interstitium, these particles accumulate in the macrophages of the lymph nodes. Twenty-four hours after intravenous administration,

3.6% of the injected USPIO dose was found in lymph nodes.

Macromolecular T_1 labels are also under development for lymph node imaging. These agents are synthesized by grafting dextran onto a polymeric Gd-DTPA-containing backbones such as poly-L-lysine. Initial data suggest that the dextran coating of these particulates is important in the high lymphatic accumulation. After IV administration of a prototypic agent, blood half-life was 2–3 h in rats. High concentrations (10–40% of injected dose per gram of tissue depending on nodal group) of agent were found in lymph nodes 12–24 h after IV administration.

Extensive prelinical trials are necessary to compare lymphotropic T_2 and T_1 agents. Efficacy will be determined by the amount of agent that accumulates in nodes, the reliability of nodal deposition of different agents, and their ability to improve cancer detection in nodes.

TUMOR-SPECIFIC AND ANTIGEN-SPECIFIC ENHANCEMENT

One strategy to specifically direct magnetophamaceuticals to tumors, and other tissues, is to link them to antigen-specific monoclonal antibodies. The feasibility of this approach to tumor imaging was recently demonstrated in a well-controlled animal investigation by Göhr-Rosenthal et al. [26] in which an implanted colorectal carcinoma was significantly enhanced at 24 and 48 h after administration of 2–3 mg Gd-labeled tumor-specific monoclonal antibody (0.9 μmol Gd per animal).

Superparamagnetic particulates, with high-dose effectiveness, may represent an advantageous alternative to paramagnetic metal complexes for the labeling of monoclonal antibodies. Weissleder and his colleagues have attached MIONs to antimyosin Fab fragments to direct the contrast agent to acutely infarcted myocardium, producing negative enhancement.

The clinical feasibility of the magnetically active monoclonal antibody approach to MRI enhancement is limited by the requirement for advanced knowledge of the immunologic characteristics of the tumor or tissue in question, the high cost of monoclonal antibodies, and the need for widely separated precontrast and postcontrast imaging to assess enhancement. Radioactive labeling of monoclonal antibodies with scintigraphic imaging may offer some advantages over the MRI approach.

GASTROINTESTINAL AGENTS

The requirements for a suitable oral MR contrast agent are reliable bowel marking, high tolerance, and low expense. Confident delineation of the bowel lumen, the pancreas, and paraaortic nodes are requisite to extend abdominal MRI beyond the evaluation of the liver. A variety of formulations are in clinical trials or have been submitted to the authorities for approval. In general, oral agents may be categorized (see Table 1) into positive and negative enhancing groups and into water miscible and immiscible groups.

ACKNOWLEDGMENT

This work was supported in part by grant CA 49786 from the National Institutes of Health. The helpful suggestions of Ralph Weissleder are appreciated.

REFERENCES

1. Brasch RC (1983) Work in Progress: Methods of contrast enhancement for NMR imaging and potential applications. *Radiology* **147**: 781–788.
2. Koenig S (1991) From the relaxivity of Gd(DTPA) to everything else. In *Workshop on Contrast Enhanced MR, Napa, CA*, Brasch R (ed) pp. 12–22. Berkeley, CA: Society for Magnetic Resonance in Medicine.
3. Weinmann H-J, Brasch RC, Press WR, Wesbey G (1984) Characteristics of gadolinium-DTPA complex: A potential MRI contrast agent. *Amer J Radiol* **142**: 619–624.
4. Brasch RC, Weinmann H-J, Wesbey GE (1984) Contrast-enhanced NMR imaging: animal studies using gadolinium-DTPA complex. *Amer J Radiol* **142**: 625–630.
5. Moseley M, Vexler Z, Asgari H, Mintorovitch J, Derugin N, Rocklage S, Kucharczyk J (1991) Comparison of Gd- and Dy-chelates for T2* contrast-enhanced imaging. In *Workshop on Contrast-Enhanced Magnetic Resonance, Napa, CA*, Brasch R (ed), pp. 131–141. Berkeley, CA: Society for Magnetic Resonance in Medicine.
6. Brasch R (1991) Rationale and applications for macromolecular Gd-based contrast agents. *Magn Reson Med* **22**: 282–287.
7. Schmiedl U, Moseley ME, Ogan MD, Chew WM, Brasch RC (1987) Comparison of initial biodistribution patterns of Gd-DTPA and albumin-(Gd-DTPA) using rapid spin echo MR imaging. *J Comput Assist Tomogr* **11**: 306–313.
8. Weiner E, Brechbiel M, Brothers H et al. (1994) Dendrimer-based metal chelates: a new class of magnetic resonance imaging contrast agents. *Mag Reson Med* **31**: 1–8.
9. Wang SC, Wikstrom MG, White DL, Klaveness J, Holtz E, Rongved P, Moseley ME, Brasch RC (1990) Evaluation of Gd-DTPA-labeled dextran as an intravascular MR contrast agent: imaging characteristics in normal rat tissues. *Radiology* **175**: 483–488.

10. Wolfe CL, Moseley ME, Wikstrom MG, Sievers RE, Wendland MF, Dupon JW, Finkbeiner WE, Lipton MJ, Parmley WW, Brasch RC (1989) Assessment of myocardial salvage after ischemia and reperfusion using magnetic resonance imaging and spectroscopy. *Circulation* **80**: 969–982.

11. Berthezene Y, Vexler V, Jerome H, Seivers R, Moseley M, Brasch R (1991) Differentiation of capillary leak and hydrostatic pulmonary edema using a macromolecular MRI contrast agent. *Radiology* **181**: 773–777.

12. Vexler V, Berthezene Y, Clément O, Muehler A, Moseley M, Brasch R (1992) Contrast-enhanced MRI of rat kidney: comparison of Gd-DTPA and two macromolecular contrast agents in detection of zonal renal ischemia. *J Magn Reson Imaging* **2**: 311–319.

13. Wikstrom MG, Moseley ME, White DL, Dupon JW, Winkelhake J, Kopplin J, Brasch RC (1989) Contrast enhanced MRI of tumors: Comparison of Gd-DTPA and a macromolecular agent. *Invest Radiol* **24**(8): 609–615.

14. Aicher KP, Dupon JW, White DL, Aukerman SL, Moseley ME, Juster R, Rosenau W, Winkelhake JL, Brasch RC (1990) Contrast-enhanced magnetic resonance imaging of tumor-bearing mice treated with human recombinant tumor necrosis factor alpha. *Cancer Res* **50**: 7376–7381.

15. Shames D, Kuwatsuru R, Vexler V, Muehler A, Brasch R (1993) Measurement of capillary permeability to macromolecules by dynamic magnetic resonance imaging: A quantitative non-invasive technique. *Magn Reson Med* **29**: 616–622.

16. Higgins C, Saeed M, Wendland M (1991) Contrast enhancement of the myocardium. In *Workshop on Contrast Enhanced Magnetic Resonance, Napa, CA,* Brasch R (ed). pp. 272–289. Berkeley, CA: Society for Magnetic Resonance in Medicine.

17. Pomeroy O, Wendland M, Wagner S, Derugin N, Holt W, Rocklage S, Quay S, Higgins C (1989) Magnetic resonance imaging of acute myocardial ischemia using a manganese chelate, Mn-DPDP. *Invest Radiol* **24**: 531–536.

18. Hamm B, Wolf K, Felix R (1987) Conventional and rapid MR imaging of the liver with gadolinium-DTPA. *Radiology* **164**: 357–362.

19. Schuhmann-Giampieri G, Schmitt-Willich H, Press WR, Nigishi C, Weinmann H-J (1992) Preclinical evaluation of Gd-EOB-DTPA as a contrast agent in MR imaging of the hepatobilliary system. *Radiology* **183**: 59–64.

20. Clément O, Mühler A, Vexler V, Berthezène Y, Brasch R (1993) Gd-EOB-DTPA, a new liver-specific MR contrast agent: relaxivity, kinetics, and enhancement patterns in normal rats. *J Magn Reson Imaging* **3**: 71–77.

21. Weissleder R, Reimer P, Lee AS, Wittenberg J, Brady TJ (1990) MR receptor imaging: ultrasmall iron oxide particles targeted to asialoglycoprotein receptors. *Am J Radiol* **155**: 1161–1167.

22. Reimer P, Weissleder R, Lee AS, Wittenberg J, Brady TJ (1990) Receptor imaging: application to MR imaging of liver cancer. *Radiology* **177**: 729–734.

23. Unger EC, MacDougall P, Cullis P, Tilcock C (1989) Liposomal Gd-DTPA: effect of encapsulation on enhancement of hepatoma model by MRI. *Magn Reson Imaging* **7**: 417–723.

24. Stark DD, Weissleder R, Elizondo G, Hahn PF, Saini S, Todd LE, Wittenberg J, Ferrucci JT (1988) Superparamagnetic iron oxide: clinical application as a contrast agent for MR imaging of the liver. *Radiology* **168**: 297–301.

25. Weissleder R, Elizondo G, Josephson L, et al (1989) Experimental lymph node metastases: enhanced detection with MR lymphography. *Radiology* **171**: 835–839.

26. Weissleder R, Elizondo G, Wittenberg J, Lee AS, Josephson L, Brady TJ (1990) Ultrasmall superparamagnetic iron oxide: an intravenous contrast agent for assessing lymph nodes with MR imaging. *Radiology* **175**: 494–498.

27. Göhr-Rosenthal S, Schmitt-Willich H, Ebert W, Gries H, Vogler H, Weinmann H-J (1991) An immunoselective contrast medium for MRI: detection of colorectal tumor transplants in mice with a Gd-labeled monoclonal antibody. *SMRM 10th Annual Scientific Meeting, San Francisco, CA.* SMRM **1**: 356.

MR and the pathogenesis of musculoskeletal disease

John V. Crues III

Cedars-Sinai Medical Center, Los Angeles, CA 90048, USA

NMR imaging has become an important diagnostic tool in the evaluation of musculoskeletal disease. However, its ability to evaluate pathogenic mechanisms of disease may eventually have even a greater impact on patient care. NMR imaging has significantly affected our understanding of the clinical significance of meniscal tears and appropriate patient management. It has also extended our understanding of the prevalence and importance of X-ray and arthroscopically occult bone, tendon, and ligament injuries. By knowing the pathogenic mechanisms of disease, we can more reliably diagnose and treat pathology. In particular, many horizontal degenerative tears in older patients may be asymptomatic and are best left in place. Many acute tears may be best treated with immediate meniscal repair. Magnetic resonance (MR) imaging can reliably differentiate these tear types with noninvasive imaging. The ability of MR to detect bone injuries may lead to aggressive early non-weight-bearing therapy on injured bone, thereby preserving the subchondral bone from collapse and the joint from secondary osteoarthrosis. The ability of MRIs to detect and stage degenerative tendonosis of tendons and ligaments, such as the rotator cuff, may lead to arthroscopic decompression or debridement which provides symptomatic relief and may preserve and protect the intact cuff.

Keywords: MRI, meniscal tears, tendonosis, tendonitis, spontaneous osteonecrosis, rotator cuff tears.

INTRODUCTION

Since its clinical introduction in the early 1980s, Magnetic resonance imaging (MRI) has made enormous inroads as a diagnostic tool in the investigation of musculoskeletal and joint diseases [1, 2]. There is, however, a much less heralded but potentially much more important aspect of MRI as an application in musculoskeletal diseases. MR has become a uniquely important tool in the evaluation of the pathogenic mechanisms of joint and soft tissue injuries.

MR has been particularly important in our understanding of three important disease processes: symptomatology associated with meniscal tears of the knee, the incidence and significance of X-ray and arthroscopically occult bone injuries, and the pathogenesis of ligament and tendon degenerative disease.

MENISCAL TEARS

We have learned much about meniscal disease since the first surgical meniscectomy was described in the

Address for correspondence: Cedars-Sinai Imaging, 8700 Beverly Blvd., Los Angeles, CA 90048, U.S.A.

mid-1800s [3, 4]. Until the mid-20th century, knee menisci were believed to be superfluous. During the last 30 years growing evidence is teaching us that the menisci are essential structures for long-term functionality of the knee in active individuals [5–7]. Recent data suggest that the long-term prognosis in patients with meniscal tears is strongly dependent on preservation of as much of the peripheral two-thirds of the meniscus as possible, even if the preserved meniscal tissue is degenerated [7]. The peripheral two-thirds of the meniscus is important in protecting the joint from repetitive microtrauma and degenerative joint disease. This has led to the popularity of meniscal-sparing surgical techniques, such as primary meniscal repair in lieu of partial meniscectomy. Primary meniscal repair is now believed to be very important for the young patient with vertical longitudinal tears for which a significant portion would have to be removed if a partial meniscectomy were to be performed. MR imaging is an accurate technique to evaluate the type and extend of tear for optimal planning of surgical intervention [5, 6]. Acute tears, especially vertical tears in the peripheral third of the meniscus or bucket-handle tears, are usually best treated immediately with primary meniscal repair. Thus, the ability of MR to differentiate between acute and chronic tears can help the orthopedist and patient plan appropriate intervention.

It has also only recently become recognized that many, if not most, meniscal tears are minimally symptomatic or asymptomatic and may not warrant surgical intervention [6, 8]. At least four lines of reasoning have led us to this conclusion. First, it was over 100 years from the first description of a meniscectomy as a surgical procedure and the first description of the most common tear, the horizontal cleavage degenerative tear, by Smillie in the 1960s [9, 10]. This delay may be due, in part, to many horizontal degenerative tears not having been sufficiently symptomatic to have warranted surgery in the prearthroscopic era. Second, studies have revealed that a high prevalence of asymptomatic meniscal tears (60%) may be seen in the autopsied population [11]. Third, clinical findings have shown two groups of patients after arthroscopic partial meniscectomy. One group has immediate relief of symptoms after surgery, and the other a delay in symptom relief of several weeks. The latter group may be symptomatic from other etiologies, such as X-ray occult bone injuries to be discussed below. Finally, MR studies in asymptomatic individuals have revealed a 20% prevalence of asymptomatic meniscal tears in patients over 50 years of age [8]. Because of these findings, the interpreter of MR images of the knee must be cautious in concluding that degenerative-type horizontal cleavage tears are the etiology of patients' complaints. With a greater than 20% prevalence of asymptomatic meniscal tears in the older patient group, other joint pathology may masquerade as symptomatic meniscal tears. In particular, X-ray and arthroscopically occult bone injuries may be a frequent cause of posttraumatic knee pain [12–17].

X-RAY AND ARTHROSCOPICALLY OCCULT BONE INJURIES

With the introduction of MRI as a clinical tool in the evaluation of meniscal tears in the mid-1980s, investigators were surprised to detect a high incidence of abnormally low signal within the medullary space of the bones around the knee on short TE spin-echo images. These lesions were hyperintense on long TR/long TE, STIR, and fat-saturated images [14, 18]. These findings are now believed to be primarily due to trabecular fractures with intramedullary hemorrhage and bone marrow edema [14–17].

We have found X-ray occult bone injuries to be frequently associated with posttraumatic pain on weight-bearing [14]. Older individuals with degenera-

tive horizontal cleavage tears and bone injuries of the underlying weight-bearing subchondral bone may be followed with conservative non-weight-bearing therapy for 3 weeks [7]. Many patients when reassessed at this time become asymptomatic [19]. Many patients' symptoms will be relieved with bone healing without surgical intervention for the meniscal tear.

The concept of spontaneous osteonecrosis of the knee has undergone considerable revision under the scrutiny of MRI [5]. Originally described by Ahlback et al., it was thought most likely to be secondary to a primary interruption of vascular supply [20]. A traumatic etiology was initially thought less likely, in part because of the usual lack of a clear history of trauma but more importantly because of the common association of initially negative-plane radiographs with this entity. We now know that radiographs are exceedingly insensitive to trabecular bone trauma and the MR appearance on classic cases of "spontaneous osteonecrosis" appear indistinguishable from trabecular fractures without the presence of a "double line sign" of osteonecrosis. MR findings support Norman's contention that this condition was of traumatic etiology [21]. The association with osteoporosis and typical healing pattern as well as characteristic histologic features of fracture strongly support stress fracture as the most likely etiology of "spontaneous osteonecrosis" [5].

TENDON DEGENERATION

Before the era of MRI we did not fully recognize the importance of X-ray occult trabecular injuries because we lacked a definitive way to establish the diagnosis. Biopsy was too invasive and subject to misinterpretation. Similarly, before MRI we were unable to visualize internal pathology within tendons and ligaments. Many people think of a rotator cuff tear as simply an acute tear of a big tendon. This concept has been fostered in part because of the custom of defining the pathology with arthrography. Arthrography can only detect disruption of the tendon surface. It cannot detect isolated internal changes and biochemical alterations.

With the advent of MRI a spectrum of signal changes were detected in tendons [22–26]. Not all of them correlated with arthroscopically and arthrographically detectable disease. Consequently, confusion ensued over the utility of MRI in the evaluation of ligament and tendon injuries [27]. Hyperintensity on short TE MR imaging (whether with spin-echo or gradient-echo techniques) is exquisitely sensitive to early collagen degeneration, which occurs with the incomplete healing of recurrent microscopic collagen tears [23]. High signal on long TR/long TE T_2-weighted spin-echo images are more specific for clinically significant degeneration, partial and complete tears [23, 24]. Commonly recognized tendon and ligament "tendonitis" is rarely an acute inflammatory condition, but it is a chronic degenerative condition that slowly worsens over years of abuse. As the degenerative disease or "tendonosis" progresses, the tendons and ligaments lose mechanic integrity; thus becoming increasingly susceptible to traumatic rupture. As the cross-collagen fibers between type 1 fibers breakdown with severe degeneration, longitudinal type 1 fibers may slip with respect to one another when the tendon is stretched, leading to pain in the absence of an arthrographically detectable complete tear. Hyperintensity within tendons on T_2-weighted long TE images is an excellent indicator of clinically significant tendon injury. Arthroscopic debridement may induce a fibroblastic response which may stabilize the collagen fibers and lead to symptomatic improvement [28].

MR imaging may also be helpful in detecting abnormalities which increase the risk of tendonosis [23]. Abrupt bony margins may impinge upon tendons [29]. Normal joint motion may cause the tendon to chronically rub against a bony prominence, leading to recurrent trauma and progression of tendon degeneration [30, 31]. This mechanism is believed to be a common cause of pain and tearing of the supraspinatus tendon of the shoulder. MR can assess the anatomic risk for subacromial impingement with detail not available with other techniques [23, 29, 32, 33].

SUMMARY

Although MRI has become an important diagnostic tool in the evaluation of joint diseases, its ability to investigate pathogenic mechanism of disease is beginning to uncover a rich field for scientific investigation. Partly with the help of NMR imaging, we now suspect that many meniscal tears, especially in older patients, are best left alone, and MRI is helpful in evaluating the bones for occult injuries. Aggressive non-weight-bearing treatment may preserve the subchondral bone from collapse during trabecular healing and improve significantly the outcome in patients with trauma and "spontaneous osteonecrosis." Finally, by understanding that tendon and ligament disease is a chronic degenerative progression, we may be able to intervene earlier to minimize the trauma of impingement and induce fibroblastic repair before a complete tendon rupture occurs.

REFERENCES

1. Mink JH, Reicher MA, Crues JVI, Deutsch AL (1993) *MRI of the Knee*, 2nd ed. p. 474. New York: Raven Press.
2. Stoller DW (1993) *Magnetic Resonance Imaging in Orthopaedics & Sports Medicine*. p. 1127. Philadelphia: Lippincott.
3. Kroiss F (1910) Die Verletzungen der Kniegelenkoszwischenknorpel und ihrer Verbindungen. *Beitr Klin Chir* **66**: 598–801.
4. Oberholzer J (1938) Archiv und Atlas der normalen und pathologischen Anatomie in typischen Rontgenbildern. In *Rontgendiagnostik der Gelenke mittels Doppelkontrastmethode*. Leipzig: Thieme.
5. Crues JV, Ryu R (1992) Knee. In *Magnetic Resonance Imaging* (Stark DD, Bradley WG, Jr., ed) pp. 2355–2423. St. Louis: Mosby Year Book.
6. Crues JV, Stoller DW (1993) The menisci. In *Magnetic Resonance Imaging of the Knee* (Mink J, et al., ed) pp. 91–140. New York: Raven Press.
7. Newman AP, Daniels AU, Burks RT (1993) Principles and decision making in meniscal surgery. *Arthroscopy* **9**(1): 33–51.
8. Kornick J, Trefelner E, McCarthy S, Lange R, Lynch K, Jokl P (1990) Meniscal abnormalities in the asymptomatic population at MR imaging. *Radiology* **177**: 463–465.
9. Ferrer-Roca O, Vilalta C (1980) Lesions of the meniscus. Part I: Macroscopic and histologic findings. *Clin Orthop* **146**: 301–307.
10. Smillie IS (1970) Clinical features of internal derangements relative to the menisci. In *Injuries of the Knee Joint*, 4th ed. pp. 70–97. London: E. & S. Livingstone.
11. Noble J, Hamblen DL (1975) The pathology of the degenerate meniscus lesion. *J Bone Joint Surg* **57**: 180–186.
12. Ruwe PA, Wright J, Randall RL, Lynch JK, Jokl P, McCarthy S (1992) Can MR imaging effectively replace diagnostic arthroscopy? *Radiology* **183**(2): 335–339.
13. Ruwe PA, McCarthy S (1993) Cost-effectiveness of magnetic resonance imaging. In *MRI of the Knee* (Mink JH et al., ed) pp. 463–466. New York: Raven Press.
14. Lynch TCP, Crues JV, Morgan FW, Sheehan WE, Harter LP, Ryu R (1989) Bone abnormalities of the knee. *Radiology* **171**: 761–766.
15. Lee JK, Yao L (1989) Occult intraosseous fracture: Magnetic resonance appearance versus age of injury. *Am J Sports Med* **17**(5): 620–623.
16. Deutsch AL, Mink JH, Shellock FG (1989) Magnetic resonance imaging of injuries to bone and articular cartilage. *Orthop Rev* **19**(1): 66–75.
17. Blum GM, Tirman PFJ, Crues JV, III (1993) Osseous and cartilaginous trauma. In *MRI of the Knee* (Mink JH et al., ed) pp. 295–332. New York: Raven Press.
18. Stafford SA, Rosenthal DI, Gebhardt MC, Brady TJ, Scott JA (1986) MRI in stress fracture. *Am J Radiol* **147**: 553–556.

19. Hede A, Hempel-Poulsen S, Jensen JS (1990) Symptoms and level of sports activity in patients awaiting arthroscopy for meniscal lesions of the knee. *J Bone Joint Surg* **72A:** 550–552.

20. Ahlback S, Bauer GCH, Bohne WH (1968) Spontaneous osteonecrosis of the knee. *Arthritis Rheum* **11**(6): 726.

21. Norman A, Baker N (1978) Spontaneous osteonecrosis of the knee and medial meniscal tears. *Radiology* **129:** 653–656.

22. Burk DL, Karasick D, Kurtz AB et al. (1989) Rotator cuff tears: Prospective comparison of MR imaging with arthrography, sonography, and surgery. *Am J Radiol* **153:** 87–92.

23. Crues JV, Ryu R (1992) The shoulder. In *Magnetic Resonance Imaging* (Stark D, Bradley WG, eds) pp. 2424–2458. St. Louis: Mosby.

24. Fritts HM (1992) MRI and shoulder imaging. *Lippincott's Rev Radiology* **1**(3): 373

25. Mink JH (1993) The cruciate and collateral ligaments. In *Magnetic Resonance Imaging of the Knee* (Mink JH et al., eds) pp. 141–188. New York: Raven Press.

26. Zlatkin MB, Iannotti JP, Roberts MC et al. (1989) Rotator cuff tears: Diagnostic performance of MR imaging. *Radiology* **172:** 223–229.

27. Stiles RG, Otte MT (1993) Imaging of the shoulder. *Radiology* **188**(3): 603–613.

28. Snyder SJ, Pachelli AF, Del Pizzo W, Friedman MJ, Ferkel RD, Pattee G (1991) Partial thickness rotator cuff tears: Results of arthroscopic treatment. *Arthroscopy* **7**(1): 1–7.

29. Crues JV, Fareed DO (1991) Magnetic resonance imaging of shoulder impingement. *Topics Magn Res Imaging* **3**(4): 39–49.

30. Bigliani LU, Morrison DS (1986) The morphology of the acromion and its relationship to rotator cuff tears. *Proc Am Shoulder Albow Surg.*

31. Neer CS (1983) Impingement lesions. *Clin Orthop* **173:** 70–77.

32. Cone R, Resnick D, Danzig L (1984) Shoulder impingement syndrome: Radiographic evaluation. *Radiology* **150**(1): 29–33.

33. Kilcoyne RF (1993) Imaging choices in the shoulder impingement syndrome. *Appl Radiol* **22**(5): 59–62.

MRI for arthritis research: current pitfalls and future prospects

Martin E. Fry,[1] William Vennart,[1]* Richard K. Jacoby,[2] Charles W. Hutton,[3] Julia Gasson,[1]
Ian R. Summers,[1] Richard E. Ellis,[1] Elizabeth A. Moore[1] and Michael C. Keen[1]

[1]*University of Exeter, Exeter EX4 4QL, UK*
[2]*Princess Elizabeth Orthopaedic Hospital, Exeter EX4 4QL, -UK*
[3]*Mount Gould Hospital, Plymouth, UK*

Arthritis is intimately associated with the destruction of cartilage. High-resolution (100–200-μm) *in vivo* images of the finger joints have been obtained using a targeted magnetic resonance imaging (MRI) system. The study of asymptomatic subjects has enabled the normal anatomical zones of cartilage as visualised by MRI to be identified. In patients with advanced osteoarthritis features such as osteophytes and loss of cartilage are clearly demonstrated. An obvious question is whether MRI can be used to measure cartilage thickness and then whether this parameter can be utilized to quantify cartilage loss during the evolution of disease processes or response to therapy. However, there are a number of difficulties with this measurement which are discussed. It is possible that more valuable insights may be gained by careful choice of specific arthropathies to be studied—for example, acromegaly, which can lead to osteoarthritis—offers a way of observing subtle early changes that occur in the cartilage and subchondral bone.

Keywords: acromegaly, artefacts, arthritis, cartilage, targeted MRI.

INTRODUCTION

Rheumatic diseases are a major health-care problem of our time. Magnetic resonance imaging (MRI) is uniquely placed to provide *in vivo* information of benefit to rheumatological research through its ability to visualize the state of soft tissues, especially cartilage which typically comprises 70% water. In collaboration with Magnex Scientific Limited and Surrey Medical Imaging Systems Limited the authors have implemented targeted MRI systems based on small-bore superconducting magnets and PC-based imaging consoles [1]. One of these systems with a magnet bore size of 310 mm has been used to generate high-resolution (100–200 μm) images of the finger joints, where arthritis often initially presents. This approach has advantages of lower cost and improved patient comfort compared with whole-body systems.

* Address for correspondence: Department of Physics, University of Exeter, Stocker Road, Exeter EX4 4QL, UK.

DISCUSSION

The structure of cartilage is classified according to four zones or layers aligned parallel to the articular surface. Initial research focused on the interpretation of high-resolution MR images of normal distal interphalangeal joints and the identification of the cartilage zones [2–4]. The finger joints of patients with relatively advanced osteoarthritis (OA) were studied, and osteophytes, loss of cartilage, bone surface erosions, inflammation and edema, and pseudocystic regions were visualized [5, 6]. Of greater interest would be the ability to visualize early arthritic changes and make quantitative measurements. At first sight, cartilage thickness would appear to be a useful parameter to quantify. However, there are a number of difficulties in achieving this.

1. **Establishing landmarks.** Between which boundaries should the measurements be made? Where exactly do the different zones of cartilage end? Articular cartilage in contact with bone has in-

creased calcification up to the "tide mark" and these regions of MR signal void are obvious landmarks; however, reversal of the read magnetic field gradient (using a gradient-echo sequence) changes the thickness of these signal voids due to a chemical shift artifact, whereby bone marrow signal is encoded into these regions of signal void [4].

2. **Slice orientation and position.** What is the optimal slice orientation for such measurements—sagittal or coronal? Also, which slice positions should be used (off-center slices are more prone to partial volume effects than the central slice)? Both orientations are scanned using a pseudo-3D sequence, whereby a second phase-encoded gradient encodes 16, 1-mm-thick (rectangular profile) slices.

3. **Limited resolution.** Finger cartilage is typically 1 mm thick; therefore, even with a pixel resolution of 100 μm, the minimum detectable change is 10%—early arthritic changes are more subtle than this. Thus, higher resolution may be required, but there are difficulties in eliminating movement artifacts and performing the scan in a realistic time.

4. **Measurements normal to the cartilage surface.** Because joints are curved, measurements should be made normal to the cartilage surface.

5. **Tapered thinning of cartilage.** Some arthritic joints demonstrate uneven thinning of cartilage.

6. **Biological variation.** Congruity of articular cartilage surfaces varies among subjects, and for individual joints, the congruity can vary according to the slice selected.

7. **Reproducibility of slice position.** Is it possible to guarantee reproducibility of the same slice position for longitudinal studies? This is relatively easy to achieve using a set of close-fitting birdcage radio-frequency (RF) transceiver coils.

8. **Disease diversity.** Some disease processes, such as the endocrine disorder acromegaly, initiate an overgrowth of cartilage which can later lead to loss of cartilage.

9. **Total cartilage volume.** Some apparent difficulties may be overcome by considering total volume of cartilage as a more useful parameter. However, observations have shown that early changes in cartilage are often of a focal nature rather than being an overall thinning process and, thus, brings into question the usefulness of such measurements.

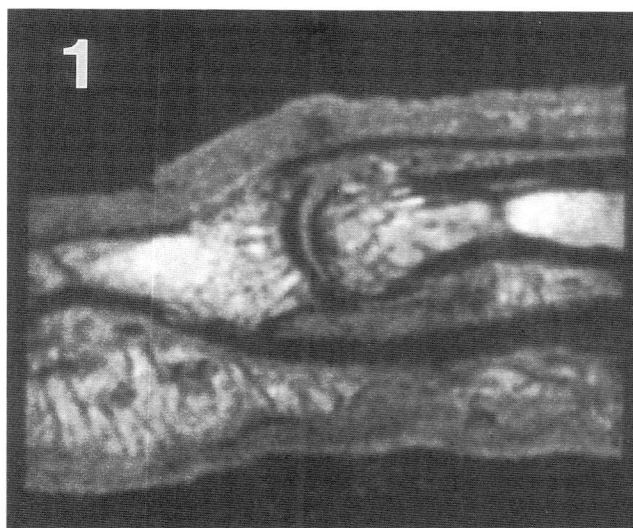

Fig. 1. Uneven cartilage thinning and early osteophyte formation.

CONCLUSIONS

The potential of MRI for arthritis research may best be exploited by careful selection of specific diseases to study—there are approximately 200 rheumatological conditions from which to choose. This philosophy has been followed by the authors' group and a few of the studies undertaken are listed here as examples. Acromegaly can lead to secondary OA; acromegalic patients may present with nonrheumatological symptoms, whereas patients with primary OA present

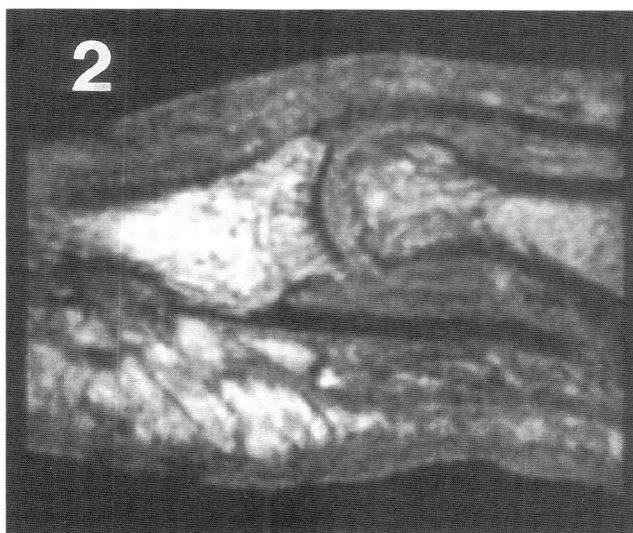

Fig. 2. Changes in the subchondral bone of the head of the medial phalanx.

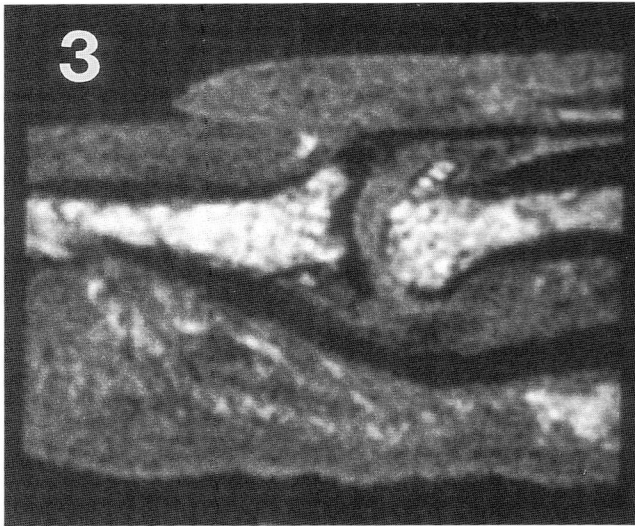

Fig. 3. Uneven cartilage thinning, osteophyte formation, and deterioration of the subchondral bone.

when the disease process is relatively advanced. Thus acromegaly offers the possibility of observing early features of OA as well as studying how acromegaly leads to OA. Another example is hemochromatosis where ferritin deposition in bone marrow has been visualized [7]. In addition, the evolution of a geode in the wrist of a patient with rheumatoid arthritis (RA) was monitored [8]. Because the metacarpophalangeal joints are often primarily effected by RA, a U-shaped

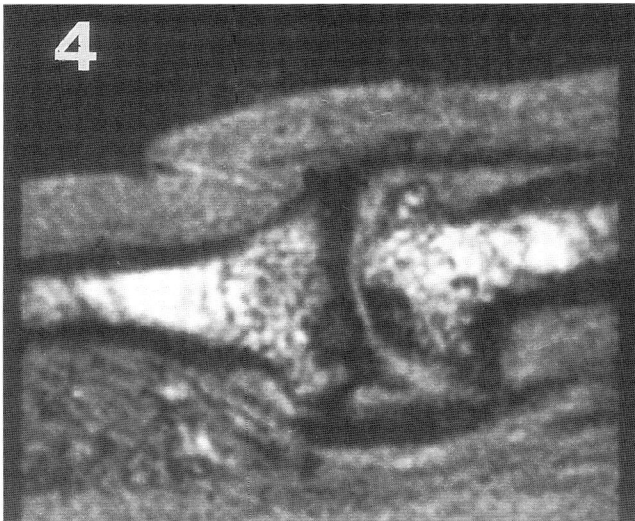

Fig. 4. Loss of cartilage, development of osteophytes, and formation of "kissing cysts" in the subchondral bone.

RF coil for imaging these joints has been developed [9].

It is also important to make very detailed investigations of one or two subjects because both OA and RA present in a number of different ways and comparison across a cohort of patients is often misleading. This systematic monitoring of the evolution of the disease in a few subjects is required if progress is to be made using MRI to study arthritis.

ACKNOWLEDGMENTS

The authors acknowledge collaborative support from Magnex Scientific Limited and Surrey Medical Imaging Systems Limited, and financial assistance from the Arthritis and Rheumatism Council for Research.

REFERENCES

1. Pittard S, Fry ME, Ellis RE, Moore EA, Vennart W (1989) A low-cost magnetic resonance imaging system. *J Phys E* **22:** 574–582.
2. Carpenter TA, Hall LD, Hodgson RJ (1990) Investigation of the distal interphalangeal joint under flexion. *8th SMRI.* Washington, DC, p. 79.
3. Cole PR, Jasani MK, Wood B, Freemont AJ, Morris GA (1990) High resolution, high field MR imaging of joints: Unexpected features in proton images of cartilage. *Br J Radiol* **63:** 907–909.
4. Fry ME, Jacoby RK, Hutton CW, Ellis RE, Pittard S, Vennart W (1991) High-resolution magnetic resonance imaging of the interphalangeal joints of the hand. *Skeletal Radiol* **20:** 273–277.
5. Fry ME, Pittard S, Ellis RE, Moore EA, Vennart W, Jacoby RK, Hutton CW (1989) Preliminary studies of arthritis using very high resolution MRI. *8th SMRM,* Amsterdam, p. 703.
6. Barry MA, Carpenter TA, Hall LD, Hazelman BL, Hodgson RJ, Tyler J (1992) High-resolution magnetic-resonance-imaging (MRI) of the normal and osteoarthritic distal interphalangeal (DIP) joints. *Arthritis Rheum* **35**(9): 134.
7. Moore EA, Vennart W, Jacoby RK, Hutton CW, Pittard S, Ellis RE (1993) Magnetic resonance imaging manifestations of idiopathic haemochromatosis in the wrist. *Br J Rheum* **32:** 917–922.
8. Moore EA, Jacoby RK, Ellis RE, Fry ME, Pittard S, Vennart W (1990) The demonstration of a geode using magnetic resonance imaging: A new light on the cause of juxta-articular bone cysts in rheumatoid arthritis. *Ann Rheum Dis* **49:** 785–787.
9. Gasson J, Fry ME, Febvre C, Summers IR, Keen MC, Ellis RE, Howseman A, Vennart W (1993) A novel U-shaped birdcage transceiver coil for high-resolution imaging of the MCP joints. *10th ESMRMB,* Rome, p. 429.

Magnetic resonance imaging of peripheral vascular disease and muscle atrophy in diabetes

John E. Foster,[1] Robin A. Damion,[1] William Vennart,[1]* Ian R. Summers,[1] Richard E. Ellis,[1] Peter Brash[2] and John Tooke[2]

[1]Physics Department, University of Exeter, Exeter Devon EX4 4QL, UK
[2]Diabetes Research Laboratories, Royal Devon and Exeter Hospital, Exeter EX4 4QL, UK.

Knowledge of the state of tissue hydration in patients suffering from peripheral vascular disease and neuropathy as a result of diabetes is important in their treatment. Further, because magnetic resonance imaging (MRI) is uniquely able to generate information about soft tissues and their water content, it is ideal for studying disorders of this kind. The feet and hands, often affected in diabetes, are ideal for studying fundamental aspects of the disease state and the response of patients to treatment. In this preliminary study, two related areas are reported: the measurement of diffusion coefficients in the finger and the visualization of the distribution of edema and muscle atrophy in the feet of people suffering from diabetes. Diffusion coefficients of water have been measured in the normal finger as a baseline study for a current patient study. It was found that the measured diffusion coefficient increased with subject age; this is not consistent with a direct-hydration model and it is conjectured that this could be linked to structural changes in proteins. Linked to this study, we have also imaged the feet of patients suffering from diabetes. Magnetization transfer has clearly demonstrated changes in muscle tissue with atrophy caused by motor neuropathy—in general, the amount of tissue water is increased as muscle volume decreases. Further, it is evident that these changes can be related to changes in cross-linking of protein and collagen molecules as muscle fibers become thinned, thus relating these studies to the diffusion coefficient measurements. The studies of the feet have also revealed artifacts in the images, consistent with the deposition of ferrous material in tissues. It is surmised that this is caused by hemosiderin deposits at ulcer sites associated with progress of the disease. MRI could be a useful tool for monitoring the distribution of ulcers below the skin surface and provide a means of determining the response of patients to treatment.

Keywords: MRI, diabetes, muscle atrophy.

INTRODUCTION

Diabetes causes a number of complications, including changes in soft tissues of the foot and hand, for example, impairment of muscle function as a result of motor neuropathy and alterations to tissue drainage caused by increased membrane permeability. Magnetic resonance imaging (MRI) with its exquisite soft-tissue contrast provides an accurate means for localizing abnormal tissue and quantifying tissue-water parameters [1, 2]. These changes in tissues often result in an increase in tissue water, leading to edema.

Further, changes in tissues (e.g., muscle breakdown) will also lead to disruption of water-binding sites to biological molecules, for example, proteins. MRI is ideally suited for monitoring edema (proton density) and changes in water binding through diffusion-coefficient and magnetization transfer measurements. The majority of research to date on diffusion coefficients has concentrated on brain tissues which have relatively long spin–spin relaxation times; it is also quite difficult to generate the necessary magnetic field gradients for the diffusion measurement. Both the fingers and the plantar part of the foot (tissues surrounding the metatarsal head) are ideal structures for targeted MRI measurements [3]; the radio-frequency (RF) coils used can surround the tissues of interest to produce relatively high-resolution images, and gradi-

* Address for correspondence: Physics Department, Stocker Road, University of Exeter, Exeter, Devon EX4 4QL, UK.

ent coils can be reduced in size with a consequent increase in gradient strength per unit current. In this article, some preliminary results will be reported that illustrate the potential of MRI techniques in the study of diabetes. The measurements being made not only demonstrate anatomical abnormalities but also functional differences where water exchange processes (crucial to the understanding of the disease process in diabetes) are the dominating contrast mechanism.

MATERIALS AND METHODS

Two separate imaging systems have been used incorporating SMIS consoles (Surrey Medical Imaging Systems Ltd., Surrey, UK) and Magnex Scientific 310-mm- and 560-mm-bore superconducting magnets (Magnex Scientific Ltd, Oxford, UK) operating at 0.5 T and fitted

with actively screened magnetic field gradients. The 310-mm system is used for diffusion coefficient measurements in the finger. Sagittal sections were used with a slice thickness of approximately 4 mm and pixel dimensions 300 μm^2. Diffusion gradients of 136 mT m^{-1} along the frequency-encoding direction were incorporated into a spin-echo sequence [4] with an echo time of 28 ms. To eliminate fat signal (the diffusion coefficient of which is an order of magnitude slower than tissue water), an inverting 180° pulse was applied before the beginning of the diffusion sequence. The 560-mm magnet was used to generate images of foot tissues surrounding the metatarsal joint—both sagittal and coronal images were obtained. The images were generated with a slice thickness of 2 mm and in-plane resolution of 280 μm using a specially adapted elliptical parallel solenoid RF coil. Both gradient- and spin-echo sequences were used. In addition, magnetization

(a)

(b)

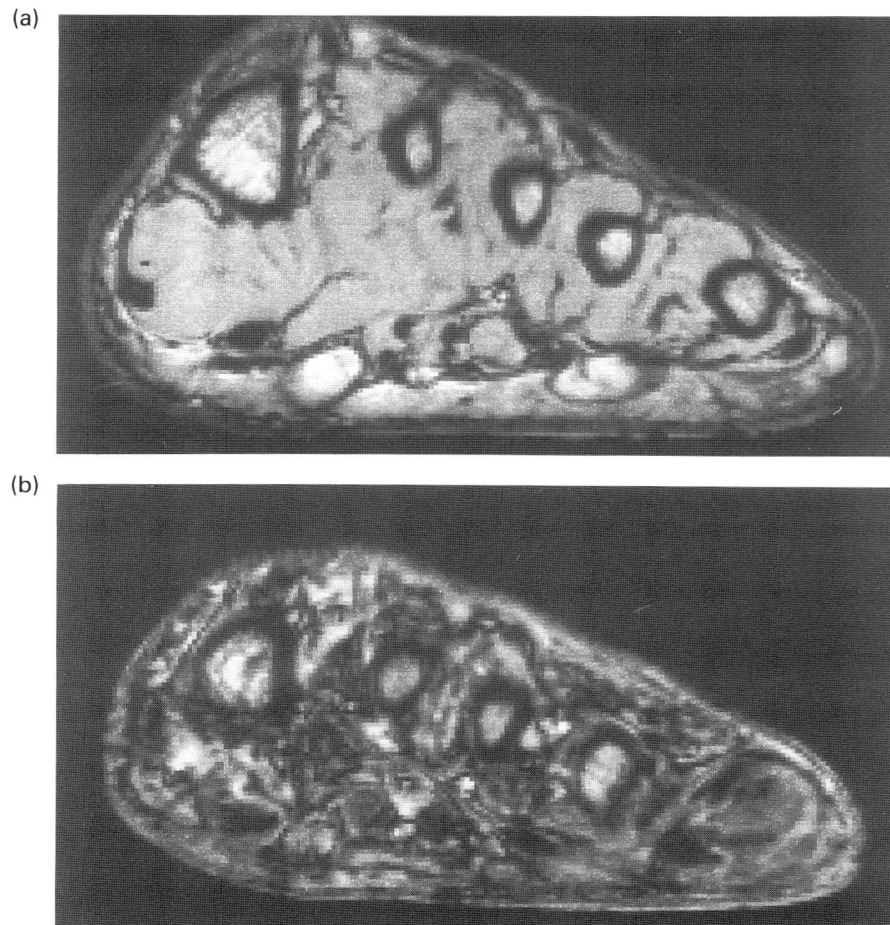

Fig. 1. (a) Axial section through a foot at the metatarsal joint demonstrating normal muscle and (b) the same section through the foot of a patient suffering from diabetes, where wasting of muscle fibers results in a mottled appearance to muscle.

transfer contrast was implemented using 65 1$\bar{2}$1 bionomial pulses of 1.5 ms overall duration and 1 ms between each pulse train.

RESULTS AND DISCUSSION

The diffusion coefficients in three regions (the finger tip, finger pulp, and bone marrow) of the distal index finger were measured in six male and six female normal volunteers whose ages ranged from 22 to 66 years; the average value was found to be 1.15×10^{-5} cm^{2}s^{-1}. The soft tissues in the finger are mainly connective tissue with a significant number of fat cells in the pulp, whereas the bone marrow diffusion coefficient is mainly associated with water in connection with fat. It has found that for males the diffusion coefficient increased with age ($p < 0.05$) in finger pulp, whereas for females this occurred only in bone marrow and the finger tip. It has been concluded that a likely cause of this increase with age is a result of changes in proteins, for example, glycosylation, especially collagen, such that the obstruction effect to water diffusion is reduced by a decrease in the size of protein molecules. This is an important finding because diabetes has been found to increase age-related changes such as glycosylation [5].

Gradient-echo images of the foot (Fig. 1) in transverse section clearly demonstrate the effect of motor neuropathy on muscle tissue where atrophy is evident and thinned muscle is replaced by tissue water. If this condition is investigated further using magnetization transfer (MT) sequences, it is clear that muscle which has undergone denervation and atrophy also has changes in protein structure (possibly cross-linkaging)

because it no longer shows exchange of water between bound and free water sites; that is, no MT is demonstrated.

A further interesting case has also been found where deposits of iron (possibly in the form of hemosiderin) have been visualized through loss of signal using a gradient-echo sequence in certain areas of the foot that is restored using spin-echo sequences. This is an exciting development that opens up the possibility of using MRI to monitor the formation of neuropathic ulcers deep in tissue. This work is also related to the role of callus formation over the metatarsal head and the distribution of pressure in soft tissues of the foot.

REFERENCES

1. Moore TE, Yuh WTC, Kathol MH, El-Khoury GY, Corson JD (1991) Abnormalities of the foot in patients with diabetes mellitus: Findings on MR imaging. *Am J Radiol* **157:** 812–816.
2. Durhan JR, Lukens ML, Campanini DS, Wright JG, Smead WL (1991) Impact of magnetic resonance imaging on the management of diabetic foot infections. *Am J Surgery* **162:** 151–154.
3. Pittard S, Fry ME, Ellis RE, Moore EA, Vennart W (1989) A low-cost magnetic resonance imaging system. *J Phys E: Sci Instrum* **22:** 574–582.
4. Le Bihan D, Bretan E, Lallemond D, Aubin ML, Viguand J, Laval-Jeantet M (1988) Separation of diffusion and perfusion in intravoxel incoherent motion MR imaging. *Radiology* **168:** 497–505.
5. Richard S, Tamas C, Sell DR, Monnier VM (1991) Tissue-specific effects of aldose reductase inhibition of fluorescence and cross-linking of extracellular matrix in chronic galactosemia. *Diabetes* **40:** 1049–1056.

A comparison of the proton relaxation in human epithelial tumors and associated uninvolved tissue

Paola Fantazzini[1]* and Alberto Sarra[2]

[1]*Dipartimento di Fisica, Università di Bologna, Bologna, Italy*
[2]*Ospedale Civile Santa Chiara, Trento, Italy*

Longitudinal and transverse proton relaxation from several sets of paired surgical samples of human epithelial tumors and associated histologically uninvolved tissues were studied at 37°C and at 20 MHz. Broad distributions of exponential terms fit all T_1 and T_2 decays well. The tumor times showed over twice the scatter of the associated tissue times but no clear trends. Although the nontumor relaxation show little variability, the tumor curves can have either longer or shorter times and different shapes.

Keywords: NMR proton relaxation, multiexponential data, adenocarcinoma, uninvolved tissue.

INTRODUCTION

Nuclear magnetic resonance relaxation of ^{1}H nuclei has been widely used to study biological tissues [1]. Relaxation curves have often been fitted to single-exponential decay functions despite the heterogeneity of some systems that might otherwise give sums or continuous distributions of exponential terms. Reports of multicomponent decay of pathological tissues are scarce, and the nonuniqueness of multiexponential analysis is a possible source of scatter in published relaxation times.

In this study longitudinal (T_1) and transverse (T_2) proton relaxation data have been analyzed for several sets of paired surgical samples of human epithelial tumors and associated histologically uninvolved tissue. This experiment simulates what happens in magnetic resonance imaging, where the patient serves as his own control, but it permits more detailed multiexponential analysis. Carcinoma that originates in the mucosa of the alimentary canal has been chosen because it is one of the most prevalent malignant tumor encountered in current practice.

---

* *Address for correspondence: Dipartimento di Fisica, Università di Bologna, Via Irnerio 46, 40126 Bologna, Italy.*

MATERIALS AND METHODS

Specimens obtained from adenocarcinomas of the stomach and intestine and from associated uninvolved tissue were taken during surgery, frozen in liquid nitrogen, and stored at −80°C. NMR measurements were performed within a few days, using a low-resolution spectrometer (20 MHz) [2]. Add/subtract phase-cycled pulse sequences were used with both inversion recovery (IR) (T_1, with 126 logarithmically spaced recovery times) and Carr–Purcell–Meiboom–Gill (CPMG) (T_2) sequences. A suitable IR signal delay prevented response to macromolecules with T_2* of the order of 20 μs. CPMG echo spacings were $2\tau = 1$ ms, with a single data point at the center of each echo. NMR measurements were begun after the sample temperature equilibrated with that of the probe (37°C), and great care was taken to prevent evaporation. Recommendations of Ref. 3 have been followed. Samples were subsequently placed in formalin for histological inspection.

Relaxation curves were fitted by nonlinear iterative procedures to stretched-exponential and multiexponential functions and to continuous distributions of relaxation times, as described elsewhere [2]. The stretched-exponential representation is $y(t) = \exp[-(t/T_{js})^{\alpha j}]$, where $y(t)$ is the normalized nuclear magnetization and $j = 1$ for T_1 and $j = 2$ for T_2. In the discrete representation $y(t) = \Sigma_{i=1,n}\ p_{ji}\ \exp(-t/T_{ji})$, where p_{ji}

are the fractions of the signal with relaxation time T_{ji}. In the continuous distribution analysis, $y(t) = \int S(T_j) \exp(-t/T_j) \, d(\ln T_j)$, where $S(T_j)$ is the signal density function [2] for a logarithmic time scale. Measurements on $CuSO_4$-doped water, used as controls for both measurement and data fitting, always showed single exponentials, with stretch parameters $\alpha = 1.00 \pm 0.01$ for T_1 or T_2.

RESULTS AND DISCUSSION

Relaxation curves for all samples (13 tumors and 13 nontumors) were non-single-exponential. For example, T_1 and T_2 continuous distributions are shown

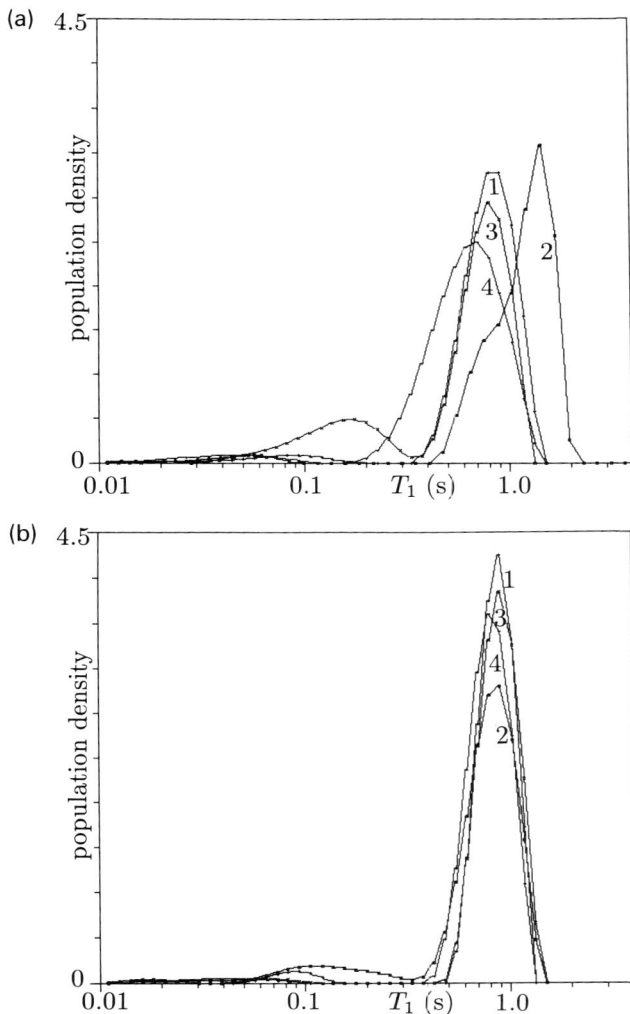

Fig. 1. Plot of population density, normalized to a unit area, of longitudinal relaxation times obtained by continuous distribution analysis for four pairs of samples. (a) Tumor samples; (b) associated histologically uninvolved samples.

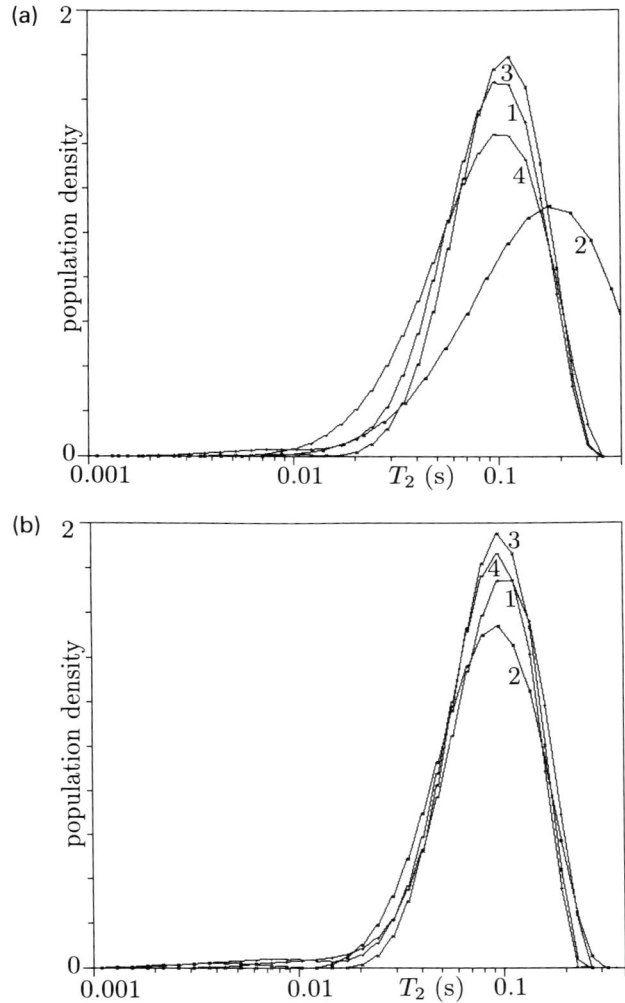

Fig. 2. Plot of population density, normalized to a unit area, of transverse relaxation times obtained by continuous distribution analysis for the samples of Fig. 1. (a) Tumor samples; (b) associated histologically uninvolved samples.

in Figs. 1 and 2 for four pairs of tumor and nontumor samples, respectively. T_1 distributions show a broad peak, accounting for the major fraction of the signal, centered near 1 s and also a tail or additional peak at shorter times. Equation (7) of Ref. 4 shows that the main peaks for both T_1 and T_2 have significant width and are not compatible with single lines. T_2 distributions tend to be broader than T_1 distributions. The root-mean-square scatter between the data and the fitted curves is in all cases a few parts per thousand, relative to the relaxing signal. Discrete multiexponential analysis gives good fits with two components for T_1 and three for T_2. The two T_1 components are in good accord with the peaks shown in Fig. 1. The three T_2 components do not represent resolved lines, as can

Table 1. Averages and standard deviations of the parameters obtained by different inversion methods for longitudinal and transverse relaxation curves.

Samples	T_{1g} [ms]	$T_{1\ continuous\ distribution}$ [ms]	T_{1s} [ms]	α_1	T_{2g} [ms]	$T_{2\ continuous\ distribution}$ [ms]	T_{2s} [ms]	α_2
Tumors	752 ± 160	840 ± 170	812 ± 170	0.91 ± 0.05	98 ± 31	116 ± 50	102 ± 34	0.83 ± 0.06
Nontumors	718 ± 69	797 ± 70	773 ± 76	0.91 ± 0.03	86 ± 13	95 ± 14	85 ± 15	0.80 ± 0.05

be seen from the criteria given in Refs. 4 and 5. We use the discrete components to compute the geometric mean, defined as $T_{jg} = \exp(\Sigma_{i=1,n}\ p_{ji} \ln T_{ji})$. The stretched-exponential computation gives T_s and α, where $1 - \alpha$ can be taken as an index of the deviation from single exponentials. For continuous distribution analysis, the time average, $\int S(T_j)T_j\ d\ (\ln T_j)$ is used, emphasizing longer times.

Table 1 compares the mean parameters obtained by the different inversion methods used. The differences in the means of the tumor and nontumor times and α's are not significant or are of marginal significance. The clearest differences in Table 1 are in the scatter of the data. Relative scatter is 20% for T_1 and 30–40% for T_2 in the tumor group, and less than half these amounts for the nontumor group.

In summary, both adenocarcinomas and the associated uninvolved tissue, as determined histologically, show non-single-exponential T_1 and T_2 proton relaxation, well fitted by broad distributions of exponential terms. The nontumor samples give very similar T_1 and T_2 distributions, whereas the tumor samples can give either longer or shorter times and can show shape differences. The wider distributions for T_2 than for T_1 is consistent with observations in other biological systems [6], as well as in natural and artificial porous media [2]. This may be partly explained by the shorter times for diffusion, leading to less diffusional averaging. With these wide distributions, different computations can lead to different results, especially if data sampling is inadequate, probably contributing to scatter among published results. However, we have shown that, even with the *same experimental conditions and computations,* relaxation for epithelial tumors shows

wider variation than the associated uninvolved tissue, indicating a variability of the tumor tissue, possibly involving some necrotic components and varied events in the history of a malignancy.

ACKNOWLEDGMENT

This work was supported by MURST grants.

REFERENCES

1. Bottomley PA, Hardy CJ, Argersinger RE, Allen-Moore G (1987) A review of ^{1}H nuclear magnetic resonance relaxation in pathology: Are T_1 and T_2 diagnostic? *Med Phys* **14:** 1–37, and references therein.
2. Borgia GC, Bortolotti V, Brown RJS, Castaldi P, Fantazzini P, Soverini U (1994) A comparison among different inversion methods for multiexponential NMR relaxation data. *Magn Reson Imaging* **12:** 209–212, and references therein.
3. EEC Concerted Research Project "Identification and Characterization of Biological Tissues by NMR" (F. Podo Project leader) (1988) II. A Protocol for in vitro proton relaxation studies. *Magn Reson Imaging* **6:** 179–184.
4. Brown RJS (1989) Information available and unavailable from multiexponential relaxation data. *J Magn Reson* **82:** 539–561.
5. Brown RJS, Borgia GC, Fantazzini P, Mesini E (1991) Problems in identifying multimodal distributions of relaxation times for NMR in porous media. *Magn Reson Imaging* **9:** 687–693.
6. Menon RS, Rusinko MS, Allen PS (1991) Multiexponential proton relaxation in model cellular systems, *Magn Reson Med.* **20:** 196–213.

Magnetic resonance imaging in obstetrics and gynecology: progress and limitations

B.S. Worthington

Sub-Department of Academic Radiology and Magnetic Resonance Centre, University of Nottingham, Nottingham NG7 2RD, UK

The introduction of phase-array coils, fast spin echo, and certain other pulse sequences together with use of contrast agents has refined the application of magnetic resonance imaging (MRI) in pelvic disease. It makes management decisions in a number of benign conditions including uterine anomalies, adenomyosis, and leiomyomas of the uterus and endometriosis, especially in the context of infertility; it facilitates identification and characterisation of adnexal masses. In uterine malignancy, the multiplanar capability and excellent soft tissue contrast permit accurate assessment of depth of tumor invasion, tumor volume, and extension to adjacent structures. Its precise role in the management of primary and recurrent ovarian cancer remains to be decided. In pelvic malignancy, contrast facilitates identification of viable tumor but does not improve tissue specificity. In obstetrics, MRI is an attractive alternative to X-ray pelvimetry and assists in the evaluation of associated uterine and pelvic pathology. The use of echo-planar imaging eliminates movement artifact and has the potential to complement ultrasound in the assessment of fetal abnormalities and provide a method of identifying growth retardation from volume measurements of body organs.

Keywords: infertility, tumor, uterus, ovary, fetus, echo-planar imaging.

INTRODUCTION

There is now an extensive knowledge base documenting the magnetic resonance appearances of most pathological conditions that occur in the female pelvis and this is constantly being extended and refined as improvements in image quality follow on advances in technique. In the present cost-conscious climate radiologists have to recommend to their clinical colleagues those applications that are most likely to significantly influence patient management, being mindful of the advances that have occurred in ultrasound, particularly when carried out with a vaginal transducer, as this in most instances will be the primary method of investigation of pelvic pathology. They must also recognize the current limitations of magnetic resonance imaging and how these might be addressed.

Address for correspondence: Professor B.S. Worthington, Sub-Department of Academic Radiology and Magnetic Resonance Centre, University of Nottingham, Nottingham NG7 2RD, UK.

TECHNIQUE

The most significant recent developments have been the advent of multicoil phase-array systems and endovaginal coils [1], providing improvements in signal to noise, and the fast spin-echo-based pulse sequences which together provide images with improved spatial resolution and excellent T_2 weighting in a much reduced scan time. The improved performance of nonresonant gradient systems will permit further reductions in imaging time without sacrifice of image quality. The use of the intravenous contrast agent gadolinium-DTPA, although giving no improvement in tissue specificity, has nonetheless provided a better display of tumor architecture in malignant disease and, in certain instances, improves the assessment of tumor spread. There remains a need for an oral contrast agent that would provide reliable mapping of the bowel lumen while giving clear delineation of the wall to facilitate identification of pelvic tumor deposits.

BENIGN PELVIC PATHOLOGY

Magnetic resonance has been shown to be valuable in a group of benign structural pelvic disorders which can present with a variety of different symptoms but may all be encountered during the investigation of infertility.

CONGENITAL ABNORMALITIES

From the standpoint of clinical management the essential distinction between those anomalies where pregnancy remains possible, with or without surgical intervention, and those in which it is precluded must be made. Complete or partial agenesis of the vagina or uterus can be accurately diagnosed. Analysis of the spectrum of genital anomalies resulting from failure of Mullerian duct fusion has been carried out conventionally by hysterosalpingography supplemented by laparoscopy to study the external contour of the uterus. By means of a series of images taken parallel to and at right angles to the long axis of the uterus, both the internal anatomy and external contour can be displayed. In particular, the commoner anomalies of septate and subseptate uteri can be accurately distinguished from a bicornuate uterus [2]. Laparoscopy is now a redundant procedure in this context.

LEIOMYOMA AND ADENOMYOSIS OF THE UTERUS

Leiomyoma is the commonest uterine tumor occurring in up to one-third of women in their reproductive years. Leiomyomas can be associated with reduced fertility by producing obstruction to the fallopian tubes and submucosal leiomyomas, which can be treated hysteroscopically, are associated with spontaneous abortion. Magnetic resonance imaging (MRI) can accurately define the number, location, and size of the tumors and is valuable as a prelude to myomectomy in order to determine whether sufficient myometrium can be spared during resection to permit future pregnancy. Magnetic resonance imaging can also be used to monitor medical treatment of leiomyomas by gonadotropic-releasing hormone analogs which produce a hypoestrogenic state that leads to atrophy. In this context, the recent identification of a highly cellular subgroup of tumors by magnetic resonance criteria [3] is of interest because this group responds well to medical treatment. It is important to distinguish between leiomyoma and adenomyosis as a

cause of uterine enlargement, as the only therapy currently available for the latter is a hysterectomy. On T_2-weighted images, focal adenomyosis is seen as oval or elongated areas of low signal intensity with ill-defined margins abutting on the junctional zone; diffuse adenomyosis results in thickening of the junctional zone to a width of greater than 5 mm. The small high-intensity areas within some of the lesions on both T_1- and T_2-weighted images represent areas of old hemorrhages. A recent study [4] has confirmed the superiority of magnetic resonance over transvaginal ultrasound in the diagnosis of adenomyosis.

ENDOMETRIOSIS

This is a common disorder mostly occurring in young nulliparous women and usually confined to the pelvis. The ovaries, rectovaginal pouch, parametria, and posterior vaginal fornix are the commonest sites of implantation, although the bladder and bowel may be implicated. In a review of 30 patients in Nottingham with suspected endometriosis studied by MRI [5], the diagnosis was confirmed by laparoscopy in 25 patients, and 13 of these had cystic tumors; the remaining 6 patients were normal. The most useful pulse sequences were found to be the STIR sequence and a very heavily T_2-weighted sequence with overall results for magnetic resonance imaging of 92% sensitivity and 83% specificity. It was noteworthy, however, that magnetic resonance often underestimated the amount of disease present—in particular, the extent of fibrous adhesions and the presence of pinpoint implants. This indicates that laparoscopy will continue to be required for staging, but magnetic resonance imaging is the best technique to confirm a clinical diagnosis and is useful in monitoring treatment whether by surgery or hormonal therapy.

MALIGNANT PELVIC PATHOLOGY

Endometrial carcinoma

The uterus has a distinctive trilaminar appearance on heavily T_2-weighted sequences: a low-intensity band separating the high signal of the endometrium from the main bulk of the myometrium. Although a nonspecific finding, endometrial carcinoma must be considered when the thickness of the endometrium exceeds 10 mm in a premenopausal woman and 5 mm in a postmenopausal woman. Absence of thinning of the low intensity band is a valuable sign of myometrial invasion in endometrial adenocarcinoma, and the multiplanar capability of magnetic resonance facilitates assessment of tumor volume [6]. The importance of the depth of myometrial invasion is emphasized by the incidence of pelvic lymph node metastases, which is less than 5% when this is superficial but can approach 50% for deep invasion. Contrast enhancement can facilitate estimation of myometrial invasion [7] and allows the better distinction between viable and necrotic tumors. Although surgical staging is usually carried out after confirming the diagnosis by dilatation and curettage in a patient with postmenopausal bleeding, magnetic resonance can substitute for this in patients with high-grade tumors who are best treated with radiotherapy and also when the general medical condition precludes surgery.

Carcinoma of the cervix

This is the second most common gynecological cancer in the United Kingdom. The prognosis is determined by the disease stage at the time of diagnosis with an overall 5-year survival rate of 50% in those with an invasive tumor. It is now accepted that magnetic resonance imaging is the primary technique for staging carcinoma of the cervix. In stages I and II, where other techniques have known limitations, magnetic resonance imaging can readily demonstrate distortion of normal cervical anatomy, spread of tumor to involve the vagina, and the critical feature of parametrial involvement, which precludes treatment by surgery in favor of radiotherapy [8]. Magnetic resonance imaging has now been shown to be superior to computed tomography in assessment of overall tumor volume and in demonstrating extension of tumor to the pelvic wall in stage III disease and involvement of the bladder and rectum in stage IV disease. Use of intravenous contrast does not improve tumor detection; indeed, overestimation of tumor size due to enhancement within peritumoral edema can occur [9]. A recent report [10], on a small series of patients, suggests that this problem may be obviated by rapid dynamic scanning after bolus injection of contrast. In advanced disease, contrast studies will facilitate assessment of tumor architecture and the recognition of bladder or rectal involvement. Assessment of nodal metastases remains based on size and morphology of the nodes. A recent study [11] has demonstrated that the most appropriate size criterion is the minimum axial diameter using a threshold of 1 cm to discriminate between normal and abnormal nodes. No difference was noted in the degree of contrast enhancement seen in true positive nodes as compared to false positive nodes.

Ovarian carcinoma

This is the commonest malignancy of the female genital tract in most Western countries. Because ovarian cancer is frequently asymptomatic, widely disseminated diagnosis is usually late in the natural history when prognosis is poor; indeed, most early-stage tumors represent incidental findings on routine pelvic examination. Although ultrasound is the initial technique for investigating such masses, when these are large, difficulties are occasionally encountered in identifying the organ of origin and magnetic resonance imaging is useful for clarification. There is considerable overlap in the appearances of histologically different ovarian tumors. Efforts to define criteria for distinguishing between benign and malignant tumors have been assisted by the advent of contrast media because enhancement allows the better visualization of intratumoral architecture and spread beyond the tumor capsule [12]. Prognosis is closely related to the stage of disease at presentation, and appropriate treatment depends on determining the histological type and accurate surgical staging using the revised classification of the International Federation of Obstetrics and Gynaecology. Imaging can assist when diagnosis is uncertain and it is sometimes used to define the extent of disease so as to plan for optimal surgery. Currently, computed tomography remains the best technique for this purpose with a staging accuracy of between 70% and 90% [13]. In a recent study in Nottingham [14], 58 patients with suspected ovarian carcinoma were examined by MRI in at least two orthogonal planes employing a variety of T_1- and T_2-weighted pulse sequences and the STIR sequence. Ovarian carcinoma was confirmed in 32 patients at laparotomy, 7 had metastatic disease in the ovary, which was indistinguishable at surgery, and 10 had a variety of benign ovarian tumors. Four primary bowel tumors, a chronic abscess, a liposarcoma, and three normal patients were correctly identified. Magnetic resonance imaging showed the solid and cystic components of the tumors and the presence of hemorrhage; only occasionally did the pattern allow the cell type to be suggested. Twenty-one out of the 32 patients were correctly staged as defined by the FIGO classification. T_2-weighted and STIR images in the sagittal and transverse axial planes gave optimal demonstration of the bladder, rectum, and pelvic side wall for which tumor involvement was demonstrated with an accuracy of 87%, 56%, and 97%, respectively. The principal shortcoming of MRI was the demonstration of bowel involvement, in particular peritoneal metastases, which was shown down to 1 cm in size but smaller deposits were missed. The use of fast-imaging strategies combined with a reliable bowel contrast agent and intravenous contrast may lead to magnetic resonance supplanting computed tomography for studies carried out prior to surgery. Patients treated with adjuvant chemotherapy are followed up with serum tumor markers and imaging to assess response, relapse, and end point of treatment. Magnetic resonance is valuable in evaluating patients with suspected recurrent or residual disease, and in a recent study of 31 patients in Nottingham [15] it was found to have a sensitivity of 87% and a specificity of 55%, the chief limitation being the detection of small volume disease.

OBSTETRICS

The introduction of diagnostic ultrasound in the 1950s revolutionized obstetric practice. Magnetic resonance imaging, which provides a wide field of view of both maternal and fetal anatomy, can complement the use of ultrasound in situations where it has known limitations. It is also to be preferred in the investigation of several acute medical emergencies occurring during pregnancy, such as spinal cord compression, where the only alternative method of investigation is a procedure using ionizing radiation. No mutagenic or oncogenic effects have been demonstrated during exposure of appropriate biological test systems to the conditions encountered in magnetic resonance imaging using commercially available scanners.

Although the use of X-ray pelvimetry has markedly declined, many obstetricians still request it in the management of a persistent breech presentation. Magnetic resonance has been shown to be a suitable alternative, in that all the relevant bony landmarks can be identified and, in addition, there is an excellent view of the relevant soft tissue anatomy.

Ultrasound is extremely accurate in the assessment of placental anatomy and site, but occasionally there are difficulties, particularly with posteriorly placed placentas lying close to the cervix. MRI can provide clarification in such equivocal examinations [16].

Magnetic resonance imaging is the method of choice for assessing the size and tissue characteristics of pelvic masses that could interfere with the normal progression of pregnancy [17]. Cervical dystocia and incompetence are important conditions, the underlying mechanisms of which are incompletely understood. MRI now provides the opportunity for studying the pathological cervix [18] and has the potential to permit the course of cervical ripening to be studied.

Gestational trophoblastic neoplasia is an uncommon complication of pregnancy. The high signal of the normal placenta on T_2-weighted images is seen in its neoplastic counterpart, and areas of hemorrhage are readily identified [19] on T_1-weighted sequences. Magnetic resonance has been shown to be valuable in the follow-up of patients with choriocarcinoma treated with chemotherapy.

Several reports have now been published documenting the utility of magnetic resonance imaging in clarifying the ultrasound appearances in a variety of congenital abnormalities. In this regard, the use of ultra-high-speed echo-planar imaging completely eliminates obtrusive movement artifacts [20] and allows a clear depiction of congenital anomalies.

It has now been established that in the management of high-risk pregnancy mortality rates show a closer correlation to birth weight than gestational age. Fetal macrosomia is associated with brachial plexus injuries and shoulder dystocia, whereas growth retardation is associated with an increased perinatal morbidity. In a recent study [21], fetal volume was estimated close to term by computer planimetry of contiguous echo-planar images containing fetal parts. A linear relationship was obtained between fetal volume and birth weight ($R = 0.97$) and the results suggest the method can provide a more accurate estimate of fetal weight during gestation than ultrasound.

Further extensions of this work can be anticipated to assist in the assessment of compromised fetal development so as to better make the difficult management decisions which frequently have to be made.

REFERENCES

1. Milestone B, Schnall MD, Lenkinski RE, Kressell H (1991) Cervical carcinoma; MR imaging with an endorectal surface coil. *Radiology* **180:** 91–95.
2. Pellerito JS, McCarthy SM, Doyle MD et al. (1992) Diagnosis of uterine anomalies: relative accuracy of MR imaging; endovaginal sonography and hysterosalpingography. *Radiology* **183:** 795–800.
3. Yamashita Y, Torashima M, Takahashi M et al. (1993) Hyperintense uterine leiomyomata at T2 weighted imaging: differentiation with dynamic enhanced MR imaging. *Radiology* **189:** 721–725.
4. Asher SM, Arnold LL, Patt RH et al. (1994) Adenomyosis: prospective comparison of MR imaging and transvaginal sonography. *Radiology* **190:** 803–806.
5. Mitchell A, Worthington BS, Powell MC, Symonds EM (1993) The role of MRI in the evaluation of endometriosis. *Br J Radiol* **66:** 41–42.
6. Powell MC, Womack C, Worthington BS, Symonds EM (1986) Pre-operative magnetic resonance imaging of stage I endometrial carcinoma. *Br J Obstet Gynaecol* **93:** 353–360.
7. Sironi S, Colombo E, Villa G (1992) Myometrial invasion

by endometrial carcinoma: assessment with plain and Gadolinium enhanced MR imaging. *Radiology* **185**: 207–212.

8. Powell MC, Worthington BS, Sokal M et al. (1986) Magnetic resonance imaging: its application to cervical carcinoma. *Br J Obstet Gynaecol* **93**: 1276–1285.

9. Sironi S, De Cobelli F, Scarfone G et al. (1993) Carcinoma of the cervix: value of plain and Gadolinium enhanced MR imaging in assessing degree of invasiveness. *Radiology* **188**: 797–801.

10. Yamashita Y, Takahashi M, Sawada T (1992) Carcinoma of the cervix: dynamic MR imaging. *Radiology* **182**: 643–648.

11. Kim SH, Kim SC, Choi BI et al. (1994) Uterine cervical carcinoma: evaluation of pelvic node metastasis with MR imaging. *Radiology* **190**: 807–811.

12. Stevens S, Hricak H, Stern JL (1991) Ovarian lesions: detection and characterization with Gadolinium enhanced MR imaging. *Radiology* **181**: 481–488.

13. Amindola MA (1985) The role of CT in the evaluation of ovarian malignancy. *Crit Rev Diagnost Imaging* **24**: 329–368.

14. Hanley P, Worthington BS, Powell MC, Symonds EM (1989) An assessment of the accuracy of magnetic resonance imaging in the diagnosis and staging of suspected primary ovarian carcinoma. *Br J Radiol* **62**: 585.

15. Kerslake RW, Worthington BS, Powell MC et al. (1990) A prospective comparison of MRI and immunoscintigraphy with Oc125 in detecting recurrent ovarian carcinoma. *Radiology* **177**: (P)242.

16. Worthington BS, Powell MC, Buckley J, Symonds EM (1985) The assessment of placental site and geometry by magnetic resonance imaging. *Radiology* **157**: (P)323.

17. Kier R, McCarthy SM, Scoutt LM et al. (1990) Pelvic masses in pregnancy: MR imaging. *Radiology* **176**: 709–713.

18. Hricak H, Chang YC, Cann CE, Paner JT (1990) Cervical incompetence: preliminary evaluation with MR imaging. *Radiology* **174**: 821–826.

19. Powell MC, Buckley J, Worthington BS, Symonds EM (1986) Magnetic resonance imaging and hydatidiform mole. *Br J Radiol* **59**: 561–564.

20. Johnson IR, Stehling MK, Blamire AM et al. (1990) A study of the internal structure of the human fetus in-utero by echo planar magnetic resonance imaging. *Am J Obstet Gynaecol* **163**: 601–607.

21. Baker PN, Johnson IR, Gowland P et al. (1994) Accurate in-utero weight estimation using echo planar imaging. *Lancet* **343**: 644–645.

Clinical role of diffusion-weighted imaging: neonatal studies

J.M. Pennock,[1] F.M. Cowan,[2] J.E. Schweiso,[1] A. Oatridge,[1] M.A. Rutherford,[2] L.M.S. Dubowitz[2] and G.M. Bydder[1]*

[1]Robert Steiner Magnetic Resonance Unit, Department of Diagnostic Radiology and [2]Department of Paediatrics and Neonatal Medicine, Hammersmith Hospital, Royal Postgraduate Medical School, London W12 0HS, UK

The application of diffusion-weighted imaging to the early diagnosis of neonatal cerebral infarction and hypoxic ischemic encephalopathy is illustrated. Diffusion-weighted images showed early infarction before conventional imaging in both cases. These were subsequently seen with conventional imaging on follow-up. In four cases of grades I and II hypoxic–ischemic encephalopathy (HIE) no abnormality was seen with either diffusion-weighted or conventional imaging. In four other cases of grades II and III HIE, much more extensive changes were seen with diffusion-weighted imaging than with conventional imaging. Follow-up scans with conventional imaging confirmed the abnormalities in the two surviving infants. Diffusion-weighted imaging may be particularly useful for the early diagnosis of ischemic–anoxic injury in infants.

Keywords: magnetic resonance imaging, diffusion-weighted imaging.

INTRODUCTION

Imaging techniques have an important role in the diagnosis of brain damage in the newborn infant because they may demonstrate abnormalities long before their clinical effects are manifest. Cranial ultrasound is the most readily available technique, but magnetic resonance imaging (MRI) is often more sensitive and more specific.

Over the last 4 years, diffusion-weighted MRI in which contrast is determined primarily by differences in the molecular motion of water rather than T_1 or T_2 has been developed for clinical use and applied to pediatric studies [1, 2].

Of particular interest has been the possibility of using diffusion-weighted imaging for the diagnosis of ischemic damage in the newborn, but because of the difficulties of managing and monitoring acutely ill infants within magnetic resonance systems this has only recently become possible.

ANIMAL MODELS OF STROKE AND GLOBAL ISCHEMIA

There have now been several cat and rat studies performed on models of middle cerebral artery infarction (stroke) in which it has been demonstrated that diffusion-weighted MRI shows effects attributable to a net reduction in the molecular motion of water in regions of infarction before changes in T_1 and T_2 are detectable [3].

The effect of the reduction in net molecular motion is seen as a relative increase in signal on the diffusion-weighted images after only a few minutes, whereas conventional T_1- and T_2-weighted sequences typically require 6–8 h for cerebral infarction to become apparent. Similarly, in a model of global ischemia produced by bilateral carotid artery occlusion in the gerbil, diffusion-weighted imaging has shown changes within 2.5 min of the onset of ischemia [4].

CEREBRAL INFARCTION AND HYPOXIC–ISCHEMIC ENCEPHALOPATHY

Anoxic–ischemic cerebral injury in term newborn infants may produce focal damage in a specific arterial distribution (infarction) or more global injury (hypoxic–ischemic encephalopathy, HIE). Focal infarction may be asymptomatic but generally presents with subtle seizures or episodes of apnoea. It usually has a relatively good outcome. HIE more commonly produces reduction in consciousness, changes in tone or tonic–clonic fits, and may have a very poor outcome. Distinction between the two conditions is of considerable prognostic importance but is difficult because some symptoms and signs such as tonic–clonic fits occur in both conditions.

---

* Address for correspondence: Robert Steiner MR Unit, Hammersmith Hospital, Du Cane Road, London W12 0HS, UK.

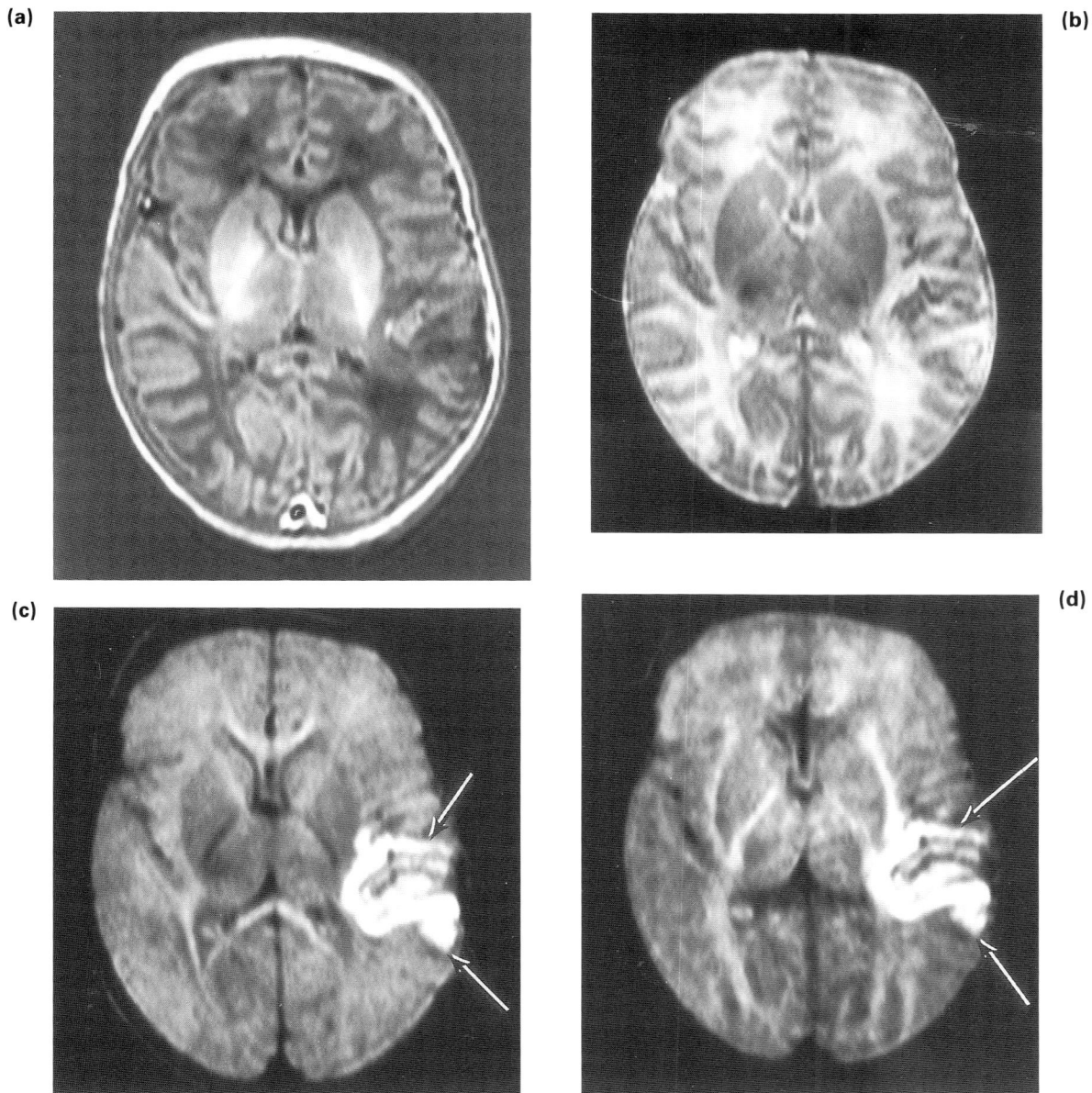

Fig. 1. Cerebral infarction: Transverse T_1-weighted spin echo (SE 720/20) (*A*), T_2-weighted spin echo (SE 3000/120) (*B*), diffusion-weighted (SE pulse interval/200 ms through plane sensitization, $b = 600$ s mm^2) (*C*), and diffusion-weighted (SE pulse interval/200 left-right sensitization, $b = 600$ s mm^2) (*D*) images. The abnormality is difficult to recognize on (*A*) and (*B*) but is readily apparent as a high-signal region in (*C*) and (*D*) (arrows).

Lack of oxygen and blood supply to the brain may result in primary energy failure which is manifest as depletion of the high-energy compounds phosphocreatine and adenosine triphosphate (ATP). Although resuscitation may produce quick restoration of some of these biochemical disturbances, a cascade of chemical reactions is set in motion, resulting in breakdown of the cell membrane, mitochondrial damage, and ultimately cell death [5].

Mitochondrial dysfunction typically occurs 8–24 h after the resuscitation from primary insult and results in a decrease in phosphocreatine and ATP levels. This has been called secondary energy failure. The period of about 5–8 h between resuscitation and secondary energy failure provides a window of opportunity where it may be possible to use drugs or hypothermia to stop the cascade of reactions leading to secondary energy failure and, therefore, improve the outcome of HIE.

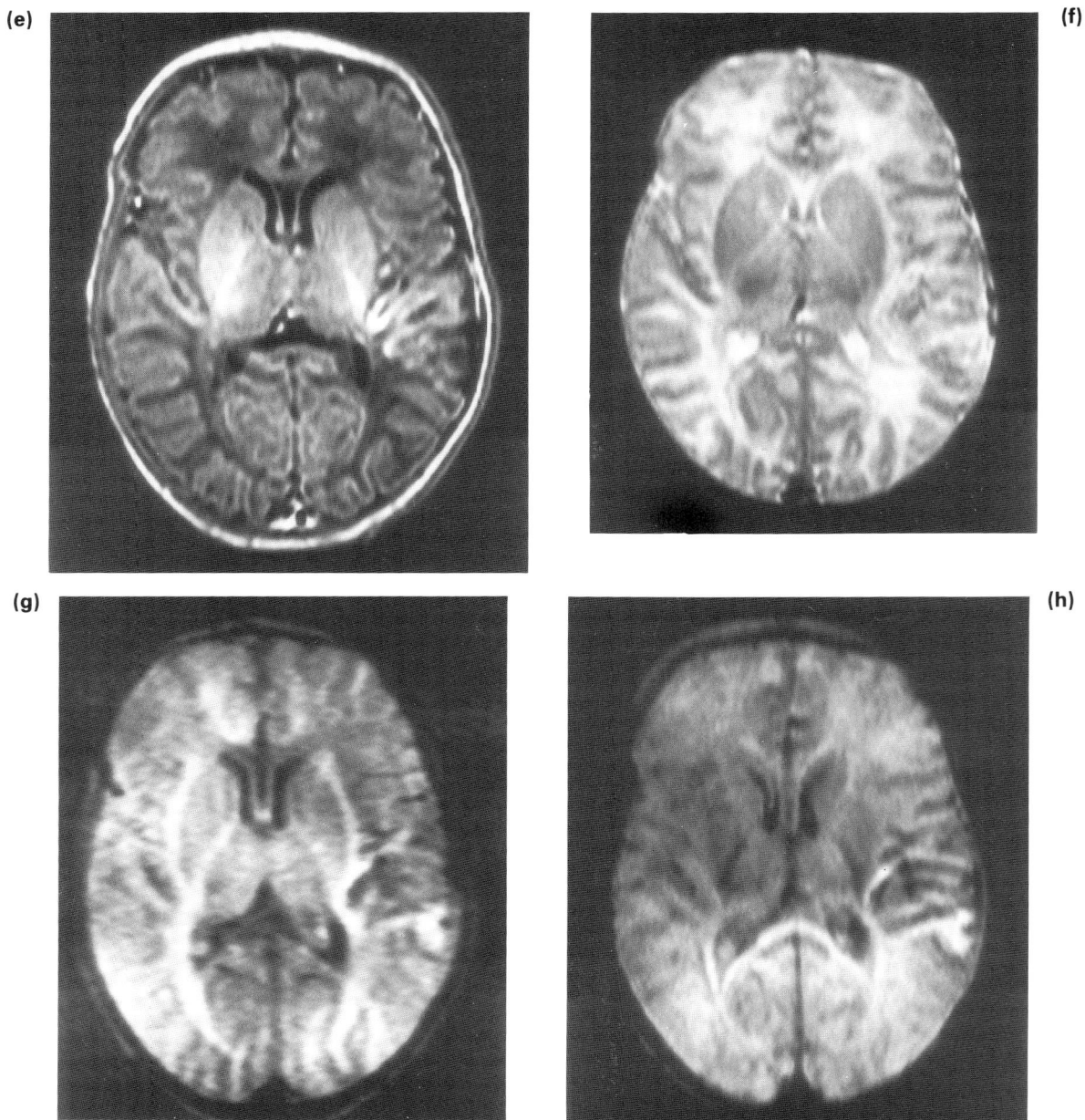

Fig. 1. (Continued) Follow-up T_1-weighted spin echo (SE720/20) (*E*) and T_2-weighted spin echo (SE3000/120)(*F*) diffusion-weighted (SE pulse interval/200 ms through plane sensitization) (*G*) and diffusion-weighted (SE pulse interval/200 ms left-right sensitization, $b = 600s$ mm^2) (*H*) images obtained six days later. Areas of abnormality seen in (*C*) and (*D*) are now seen on (*E*) and (*F*) and are reduced on (*G*) and (*H*).

MAGNETIC RESONANCE STUDIES IN ACUTE CEREBRAL INFARCTION AND HYPOXIC–ISCHAEMIC ENCEPHALOPATHY

The animal studies of focal and global ischemia described above suggested that diffusion-weighted MRI might be of particular value in the early diagnosis of ischemic damage in the newborn. We therefore performed studies on 10 infants with suspected ischemic-anoxic damage.

All magnetic resonance (MR) studies were performed on a Picker (Cleveland, OH, USA) HPQ Vista scanner operating at 1.0 T. Conventional MRI examination consisted of a T_1-weighted spin echo (SE 720/20

(a)

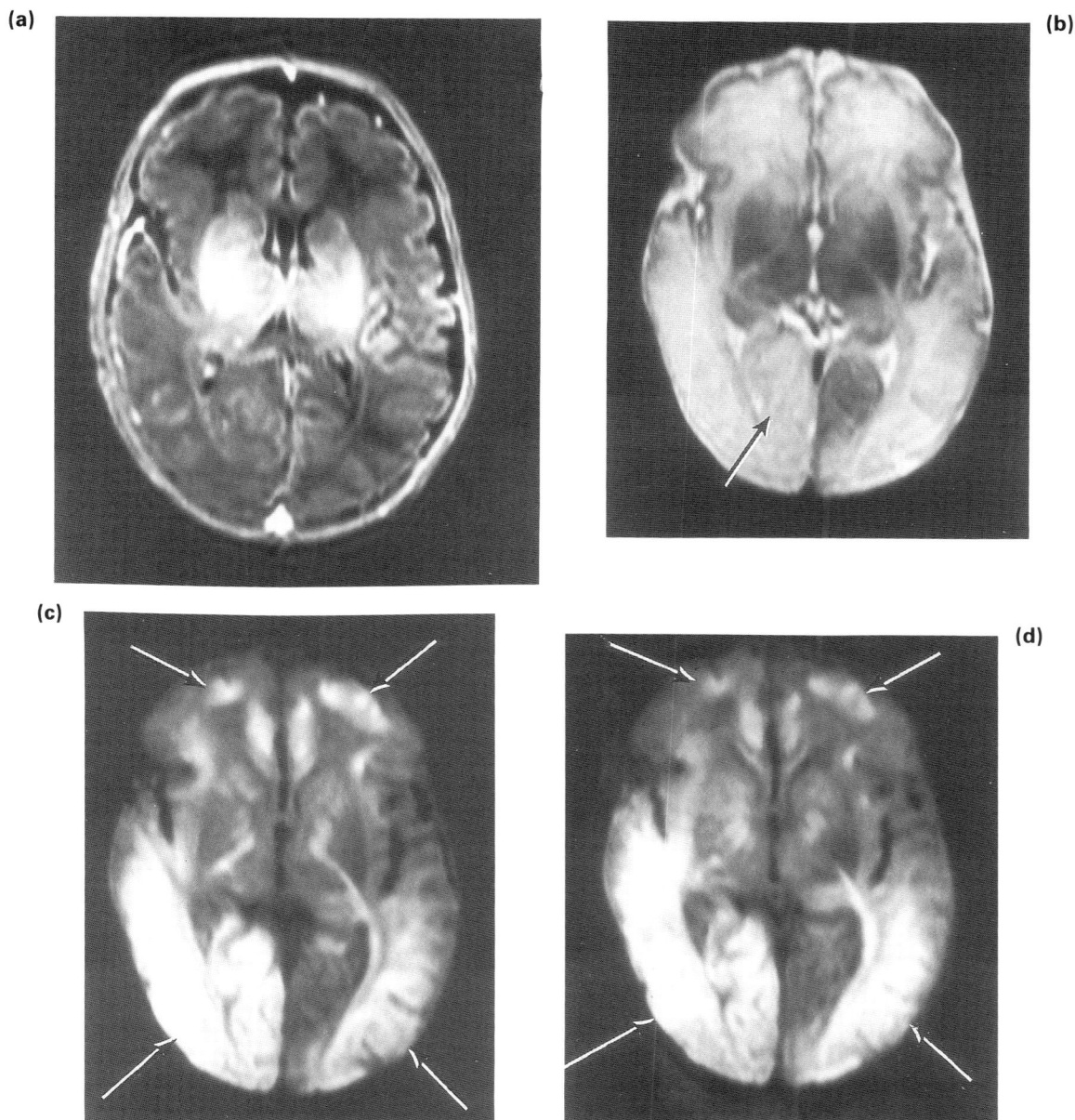

(b)

(c)

(d)

Fig. 2. Hypoxic–ischemic encephalopathy: Transverse T_1-weighted spin echo (SE 720/20) (A), T_2-weighted spin echo (SE 3000/120) (B), diffusion-weighted (SE pulse interval/200 ms, antero-posterior sensitization, b = 600 s mm²) (C), and diffusion-weighted (SE pulse interval/200 ms through plane sensitization) (D). High signal is seen in the medial right occipital lobe in (B) (arrow), but much more extensive abnormalities are seen in the frontal temporal and occipital lobes using diffusion-weighted

imaging in (C) and (D) (arrows). Follow-up T_1-weighted spin echo (SE 720/20) (E), T_2-weighted spin echo (SE 3000/120) (F), diffusion-weighted (SE pulse interval/200 ms left-right sensitization, b = 600 s mm²) (G), and diffusion-weighted (SE pulse interval/200 ms through plane sensitization) (H) images obtained 20 days later. Areas of abnormality seen in (C) and (D) are now highlighted in (E) (arrows) probably due to the presence of hemorrhage. The diffusion-weighted images show less change on follow-up.

ms), inversion recovery (IR 3000/30/950 ms), and T_2-weighted spin echo (SE 3000/120 ms).

The diffusion-weighted images use a gated pulsed gradient spin-echo sequence (SE pulse interval/200

ms) with a diffusion sensitivity parameter, b [6], of 600 s mm² with four data acquisitions in x, y, and z axes.

Diffusion-weighted MRI scans were graded by two experienced observers. Particular attention was paid

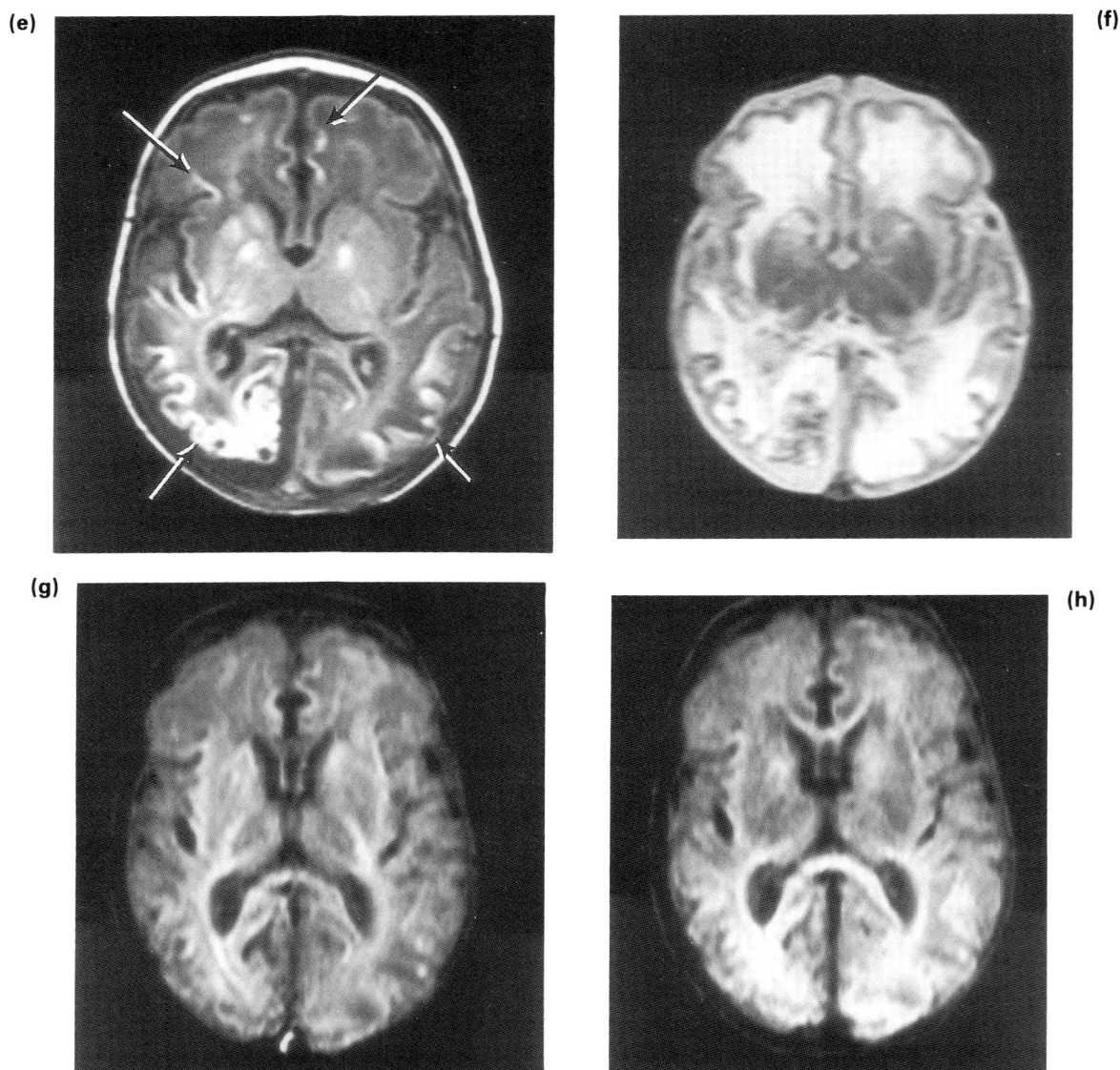

Fig. 2. (Continued) Follow-up T_1-weighted spin echo (SE720/20) (*E*) and T_2-weighted spin echo (SE3000/120)(*F*) diffusion-weighted (SE pulse interval/200 ms through plane sensitization), (*G*) and diffusion-weighted (SE pulse interval/200 ms left-right sensitization, b = 600s/mm^2), (*H*) images obtained six days later. Areas of abnormality seen in (*C*) and (*D*) are now seen on (*E*) and (*F*) and are reduced on (*G*) and (*H*).

to gray and white matter changes, including those in named tracts and the presence or absence of aniso-tropic change.

RESULTS

Two infants with infarction and eight infants with grades I to III HIE [7] were examined. The two areas of infarction were seen on days 4 and 6 with diffusion-weighted imaging before conventional MR imaging showed any significant change (Fig. 1). The areas of abnormality matched the changes that were seen later with conventional magnetic resonance images.

Four infants with grades I or II HIE showed no abnormality with diffusion-weighted or conventional imaging. Another four infants with grades II or III HIE showed much more extensive abnormality with diffusion-weighted imaging (Fig. 2). Follow-up in the two survivors showed changes with conventional imaging in the areas first shown as abnormal with diffusion-weighted imaging (Fig. 2).

DISCUSSION

Early diffusion-weighted imaging showed abnormalities that could not be seen with conventional MRI in the first 5 days after birth and distinguished focal infarction from HIE. The diffusion-weighted changes were only seen for a few days after the onset of symptoms but accurately predicted the extent of the involvement seen later with conventional MR and at postmortem.

In diffusion-weighted MRI, image contrast depends mainly on differences in the molecular motion of water rather than changes in T_1 or T_2. The early changes in infarction and HIE have been attributed to a reduction in intracellular transport, influx of water into the intracellular space, decrease in brain pulsatility, and other mechanisms [8]. Increases in T_1 and T_2 appear later and probably require the presence of vasogenic edema.

Our findings are consistent with animal data though the time scale of changes is slower. With animal experiments the injury is accurately timed, whereas with our infant data the injury may have occurred slowly or intermittently and no definite timing of the actual events was possible. This was true for both focal infarction and global injury.

Animal studies have shown a reduction in the extent of the abnormality detected with diffusion-weighted imaging in stroke models following treatment with cerebroprotective agents [9–11]. Diffusion-weighted MRI may be of critical importance in diagnosis and monitoring therapeutic effectiveness if new therapies of this type are used for treatment of HIE.

REFERENCES

1. Rutherford MA, Cowan FM, Manzur AY, Dubowitz LMS, Pennock JM, Hajnal JV, Young IR, Bydder GM (1991) MR imaging of anisotropically restricted diffusion in the brain of neonates and infants. *J Comput Assist Tomogr* **15**: 188–198.

2. Sakuma H, Nomura Y, Takeda K, Tagami T, Nakagawa T, Tamagawa Y, Ishii Y, Tsukamoto T (1991) Adult and neonatal human brain diffusion anisotropy and myelination with diffusion-weighted MR imaging. *Radiology* **180**: 229–233.

3. Moseley ME, Kucharczyk J, Mintovitch J et al. (1990) Diffusion weighted MR imaging of acute stroke: correlation with T2 weighted and magnetic susceptibility enhanced MR imaging in cats. *Am J Nucl Reson* 423–429.

4. Busza AL, Allen KL, King MD et al. (1992) Diffusion weighted imaging studies of cerebral ischemia in gerbils. Potential relevance to energy failure. *Stroke* **23**: 1602–1612.

5. Azzopardi D, Wyatt JS, Cady EB et al. (1989) Progress of newborn infants with hypoxic–ischaemic brain imaging assessed by phosphorus magnetic resonance spectroscopy. *Pediatr Res* **25**: 445–451.

6. Le Bihan D, Breton E, Lallemand D, Grenier P, Cabanis EA, Laval-Jeantet M (1986) MR imaging of intravoxel incoherent motions: application to diffusion and perfusion in neurological disorders. *Radiology* **161**: 401–407.

7. Sarnat HB, Sarnat MS (1976) Neonatal encephalopathy following fetal distress. *Arch Neurol* **33**: 696–705.

8. Le Bihan D, Turner R, Douek P, Patronovs N (1992) Diffusion MR imaging: clinical applications. *Am J Radiol* **159**: 591–599.

9. Haraldseth O, Jones RA, Muller JB, Unsgard G, Ring PA, Oskendal AW (1993) Comparison of MR "perfusion" imaging and diffusion weighted imaging for *in-vivo* evaluation of cerebroprotective therapy. In *Book of Abstracts, Society of Magnetic Resonance in Medicine (SMRM) Twelfth Annual Meeting, New York.* p. 252. Berkeley, CA: Society of Magnetic Resonance in Medicine.

10. Huang NC, Quast MJ, Hillman GR, Kent TA (1993) Effects of MR-801 on ischaemic injury in rat models of permanent and temporary focal cerebral ischaemia. In *Book of Abstracts, Society of Magnetic Resonance in Medicine (SMRM) Twelfth Annual Meeting, New York.* p. 254. Berkeley, CA: Society of Magnetic Resonance in Medicine.

11. Remy C, Le Bars E, Devoulon P et al. (1993) Interest of diffusion imaging for pharmacological investigation in focal cerebral ischaemic study of a normal compound S20390. In *Book of Abstracts Society of Magnetic Resonance in Medicine (SMRM) Twelfth Annual Meeting, New York.* p. 596. Berkeley, CA: Society of Magnetic Resonance in Medicine.

The measurement of gastric motor function and transit in man by echo planar magnetic resonance imaging

J. Wright,[1]* V. Adams,[3] J. Hykin,[3] P. Gowland,[3] B. Issa,[3] P. Boulby,[3]
P. Tokarczuk,[3] D. Evans,[4] R. Spiller[2] and P. Mansfield[3]

[1]*Departments of Surgery, [2]Gastroenterology and [3]Magnetic Resonance Centre,
University of Nottingham, Nottingham, UK
[4]GI Science Research Unit, London Hospital Medical College, London, UK*

Echo-planar imaging (EPI) can be used to produce snapshot images of the human stomach and antro-pyloro-duodenal segment in real time as an alternative technique to intubation and exposure to ionizing radiation. The method has been further developed to monitor simultaneous gastric motility and gastric emptying of liquid and solid meals. The model has been utilized to study the effects of pharmacological agents on gastric function.

Eight normal subjects were imaged in a 0.5-T superconducting magnet for up to 6 h following ingestion of 800 ml tap water, followed by 500 ml porridge test meal + 500 ml tap water. A rapid multislice technique was adopted to image adjacent transverse slices (10 mm thick) through the gastric region. In addition, three subjects were orally dosed with 20 mg of the prokinetic agent Cisapride. Gastric volumes for each slice were calculated and summed to produce a measure of total gastric volume and gastric emptying. Contractile activity at the level of the antro-pyloric segment was detected using sequential 128 ms images at 3 s intervals. Alternate measurements of gastric volume and motility were made for the duration of the study.

Gastric emptying $T_{1/2}$'s (times to empty 50% of the gastric contents) of 12.9 min for water and 116 min for porridge were in agreement with results obtained by the traditional techniques of gamma scintigraphy and impedance imaging. The frequency of gastric contractions increased from 2.4 contractions per minute (cpm) to 3.2 cpm following water and from 2.9 to 3.2 cpm following porridge. The prokinetic effect of enhanced coordination of antroduodenal contractions was also observed. These studies have demonstrated that EPI can be used to detect and image gastro-duodenal function in man, totally noninvasively, and can be used to study the effects of drugs acting on the gastrointestinal tract.

Keywords: echo planar, stomach, motility, stomach emptying.

INTRODUCTION

One of the major functions of the human stomach is as a reservoir for food prior to digestion and absorption. Food can remain in the stomach for many hours after ingestion, during which time it is reduced to a fine particulate matter by the contractile activity of the gastric muscle wall. Established methods for measurement of gastric function are gamma scintigraphy and radiological techniques for transit and manometry for contractile activity. All methods rely on either administration of radioisotopes or X-rays or intubation, making them invasive and uncomfortable for patients and of limited use in multiple studies. There is clearly scope for a hazard-free, noninvasive method of measuring simultaneous gastrintestinal transit and motility.

There have been considerable technical improvements in magnetic resonance imaging in recent years [1] and it has now become an established diagnostic tool in clinical medicine. The method has been further developed to produce snapshot images of the gastrointestinal (GI) tract in real time using the ultrafast

* Address for correspondence: Department of Surgery, Floor E West, University Hospital, Clifton Boulevard, Nottingham NG7 2UH, UK.

imaging technique MBEST (modulus blipped echo-planar single-pulse technique) [2] and its accuracy validated against manometric techniques [3].

We have further developed the method to monitor gastric emptying and motility following solid and liquid test meals.

MATERIALS AND METHODS

Technique—EPI

Gastrointestinal images were obtained using a 0.52-T, purpose-built superconducting magnet incorporating the high-speed echo-planar imaging (EPI) technique MBEST in which 128×128 pixel images are collected in 128 ms. Signals from tissue with a short T_2 (gut wall) experience significant decay and appear dark, whereas free water (luminal content), with a long T_2, appear as a bright image. This technique, in conjunction with voluntary respiratory gating, produces images of organs with aperiodic motion which are free from movement artifact. Data sets consisting of 100 images with a sampling interval of 3 s were collected for the duration of the study.

Technique—Volume

A rapid multislice technique was used to image 20 adjacent, 10-mm-thick, transverse slices through the gastric region at a sampling interval of 128 ms. Following image reconstruction, the stomach was identified in each slice, and a region-of-interest analysis was used to measure the gastric volume. The slice volumes were then summated to produce a measure of total gastric volume. Volume measurements were made at 10-min (water) and 20-min (solid) intervals, enabling changes in gastric volume against time to be assessed throughout the study.

Technique—Motility

Antroduodenal motility was observed in each dataset comprising 100 images taken at 3-s intervals. Gastric wall movement was visually assessed in consecutive images by at least two observers. A fixed point on the image in the antropyloric region was used to measure the start of each contraction. The number of contractions passing this point was counted and the frequency of contractions occurring within each dataset calculated.

SUBJECTS AND PROTOCOL

Eight normal male volunteers with no history of GI disease were imaged for up to 6 h in the supine position following the ingestion of 800 ml water followed by 500 ml porridge plus 500 ml water. Volume measurements were alternated with those of motility with the time between imaging spent seated outside the scanner. In three subjects, a prokinetic agent (20 mg Cisapride) was administered during the feed period.

RESULTS

Echo-planar imaging (EPI) was clearly able to differentiate between the liquid and solid components of a test meal (Fig. 1). The gastric emptying of water followed an exponential pattern with 50% of the stomach contents ($T_{1/2}$) emptying in 12.9 (±2.27 SE) min. The emptying of the solid meal was longer with a $T_{1/2}$ of 100 (±13.17) min. These results were found to be in agreement with similar studies using the traditional techniques of gamma scintigraphy and electrical impedance tomography (Fig. 2).

Gastric contractile activity was present in all subjects following feeding. The frequency of contractions following water increased from 2.37 (±0.06) contractions per minute (cpm) to a maximum of 3.22 (±0.08) cpm 40 min later. Similar increases were seen following porridge: from 2.85 (±0.04) cpm to a maximum of 3.24 (±0.08) cpm at 60 min.

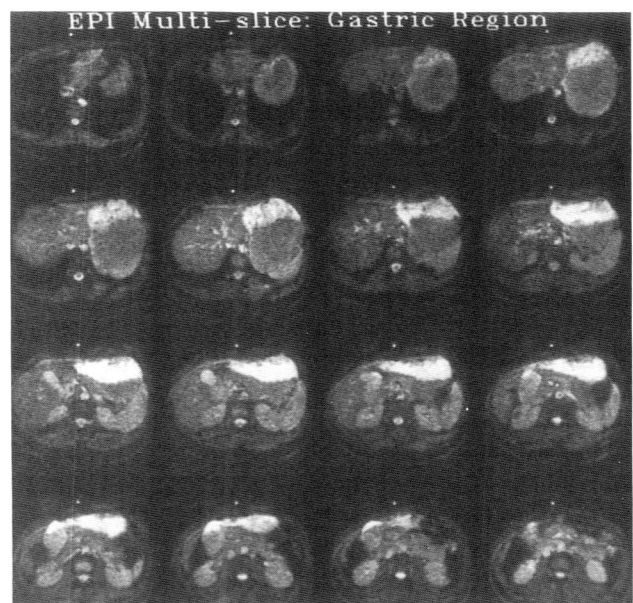

Fig. 1. Sequential, transverse MBEST images of the gastric region taken at 128-ms intervals. The bright image of the water can be clearly seen as a layer on top of the darker porridge image.

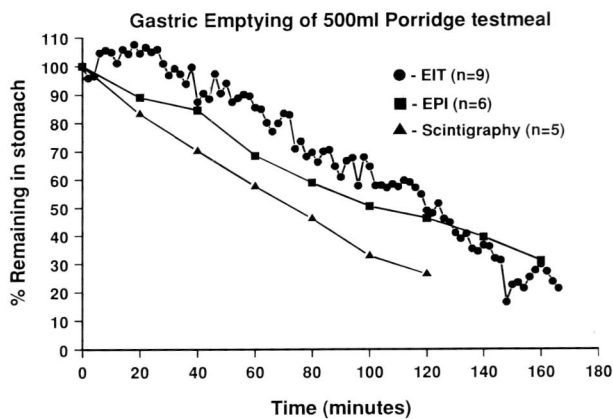

Fig. 2. Gastric emptying curve of a 500-ml porridge test meal highlighting the comparability of results obtained with echo-planar imaging, electrical impedance tomography, and gamma scintigraphy.

Cisapride had no effect on the frequency of gastric contractions, but it did, however, increase antroduodenal coordination, with 97% of contractions propagating from the antrum to the duodenum as compared to control values of 75% following food.

CONCLUSIONS

These studies have demonstrated that EPI can be used to detect and image gastro-duodenal function in man, totally noninvasively, and can be used to study the effects of food and drugs acting on the gastrointestinal tract. The gastric emptying $T_{1/2}$ times measured by EPI compared well with those reported by other methods,

and the images produced clearly showed the distinction between the solid and liquid phases of the test meal, highlighting the layering of water on top of the solid component. Frequency changes in gastric contractile activity following mixed test meals have previously been detected by ultrasound [4] and electrogastrography [5]. EPI while confirming these results has, in addition, demonstrated an increase in coordination of antro-duodenal contractions following prokinetic administration. We believe this technique will help to improve our understanding of the gastrointestinal motility and may be of use in the future for investigation of patients with motility disorders.

REFERENCES

1. Mansfield P (1988) Imaging by nuclear magnetic resonance. *J Phys E Sci Instrum* **21:** 18–30.
2. Stehling MK, Evans DF, Lamont G, Ordidge RJ, Howseman AM, Chapman B, Coxon R, Mansfield P, Hardcastle JD, Coupland RE (1989) Gastrointestinal tract: Dynamic MR studies with echo-planar imaging. *Radiology* **171:** 41–46.
3. Evans DF, Wright JW, Gowland P, Mansfield P (1993) Validation of antro-duodenal motility and gastric emptying by echo planar magnetic resonance imaging. *Gut* **34**(Suppl 1): S54.
4. Brown BP, Schulze-Delrieh S, Schrier JE, Abu-Yousef MM (1993) The configuration of the human gastroduodenal junction in the separate emptying of liquids and solids. *Gastroenterology* **105:** 433–440.
5. Geldof H, van der Schee EJ, van Blankenstein M, Grashuis JL (1986) Electrogastrographic study of gastric myoelectrical activity in patients with unexplained nausea and vomiting. *Gut* **27:** 799–808.

Measurement of GI water content using EPI at 0.5 tesla

J. Hykin,[1] A. Freeman,[1] P. Gowland,[1] R. Bowtell,[1] B. Worthington,[2] R. Spiller,[3] and P. Mansfield[1]*

[1]Magnetic Resonance Centre and Departments of [2]Radiology and [3]Medicine, Nottingham University, Nottingham NG7 2RD, UK

Recent work has shown that echo-planar magnetic resonance imaging has the potential to become a useful tool in the assessment of gastrointestinal (GI) tract motility, gastric emptying, and food rheology. This work extends this role to the measurement of water absorption in the GI tract, an important clinical measure. Currently, this involves intestinal intubation and considerable discomfort. By using multislice echo-planar magnetic resonance imaging, we can acquire a set of images covering the whole abdominal cavity in under 30 s. By suitable scaling of the pixel intensities in the small bowel and by planimetry of the areas of water in the stomach it is possible to estimate the total volume of water in the GI tract. By comparing the amount of water lost by the stomach and the amount gained by the small bowel following a test meal it is then possible to create water absorption curves. Using this method, we have shown a difference in water absorption for various solutions (water, mannitol solution, and normal saline). In addition, by assuming very slow water absorption from saline we have been able to asses the errors in this technique to be approximately 8–30%. This work, which describes the first noninvasive measure of gastrointestinal water absorption, will give important insights into clinical malabsorption states and help in the development of more effective oral rehydration therapies.

Keywords: echo-planar MRI, GI water absorption.

INTRODUCTION

We have shown previously that echo-planar imaging (EPI) is a useful tool in the assessment of gastrointestinal (GI) physiology [1, 2]. This early work on motility has been recently extended to the assessment of the effect of prokinetic drugs on GI motility and gastric emptying rates and in the investigation of the rheology of gastric contents [3]. In this article, we extend the role of gastrointestinal EPI to the measurement of GI water content.

The measurement of the rate of water absorption from the GI tract is important clinically, for example, in malabsorption states, inflammatory bowel disease, and the design of oral rehydration therapy solutions. In particular, in cases of dehydration following infective gastroenteritis, a common cause of morbidity and mortality in children worldwide, the need for fast effective water absorption from oral rehydration solutions is essential. The ideal composition of these solutions, is however, still a matter of much debate [4].

Current methods of investigating GI water absorption involve either resected animal gut segments or intubation studies. These studies are invasive and nonphysiologic and have limited relevance to the intact complete GI tract *in vivo* because they measure absorption from a small part of the bowel only, not the entire GI tract. An accurate and noninvasive method for measuring water absorption by the whole GI tract from various solutions and in various disease states is, therefore, required. The results of this pilot study suggest that EPI of the GI tract may fulfill this role.

AIMS

The aim of this study was to asses the potential of EPI to accurately determine the content of GI water and to quantify the error in this measurement.

Correspondence and reprint requests to: Sir Peter Mansfield, Magnetic Resonance Centre, University of Nottingham, Nottingham, NG7 2RD.

METHOD

Three test meals were chosen. These were 1 L each of pure water, saline (0.9% w/v), and mannitol solution (50 g L^{-1}). These solutions were chosen because they are known to have a wide spectrum of differing water absorption profiles.

All images were obtained on a dedicated EPI scanner at 0.5 T. All EPI scans were obtained using the MBEST sequence [5]. An effective gradient echo time of 32 ms was used. By using multislice acquisition a volume data set covering the complete GI tract was obtained in under 30 s. Imaging was performed immediately before the meal and then at 2-min intervals for the following 20 min.

The first step in the estimation of water content is to extract pixels containing water from pixels containing GI tissue. This was carried out in two ways:

1. The images were regioned manually to remove major organs and vessels
2. The remaining image was thresholded above a level chosen to exclude pixels with low signal from intestinal gas and from short T_2^* tissues, for example, muscle, fibrous tissue, and fat, assuming that these pixels contained no water.

It was assumed, therefore, that the remaining pixels contained only water and the signal intensity was directly proportional to the water content. A reference phantom was used to determine the maximum intensity (I_{max}) of a pixel corresponding to 100% water; thus, for n pixels with intensity I_n, the total GI water content V_{tot} is given by

$$V_{tot} = \frac{V_p}{I_{max}} \sum_{i=1}^{n} I_i$$

where V_p is the pixel volume.

The content of water in the stomach was measured using regioning and area summation [6]. In this way, following test meal solutions, it was possible to measure the water lost by the stomach and the water gained by the small bowel during an interval of time; by comparing these values, it was possible to estimate the water absorbed during this time. By repeating these measurements at 2-min intervals, water absorption curves were created.

RESULTS

The water absorption curves for the three test solutions are shown in Fig 1. The results are in close agreement with those from the literature with pure

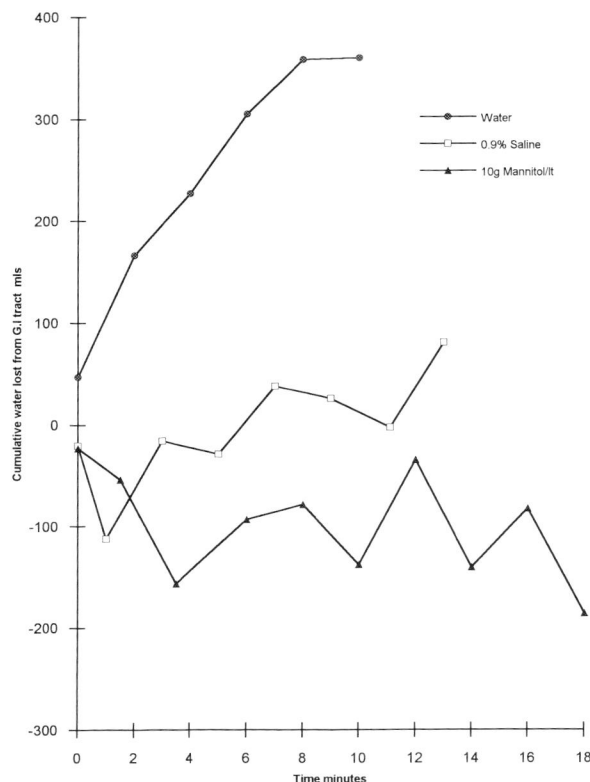

Fig. 1. Graph showing water absorption curves for three different test meal solutions measured using EPI of the GI tract.

water showing fast water absorption. Saline showing little or no absorption due to its isotonicity and mannitol showing negative absorption, that is, it draws water into the gut, due to its hypertonicity and low sodium content.

It can be assumed that for the period of the experiment (20 min) the absorption of water from saline is negligible. The difference between water lost from the stomach and that gained by the small bowel can, therefore, be used as an assessment of the error in the technique. The mean error was −10 ml and the standard deviation of the errors was 65 ml. This represents a percentage error of between 8% and 30% depending on the total volume of GI water.

CONCLUSIONS

This study represents the first use of magnetic resonance imaging to measure water absorption from the GI tract. The results of this pilot study suggest that this technique appears reliable in demonstrating differences between water absorption profiles from different solutions.

The errors in this technique are due to inadequate differentiation between GI water and GI tissue. This may be improved by optimising the echo time or by varying the T_1 contrast using inversion recovery EPI.

ACKNOWLEDGMENTS

We should like to thank the Medical Research Council for funding the 0.5-T EPI program.

REFERENCES

1. Stehling M, Evans D, Lamont G, Ordidge R, Howseman A, Chapman B, Coxon R, Mansfield P, Hardcastle J, Coupland R (1989) Gastrointestinal tract: Dynamic MR studies with echo-planar imaging. *Radiology* **171**(1): 41–46.
2. Evans D, Lamont G, Stehling M, Blamire A, Gibbs P, Coxon R, Hardcastle J, Mansfield P (1993) Prolonged monitoring of the upper GI tract using echo-planar MRI. *Gut* **34**: 848–852.
3. Wright J, Freeman A, Adams V, Hykin J, Gowland P, Harvey P, Evans D, Mansfield P (1994) Gastric emptying, motility and flow measured by echo-planar MRI. *Gut* (in press).
4. Carpenter C, Greenough W, Pierce N (1988) Oral rehydration therapies: the role of polymeric substrates. *New Engl J Med* **319**: 1346–1348.
5. Howseman AM, Stehling MK, Chapman B, Coxon R, Turner R, Ordidge RJ, Cawley MG, Glover P, Mansfield P, Coupland RE (1988) Improvements in snapshot NMR imaging. *Br J Radiol* **61**: 822–828.

ABSTRACTS OF INVITED PAPERS

P02

Functional magnetic resonance imaging (fMRI) of the brain

T.J. BRADY

Massachusetts General Hospital, NMR Center, Charlesworth, Massachusetts, USA

It is well known from anatomical, physiological, and cognitive studies that the brain possesses anatomically distinct processing regions. During cognitive psychological testing, regional alterations in neuronal activity induces local changes in cerebral metabolism and blood flow, which can be used to map the functional foci of mental activity. Similarly, changes in metabolism and blood flow frequently accompany pathological processes involving the brain.

The initial fMRI approach used exogenously administered contrast agents (e.g., Gd-DTPA), together with EPI, to evaluate its time course and regional distribution through the entire brain. Studies have demonstrated that fMRI blood volume mapping is useful in the classification of gliomas, in selecting biopsy sites; in separating radiation necrosis from recurrent tumor, and in the planning of radiotherapy and has applications in patients with cerebrovascular disease and dementia.

The second approach uses the body's own contrast agent, deoxyhemoglobin. Increased blood flow with much smaller increases in oxygen utilization results in a higher oxygen content of the capillary and venous blood. As the blood oxygen level increases, the endogenous susceptibility effect of deoxyhemoglobin is reduced, resulting in an increase in MR signal in the brain regions with increased flow. This effect is small, $\sim 2\%$ at 1.5 T, but increases at larger magnetic field, $\sim 7\%$ at 4.0 T. Also, the effect is influenced by the vessel size and pulse sequence with spin-echo sequences selectively sensitive to the microvasculature. This technique is used worldwide for a variety of task-activation paradigms including primary sensory-motor and higher-order studies and is being applied clinically both in psychiatry and operative planning in neurosurgery. Using EPI, hemodynamic changes associated with brain activity can be measured at a temporal resolution of ~ 100 ms per two-dimensional image. The latency of the hemodynamic response sets the ultimate limit on temporal resolution of this method.

C11

Turboflash (TF) sequence optimization for pulmonary parenchymal MRI

A. MOODY, S. BOLTON and M. HORSFIELD

Department of Radiology, University of Leicester, Leicester Royal Infirmary, Leicester LE8 OGG, UK

Introduction: Pulmonary MRI is made difficult by low proton density, high susceptibility effects, and respiratory and cardiac motion. The purpose of this study was to optimize a breath-held gradient-echo technique for imaging lung parenchyma.

Method: Scans were performed using a Siemens 1-T imager with a 50-cm body coil and 10-mT m^{-1} gradients. Comparison was made between a magnetization-prepared turbo-FLASH (TR/TE/FA: 8/4/15 or 4/2/15), a short TE spin-echo (1000/10/90), and a FLASH (10/4/15) sequences. Five normal volunteers were scanned. A single slice was obtained in inspiration, expiration, and suspended respiration. Slice thickness was varied between 10, 15, and 20 mm. The S/N was calculated for each slice. Respiratory and cardiac motion artifact and detection of vessels and airways were scored for each sequence.

Results and discussion: Pulmonary signal improves with increasing proton density or reducing susceptibility effects. Susceptibility is decreased by reducing B_0, TE, or the alveolar–air interfaces within the lung. Reducing TE from 4 to 2 ms doubled the lung S/N using the TF sequence. The signal was further raised by increasing the acquisitions and slice thickness. Full lung expansion produced a marked S/N decrease (inspiratory image S/N < 1). The TF sequence demonstrated the expected antero-posterior increase in signal intensity. Combining these optimized factors produced a S/N of 8.8 compared with 10.9 for the SE sequence. The FLASH sequence had signal similar to TF but was degraded by cardiac motion. The TF sequence was unaffected motion. Vessels were seen to the mid-third of the lung, but airways were poorly seen.

Conclusion: Despite using a gradient-echo technique, a useful signal can be obtained from the lung when TF sequences are optimized. The ability to visualize the lung of altered aeration and density suggests this sequence will be useful in detecting and characterizing pulmonary parenchymal disease with the added advantage of rapid breath-held acquisition and absence of motion artifact.

C12

MR cine imaging and velocity mapping of complications following surgery for transposition of the great arteries

C. SAMPSON, P. KILNER, R. HIRSCH, S. REES, J. SOMERVILLE, and R. UNDERWOOD
MRI Unit and Grown Up Congenital Heart Unit, Royal Brompton Hospital. London, UK

MRI spin-echo and short-echo (TE6) gradient-echo sequences with velocity mapping were used for the detection of obstruction of the veno-atrial pathways and Baffle leak which are late complications following Mustard's operation for transposition of the great arteries. The findings were compared with other imaging methods.

Twenty-one patients were studied by MRI: 20 had transthoracic echocardiography (TTE), 19 had X-ray angiocardiography, and 5 had transesophageal echocardiography (TOE).

MRI found no obstruction in nine patients. This was confirmed by angiocardiography in seven and postmortem examination in 1. In one case, MRI demonstrated a leak at the baffle suture line.

In 12 studies in which MRI reported obstruction of the veno-atrial pathways, 9 were confirmed by angiocardiography or surgery. There were two false positive MRI studies, one false negative angiocardiogram, and one case in which there was no conclusion. Nine of the 20 TTE studies were inconclusive.

We conclude that with the addition of gradient-echo cine imaging and velocity mapping to spin-echo imaging, MRI is an important noninvasive method of investigating late complications following Mustard's operation.

C50

BMS 180549: a new superparamagnetic iron oxide MR contrast agent

S.J. McLACHLAN and M. MORRIS
Squibb Diagnostics, Princeton, New Jersey, USA

BMS 180549 is a new MR contrast agent consisting of biodegradable superparamagnetic iron oxide particles coated with a low-molecular-weight dextran. These particles have an iron oxide core of 4–6 nm and an overall particle size of 17–21 nm. The relaxivity of BMS 180549, measured at 39°C and 20 MHz, are $R1 = 24.5$ $(\text{nM s})^{-1}$ and $R2 = 52$ $(\text{nM s})^{-1}$. Preclinical animal studies have shown T_1 and T_2 enhancing properties of this agent. In addition, this agent has a long blood half-life (> 200 min) and is eventually taken up by elements of the reticuloendothelial system including lymph nodes.

Clinical studies confirm the unique biodistribution of BMS 180549. Early imaging, within 60 min of drug administration, provides enhancement of the vasculature and well-perfused organs. Late imaging, 24 h after drug administration, shows enhancement of lymph nodes.

This contribution will present preliminary results of the clinical evaluation of this agent and its biodistribution and imaging properties.

Magnetic resonance functional imaging of the brain at 4 T

R. Turner[1]* and P. Jezzard[2]

[1]*Institute of Neurology, Queen Square, London, UK*
[2]*National Institutes of Health, Bethesda, MD, USA*

Blood Oxygenation Level Dependent (BOLD) contrast imaging of human brain function using echo-planar imaging at 4 T gives good freedom from motion artifact, high signal-to-noise ratio/unit time, and adequate spatial resolution. Studies were made of brain activation associated with perceptual and cognitive tasks of several minutes duration.

Several cortical areas show task-dependent activity consistent across subjects, in images with a spatial resolution of 2.5 mm $\times$ 2.5 mm $\times$ 5 mm and a temporal resolution of up to 1 s. Multislice data were obtained at a rate of up to five slices per second. At 4 T, fractional changes of magnetic resonance (MR) image intensity up to 25% were observed.

Novel cross-correlation methods, including the effect of the temporal point-spread function associated with the relatively slow hemodynamic response of the brain, allow activation maps of the brain to be generated with statistically meaningful thresholds.

With appropriate data analysis, it is clear that oxygenation changes in large draining veins distant from active neural tissue do not dominate the changes observed, especially when brain tasks activating only a limited volume of gray matter are chosen. This is consistent with downstream dilution of blood oxygenation changes and direct optical observations of functional brain activity in animals.

Keywords: brain mapping, functional MRI, BOLD contrast, 4 Tesla, EPI.

INTRODUCTION

The brain is the most complicated organ in the body, in terms of significant anatomy at every distance scale above 5 μ. On computer tomography (CT) scans and conventional MRI scans much of the functional specificity of regions of the brain is not apparent. Typical image segmentation algorithms partition magnetic resonance (MR) images of brain tissue into gray and white matter, and perhaps basal ganglia. Although they perform widely differing tasks, cortical regions cannot be distinguished by image intensity in anatomical scans, except for striate visual cortex [1], and their specific physiological role is normally deduced from location. Common landmarks can be identified fairly easily in most human brains, such as the Sylvian fissure (separating the frontal and temporal lobes), the calcarine fissure (housing the primary visual cortex), and the central sulcus (separating the primary motor and somatosensory cortices). It is only on the level of cellular architecture that obvious differences can be observed, using optical microscopy, between regions of gray matter serving different purposes, as studied by Brodmann [2] and subsequent researchers [3]. Even at this level it can be very difficult to characterize cytoarchitectural differences precisely [4], and, of course, it is not possible to perform this kind of study on living human subjects. What these studies reveal [3] is that the cortical folding pattern, into gyri and sulci, is by no means an infallible guide to the location of cytoarchitectonically different, and thus by inference functionally different, regions.

One of the major goals of neuroscience is to understand the cortical division of labor. What are the primary functions subserved by particular groups of neurons, and how are these disparate groups recruited, coordinated, and reorganized in the performance of more complex brain operations? Pursuit of this goal has led to the development of a number of techniques for functional brain mapping, including positron emission tomography (PET), single-photon emission tomography (SPET), electroencephalogra-

---

* Address for Correspondence: RCS Biophysics Unit, Institute of Child Health, 30 Guildford Street, London WC1N 1EH, UK.

phy (EEG), and magnetoencephalography (MEG). Without going into technical details, it is enough to say that each of these techniques has clearly defined intrinsic limitations. Dosage restrictions on the radio-isotopes used in PET and SPET and geometrical factors regarding the arrangement of particle detectors limit their spatial resolution to about 125 mm^3. Even with recent technical advances (e.g., Ref. 5) no more than about six PET scans can be performed on a single subject at any one time, and longitudinal studies require long interscan periods of six months or more. Temporal resolution, determined by the isotope half-life, is on the order of minutes.

MEG and EEG are far less invasive than PET, relying only on the residual electric or magnetic fields which can be detected outside the skull resulting from coherent neural activity taking place in a well-defined cortical region. Temporal resolution is excellent, to about 10 ms or less. Repeated single-subject studies are easy to perform. However, spatial resolution is extremely poor, except for tasks in which it is known that only a very small number of small cortical areas are active (e.g., Ref. 6). In general, the inverse problem has no solution; any observed electric or magnetic field configuration observed on the scalp can be accounted for by an infinite number of intracranial current sources.

Thus, the new techniques [7–10] of magnetic resonance functional neuroimaging (MRFN), which promise spatial resolution better than 10 mm^3, temporal resolution of 1 s, and the possibility of exhaustive single-subject studies, have aroused intense interest among neuroscientists. This article will discuss the MRI method that appears to allow the most rapid volumetric imaging of brain function, with the greatest freedom from distributed motion artifact, and the most sizable and robust image intensity changes directly associated with regional neural activity. The technique in question is echo-planar imaging (EPI), proposed by Mansfield [11]. Most of the work described here has been performed at the unusually high static magnetic field of 4 T, 2.7 times larger than the common commercial MRI field strength of 1.5 T. This has advantages and difficulties, which will be analyzed in some detail.

BOLD CONTRAST

For several years, contrast-enhanced MRI scans have been performed with the aid of a paramagnetic intravascular contrast agent, Gd-DTPA, which is injected into a leg vein and gives rise to enhancement in

T_1-weighted scans in regions of compromised blood-brain barrier and loss of signal in T_2- or T_2^*-weighted scans. If injected as a rapid bolus and imaged with a rapid imaging technique, with image acquisition time of 2 s or less, its first-pass passage through the brain can be monitored and relative blood volume maps can be calculated, showing areas of higher blood volume associated with regional functional activity [12]. It was the work of Ogawa [13] and Turner [14], drawing on earlier studies by Thulborn [15] and Brooks [16], which demonstrated that deoxygenated blood itself could function as a natural MRI paramagnetic contrast agent. Initial studies were made on animal models, in which the arterial oxygenation could be manipulated by respiratory challenges [14] or the venous oxygenation by changing levels of glycemia [13]. Gradient-echo MRI images showed a loss of signal in tissue surrounding vessels, the time course of which could be monitored [14]. Further studies with a feline model, where hemoglobin oxygen saturation was independently measured via a cranial window by optical methods [17] while MRI acquisition was taking place during a respiratory challenge, suggested that the change of signal (expressed as a change of T_2^* relaxation rate) was proportional to the change in total deoxyhaemoglobin in the image voxel.

Meanwhile Kwong [7] succeeded in showing, using a 1.5-T MRI system, that when human volunteers were given visual stimulation, the gradient-echo MRI signal in the primary visual cortex increased in amplitude. This corresponds to a relative decrease in tissue deoxyhemoglobin content, consistent with the work of Fox and Raichle [18], who showed using PET that oxygen uptake during regional brain activation was proportionately much less than the increase of blood flow, which would result in dilution of deoxyhemoglobin. Frostig et al. [19], using far-red micrography of cat and monkey visual cortex via cranial windows, also demonstrated a decrease of deoxyhemoglobin within a few seconds of the onset of visual stimulation.

Results similar to those of Kwong et al. were shown by Ogawa et al. [8], using a somewhat different MRI acquisition sequence but still sensitive to T_2^* contrast. This group used the very high-MRI field of 4 T and were rewarded by the observation of much larger signal changes associated with functional activity of the visual cortex. A dependence on field strength which is at least linear is to be expected from an effect that depends on changes in susceptibility of blood [20, 21]. A direct comparison using the same volunteer, the same visual stimulus, and, as nearly as possible, the same region of interest was made by Turner et al. [22], between the field strengths of 1.5 T and 4 T, which showed a faster than linear increase in fractional change of signal with field.

MRI DATA ACQUISITION

Given the relative ease with which MR brain images can show functionally related changes in intensity in active cortex, the question arises, "What is the best field and type of data acquisition to use?" Here we must digress a little to discuss the principles of MRI data acquisition.

As is well known [23], MRI data is obtained by sampling the NMR signal from the object while the imposition of imaging gradients causes the sampling point to trace out a trajectory in a space corresponding to the diffraction pattern of the object, known as k-space and familiar in X-ray crystallography. Here the reciprocal space variable **k** is defined by

$$\mathbf{k} = \gamma \int_0^t \mathbf{G}(t') \, dt' \qquad (1)$$

where $\mathbf{G}(t)$ describes the magnetic field gradients imposed after radio-frequency (RF) excitation of the nuclear spins and γ is the magnetogyric ratio. The entirety of a region of this space centered about the origin must be sampled in order to provide an accurate image of the selected slice of the object when the data have been Fourier transformed. The crucial insight was provided by Mansfield [11], who realized that the entire space could be adequately sampled following only one RF excitation pulse, provided that the magnetic field gradients creating the sampling trajectory could be switched rapidly enough and with sufficient magnitude. It then became possible to consider intermediate strategies for sampling k-space in several segments and to analyze the comparative efficiency of various such methods.

There is some divergence of opinion regarding nomenclature. As originally conceived, the term "echo-planar imaging" (EPI) should apply strictly to techniques where a series of gradient reversals leads to the formation of a number of gradient echoes. However, by a simple extension, it can equally apply to any other method of scanning k-space in one pass following a single RF excitation, such as spiral scanning [23, 24]. By another extension, it has been applied to segmented or interleaved trajectories in k-space—MESH, MOSAIC [25], Interleaved Gradient-echo Echo-Planar Imaging (IGEPI) [26]. The common feature in all these methods of MRI data acquisition is the traversal of an area, rather than a line, of k-space for each RF excitation. Thus, Gradient And Spin Echo (GRASE) [27], in which, after an initial 90° RF excita-

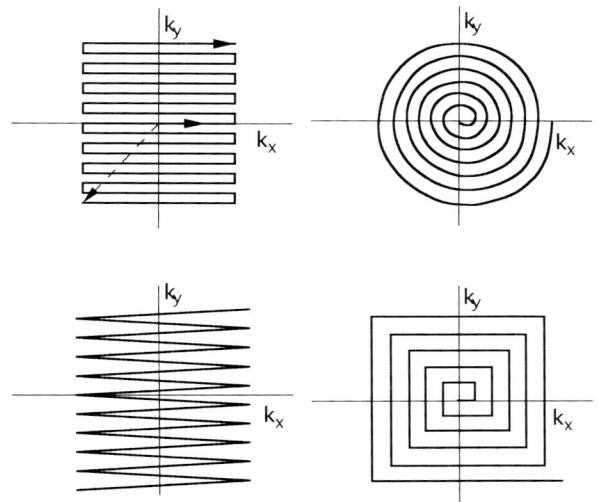

Fig. 1. Varieties of trajectories covering k-space after a single RF excitation.

tion pulse, 180° refocusing pulses are separated by several read gradient reversals, can also be described as a type of EPI. Fig. 1 shows a number of possible trajectories in k-space involving relatively simple gradient switching sequences, and Fig. 2 shows typical EPI sequences.

The chief advantages of EPI, as compared with MRI methods acquiring only a line of data in k-space for each RF excitation pulse, are speed of acquisition [28] and comparatively good signal-to-noise ratio (S/N). For the same receiver bandwidth, EPI is inherently faster than Fast Low-Angle SHOT (FLASH) or Gradient-echo Acquisition in Steady-State (GRASS) because there is no need to perform a fresh RF excitation, with slice selection and refocusing gradients, between acquisitions of each line of k-space. Furthermore, for an EPI image repeat time as short as 1 s most of the object's nuclear magnetization is available for each RF pulse, whereas for this image acquisition time, a flip angle of less than 10°, exciting less than 20% of the total magnetization, is optimal for FLASH or GRASS. The comparison with low-angle RF pulse methods becomes even more favorable to EPI in collection of volume data. EPI can obtain 10 slices per second, with 128 × 128 pixel resolution, whereas 3D low-flip-angle methods struggle to obtain 32 slices in 20 s. The lower S/N of EPI in this case can be compensated easily by image averaging if need be. A further option, 3D EPI, in which a thick slice is selected and a phase encode gradient is applied in the slice select direction [25], offers both good S/N and rapid image acquisition, at the cost of no longer truly being a single-shot technique.

a) Gradient-echo EPI sequence

b) Spin-echo EPI sequence

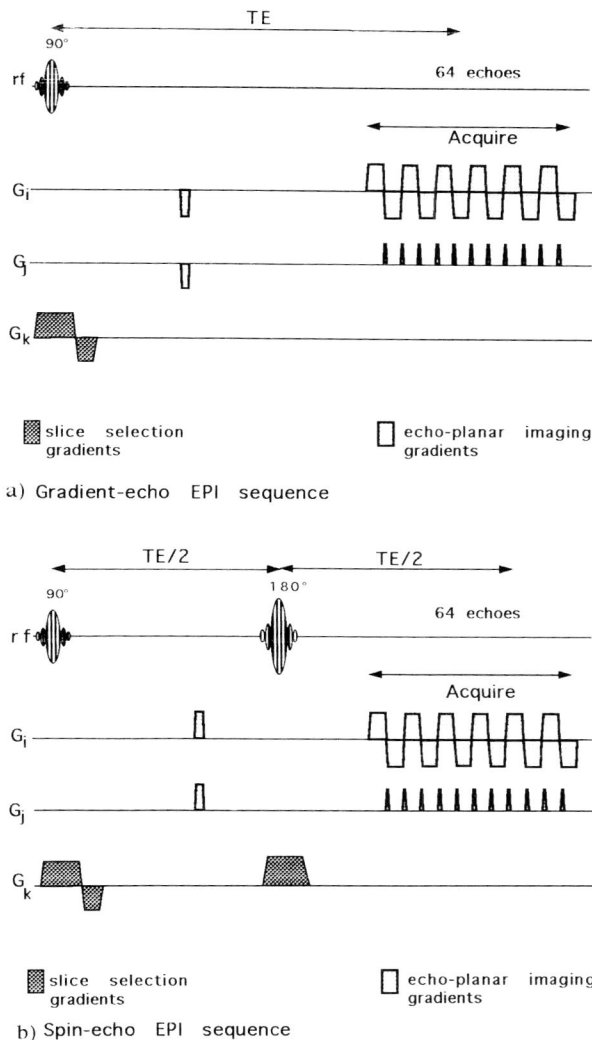

Fig. 2. Spin-echo and gradient-echo EPI sequence diagrams.

Why is it beneficial to use single-shot MRI? Even in the brain, pulsations due to cardiac and respiratory cycles, and small involuntary head motion, can result in a distributed incoherent image ghost in the phase-encode direction, of sufficient magnitude to swamp the small image intensity changes resulting from blood oxygenation changes. Although it is possible to minimize motion artifact in low-flip-angle acquisition using motion-compensated gradients, out-of-slice motion still presents a major problem. With an EPI acquisition lasting only 40–100 ms, motion-related ghosting is never observed in the brain.

One potential disadvantage of EPI is the limited spatial resolution found with crude implementations of the technique, rarely better than 2 mm in-plane. For some neuroscientific purposes a much higher resolution would be desirable. However, for reasons to be discussed below, the nature of BOLD contrast itself may prevent a higher resolution from being obtainable.

EPI AT 4 T

Compared with other MRI methods, EPI is particularly sensitive to static field inhomogeneity. The period during which data are acquired following each RF pulse is up to 128 times longer, giving nuclear spins much more time to precess at different rates in a nonuniform field, resulting in signal loss, image distortion, and increased likelihood of severe image artifact in the form of the familiar "Nyquist" ghost halfway across the field of view (FOV) from the desired image. The first two of these image defects originate in an obvious way, but the third requires further explanation. Because the most common form of EPI (Fig. 1a) collects data while the trajectory moves in alternate directions across k-space, image processing involves an initial step of time reversal of alternate echoes. This causes the echoes to become paired up in time unless they are already equally spaced and the points about which they are time-reversed are correctly chosen. If there is severe field inhomogeneity, the echo-spacing is not consistent during the acquisition and it is not possible to find points about which to time-reverse alternate echoes correctly. The residual nonuniform pairing of echoes results in the Nyquist ghost after the data are Fourier transformed to form the image.

Unfortunately, field inhomogeneities due to variations in the magnetic susceptibility of the object, such as those around the nasal sinuses and petrous bone in the human head, have an increasingly important effect as the static field increases. If proportionately larger imaging gradients could be used, this would have no serious consequences, but the strength of the imaging gradients is dictated by gradient amplifier and coil limitations, by digitizer bandwidth limits, by the fact that too large a field will cause peripheral neural stimulation when rapidly switched [28], and by loss of S/N as receiver bandwidth is increased. (In practice, if a head gradient coil is used which restricts the gradients to the region of the head, a gradient of 40 mT-m^{-1} may be switched in 100 μs without complications.) Thus, it has been found, even at fields of 3 T, that regions of the brain close to the sinuses, such as the limbic system and the lower temporal lobe, are not well visualized in echo-planar images. At 4-T EPI image drop-out, distortion and ghosting in these regions are severe and slices of the brain where it is otherwise of good field homogeneity, which pass through these regions, are also seriously compromised because of the local Nyquist ghost, which is often superimposed on a better part of the image. Use of segmented *k*-space EPI, which has not yet been widely exploited, may improve image quality at the expense of a greater risk of motion artifact.

EPI BOLD-CONTRAST IMAGING of BRAIN FUNCTION

Despite the difficulties just described in obtaining good image quality, it has been possible to perform EPI imaging of the human brain at 4 T. Experience was gained previously using animal models with GE Omega MRI systems [29, 30] at 2.0 T and 4.7 T, and the EPI sequences developed by Turner and Sukumar were easily transferred to the GE/Bruker Omega MRI console driving the 4.0-T whole-body MRI system at the National Institutes of Health. With the aid of a *z*-axis local gradient coil providing up to 42 mT-m^{-1}, driven by a series pair of 100-A Techron gradient power supplies, coronal and sagittal EPI images with FOV of as little as 12 cm with 64 × 64-pixel resolution, were obtained with a total acquisition time of 41 ms. Generally, the FOV was 16 cm and slice thickness 5 mm. For most studies a gradient-echo EPI sequence was used, with effective TE of 25 ms. An RF trasmit/ receive surface coil was used, as it proved impossible to install a whole-head RF coil inside the local gradient coil because of severe RF loading. With a 20-cm-diameter loop RF coil, about half of the brain could be imaged with adequate S/N, allowing studies of mid-line structures in sagittal views and visualization of the entire cerebellum in coronal views with the coil placed on the occiput.

Typically eight contiguous slices were obtained in each TR interval of 3–4 s, and 64 images were obtained of each slice image, giving experimental runs of 3–4 min. During this time, depending on the study, a variety of stimuli or tasks were presented to the subject, generally for 30 s at a time, interspersed by rest periods or contrasting stimuli/tasks. Visual stimuli were introduced either by the use of GRASS photic stimulator goggles, fitted with arrays of red LEDs with a controllable flicker rate, or with a video LCD projector, clad with thin steel to provide partial magnetic shielding for the mechanical fan within, which displayed video or computer images on a translucent screen mounted on the patient bed at the subject's feet.

The subjects' heads were immobilized using foam pads inserted firmly between the gradient coil and the sides of the head. Care was taken to ensure that the subject was comfortable and, thus, not inclined to move to relieve local pressure. Inspection of EPI data showed that in most cases movements of more than 1 mm were rare.

DATA ANALYSIS

The simplest method for characterizing local changes in image intensity which might be associated with cortical activity is to subtract images obtained during rest or a control task from images during the experimental task or stimulus. The image difference can be expressed as a percentage or fraction of the "rest" image. Commonly, areas of the image such as the large venous sinuses, which naturally have a large variance but show no intensity changes associated with brain activity, show up on such difference maps by chance. To filter out such regions it is simple to construct a "z-map" by dividing the difference between experimental image and control in each pixel by the standard deviation of that pixel, as determined from several control images obtained before any task or stimulus is begun [31, 32]. The z-map, suitably thresholded (usually at a value between 1 and 2), can be superimposed in color on a gray-scale reference image to give a plausible image of active cortical areas.

This ad hoc procedure, although often giving a good indication of which cortical areas might be changing in correlation with the task, has several pitfalls. The first is that the value of z thus calculated has little statistical significance, as it does not take into account the spatial and temporal smoothness of the data. The temporal smoothness is the major factor which requires a different approach—changes in BOLD contrast typically occur over about 10 s, corresponding to the hemodynamic response time in the brain and many fMRI studies use an image repetition time considerably shorter than this. Temporal and spatial smoothness can be given appropriate statistical treatment by correlating the time dependence of the signal in each pixel with a smoothed contrast function. This allows correctly thresholded activation maps to be generated [33].

A second pitfall is that artifact caused by misregistration of successive images, brought about by involuntary head motion or pulsatile brain motion, can easily masquerade as significant activation in z-maps. Normally, such an artifact is obvious, showing up as a double light and dark line along features with abrupt change in contrast, such as the edge of the brain. Most functional MRI (fMRI) researchers have carefully excluded images with such obvious artifact from further analysis, but in exceptional circumstances motion may be such as to selectively enhance a region which could be mistaken for activated cortex [34]. Robust, flexible, and computationally efficient algorithms (e.g., Ref. 35) are essential for retrieving data obviously flawed by such artifact, or even merely suspect.

DRAINING VEINS

A further potential source of artifact is the fact that changes in the oxygenation state of blood flowing through active neural regions will be passed on downstream to the veins draining the cortex. It has been shown by several authors [20, 36, 37] that with a gradient-echo sequence a given concentration of paramagnetic contrast agent in the blood will affect the MRI signal from surrounding tissue to a degree almost independent of vessel size. Observations by Haacke [38] and Menon [21] show activated regions, which look very like veins, in the same location as veins found on venograms. Direct observation of the surface of the brain during widespread seizure activity shows poorly mixed hyperoxygenated blood flowing alongside deoxygenated blood from inactive regions [39].

However, there are many fMRI observations that are very hard to explain in terms of large vessels. For instance, the retinotopic data of De Yoe et al. [40], and Tootell [41] indicate no major involvement of the calcarine vein downstream from the more anterior area activated by peripheral field visual stimulation. In sagittal images of the hand representation, activation appears only in slices 30–40 mm from the brain midline, and more medial activation, corresponding to the vein draining the central sulcus into the superior venous sinus, is never seen. Furthermore, because activity-dependent control of blood flow is localized to the arterioles supplying a given cortical region, it would be surprising to see changes far downstream in a large vessel, as the effects of oxygenation or flow changes in a small portion of the vasculature would surely be rapidly diluted.

The resolution of this problem comes from direct optical observation of localized blood oxygenation changes in experimental animals via a cranial window. Here, by using an appropriate light wavelength (605 nm), changes in hemoglobin saturation can be mapped with a spatial resolution of 5 μ and a temporal resolution of 200 ms [19]. Because the changes in the color of hemoglobin are caused by the same rearrangement of electrons on molecular energy levels which creates the susceptibility difference between oxyhemo-

globin and deoxyhemoglobin, the techniques are beautifully comparable. Preliminary results indicate that if the area of activated cortex is small, say 1 cm^2, the overlap of draining veins from this region is no more than about 2 mm.

RESULTS

A wide variety of sensory stimuli and cognitive tasks have been used successfully to elicit changes in BOLD contrast brain intensity in cortical regions that are broadly consistent with the earlier findings of PET and single-electrode recording. In this article we mention four experiments, for each of which at least four volunteer subjects have been studied. The data shown here had little or no misregistration artifact.

The first of these [22] is simple visual stimulation, applied with GRASS SV106 photic stimulator goggles, consisting of an array of red LEDs with a flicker rate of 16 Hz. Coronal echo-planar images through the occipital lobe were acquired at 3-s time intervals, and the goggles were switched on and off at 30-s intervals. The time course for a pixel adjacent to the calcarine sulcus is shown in Fig. 3. The smooth variation of signal intensity, with a rise time of about 10 s, is noticeable. Related experiments dealing with mental imagery have also been successful [30].

A second experiment [42] provided auditory stimulation in the form of a single musical note played repetitively at 1-s intervals for a period of 30 s, followed by 30 s rest, for three episodes. Despite the potential interference by the loud noise produced by the imaging gradients, discrete areas of the brain on the superior surface of the temporal lobe, corresponding to the auditory cortex, showed intensity changes well correlated with the stimulus, as shown in Fig. 4.

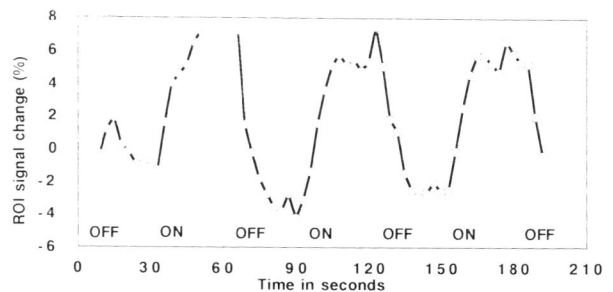

Fig. 3. Time course of the mean EPI intensity in a four-voxel ROI in the primary visual cortex of a volunteer experiencing photic stimulation. Field strength 4 T, TE 27 ms.

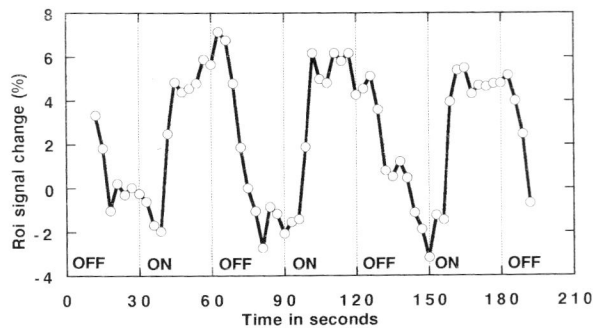

Fig. 4. Time course of the mean EPI intensity in a two-voxel ROI in the auditory cortex of a volunteer experiencing auditory stimulation. Field strength 4 T, TE 27 ms.

A further experiment, needing no presentation equipment, examined the response of the frontal and temporal cortex in a task requiring the subject to generate silently as many words as possible in a period of 30 s following a cue consisting of the initial letter [43]. The experimenter provided the initial letter aurally from the side of the subject's bed. Sagittal images of eight slices were obtained through the left side of the brain. The control task was either to imagine a night sky or to generate words automatically, for instance the days of the week. In either case, the result was the same, as shown in Fig. 5. Here the

active areas, shown in color on the original image, have been outlined for ease of identification. EPI difference image data were superimposed on a high-resolution Gradient-Recalled Echo (GRE) reference scan. The time course of activity in Broca's area is also shown. For this task, a complex functional network of cortical areas is apparently deployed, the components of which have not yet been fully identified.

Finally, a motor task was studied, in which the subject was required either to tap fingers successively to thumb or to remain passive while his fingertips were stroked lightly with gauze. Here the reference scan was itself an EPI image. Figure 6a shows the activated area for the passive stimulation, whereas Fig. 6b shows the response to the active motor task. An area deep in the central sulcus showing a highly significant difference between the two conditions can be identified with the M1 primary motor cortex driving the finger movement.

DISCUSSION

BOLD contrast functional MRI provides detailed visualizations of cortical areas responsible for many brain tasks. Other areas studied at the National Institutes of Health have been cerebellum (motor tasks), extrastri-

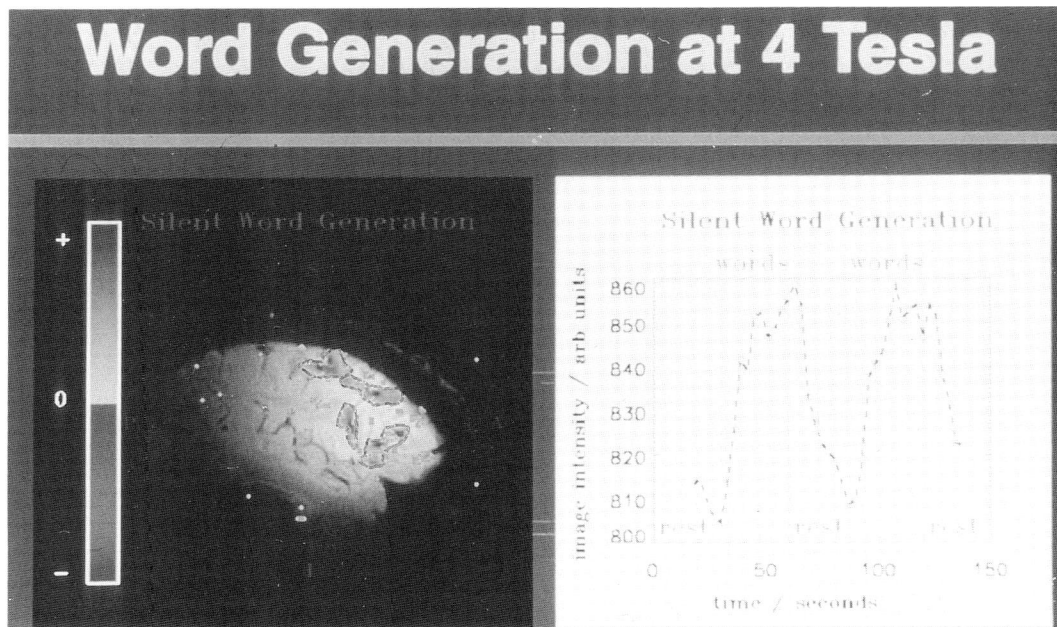

Fig. 5. Activation *z*-map of a sagittal slice 45 mm left of midline in a volunteer silently generating words. EPI data (64 × 64-pixel resolution) overlaid on high-resolution GRE reference scan (128 × 256-pixel resolution). Activated areas are outlined. Field strength 4 T, slice thickness 5 mm, TE 27 ms.

(a)

(b)

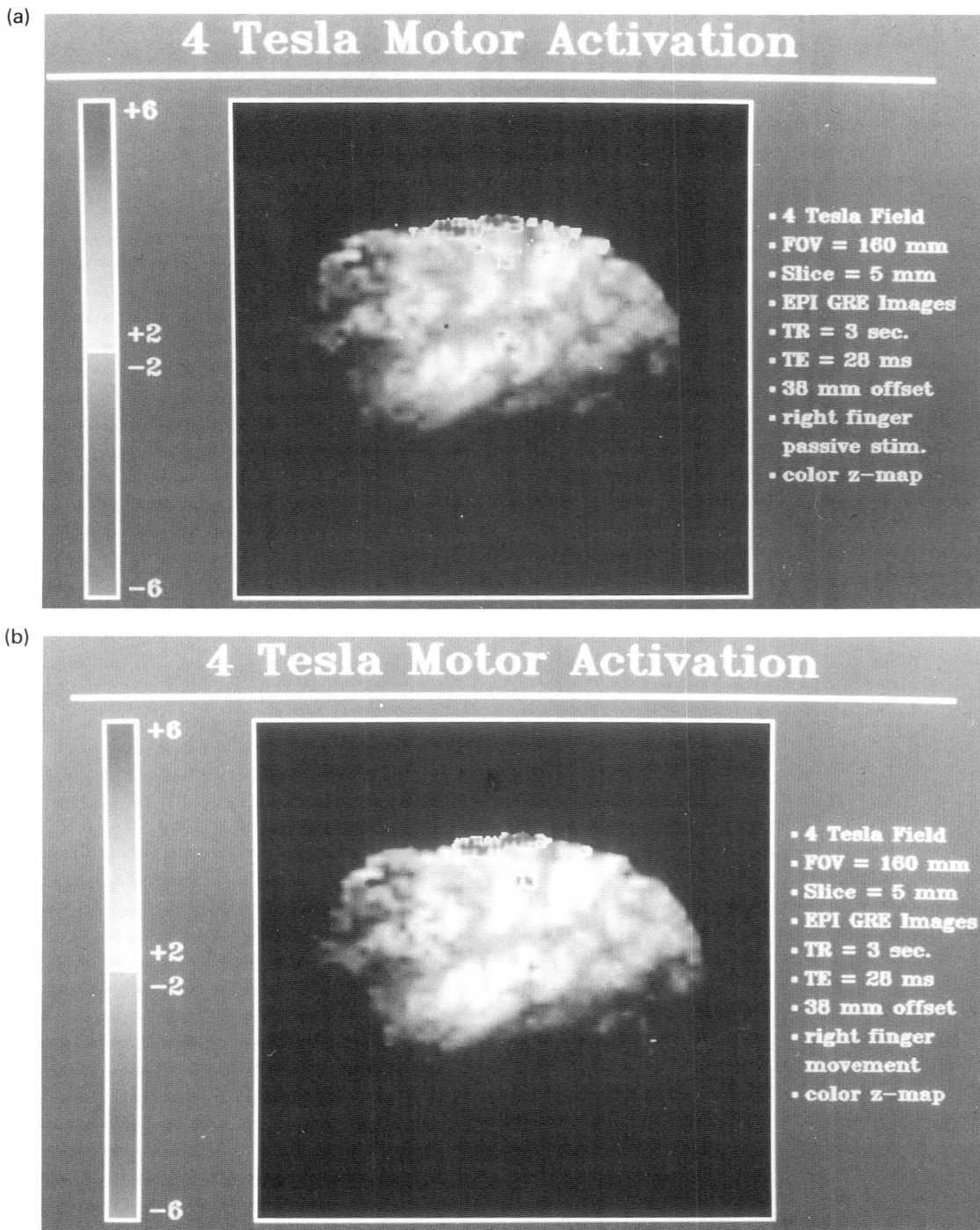

Fig. 6. (a) Activation *z*-map of a sagittal slice 35 mm left of midline in a volunteer experiencing passive finger stimulation. EPI *z*-score data overlaid on EPI reference scan. (b) Activation *z*-map (same experimental run) with volunteer actively tapping fingers to thumb. Field strength 4 T, slice thickness 5 mm, TE 27 ms.

ate cortex, somatotopy along the motor strip (from tongue to foot), supplementary motor area, and parietal cortex. For most of the tasks used, the areas of activation are not large, and contamination by large draining veins is not likely to be serious. Because of the high magnetic field used, the changes in signal are normally 5% or more, even for subtle cognitive tasks, whereas image S/N is often better than 200, offering a highly robust experimental situation. The major problem is image distortion and drop-out near the sinuses and petrous bone, which has prevented any serious attempts to seek activation in subcortical structures.

REFERENCES

1. Clark VP, Courchesne E, Grafe M (1992) In vivo myeloarchitectonic analysis of human striate and extrastriate cortex using magnetic resonance imaging. *Cerebral Cortex* **2**: 417–424.

2. Brodmann K (1909) *Vergleichende Lokalizationslehre der Grosshirnrinde in ihren Prinzipien dargestellt auf Grund des Zellenbaues.* Leipzig: Barth.

3. Rademacher J, Caviness VS, Steinmetz H, Galaburda AM (1993) Topographical variation of the human primary cortices: implications for neuroimaging, brain mapping, and neurobiology. *Cerebral Cortex* **3**: 313–329.

4. Chiavaras M, Petrides M, Pandya DN (1993) Cytoarchitectonic investigation of the human prefrontal cortex (Abstract). *Society for Neuroscience, Annual Meeting, Washington DC.* p. 1212.

5. Friston KJ, Frith CD, Liddle PF, Frackowiak RSJ (1993) Functional connectivity: the principal-component analysis of large PET data sets. *J Cereb Blood Flow Metab* **13**: 5–14.

6. Supek S, Aine CJ (1993) Simulation studies of multiple dipole neuromagnetic source localization: model order and limits of source resolution. *IEEE Trans Biomed Eng* **BE-40**: 529–540.

7. Kwong KK, Belliveau JW, Cheslar DA, Goldberg IE, Weisskoff RM, Poncelet BP, Kennedy DN, Hoppel BE, Cohen MS, Turner R, Cheng H-M, Brady TJ, Rosen BR (1992) Dynamic magnetic resonance imaging of human brain activity during primary sensory stimulation. *Proc Natl Acad USA* **89**: 5675–5679.

8. Ogawa S et al. (1992) Intrinsic signal changes accompanying sensory stimulation—functional brain mapping with magnetic resonance imaging. *Proc Natl Acad Sci USA* **89**: 5951–5955.

9. Bandettini PA et al. (1992) Time course EPI of human brain function during task activation. *Magn Reson Med* **25**: 390–397.

10. Turner R (1992) Magnetic resonance imaging of brain function. *Am J Physiol Imag* **3/4**: 136–145.

11. Mansfield P (1977) Multiplanar image formation using NMR spin echoes. *J Phys C* **10**: L55–L58.

12. Belliveau JW et al. (1991) Functional mapping of the human visual cortex by magnetic resonance imaging. *Science* **254**: 716–719.

13. Ogawa S, Lee T-M, Nayak AS, Glynn P (1990) Oxygenation-sensitive contrast in magnetic resonance image of rodent brain at high magnetic fields. *Magn Reson Med* **14**: 68–78.

14. Turner R, Le Bihan D, Moonen CTW, Despres D, Frank J (1991) Echo-planar time course MRI of cat brain deoxygenation changes. *Magn Reson Med* **22**: 159–166.

15. Thulborn KR, Waterton JC, Matthews PM, Radda GK (1982) Oxygenation dependence of the transverse relaxation time of water protons in whole blood at high field. *Biochim Biophys Acta* **714**: 265–270.

16. Brooks RA, Di Chiro G (1987) Magnetic resonance imaging of stationary blood: a review. *Med Phys* **14**: 903–913.

17. Jezzard P, Heineman F, Taylor J, DesPres D, Wen H, Balaban RS, Turner R (1994) Comparison of EPI gradient-echo contrast changes in cat brain caused by respiratory challenges with direct simultaneous evaluation of cerebral oxygenation via a cranial window. *NMR Biomed.* (in press).

18. Fox PT, Raichle ME (1986) *Proc Natl Acad Sci USA* **83**, 1140.

19. Frostig RD, Lieke EE, Ts'o DY, Grinvald A (1990) Cortical functional architecture and local coupling between neuronal activity and the microcirculation revealed by in-vivo high-resolution optical imaging of intrinsic signals. *Proc Natl Acad Sci USA* **87**: 6082–6086.

20. Weisskoff RM (1993) Endogenous susceptibility contrast: principles of relationship between blood oxygenation and MR signal change. In *Syllabus, SMRM/SMRI Workshop on Functional MRI of the Brain, Arlington, VA.* Berkeley, CA: Society of Magnetic Resonance in Medicine, p. 103.

21. Menon R, Ogawa S, Tank DW, Ugurbil K (1993) 4 tesla gradient recalled echo characteristics of photic stimulation-induced signal changes in the human primary visual cortex. *Magn Reson Med* **30**: 380–386.

22. Turner R, Jezzard P, Wen H, Kwong KK, Le Bihan D, Zeffiro T, Balaban RS (1993) Functional mapping of the human visual cortex at 4 tesla and 1.5 tesla using deoxygenation contrast EPI. *Magn Reson Med* **29**: 281–283.

23. Ljunggren S (1983) A simple graphical representation of Fourier-based imaging methods. *J Magn Reson* **54**: 338–343.

24. Meyer CH, Hu BS, Nishimura DG, Macovski A (1992) Fast spiral coronary artery imaging. *Magn Reson Med* **28**: 202–213.

25. Cohen MS, Weisskoff RM (1991) Ultra-fast imaging. *Magn Reson Imaging* **9**: 1–37.

26. McKinnon G (1993) Ultrafast interleaved gradient-echo-planar imaging on a standard scanner, *Magn Reson Med* **30**: 609–616.

27. Oshio K, Feinberg DA (1991) Fast T2 weighted MRI using novel gradient and spin echo (GRASE) imaging. *Magn Reson Med* **20**: 344–348.

28. Stehling MK, Turner R, Mansfield P (1991) Echo-planar imaging: magnetic resonance imaging in a fraction of a second. *Science* **254**: 43–50.

29. Turner R, von Kienlin M, Moonen CTW, van Zijl PCM (1990) Single-shot localized echo-planar imaging (STEAM–EPI) at 4.7 tesla. *Magn Reson Med* **14**: 401–408.

30. Turner R, Le Bihan D (1990) Single-shot diffusion imaging at 2.0 tesla. *J Magn Reson Med* **86**: 445–452.

31. Le Bihan D, Jezzard P, Turner R, Cuenod CA, Pannier L, Prinster A (1993) Practical problems and limitations in

using z-maps for processing of brain function MR images. *Proc. SMRM, 12th Annual Meeting,* p. 11.

32. Le Bihan D, Turner R, Zeffiro T, Cuenod C-A, Jezzard P, Bonnerot V (1993) Activation of human primary visual cortex during visual recall: an MRI study. *Proc Natl Acad Sci USA* **90:** 11802.

33. Friston K, Jezzard P, Turner R (1994) The analysis of functional MRI time series. *Human Brain Mapping* **1:** 1–19.

34. Hajnal JV, Oatridge A, Schwieso J, Cowan FM, Young IR, Bydder GM (1993) Cautionary remarks on the role of veins in the variability of functional imaging experiments. *Proc. SMRM, 12th Annual Meeting,* p. 166.

35. Woods RP, Cherry SR, Mazziotta JC (1992) Rapid automated algorithm for aligning and reslicing PET images. *JCAT* **115:** 565–587.

36. Ogawa S, Menon RS, Tank DW, Kim S-G, Merkle H, Ellermann JM, Ugurbil K (1993) Functional brain mapping by blood oxygenation level-dependent contrast magnetic resonance imaging. *Biophys J* **64:** 803–812.

37. Kennan RP, Zhong J, Gore JC. (1994) Intravascular susceptibility contrast mechanisms in tissues. Magn. Reson. Med. **31,** 9–21.

38. Lai S, Hopkins AL, Haacke EM, Wasserman BA, Buckley P, Friedman L, Meltzer H, Hedera P, Friedland R (1993) Identification of vascular structures as a major source of signal contrast in high resolution 2D and 3D functional activation imaging of the motor cortex at 1.5 T: preliminary results. *Magn Reson Med* **30:** 387–392.

39. Penfield W (1933) The evidence for a cerebral vascular mechanism in epilepsy. *Ann Intern Med* **7:** 303–310.

40. De Yoe EA, Neitz J, Miller D, Wieser J (1993) Functional magnetic resonance imaging (FMRI) of visual cortex in human subjects using a unique video graphics stimulator. *Proc. SMRM, 12th Annual Meeting,* p. 1394.

41. Tootell R. (1994) Personal communication.

42. Turner R, Jezzard P, Le Bihan D, Prinster A, Pannier L, Zeffiro T (1993) BOLD contrast imaging of cortical regions used in processing auditory stimuli. *Proc. SMRM, 12th Annual Meeting,* p. 1411.

43. Rueckert L, Appollonio I, Grafman J, Jezzard P, Johnson R, Le Bihan D, Turner R (1994) MRI functional activation of left frontal cortex during covert word production. *J Neuroimaging* **4:** 67–70.

Echo-volumar imaging

P. Mansfield, P.R. Harvey and M.K. Stehling

Magnetic Resonance Centre, University of Nottingham, Nottingham, NG7 2RD, UK

Echo-volumar imaging is a hyperfast technique capable of producing volumetric magnetic resonance images in times of the order of 100 ms. By increasing the gradient strengths and introducing real-time processing and display, we have been able to produce the first $16 \times 16 \times 16$ voxel snapshot head images on volunteers.

Keywords: hyperfast MRI, 3D MRI, echo-volumar imaging.

INTRODUCTION

Although echo-volumar imaging (EVI) was proposed some time ago by Mansfield [1], the first experimental work was restricted to an initial evaluation using phantoms [2]. Considerable improvements have been implemented both in terms of the details of the EVI technique and in the software implementation. It is now possible to acquire data and display the full volume set essentially instantaneously as in echo-planar imaging (EPI). This facility allows correct setting up procedures on the fly. Ghosting artifact and homogeneity distortion effects can, therefore, be minimized extremely rapidly.

MATERIALS AND METHODS

All data were obtained on a 0.5-T in-house-built whole-body scanner. The data were acquired using a head coil with an object field of $196 \times 196 \times 196$ mm^3. A thick transaxial slice is initially excited in the G_z gradient to create a free-induction decay (FID) of active spins. At the beginning of the FID a large gradient G_y is modulated in a trapezoidal manner at frequency f_y. Simultaneously G_x is modulated in a trapezoidal manner at frequency f_x and a smaller gradient G_z is applied in a steady fashion. The pulse timing diagram is shown in Fig. 1a. The signal data are acquired in the form of a series of modulated spin

Address for correspondence: Magnetic Resonance Centre, University of Nottingham, Nottingham NG7 2RD, UK.

echoes. In a particular two-pass version of EVI, the starting phase of G_x is reversed in the second pass and alternate lines, corresponding to the G_y modulation period, are time reversed. The time data from the two sets are spliced and suitably reordered and a Fourier transform of total time data obtained using an fast Fourier transform. The frequency or image data are then ordered into a set of 16 images, each image comprising 16×16 pixels. The equivalent 3D k-space trajectory is shown in Fig. 1b.

The fastest switching rates used in the acquisition of head and body images were well below the level outlined in the NRPB Guidelines [3].

RESULTS

Figure 2 shows a complete volume data set displayed as 16 transaxial images through the head of a volunteer. The total image set was obtained in two passes each of 64 ms. The voxel size was $12 \times 12 \times 12$ mm^3. Although relatively coarse, these data can be spatially averaged to bring out gross features such as the ventricles, orbits and cerebellum as indicated in Fig. 3.

DISCUSSION AND CONCLUSIONS

Although at an embryological stage in its development, we have demonstrated that EVI can produce rapid, though so far coarse, anatomical images of the head. Other images showing whole-body anatomy

E.V.I. SEQUENCE A

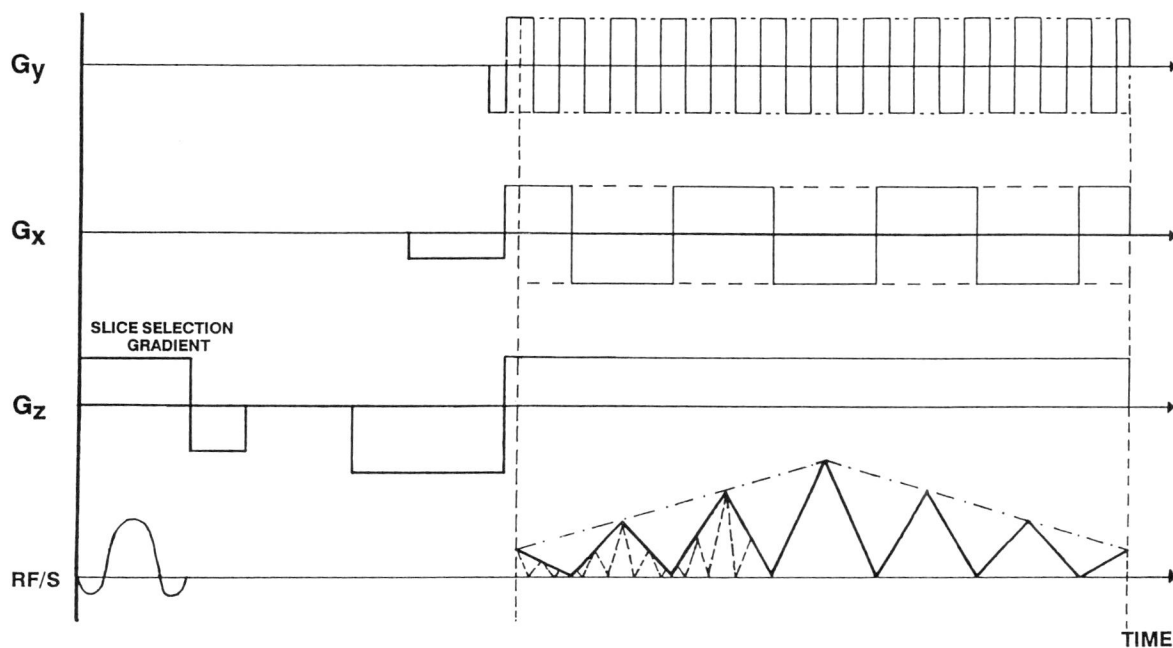

3D K-SPACE TRAJECTORY

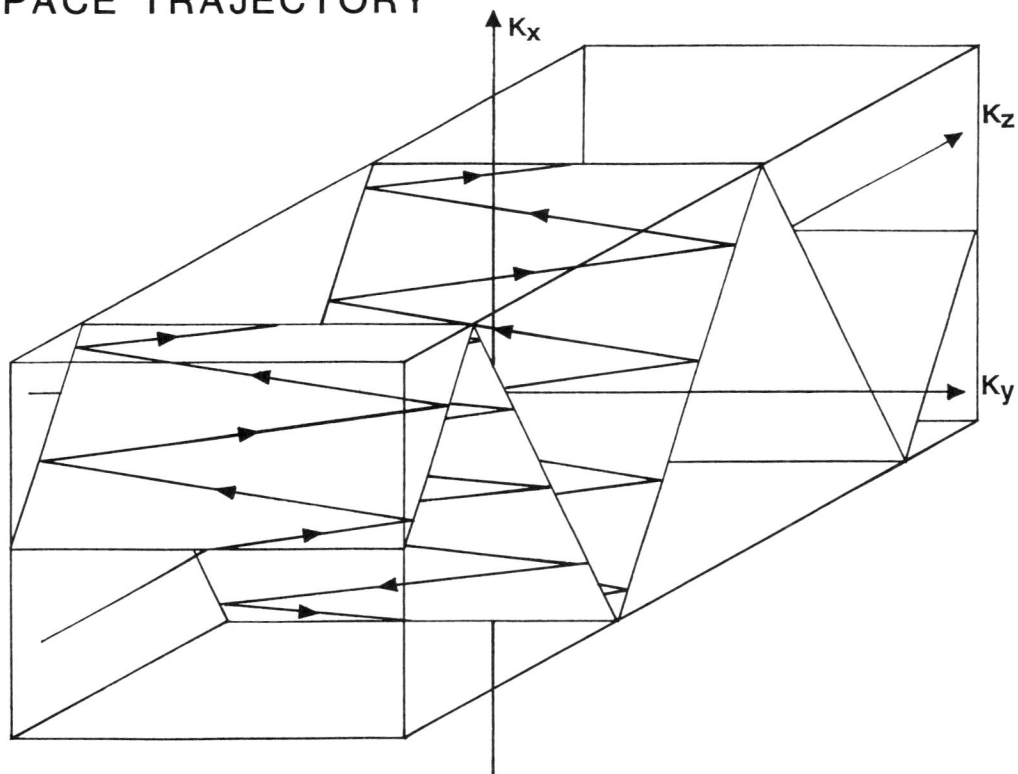

Fig. 1. (a) Timing sequence for EVI together with sketch of signal evolution in the presence of the modulated gradients G_x, G_y and G_z. (b) The EVI equivalent 3D k-space trajectory for the timing diagram in (a).

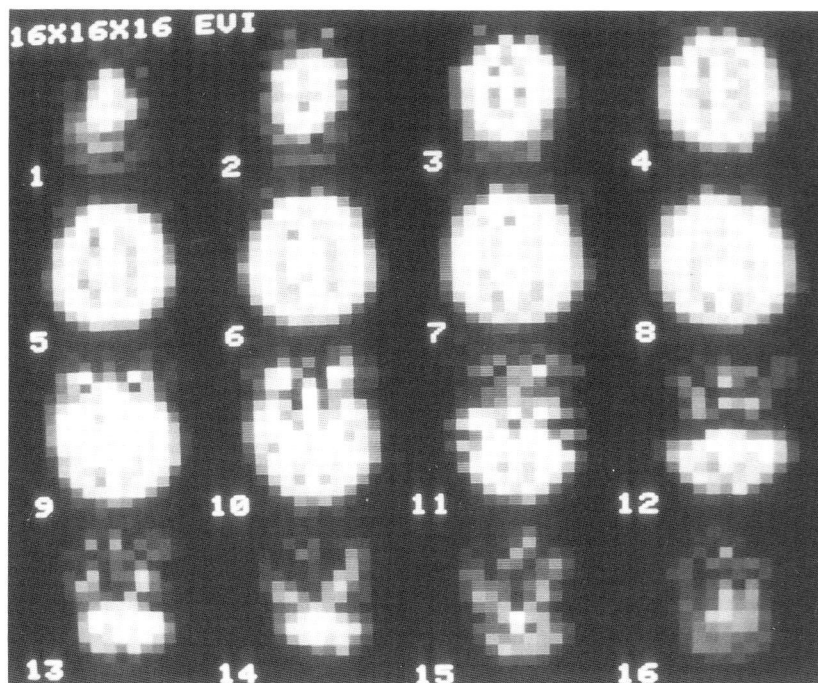

Fig. 2. Head images obtained using a two-pass EVI sequence. Each pass was obtained in 64 ms. The total array size in this example comprises 16 × 16 × 16 voxels with a spatial resolution of 12 mm. The images correspond to transaxial planes through the head and although coarse reveal structural details in the brain.

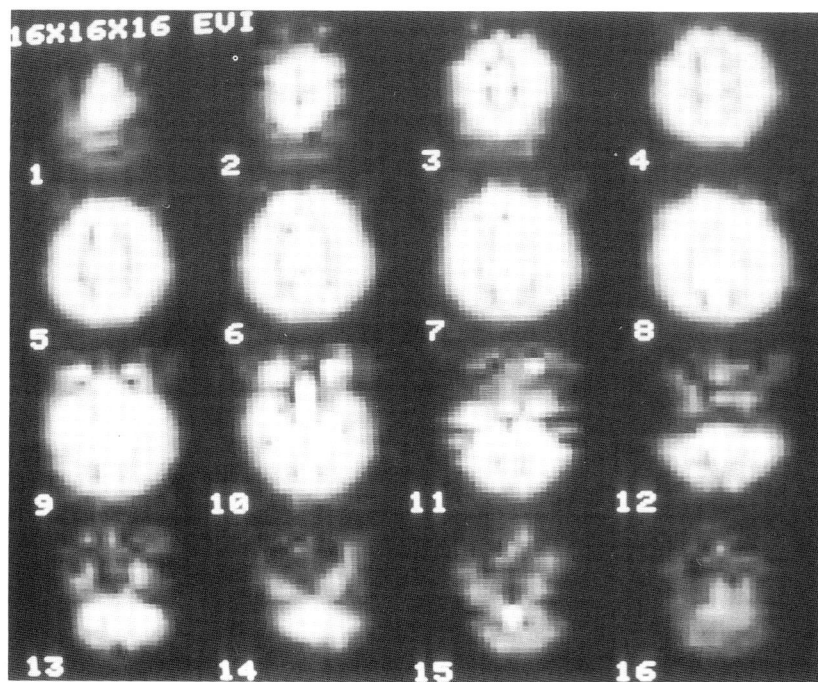

Fig. 3. Spatially smoothed EVI data of Fig. 2. The small degree of smoothing shows more clearly the structural details in the brain. The ventricles are clearly visible as are the orbits and cerebellum.

will be presented elsewhere. With the advent of neurofunctional brain imaging at high magnetic field strengths, EVI could find initial application in this area despite the poor resolution. EVI spatial resolution is currently similar to that achieved by PET but with much faster acquisition.

The NRPB Guidelines leave some room for maneuver regarding resolution improvement. However, at present, resolution is limited by a number of technical problems which include the generation of large, fast rise gradients and the reduction of associated high levels of unwanted acoustic noise, especially at 3.0 T.

ACKNOWLEDGMENT

We are grateful to the Medical Research Council for support of the high-speed EPI and EVI programs.

REFERENCES

1. Mansfield P (1977) Multi-planar image formation using NMR spin echoes. *J Phys C* **10**: L55–L58.
2. Mansfield P, Howseman A, Ordidge R (1989) Volumar imaging using NMR spin echoes: echo-volumar imaging (EVI). *J Phys E* **22**: 324–330.
3. NRPB Revised Guidelines for Clinical Imaging (1983) *Br J Radiol* **56**: 974.

Gastric motility by tagged EPI

B. Issa,* A. Freeman, P. Boulby, J. Wright,[1] P. Gowland, R. Bowtell, R. Spiller[2] and P. Mansfield

Magnetic Resonance Centre, University of Nottingham and Departments of [1]Surgery and [2]Therapeutics, University Hospital, Nottingham, NG7 2RD, UK

The high speed echo-planar NMR imaging technique is particularly suitable for visualizing human gut motility and transit. To enable a quantitative study of the rheology of the stomach contents, the magnetization can be prepared using a SPAMM (SPAtial Modulation of Magnetization) tagging sequence prior to imaging. Movement of stomach contents has been measured and analyzed temporally and in the Fourier domain and correlated with stomach motility. Increased stomach activity combined with retropulsive motion were observed at about 25 min following a porridge meal, indicating mixing of the meal and inhibition of gastric emptying.

Keywords: hyperfast MRI; EPI MRI; tagged MRI; gastric motility.

INTRODUCTION

Real-time monitoring of gut motility and transit has been previously demonstrated [1–3] using the magnetic resonance echo-planar imaging (EPI) technique, with which images of 128×128 pixels are acquired within 130 ms overcoming motion artifacts. The noninvasive nature of magnetic resonance (MR) imaging offers a significant advantage over conventional methods of monitoring the gastrointestinal tract, such as manometry and nuclear medicine. In this article, a new application of the SPAMM (SPAtial Modulation of Magnetization) tagging sequence to the study of the movement and mixing of stomach contents is described.

The tagging sequence SPAMM [4, 5] was applied prior to echo-planar imaging module and consisted of the simultaneous application of four hard radio frequency (RF) pulses of equal duration (100 μs) with relative amplitudes chosen according to the binomial sequence (1-3-3-1) and a linear conventional G_x field gradient. The phase acquired by the spins during the application of the magnetic field gradient produces a variation of the longitudinal magnetization component along the direction of the gradient, which is sharper than the sinusoidal variation associated with just two RF pulses. For stationary spins, straight lines, or tags, of low intensity will appear orthogonal to the

direction of magnetic field gradient. Any motion of spins between the SPAMM preparation module and the EPI imaging module causes the tag lines to be deflected. The technique was used to study the rheology of the stomach contents as shown in Fig. 1; movement of fluid across the antrum was demonstrated clearly by the deflection of the tags.

METHOD

All images were acquired using the MBEST (Modulus Blipped Echo-planar Single Pulse Technique) echo-planar imaging sequence at a field strength 0.5 T. The strength of the magnetic field gradient used in SPAMM was 1.4 mT m^{-1} with each pulse applied between the RF pulses lasting for 0.84 ms. This produced a tag separation of eight pixels corresponding to 2 cm. The gradient is applied in the conventional x direction (horizontal in a transaxial image). The tagged images are then converted to tag maps using minimization and threshold detection, noise pixels were assigned zero deflection. Tag line deflections are easily measured on these maps allowing convenient calculation of the speed and direction of stomach content movement. The sum of deflections (positive and negative) along each tag (which represents average velocity when divided by the number of pixels) was then used as a single parameter to be analyzed in detail both spatially and temporally. The sum of modulus deflections can also be used which is a measure of turbulence. A selected portion of 25 pixels length was

---

* Address for correspondence: Magnetic Resonance Center, University of Nottingham, Nottingham NG7 2RD, UK.

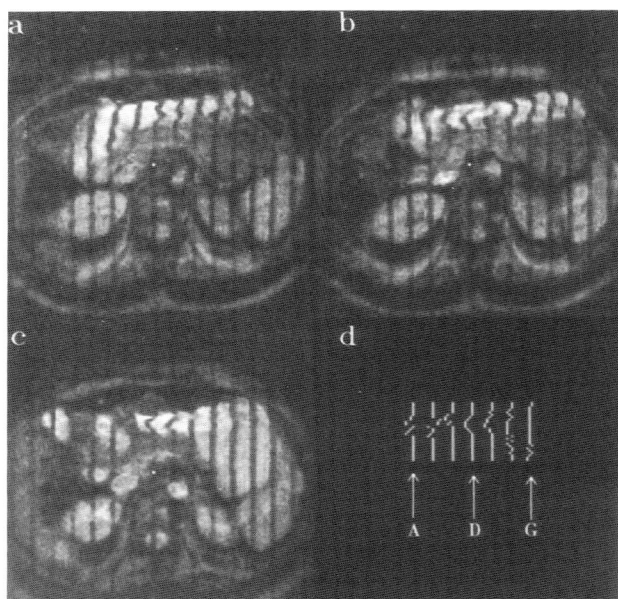

Fig. 1. Two tagged EPI images showing water and porridge filled stomach. (d) is a tag map produced from a water filled stomach image (c).

analyzed in detail along 7 central tag lines, these were labeled A, B, . . ., G from left to right.

RESULTS

The sum of deflections along the central tag (D) (see Fig. 1d) is plotted as displacement in pixels versus time as shown in Fig. 2. Negative displacements are to the left (down the gastrointestinal tract), positive displacements indicate retropulsive movement. At early times (Fig. 2a b), the porridge displacement amplitude (Fig. 2b) is smaller than for the water (Fig. 2a), indicating lower fluid velocities. At later times for porridge (Fig. 2c) a marked increase in activity is seen which suggests that the porridge is being mixed. Some positive displacement was also observed at later times, indicating backward retropulsive motion confirming the mixing and inhibition of gastric emptying. The Fourier transform of the displacement–time curves was calculated and the Fourier components for three central tags are shown in Fig. 3. At earlier times (0–6 min), little activity is seen except at tag C, which may suggest that the contraction is stronger at position C. This has a frequency component at the expected contraction rate of one every 20 s. The increased stomach activity, shown in Fig. 2, is reflected by the higher-frequency components evident at later times in the study. In contrast with earlier times, this component exists at all three tag positions. Furthermore, the

dc (zero frequency) component, which represents the average spatial–temporal displacement of the tag, is increasing progressively from tag E to tag C. This indicates larger velocities for the leftmost tag, which lays over the narrowest section of the antrum.

CONCLUSIONS

The study of gastric motility using EPI has so far been hampered by the large amount of data produced and the problems of quantification. Tagged EPI has a great potential to solve these problems. Temporal analysis of tag displacement has shown increased stomach

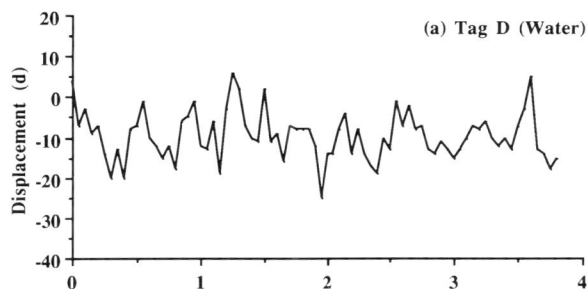

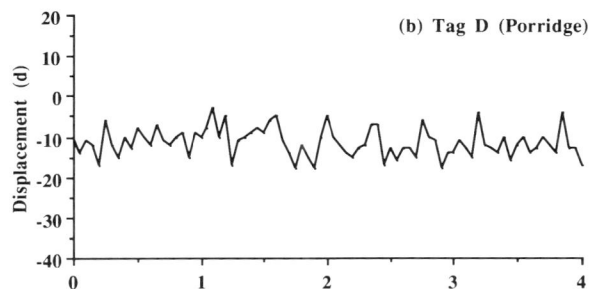

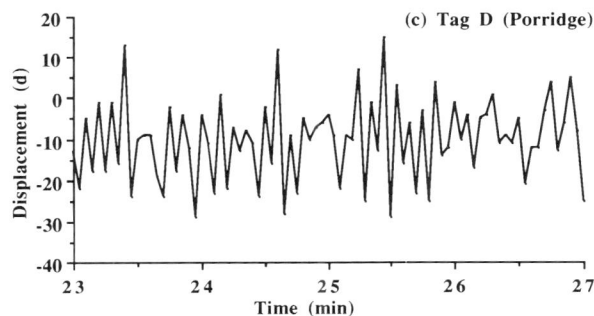

Fig. 2. The sum of deflections along the central tag (D) is plotted against time (a) for water and (b) and (c) for porridge.

FOURIER ANALYSIS

0-6 min   **23-29 min**

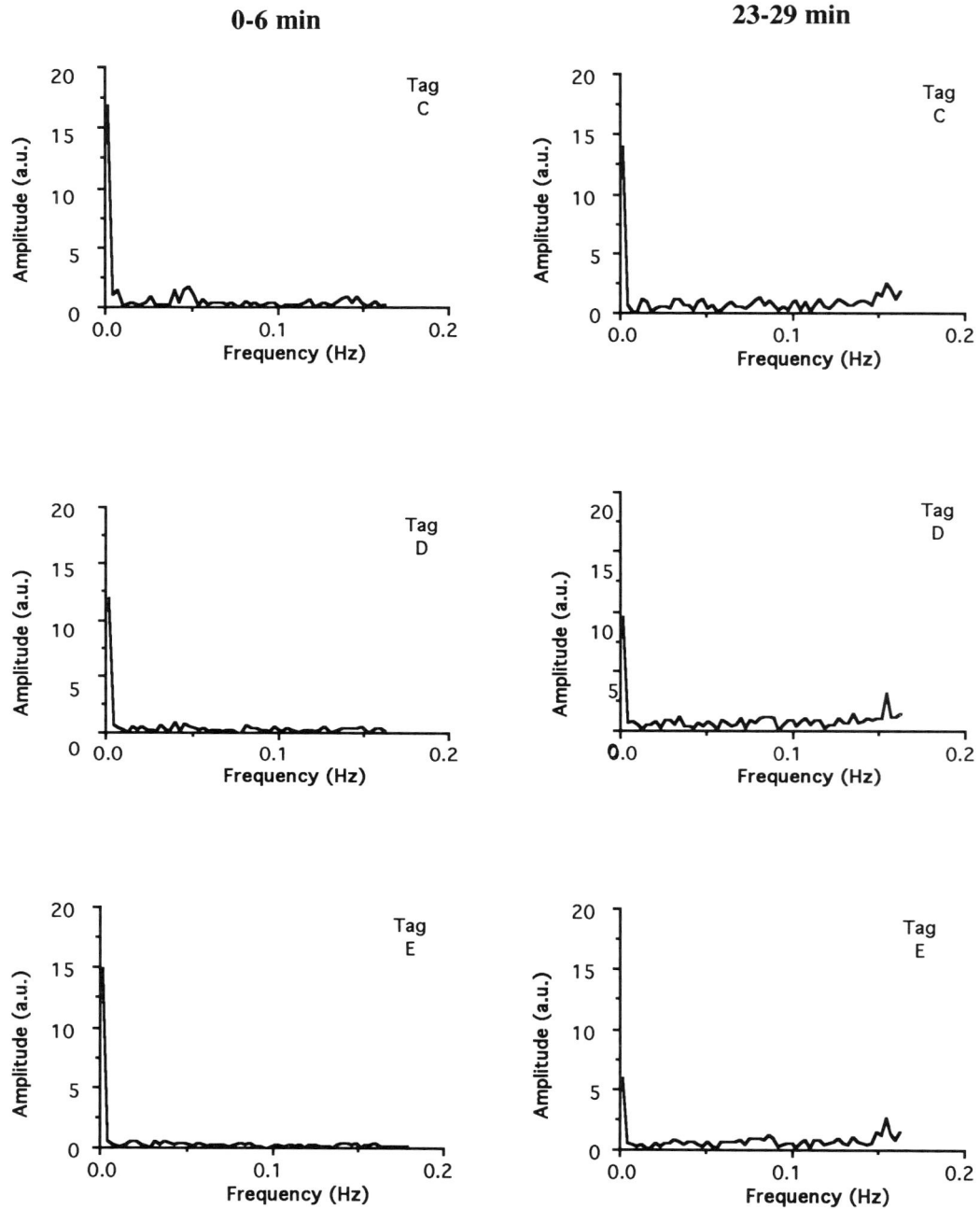

Fig. 3. Fourier analysis for three central tag lines at two different times for porridge.

activity with time following a porridge meal. This increase is represented by larger displacement amplitudes and more rapid fluctuations. Retropulsion and inhibition of gastric emptying is also observed at later times and can be studied further using meals of varying energy content. Fourier analysis has been used to determine the frequency components of the tag displacements and offers a more compact way of data analysis and presentation. The technique can be improved further by extending tagging into two orthogonal directions and by improved spatial and temporal resolution. Better resolution of the tags (narrower) is possible by the use of larger number of RF pulses. Quantification of emptying rates can be achieved by performing tagging with multislice imaging. Correlation of contractions with food volumes movements through the gut will aid in understanding the mechanism of food mixing, movement, and grinding in the stomach.

REFERENCES

1. Stehling M, Evans D, Lamont G, Ordidge R, Howseman A, Chapman B, Coxon R, Mansfield P, Hardcastle J, Coupland R (1989) Gastrointestinal tract: dynamic MR studies with echo-planar imaging. *Radiology* **171**: 41–46.
2. Evans D, Lamont G, Stehling M, Blamire A, Gibbs P, Coxon R, Hardcastle J, Mansfield P (1992) Prolonged monitoring of the upper gastrointestinal tract using echo planar magnetic resonance imaging. *Gut* **34**: 848–852.
3. Gowland P, Wright J, Evans D, Mansfield P (1992) A study of stomach emptying using echo planar imaging. *Proc. 11th meeting of the SMRM*, p. 109.
4. Axel L, Dougherty L (1989) MR imaging of motion with spatial modulation of magnetization. *Radiology* **171**: 841–845.
5. Axel L, Dougherty L (1989) Heart wall motion: improved method for spatial modulation of magnetization for MR imaging. *Radiology* **172**: 349–350.

Near real-time MRI of interstitial laser photocoagulation of *in vivo* rat liver

M. Clemence,[1]* H.R.S. Roberts,[1] M. Paley,[2] G. Buonaccorsi,[1]
M.A. Hall-Craggs,[2] S.G. Brown[1] and W.R. Lees[2]

[1]*National Medical Laser Centre, University College London, London, UK*
[2]*Middlesex Hospital, UCL Hospitals Group, London, UK*

Magnetic resonance imaging (MRI) is showing considerable promise as a monitor for interventional procedures. Laser surgery is "MRI compatible," and temperature-sensitive imaging techniques can be usefully applied to these procedures. We have been investigating T_1-derived temperature-dependent imaging as a monitor for interstitial laser photocoagulation (ILP) in rat liver. *In vitro* experiments suggested that temperature calibration may be achieved. We have investigated ILP *in vivo* using short TR spin-echo imaging sequences taking one set of images every 30 s during and after the procedure. Our results *in vivo* suggest that this simple model may be inadequate for temperature mapping as the biological reaction to the ILP is on a similar time scale to that of the procedure. Nonetheless, MRI shows well-defined, repeatable signal changes that can be related to histological borders.

Keywords: MRI, laser surgery, ILP, real-time, rat liver.

INTRODUCTION

With the release of imaging systems with which access to the patient is maintained, there is an increasing interest for interventional magnetic resonance imaging (MRI). Laser surgery is a natural candidate for this approach due its intrinsic MRI compatibility. With the development of small portable semiconductor lasers, the implementation of laser procedures within a typical MRI suite is straightforward. Interstitial laser photocoagulation (ILP) [1] is a technique by which tissue within solid organs (e.g., liver, breast) may be destroyed through local heating effects. An optical fiber is introduced into the target percutaneously through a needle and low laser powers (~ 2 W) are applied for long times (typically 500 s) to induce local heating, destroying roughly spherical areas of tissue. Currently, ultrasound is used to both position the fiber and follow the procedure. Changes are produced on an ultrasound image not only from the tissue changes but by the production of microbubbles at the fiber tip.

These gradually migrate through the tissue, masking the tissue changes and so making ultrasonography less effective as the treatment progresses. Temperature-dependent contrast MRI may be used to directly image the developing lesion. There are several methods of temperature-dependent MRI, T_1 variation [2] and diffusion-weighted imaging [3] being the most common. We chose T_1-weighted imaging for our experiments, not only because we intend to use ILP–MRI in the liver and breast where diffusion imaging is difficult due to breathing motion but also as the majority of scanners can perform short TR spin-echo (SE) imaging with no modifications.

MATERIALS AND METHODS

We chose as our model male Wistar rats. Due to the difficulty in accurately targeting the liver percutaneously in small animals, the liver is exposed at laparotomy, and the optical fiber inserted. Two markers [4] are placed either side of the fiber tip to facilitate image plane location and to enable correlation between histological sample and imaging experiments.

* *Address for correspondence: National Medical Laser Centre, University College London, 5 University Street, London, UK.*

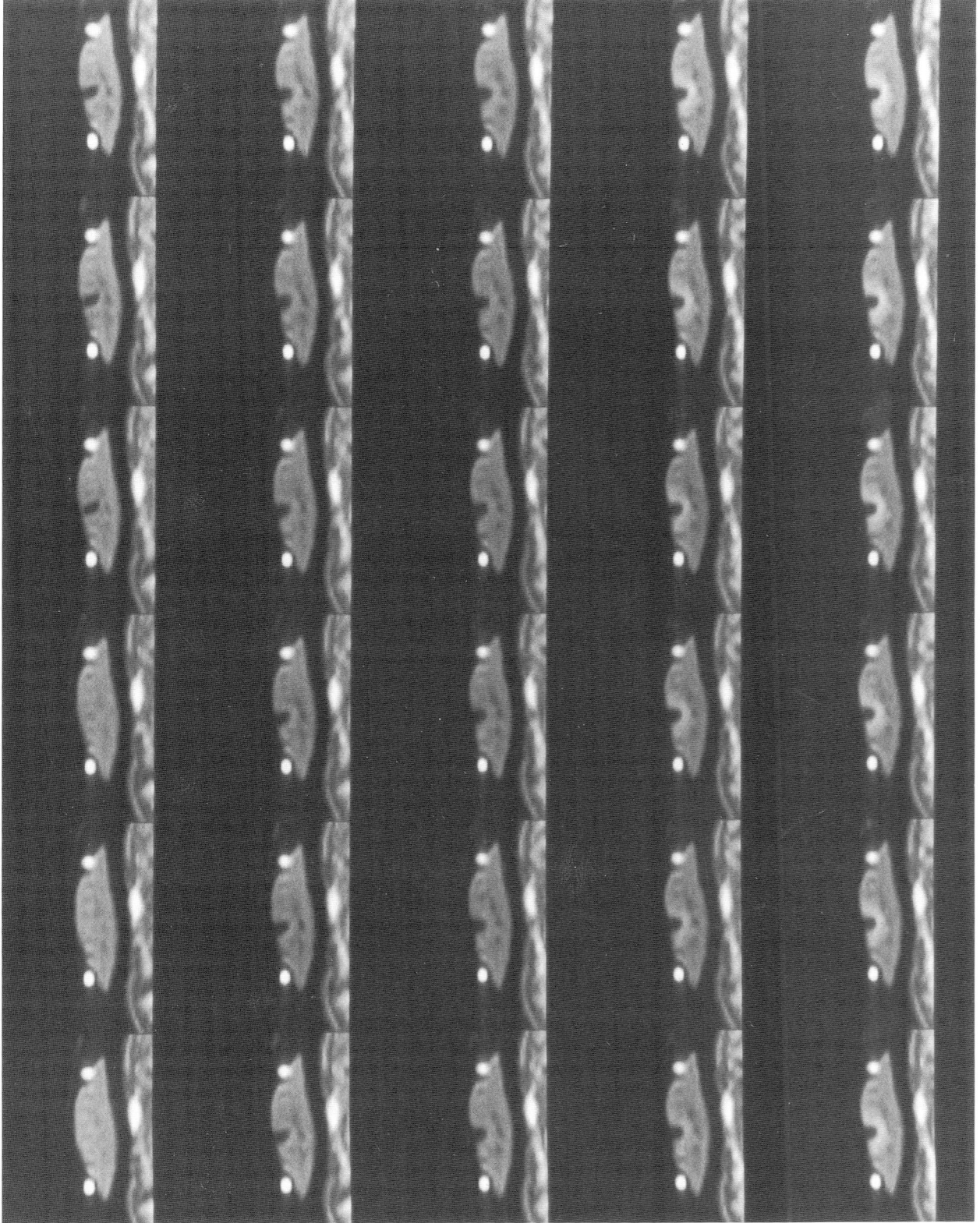

Fig. 1. SE TR = 200 ms, TE = 10 ms; 30-image set, *in vivo* ILP in rat liver. The bright dots on the upper surface of the liver are plane location markers.

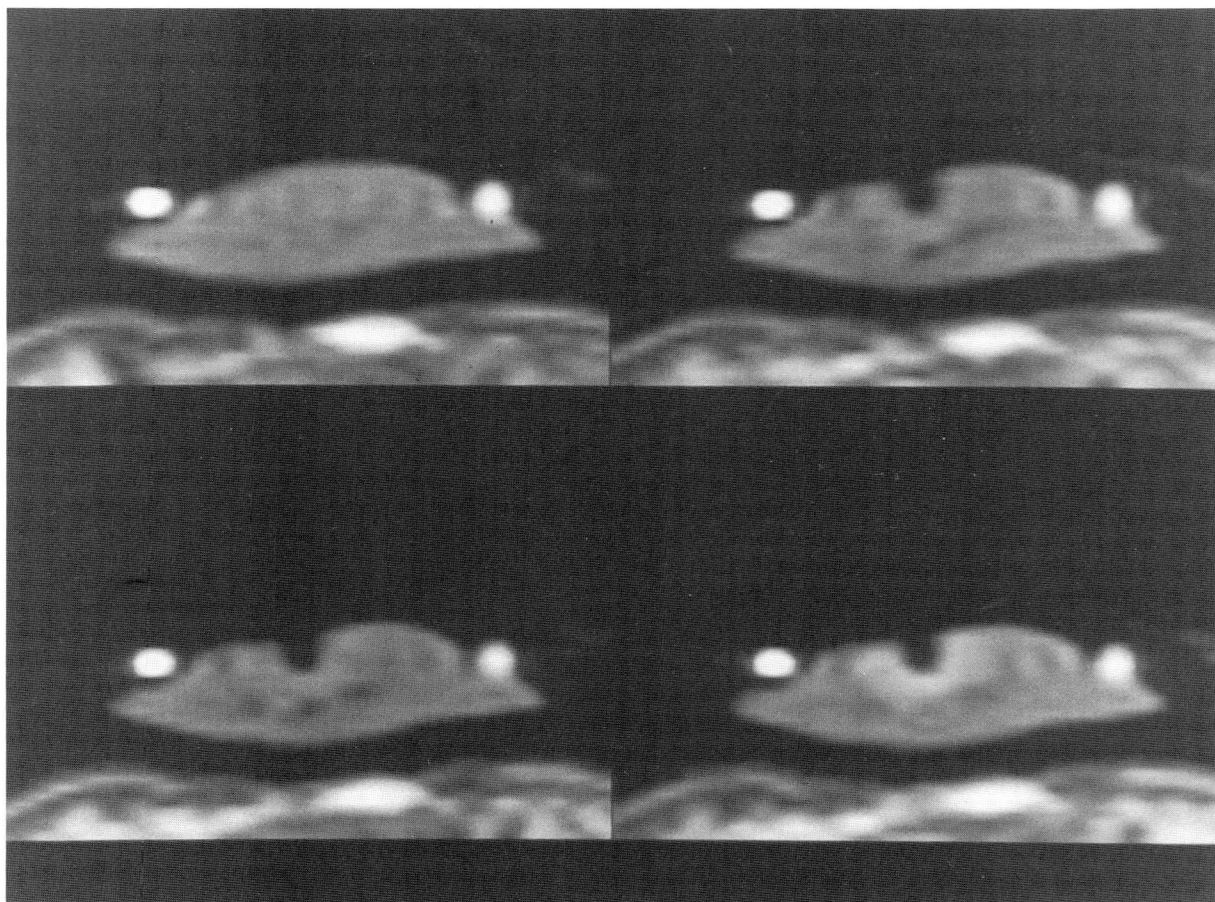

Fig. 2. Excerpts from the data set of Fig. 1 showing baseline ($t = 0$ s), mid-burn ($t = 330$ s), end burn ($t = 540$ s), and after cooling ($t = 870$ s).

The laser was a Diomed 25 semiconductor laser, wavelength 805 nm. ILP was performed using 1 W for 500 s. The animal was then sacrificed and the liver removed, sectioned, and the necrotic lesion measured.

Imaging was performed using a Siemens 1.5-T Magnetom using SE (TR 200 ms, TE 10 ms) imaging sequences with an overall repeat time of 30 s. Two sets of images were taken as a baseline, then a further 28 sets were taken, covering both temperature elevation and subsequent cooling after the laser was turned off. The optical fiber was normal to the imaging plane (3 mm slice thickness) to minimize partial volume effects.

RESULTS

Figure 1 shows a typical 30-image SE sequence. In this example, the fiber was placed high of center, leading to a cavity at the surface. The two bright dots on either side of the liver lobe are the slice plane markers. The laser is applied during images 3–19 and the remainder

show the return to equilibrium. Figure 2 shows in greater detail images 1, 12, 19, and 30. The area of signal enhancement in image 30 can be clearly seen. Figure 3 is a graph showing the time variation of intensity of four individual pixels taken from differing regions of the developing lesion from the data set of Fig. 1. For comparison purposes, Fig. 4 shows a similar set of results taken from an *in vitro* experiment, performed on fresh pig liver.

DISCUSSION

In vitro experiments, similar to that which produced the data in Fig. 4, indicated that accurate temperature correlation could be achieved in biological tissues. This graph demonstrates that even *in vitro*, additional responses complicate the model. Five millimeters from the lesion center the signal does return to the baseline value after the laser is turned off. However, closer in, permanent tissue changes have occurred (including

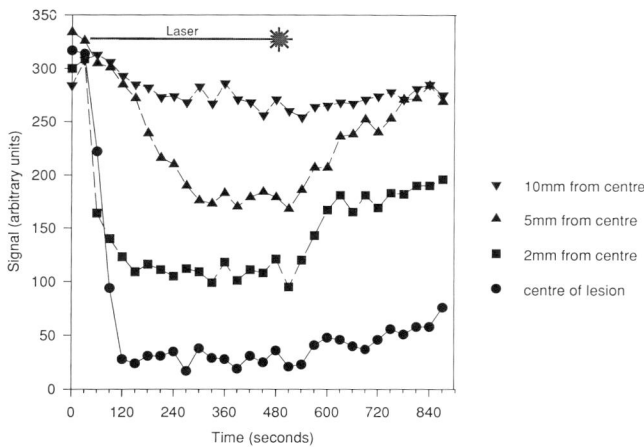

Fig. 3. Time course profiles of signal intensity taken from four pixels at differing distances from the ILP lesion center. *In vitro* pig liver sample.

possibly drying) to give lower signal at the end of the experiment. *In vivo,* the situation is complicated still more. Our studies of animals at 24 h post-ILP using MRI have indicated that, within the lesion, T_1, T_2, and proton density all increase. Images such as those in Fig. 2 show a clear enhancement of a region around the central cavity due to this effect taking place during

the laser treatment. Figure 3 demonstrates this more clearly. Indeed, it would appear that 5 mm from the cavity, where before the signal drop could be seen, the tissue reaction is now sufficient to mask any temperature-dependent signal loss, and only signal enhancement is seen once the laser is off.

CONCLUSION

Temperature correlation is unlikely to be achievable *in vivo* as the biological reaction, edema, hemorrhage, blood supply shutdown, cell death, etc., cause signal changes of a similar time scale and in opposite directions. However, MRI clearly shows a tissue change which, if it is repeatable for given organ, may be used to produce a useful real-time monitor. Even as this work stands at the present time, the image quality is superior to ultrasound and does not suffer by becoming less effective as the procedure progresses. However, in order to obviate the difficulties of working within the MR environment, as well as the extra costs involved, clear benefits in treatment effectiveness need to be demonstrated in a clinical setting. Further work is required to demonstrate the accuracy of the measurement of lesion sizes. For this purpose, rat liver is probably too small, as lesions are only 10–15 pixels across, leading to large quantization errors when measuring off the image. In addition, accidental infarct is more common, leading to large areas of necrosis not due to laser damage.

REFERENCES

1. Bown SG (1983) Phototherapy of tumours. *World J Surg* **7:** 700–709.
2. Dickinson RJ, Hall AS, Hind AJ, Young IR (1986) Measurement of changes in tissue temperature using MR imaging. *J Comput Assist Tomogr* **10**(3): 468–472.
3. Delannoy J, Chen Ching-Nien, Turner R, Levin RL, Le Bihan D (1991) Noninvasive temperature imaging using diffusion MRI. *Magn Res Med* **19:** 333–339.
4. Clemence M, Amin Z, Lees WR, Bown SG (1993) Markers for accurate MR imaging pathologic correlation following interstitial laser photocoagulation of rat liver. *Proc Society of Magnetic Resonance in Medicine 12th Annual Congress New York,* p. 164.

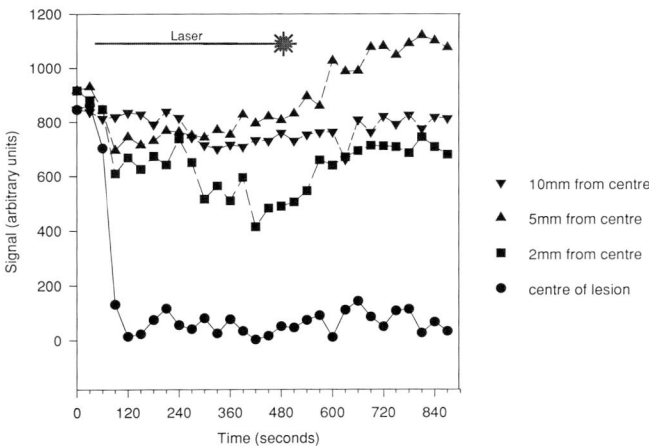

Fig. 4. Time course profiles of signal intensity taken from four pixels at differing distances from the ILP lesion center. *In vivo* rat liver model (data from Fig. 1).

Principles and applications of FLASH NMR imaging

Axel Haase

Physikalisches Institut, Universität Würzburg, Würzburg, Germany

Routine clinical NMR scanners apply low-flip-angle gradient-echo sequences as fast-imaging modalities. Fast low-angle shot (FLASH) NMR imaging is the first version of a large family of fast gradient-echo methods. It is based on the application of reduced flip angles for NMR excitation, the acquisition of magnetic field gradient echoes, and considerably shortened repetition times. Under these conditions, transverse magnetization survives. This magnetization can be destroyed in "spoiled FLASH" or used for imaging in "refocused FLASH." The measuring time of FLASH NMR images is dependent on gradient hardware and is under optimal technical conditions user selectable between less than 100 ms and 1 s. Short imaging times give the possibility to apply magnetization preparation before imaging. This technique allows the acquisition of image contrast with respect to any selected parameter, e.g. T_1, T_2, or diffusion constant. This FLASH version has been called "snapshot"-, "turbo"-, or magnetization-prepared RAGE.

Keywords: NMR imaging, fast imaging, gradient echo, FLASH, snapshot-FLASH.

INTRODUCTION

Many applications of NMR imaging focus on medical diagnosis. The inherent problem in early clinical practice was that NMR imaging was supposed to be a time-consuming technique. In 1977, a fast NMR imaging method, echo-planar imaging (EPI), was described [1]. In 1985, a further fast imaging method was described, which was immediately implemented in many clinical NMR imagers, the FLASH (fast low-angle shot) technique [2]. Both methods rely on different approaches to fast sampling of NMR image data. The purpose of this article is to present the physical principles and different versions of FLASH-based fast NMR imaging.

The purpose of FLASH NMR imaging is to reduce all kinds of motional artifacts, e.g., heart motion, breathing, and random motion by the patient. Therefore, it can study organ functions [3] and organ motion [4]. A further benefit is to acquire multiparameter data sets within shorter time intervals, e.g., three-dimensional imaging [5], flow velocity information, and NMR parameter imaging [6].

Address for correspondence: Physikalisches Institut, Universität Würzburg, Am Hubland, D-97074 Würzburg, Germany.

TECHNICAL CONSIDERATIONS

All FLASH techniques are based on two- or three-dimensional Fourier transform, first proposed as "Fourier Zeugmatography" in 1975 [7]. FLASH sequences rely on a considerable reduction of the repetition time. A reduction of the repetition time, however, has a considerable drawback. Each excitation of an NMR signal for a k-space line decreases the longitudinal magnetization to a lower value M_z. During the time interval TR, M_z recovers toward its equilibrium value M_0 by spin-lattice relaxation T_1. M_z tends to a zero level when the excitation flip angle is 90°. Furthermore, when spin-echo experiments with 180° radio-frequency refocusing pulses are used, the magnetization will dramatically reduce under short TR conditions.

The idea to reduce the repetition time TR to short values is, however, most promising. According to the above discussion, the goal can be reached when spin-echo experiments are avoided and lower flip angles are used. In 1D NMR spectroscopy low flip angles are used to speed up measuring times while retaining a high level of NMR signal. It is known for many years that for a given TR and T_1 value, an optimum flip angle, the "Ernst angle" α_E, exists, where the maximum signal strength per measuring time can be expected [8]:

$$\cos \alpha_E = \exp(-TR/T_1) \tag{1}$$

Although, an "Ernst angle" cannot be defined under imaging conditions, where many different T_1 values can be found, the idea to use a reduced flip angle is promising.

The second need, resulting from the above discussion, is to avoid spin-echo experiments. This is done in conventional 1D NMR spectroscopy by the acquisition of the FID signal. Under imaging conditions, the FID signal is acquired with the help of the inversion of one magnetic field gradient [9]. This signal is called the gradient echo. The physical content of FLASH-based fast NMR imaging sequences is, therefore, fast acquisitions of gradient echoes excited by low-flip-angle NMR excitation [2].

Because the time interval responsible to produce a gradient echo can be changed easily, the gradient echo time T_G at which the gradient echo appears is under the control of the NMR expert. The signal strength of the gradient echo is dependent on T_G and the relaxation time responsible for the FID decay, the T_2^*. T_2^* is much shorter than T_2. It is known that the relaxivity $1/T_2^*$ is composed of the sum of different contributions:

$$1/T_2^* = 1/T_2 + 1/T_{2i} + 1/T_{2s} + 1/T_{2c} + \cdots \tag{2}$$

Here T_2 is the spin–spin relaxation time, T_{2i} is given by inhomogeneities of the main magnetic field, T_{2s} is produced by magnetic susceptibility gradients, T_{2c} is due to the chemical shift dispersion of the NMR signal. Other field homogeneities and motions within the magnet can cause further relaxation paths.

Therefore, it should be emphasized that a gradient echo signal is strongly affected by magnetic field inhomogeneities. Furthermore, a gradient echo acquired at T_G always exhibits lower signal strength than a spin echo at the same spin-echo time TE.

The theoretical minimum gradient echo time TG is the sum of the time intervals of the slice-selective excitation pulse, inversion of the read gradient, and one-half of the time interval for acquisition of the gradient echo. At least two time intervals have to be reserved for the switching processes of gradients. In summary, the minimum T_G is totally hardware dependent. Minimum values of approximately 1 ms have been achieved so far. The minimum repetition time of a gradient echo imaging experiment is approximately twice as long as T_G. Therefore, measuring times of a 128 × 128-pixel image of the order of 250 ms are possible and have been reached by many groups. However, it should be noted that the measuring time, or the minimum repetition time TR, is hardware dependent. Increasing the gradient strength results in a decreased data-acquisition, phase-encoding, and slice-selection interval. The speedup of the gradient power amplifiers further reduces T_G and TR, respectively.

SIGNAL BEHAVIOR

Fast repetitions of NMR excitations with short repetition times TR and low-flip-angle RF pulses need a reconsideration of the signal behavior. It is known that a train of RF pulses with TR smaller than T_2 generate a constant NMR-signal level with an FID contribution following an RF pulse and an echolike signal before each pulse [10]. The echo part of the signal can be destroyed by various kinds of "spoiling" methods using gradient pulses [11] or phase scrambling of the RF pulses [12]. The echo part can also be refocused when all magnetic field gradient pulses are inverted in polarity after the acquisition of the gradient echo and before the next pulse [13, 14].

If we assume that any transverse magnetization has been spoiled between the RF pulses, the signal will be proportional to

$$S \sim \frac{[1 - \exp(-TR/T_1)] \exp(-TG/T_2^*) \sin \alpha}{1 - \cos \alpha \exp(-TR/T_1)} \tag{3}$$

If we consider refocused experiments, then the signal will be proportional to

$$S \sim \frac{[1 - \exp(-TR/T_1)] \sin \alpha}{\begin{array}{c} 1 - \exp(-TR/T_1) \exp(TG/T_2) \\ - [\exp(-TR/T_1) - \exp(-TG/T_2)] \cos \alpha \end{array}} \tag{4}$$

It is interesting to note how this signal behavior changes under fast-imaging conditions. Here TR and T_G will be much smaller than T_1 and T_2.

For spoiled fast gradient echo imaging and large flip angles, the signal strength will be proportional to

$$S \sim TR/T_1 \tag{5}$$

For low-flip-angle pulses, the signal is no more dependent on relaxation time differences and will be dominated by spin density.

In refocused fast gradient echo imaging using large flip angles, the signal strength is proportional to

$$S \sim T_2/T_1 \tag{6}$$

Again, the signal will be dominated by the spin-density contrast when using lower flip angles.

The application of fast gradient echo imaging has a large possibility to change the image contrast. So, "refocused" gradient echo imaging can produce T_2-weighted images, according to Eq. (6), or "spoiled" gradient echo images give T_1-weighted images, according to Eq. (5), and both techniques result in "spin-density" images using low-flip-angle pulses.

POSSIBLE IMAGE ARTIFACTS

Numerous artifacts can appear and but can also be avoided in fast gradient echo imaging. The first and not always visible artifact is a severe distortion of the slice profile. It has been known for many years that the slice profile is completely changed when using large flip angles and short repetition times [15]. In practical slice-selective imaging experiments, the flip angle varies across the slice, resulting in an often "Gaussian-shaped" slice profile. As a consequence of this effect, large flip angles are found in the center and low flip angles at the edges of the slice profile. Higher flip angles and short repetition times TR will result in a heavy saturation in the center and almost no saturation at the edges of the slice profile.

This is the case when strongly T_1-weighted fast gradient echo images are needed. The discussion shows that it is unrealistic to calculate T_1 maps from a series of T_1-weighted fast gradient echo images.

The most prominent feature of fast gradient echo imaging is the high-intensity signal of blood flowing perpendicular to the slice orientation. This is due to an in-flow of fully relaxed magnetization during TR [4]. The enhancement of the signal intensity of flowing blood depends on imaging parameters (TR, flip angle, slice thickness), T_1 of blood, and the flow velocity. Although this effect can be used to image blood vessels magnetic resonance (MR) angiography, it has a negative feature. Flowing spins accumulate a velocity- (v) dependent phase when flowing along a magnetic field gradient G, according to

$$\phi = \gamma G v t^2 / 2 \tag{7}$$

Here t is the time interval between the NMR excitation and read-out of the signal. As long as the velocity remains constant, a constant phase is obtained. However, if the velocity changes during the imaging experiment, e.g., due to pulsatile flow, different phases are accumulated, leading to severe "flow artifacts" of bright intensity in the phase-encoding direction. This artifact can be reduced by rephasing gradients giving no net phase shift due to flow velocity ("flow-compensated" gradient pulses).

All gradient echo imaging experiments suffer from the common feature of FID signals, the T_2^* relaxation. The signal intensity depends on magnetic field inhomogeneities of various sources, and chemical shift effects. If we have a magnetic field inhomogeneity given by the gradient G within a pixel of a diameter dr,

a phase spread will appear during the gradient echo time T_G:

$$\phi = \gamma G dr \text{TE} \tag{8}$$

High values of ϕ give low signal intensity in gradient echo imaging. It is clearly visible that magnetic field homogeneity effects decrease when the spatial resolution increases and/or the gradient echo time T_G decreases. Of course, this has technological limitations because the gradient strength and gradient switching time has to be improved. This effect, often called the susceptibility effect appears near air–soft tissue interphases (e.g., nasopharynx region, air-filled bowels, lung, etc.). A similar effect of signal change is observed when different chemical shift values are present in one image element. From the inspection of an FID signal containing two close frequency components, we know that a beat is observed, having oscillations of the signal during T_2^* decay. At periodic times, the signal vanishes, often called the opposed-phase signal. If the gradient echo time T_G is exactly matched to this time, no signal can be measured from a pixel where two chemical shift components with equal intensity are present. Therefore, by a careful selection of the gradient echo time T_G, "in-phase," or "opposed-phase" gradient echo images are measured.

QUANTITATIVE IMAGING

Fast NMR imaging increased the interest for well-defined image contrast or even quantitative NMR imaging of relaxation times, diffusion constants, and flow velocities. As pointed out in the above sections, it is problematic to observe a well-defined image contrast and even more difficult to image quantitative data using fast gradient echo sequences. For example, T_1 contrast suffers from slice profile artifacts, T_2 contrast is not obtainable using spoiled sequences and mixed with T_1 information using refocused methods, and flow and diffusion information needs longer gradient echo times with adverse effects due to susceptibility artifacts. This problematic situation completely changed when magnetization-prepared fast gradient echo sequences appeared. These are called snapshot-, turbo-, or MP (magnetization-prepared)- gradient echo sequences [6].

These methods gain from the fact that due to hardware improvements, short repetition times of 5 ms or less became possible in whole-body scanners. Now, the total measuring time is less than 1 s and, therefore, comparable to an average T_1 relaxation in high magnetic fields. Magnetization preparation means that the longitudinal magnetization is changed in a defined way before the acquisition of the whole snapshot image, having short TR values. The image contrast will then be dependent on the magnetization preparation because this lasts for a few T_1 intervals (typically one to three times T1). Magnetization preparation can be performed using a single inversion pulse for IR T_1-weighted images, a single 90°–180°–90° (DEFT) pulse for spin-echo T_2-weighted images, or a DEFT pulse combined with diffusion- or flow-encoding gradients for diffusion- or flow-weighted images. This technique does not suffer from all previous artifacts and gives true quantitative image data when a series of images are acquired [6].

APPLICATIONS AND CONCLUSIONS

A multitude of different applications have been described in the past 8 years since the beginning of fast gradient echo experiments. One of the most prominent applications is in the field of rapid 3D NMR imaging. Here the total measuring time can be limited to a few minutes and remains a practical investigation for medical diagnosis. Recent software and computer improvements helped to increase the importance of 3D NMR imaging.

A further principal application is in the field of "functional" NMR imaging. From the beginning, dynamic contrast media studies were very helpful in organ studies. The time resolution in fast gradient echo imaging is of the order of a few seconds. The time course of a bolus injection of an NMR contrast medium can be easily followed, and kinetic data calculated. This was first done for kidney and liver studies and later for "functional" NMR imaging in the brain. However, it should be emphasized that dynamic fast gradient echo imaging using contrast media acquires a time-dependent dynamic signal change. As discussed above, the signal of fast gradient echo images has a complex dependence on various parameters, like relaxation times, susceptibility, etc. Therefore, the signal intensity is not clearly related to the local concentration of a contrast medium and is strongly dependent on the used imaging experiment and parameters. It should be emphasized that quantitative data have to be acquired for quantitative contrast media studies.

The importance and applications of fast gradient echo sequences will—as in the past—further gain from hardware improvements. An important parameter in this respect in the gradient echo time. All adverse artifacts can be reduced and the signal intensity improved when this parameter is minimized. This improvement would also help to implement more "hybrid" fast-imaging sequences. In a few cases, hybrids between EPI and fast gradient echo imaging can be of advantage. The ultimate limit of all fast-imaging sequences, however, is not given by technological constraints but by biological effects due to nerve stimulation in rapidly switched magnetic fields.

REFERENCES

1. Mansfield P (1977) Multi-planar image formation using NMR spin echoes. *J Phys E* **10**: 55–62.
2. Haase A, Frahm J, Matthaei D, Hänicke W, Merboldt KD (1986) FLASH Imaging: Rapid NMR imaging using low flip angle pulses. *J Magn Reson* **67**: 258–266.
3. Matthaei D, Frahm J, Haase A, Hänicke W (1985) Regional physiological functions depicted by sequences of rapid MR images. *Lancet*, 893.
4. Frahm J, Haase A, Matthaei D, Merboldt KD, Hänicke W (1986) Rapid NMR imaging of dynamic processes using the FLASH technique. *Magn Reson Med* **4**: 48–60.
5. Frahm J, Haase A, Matthaei D (1986) Rapid three dimensional MR imaging using the FLASH technique. *J Comput Assist Tomogr* **10**: 363–368.
6. Haase A (1990) Snapshot FLASH MRI. Applications to T1, T2, and chemical shift imaging. *Magn Reson Med* **13**: 77–89.
7. Kumar A, Welti D, Ernst RR (1975) NMR Fourier zeugmatography. *J Magn Reson* **18**: 69–83.
8. Ernst RR, Anderson WA (1966) Application of Fourier transform spectroscopy to magnetic resonance. *Rev Sci Instrum* **37**: 93–102.
9. Edelstein WA, Hutchison JMS, Johnson G, Redpath T (1980) Spin warp imaging and applications to human whole-body imaging. *Phys Med Biol* **25**: 756–759.
10. Patz S (1989) Steady-state free precession: An overview of basic concepts and applications. *Adv Magn Reson Imag* **1**: 73–102.
11. Frahm J, Merboldt KD, Hänicke W (1987) Transverse coherence in rapid FLASH NMR imaging. *J Magn Reson* **27**: 307–314.
12. Zur Y, Bendel P (1987) A method for removing artifacts in short TR imaging. *Radiology* **156(p)**: 154.
13. Oppelt A, Graumann R, Barfuss H, Fischer H, Hartl W, Schajor W (1986) Fast imaging with steady state precession. *Electromedica* **1**: 15–18.
14. Gyngell ML (1988) The application of steady-state free precession in rapid 2DFT NMR imaging: fast and CE-FAST sequences. *Magn Reson Med* **6**: 415–419.
15. Young IR, Bryant DJ, Payne JA (1985) Variations of Slice shape and absorption as artifacts in the determination of tissue parameters in NMR imaging. *Magn Reson Med* **2**: 355–389.

Roles for paramagnetic substances in MRI: contrast agents, molecular amplifiers, and indicators for redox and pH mapping

Alan E. Fischer and Laurance D. Hall*

Herchel Smith Laboratory for Medicinal Chemistry, University of Cambridge School for Clinical Medicine, Cambridge CB2 2PZ, UK

A "molecular amplifier" is a substance which at high dilution can significantly influence the magnetic resonance (MR) properties of water; its "gain" can be controlled by varying either its chemical or magnetic properties. If the "gain" of that amplifier is sensitive to the chemical potential of its molecular environment, then it can be used as an "MRI-active chemical indicator." Three examples are described: (a) the use of the ethylenediaminetetraacetic acid-copper(II) complex to map the spatial distribution of pH; (b) the use of Fe(II)/Fe(III) ions to map redox potential and thereby reducing species such as ascorbic acid or oxidants such as perbromate ion; (c) similar use of a stable nitroxide free radical to map reducing agents. The mass transport diffusion of those species can be visualized in hydrocolloid gels and in articular cartilage by MR imaging and the diffusion coefficients measured quantitatively using the null-point MR imaging method.

Keywords: magnetic resonance imaging, pH, redox potential, paramagnetic contrast agents, diffusion, null-point imaging.

INTRODUCTION

The purpose of this article is to illustrate how some of the same fundamental concepts which led to the invention [1] of gadolinium-diethylenetriaminepentaacetate (Gd-DTPA) (*1*) enabled us to develop chemical substances that are sensitive to their chemical environment and that can act as "MR-active chemical indicators" [2]. Given that those indicators should be clearly visible by magnetic resonance imaging (MRI), yet mindful that as with traditional types of chemical indicators they must be used at low concentrations, it is also necessary to introduce the concept of a "molecular amplifier" [3].

It is instructive to place these concepts in context by reference to a simple experiment, in which MRI was used to visualize the water on a ion-exchange chromatography column, 10 cm long and 0.5 cm in diameter [3] (Fig. 1). Approximately 10^{-3} g (10^{-5} mol) of copper sulfate was added, the column developed in the usual way, and the MRI measurement repeated; this showed a loss of signal intensity from approximately 0.2 mL volume (Fig. 1c). That same volume could be visualized alone, with suppression of the water on the column (Fig. 1b), using a different MRI sequence. In the context of "molecular amplification," the copper ions used in this case have a gain of approximately 10^4. They function as they do because the spin relaxation of the protons of those water molecules that are in the solvation shell surrounding the dissolved Cu^{2+} ions is enhanced considerably as compared with those of bulk water. The weighted time average of the proton MR relaxation times of those two populations of water molecules results in a substantial enhancement of both spin–lattice and spin–spin relaxation times of the protons of the sample in the near vicinity of the copper ions.

* Address for correspondence: Herchel Smith Laboratory for Medicinal Chemistry, Robinson Way, Cambridge CB2 2PZ, UK.

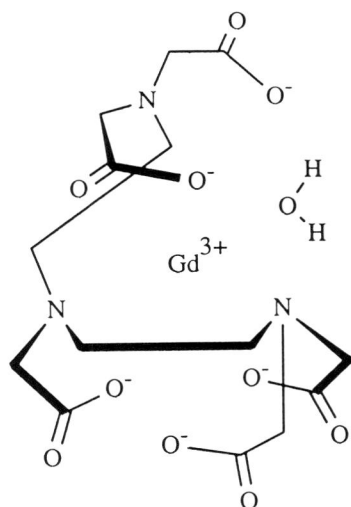

+ 2 methyl-glucamine

1

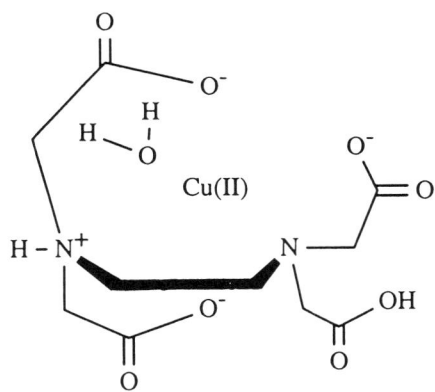

2

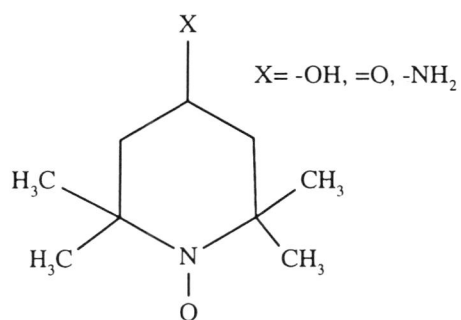

X= -OH, =O, -NH₂

3

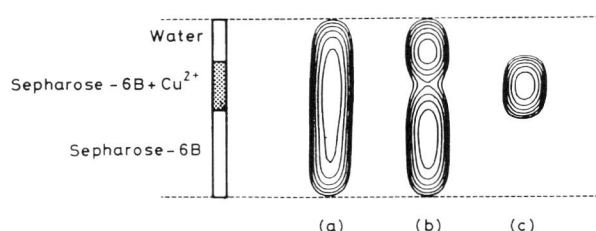

Fig. 1. Schematic magnetic resonance images of a chromatography column containing 1.5 ml "chelating-sepharose-6B" on which part of the Cu^{2+} ions are adsorbed (approximately 0.2 ml). The three images displayed were acquired using an inversion recovery sequence with different recovery delays τ. For a τ of 3000 ms (a) the image intensity is uniform, whereas a τ of 1 ms (b) and 300 ms (c) suppresses the signal from column material containing copper ions and Cu^{2+} ion-free material, respectively.

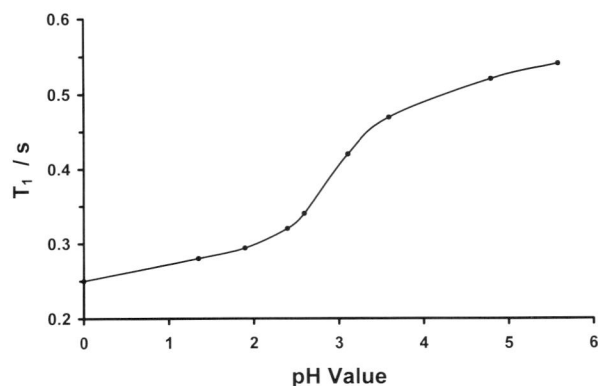

Fig. 2. Dependence of the longitudinal relaxation time (T_1) of the water protons of a 8 mM Cu-EDTA solution on the pH value of the solution.

RESULTS AND DISCUSSION

Clearly, the "gain" of that amplifier depends on both the intrinsic magnetism of the paramagnetic center and the overall number of molecules of water it influences; control of each of those parameters will then alter the appearance of a suitably sensitized MRI scan. We now give three examples that illustrate how that can be achieved and utilized.

Consider first the spin–lattice relaxation times of a 10 mM aqueous solution of copper sulfate ($T_1 = 100$ ms) or 10 mM copper-ethylenediaminetetraacetic acid (Cu-EDTA) at pH 7 (*2*) ($T_1 = 400$ ms). The fact that the latter is lower than the former reflects the decreased number of water molecules that can pass through the solvation shell of copper ions which have six solvation sites sequestered by the EDTA moieties [4]. Consider now the effect of changing the pH of the Cu-EDTA solution. Increased proton concentration of the solution will increase the protonation of the nitrogen and carboxylate moieties of the EDTA, which will decrease the extent of complexation and thereby increase the amount of free copper ions in the solution [5]; that will increase the effective molar longitudinal relaxivity of the solution which can then be visualized in a T_1-weighted MR measurement. Indeed, a classical titration curve (Fig. 2) results from a bulk MR experiment in which Cu-EDTA acts as a pH-sensitive indicator.

A simple example of an MR indicator which is sensitive to the redox potential involves the Fe(II) ↔ Fe(III) equilibrium [6]; due to the fact that Fe(II) ions have one unpaired *d* electron less, they have a molar relaxivity which is 30-fold smaller than that of Fe(III) ions. Titration curves equivalent to Fig. 2 can be produced for aqueous solutions of iron ions as a function of redox potential, albeit with the added complication that at high pH values, the iron ions can precipitate as a complex mixture of mononuclear and polynuclear aqua-hydroxy complexes. Both the examples of MR indicators discussed thus far involve paramagnetic ions and it is appropriate now to draw attention to stable nitroxide free radicals such as 4-amino-2,2,6,6-tetramethylpiperidinyloxyl (*3*). Although the molar relaxivity of nitroxides is far lower than that of paramagnetic metal ions (190 L s^{-1} mol^{-1} compared to 10 000 L s^{-1} mol^{-1} for Fe(III)), they nevertheless can be used to locate reducing agents, such as ascorbic acid.

These MR indicators can be used to study a range of phenomena, including the mass transport diffusion either of the species themselves or of chemical reagents that influence chemical potential. For example, Fig. 3 shows how the Cu-EDTA system can be used to monitor the temporal progression of pH changes which accompany the migration of protons through a gel; note the enhanced signal intensity of the image that occurs with protonation of the EDTA nitrogen atoms. Figures 4 and 5 illustrate examples based on the iron and on the nitroxide redox system, using a 1% agarose gel as the heterogenous medium.

Measurements of mass transport diffusion coefficients can be made by direct observation of the movement of the interface between the chemical reagent and the unreacted medium, as visualized by the change of image intensity. For many complex systems, the rate of change does not allow complete mapping of the reaction front. However, using the null-point method [7] the location of one particular concentration of paramagnetic species can be visual-

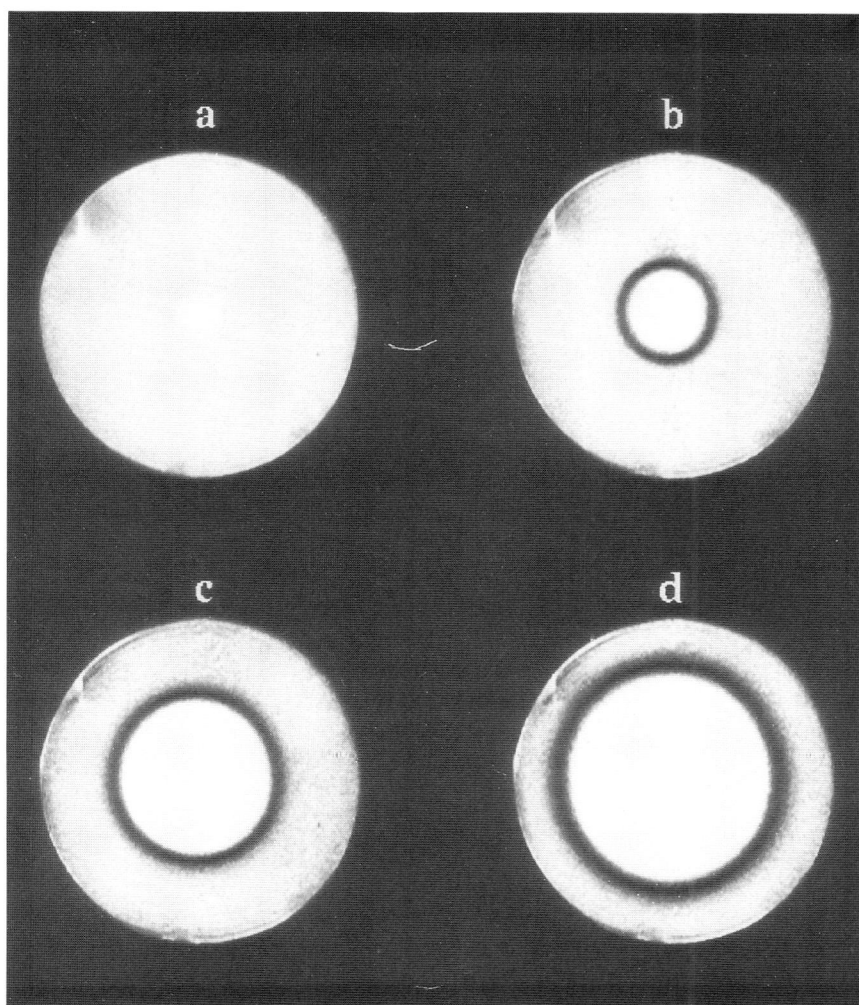

Fig. 3. Four Images of the diffusion of 1 M sulfuric acid from a central reservoir into a polyacrylamide (10%) cylinder sequestered with 10 mM Cu-EDTA solution at pH 7.0. The images were acquired immediately before the commencement of the experiment (a), then 3 min (b), 30 min (c), and 60 min (d) after exchanging the fluid in the central void with 1 M sulfuric acid; fast inversion recovery sequence (FIR 460/120/10), field of view 37 mm, the echo time 10 ms, and in-plane resolution 130 μm. The sulfuric acid concentration was kept constant by exchanging the fluid in the reservoir continuously. The recovery delay was chosen such that zero signal intensity was achieved for a pH of 1.3, which appears in the images as a black circular null contour spreading with time.

ized, which in many cases is sufficient to quantitate the diffusion rate. The null-point method makes use of the fact that the T_1 value of water is linearly dependent on the concentration of the paramagnetic species; consequently, if a calibration curve is available, then a defined value of T_1 is equivalent to a defined concentration. Given the explicit relationship between a T_1 value and the null point of an inversion recovery sequence, it follows that a null-point inversion recovery MR image can locate the spatial position of one particular concentration of a chemical species; if acqui-

sition of images with different recovery delays are interleaved, multiple concentrations can be mapped. The effectiveness of this approach is demonstrated in Fig. 3; the null-point method produces a band of low signal intensity which moves progressively behind the advancing diffusion front, which in this case shows as the region of high signal intensity.

Although we have relatively little practical experience so far, it is appropriate to end with an example of how this methodology can be used to study diffusion in intact cartilage. Figure 5a shows an MR image of an

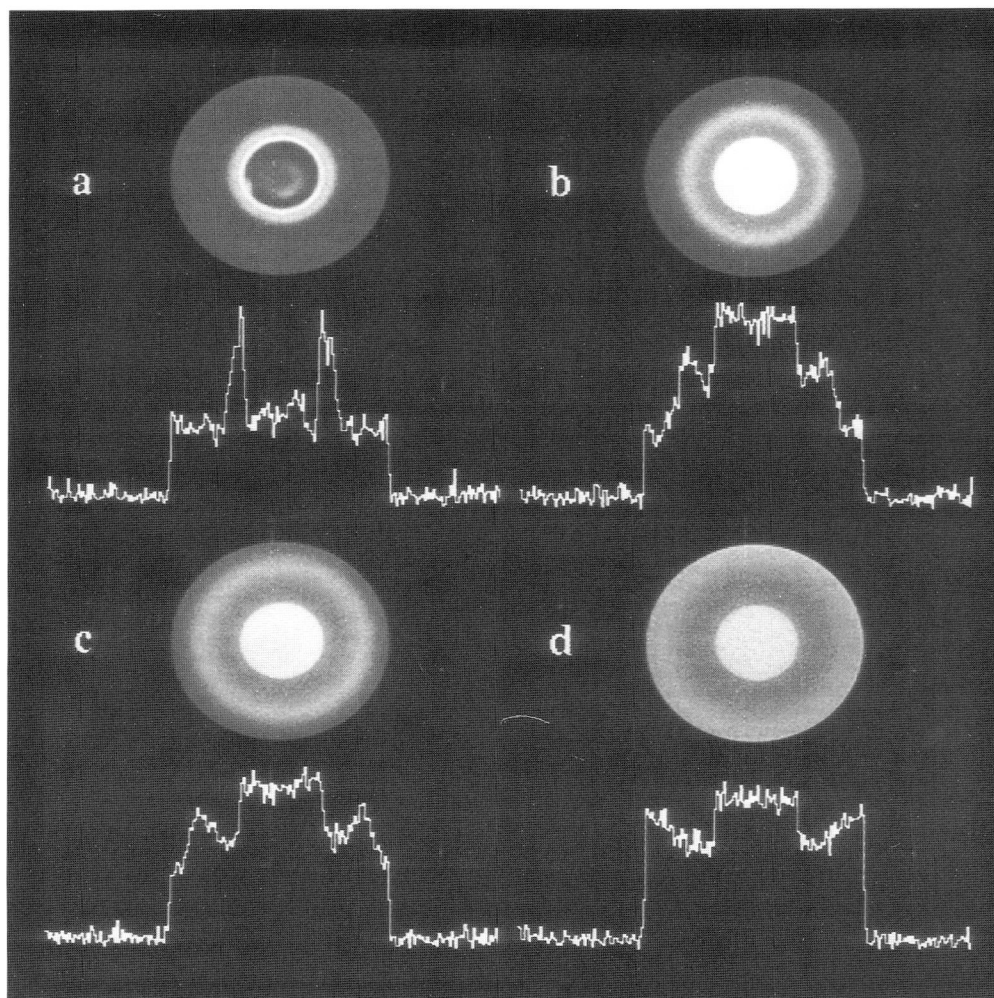

Fig. 4. Migration of sodium bromate into an agarose gel (1%) cylinder sequestered with 1 mM Fe(II)-sulfate at pH 3.0. At the commencement of the experiment, 0.1 M sodium bromate solution was added to the central void. Images were then acquired after 15 min (a), 30 min (b), 45 min (c), and 60 min (d) with a conventional spin-echo sequence (SE 500/16); field of view 50 mm, in-plane resolution 100 μm. The horizontal traces demonstrate the complexity of signal contrast within the diffusion–reaction zone, partly caused by precipitating Fe(III)-hydroxides which form at lower pH than the corresponding Fe(II)-hydroxides.

intact hen knee joint; cartilage is clearly delineated, and internal structure within the cartilage is visible. When the excised head of the femur was immersed in an aqueous solution of 4-hydroxy-TEMPO (3), the signal intensity of the cartilage was systematically depressed as the nulled concentration of (3) migrated progressively into the cartilage. An unexpected feature of this experiment was that the migration through the cartilage was followed by a slower progression through the cartilage growth plate and the marrow into the bone.

CONCLUSIONS

The concept of a substance that can be used to control the relative intensities of different regions of a magnetic resonance image, and hence the perceived contrast within that image, was first recognized by Lauterbur et al. [8]. However, it was predated by the previously documented effect [9] of paramagnetic metal ions on the nuclear relaxation times of many nuclides, especially proton and carbon-13. As a result of a major investment, Gd-DTPA (neutralized with

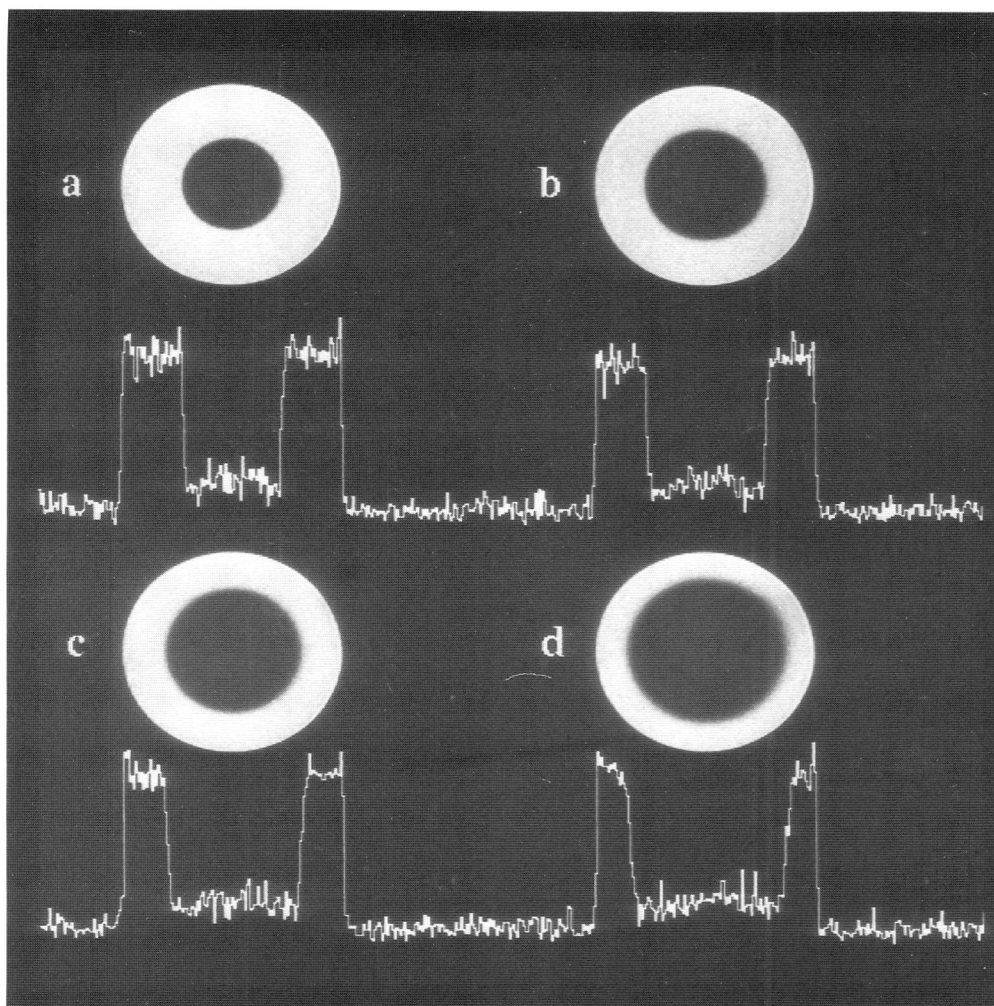

Fig. 5. Time course of the migration of ascorbic acid into an agarose gel (1%) sequestered with 50 mM 4-amino-TEMPO at neutral pH. At the commencement of the experiment, 1 M ascorbic acid was added to the central void; images were then acquired after 15 min (a), 27 min (b), 40 min (c), and 55 min (d) using a conventional spin-echo sequence (SE 500/16); field of view 50 mm, and in-plane resolution 100 μm. Horizontal traces are displayed to demonstrate the sharpness of the advancing front.

two equivalents of *N*-methylglucamine) has received international clearance for use in man [1], where it is used in conjunction with many different MRI protocols to heighten the contrast between different tissues on the basis of their relative vascularity. More recently, other classes of paramagnetic complexes have been invented [10] which can similarly alter image contrast *in vivo*; these include those based on stable nitroxide free radicals. Besides intellectual curiosity, many of those substances have been synthesized because of the recognized need to control the pharmacokinetics and tissue specificity of the contrast agents.

The present work in Cambridge has a different objective: the design of substances which are sensitive to the chemical potential of their surroundings which they can relay to the observer via their effect on the MRI properties of water. The examples chosen for this article have potential uses for both *in vitro* and *in vivo* situations. For example, with suitable modifications, metal chelate complexes can be designed to be sensitive to specific pH regimes appropriate for studies of the human gastrointestinal system. With regard to redox systems there is already precedent from the elegant work of Armstrong and coworkers [11] where

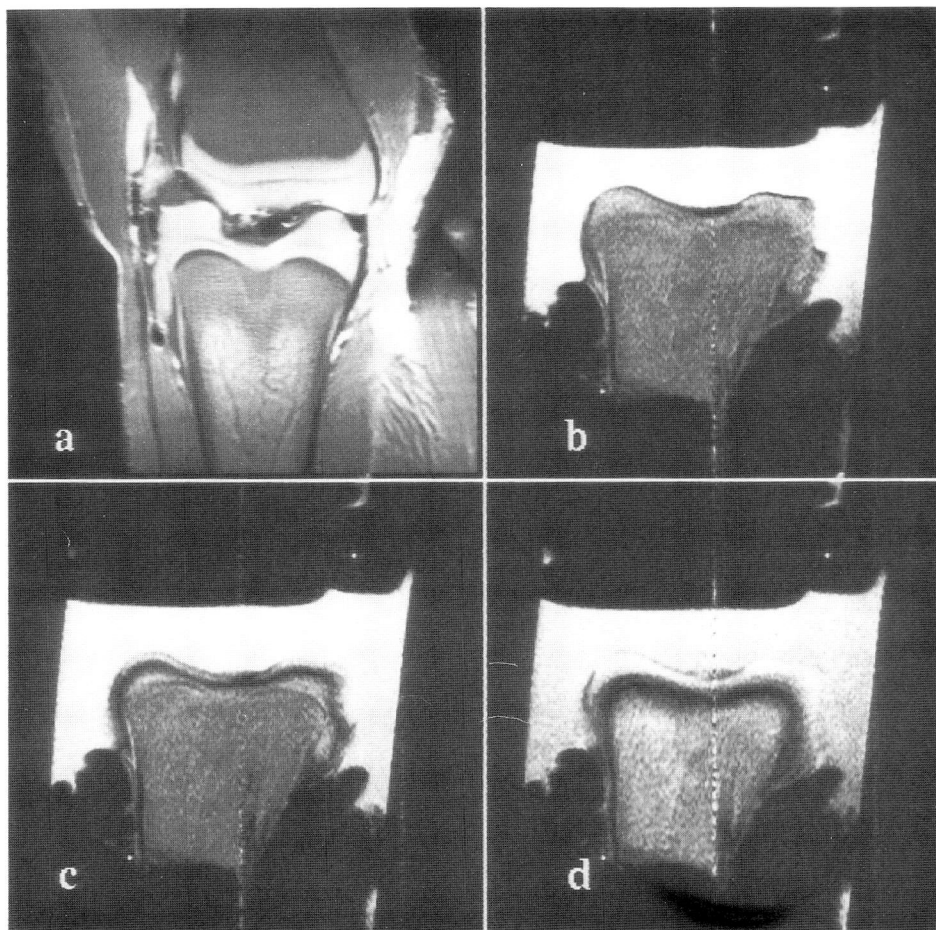

Fig. 6. Time course of the migration of 4-hydroxy-TEMPO into the femoral chondyle of an excised hen leg. The figure shows the knee joint before disarticulation (a), immediately after immersing it in 0.1 M 4-hydroxy-TEMPO solution (b), after 30 min (c), and after 6 h (d). Image a was acquired with a conventional spin-echo sequence (SE 1000/20), whereas the last three images were acquired with a fast inversion recovery sequence (FIR 460/100/10), nulling a concentration of 25 mM 4-hydroxy-TEMPO; field of view 37 mm, echo time 10 ms, and in-plane resolution 130 μm.

the equilibrium Mn(II) ↔ Mn(III) was used to follow oscillating chemical reactions *in vitro*. However, to follow changes of redox potential in man will require more subtle forms of molecular control; in that context, the use of nitroxides to detect reducing potential is particularly attractive.

ACKNOWLEDGMENTS

It is a pleasure to thank Dr. Herchel Smith for an Endowment (LDH) and for a studentship (AEF). The help of Dr. B. J. Balcom in initiating aspects of this work is appreciated.

REFERENCES

1. Schörner W, Felix R, Laniado M, Lange L, Weinmann HJ, Claussen C, Fiegler W, Speck U, Kazner E (1984) Testing the nuclear magnetic tomography contrast medium gadolinium DTPA in humans: tolerance, alteration of contrast, and first clinical results. *ROFO* **140:** 493–500.
2. Fischer AE, Balcom BJ, Carpenter TA, Hall LD (1993) NMR Imaging as an indicator of chemical potential (Abstract). *2nd International Conference on Magnetic Resonance Microscopy,* Heidelberg, p. 85.
3. Hall LD, Rajanayagam V (1985) Visualization of chromatography columns by NMR imaging. *J Chem Soc Chem Commun* **1985:** 499–501.

4. Lauffer RB (1987) Paramagnetic metal complexes as water proton relaxation agents for NMR imaging: theory and design. *Chem Rev* **87**: 908.

5. Bell CF (1977) Aminopolycarboxylic acids. In *Principles and Applications of Metal Chelation,* 1st ed. Oxford: Clarendon Press.

6. Balcom BJ, Carpenter TA, Hall LD (1992) Spatial and temporal visualization of two aqueous iron oxidation–reduction reactions by nuclear magnetic resonance imaging. *J Chem Soc Chem Commun* **1992**: 312–313.

7. Balcom BJ, Fischer AE, Carpenter TA, Hall LD (1993) Diffusion in aqueous gels. Mutual diffusion coefficients measured by one-dimensional nuclear magnetic resonance imaging. *J Am Chem Soc* **115**: 3300–3305.

8. Lauterbur PC, Mendonca-Dias MH, Rudin AM (1978) Augmentation of tissue water protein spin–lattice relaxation rates by in-vivo addition of paramagnetic ions. *Front Biol Eng* **1**: 752–759.

9. Bloch F, Hansen WW, Packard M (1948) The nuclear induction experiment. *Phys Rev* **70**: 474–485.

10. Fritzsch T, Krause W, Weinmann HJ (1992) Status of contrast media research in MRI, ultrasound and X-ray. *Eur Radiol* **2**: 2–13.

11. Armstrong RL, Tzalmona A, Menzinger M, Cross A, Lemaire C (1992) Imaging the dynamics of chemical waves: the Belousov–Zhabotinsky reaction. In *Magnetic Resonance Microscopy: Methods and Applications in Material Science, Agriculture and Biomedicine* (Blümich B, Kuhn W, eds.). Weinheim: VCH.

Effect of opsonins on the uptake of magnetic starch microspheres by rat Kupffer cells

Jean-Marie Colet and Robert N. Muller*

NMR Laboratory, University of Mons-Hainaut, B-7000 Mons, Belgium

The influence of various sera and proteins on the uptake of a superparamagnetic colloid (magnetic starch microspheres (MSM); particle size, 200 nm; crystal size, 10 nm) by the isolated and perfused rat liver has been studied. It is demonstrated that the capture of MSM is slightly reduced by the addition of rat blood to the protein-free perfusion medium but highly reduced by newborn calf serum (NCS). The SDS–PAGE (sodium dodecyl sulfate–polyacrylamide gel electrophoresis) analysis of proteins adsorbed on the nanoparticles incubated in NCS reveals major coating by albumin and IgG. The addition of bovine IgG to the perfusion fluid reduces the rate of MSM uptake in the same extent that NCS, whereas fetal calf serum that contains only traces of IgG weakly alters the MSM clearance. Finally, complemented and decomplemented NCS exhibit the same influence on the MSM hepatic extraction. It is concluded that although lectins are largely involved in the uptake of MSM administered in the absence of proteins, opsonins receptors are implicated when the perfusion medium contains relevant blood components.

Keywords: MRI contrast agents, superparamagnetic particles, opsonins, perfused liver.

INTRODUCTION

Superparamagnetic particles are promising agents for magnetic resonance imaging (MRI) contrast enhancement. They are made of ferrite cores (i.e., iron oxides) dispersed in biocompatible coating which prevents aggregation and may govern their biodistribution [1]. Magnetic starch microspheres (MSM) are such particles with an overall size of 200 ± 50 nm consisting of 10-nm magnetic crystals coated with starch [2]. After intravenous injection in animals, MSM are rapidly concentrated in the mononuclear phagocytotic system, mainly in the liver and spleen [3]. The mechanisms of recognition and clearance of these contrast agents are not yet fully understood. One remaining question is whether the recognition of MSM by Kupffer cells is mediated by opsonins.

As previously demonstrated in the isolated rat liver perfused with Krebs–Henseleit solution, the uptake of MSM by Kupffer cells is mediated by lectins [4]. However, *in vivo* recognition factors called opsonins

are known to cover exogenous materials and to promote their binding to macrophage receptors. Numerous molecules show opsonic activity, e.g., fibronectin, immunoglobulins, and complement factors. The coating depends on the nature and on the size of the foreign body. This has been well documented for liposomes [5, 6] and polyacrylstarch microparticles [7, 8].

In the presence of blood components, other mechanisms than those involving lectins are, thus, expected to participate to the clearance of MSM by the liver, as Kupffer cells contain receptors for fibronectin, immunoglobulins (IgG and IgM), and factor C3 of the complement.

In this study, the influence of blood components from various origins on the hepatic MSM uptake was evaluated and the nature of some opsonins involved in the recognition of those colloidal contrast agents was determined by electrophoresis.

MATERIALS AND METHODS

Livers from male Wistar rats (± 150 g) were isolated and perfused at 37°C with 3–4 ml min^{-1} g^{-1} of liver weight through the portal vein with 180 ml of a recirculating medium. Krebs–Henseleit solution was

* Address for correspondence: Department of Organic Chemistry and NMR Laboratory, University of Mons-Hainaut, B-7000 Mons, Belgium.

used for a control group ($n = 10$). For the other groups ($n = 8$ for each group), the perfusion fluid was supplemented with (i) 5% of rat blood from the liver donor, (ii) newborn calf serum (NCS) (Sigma, 021-06010) complemented and decomplemented by heating at 56°C for 30 min, and (iii) fetal calf serum (FCS) (Sigma, 011-06290). Two other groups of livers received 500 mg of bovine serum albumin and increasing doses (25 and 50 mg) of IgG, respectively.

MSM were added to the perfusion medium at a dose of 100 μg of iron per g of liver weight and their concentration in the perfusate was followed by proton relaxometry on aliquots of 0.3 ml at 0.47 T and 37°C on a spin analyzer (Minispec PC-120; Bruker, Karlsruhe, Germany). Knowing the r_2 relaxivity in these conditions ($177\ s^{-1}\ mM^{-1}$), the concentration was calculated from the relaxation rate R_2 of the perfusion medium. ^{31}P–NMR spectra of the perfused livers were obtained on a spectrometer (AMX-300; Bruker, Karlsruhe, Germany) with the following conditions: number of averages = 300, flip angle = 60°, and repetition time = 1 s.

In order to identify the proteins adsorbed on the particles, the MSM were suspended in Krebs–Henseleit solution supplemented with NCS. The mixture was incubated at 37°C for 1 h. The particles were then concentrated and purified by magnetophoresis and washed with sodium dodecyl sulfate (SDS) 1%. SDS–PAGE (polyacrylamide gel electrophoresis) of proteins was performed on a LKB 2050 Midget electrophoresis unit.

RESULTS AND DISCUSSION

The concentration of MSM in the Krebs–Henseleit medium delivered to the isolated and perfused rat liver progressively decreases due to their uptake by Kupffer cells (A in Fig. 1). The observed half-life is 14 min.

The clearance of MSM by the liver is slightly reduced by rat blood (C in Fig. 1) but highly decreased in the presence of NCS (D in Fig. 1). This can be attributed either to an effect of the serum components on the phagocytic capability of the liver or to an alteration of the nanoparticles.

The first hypothesis of a direct influence of serum components on the liver was evaluated and rejected by the following experiments. First, no influence of the assayed sera on the hepatic metabolism was observed in the ^{31}P–NMR spectra which evolved identically to the controls for a period of 90 min. Second, the inhibiting effect of NCS could be counteracted by a subsequent addition of rat blood (results not shown).

In order to verify the assumption of a modification of the nanoparticles, electrophoresis was performed

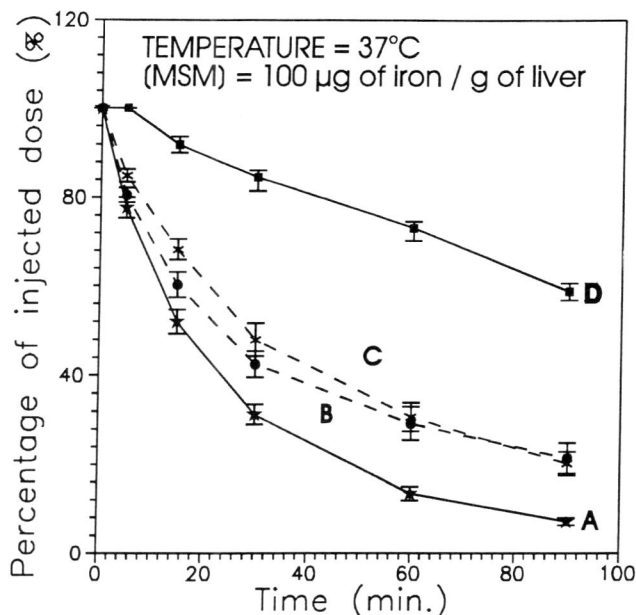

Fig. 1. Evolution of the MSM concentration in the perfusion fluid of isolated rat livers perfused with (A) Krebs–Henseleit solution, (B) fetal calf serum, (C) rat blood, and (D) newborn calf serum.

on MSM incubated in NCS. The electropherogram revealed two bands corresponding to albumin and IgG. These results give evidences for the opsonization of the nanoparticles by IgG. The weak albeit significant affinity of bovine IgG for rat Kupffer cells receptors could explain the large reduction of the MSM clearance induced by NCS with respect to rat blood. The experiment was repeated with FCS that is known to contain only traces of IgG ($7.510^{-4}\ g\ L^{-1}$) as compared to NCS ($21\ g\ IgG\ L^{-1}$). The results obtained show but a weak influence of FCS on the MSM clearance (B in Figure 1) and, thus, confirm the predominant role of IgG.

On the other hand, bovine serum albumin (BSA) has a much smaller influence than bovine IgG, which, to the contrary, has a significant and dose-dependent effect (Fig. 2). Finally, the thermal denaturation of complement factors of NCS (56°C for 30 min) does not alter its effect on MSM clearance (data not shown).

CONCLUSIONS

Previously, we have demonstrated that the endocytosis of MSM by the isolated rat liver perfused with Krebs–Henseleit solution was mediated by Kupffer cells lectins [4]. We now could show that the addition of rat serum to the perfusion fluid promotes the

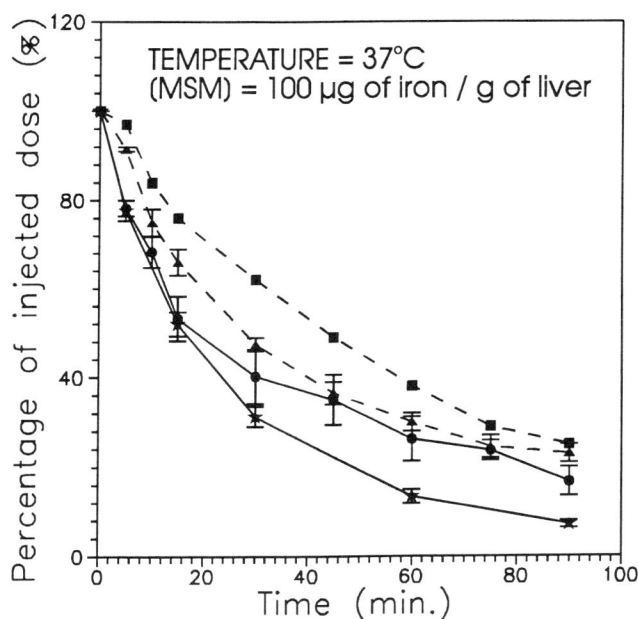

Fig. 2. Evolution of the MSM concentration in the perfusion fluid of isolated rat livers perfused with Krebs–Henseleit solution (★) and with Krebs–Henseleit solution supplemented with 500 mg of BSA (▲) or 25 mg (●) or 50 (■) of bovine IgG.

coating of the particles by IgG and albumin, leading to a shift to other receptors and to a decrease of the MSM clearance. Thus, the predominant role of IgG becomes clear. Harashima et al. [5] reported that opsonization decreased the extraction of small liposomes (0.2 μm) by the rat liver perfused *in situ* but increased the uptake of large liposomes (0.8 μm). The latter observation was supported by Artursson et al. [7, 8] who reported similar opsonization of polyacrylstarch and polyacrylmannan microparticles of about 2 μm, followed by an increase in uptake by macrophages in culture. The behavior of our colloidal system, which is characterized by a mean particle size of 0.2 μm, is thus in good agreement with the results reported by the first authors.

The binding of IgG to rat Kupffer cells receptors seems to be very specific because the coating of MSM by bovine IgG strongly prolongs the persistence of the particles in the perfusion medium. The process is reversed when nanoparticles coated with bovine IgG are opsonized with rat blood.

ACKNOWLEDGMENTS

This work was supported by the ARC Program 90/94-142 of the Communauté Française de Belgique. The authors are grateful to Prof. M. Joniau of KULAC, Kortrijk for stimulating discussions.

REFERENCES

1. Weissleder R, Papisov M (1992) Pharmaceutical Iron Oxides for MR Imaging. *Reviews of Magnetic Resonance in Medicine* 4:1.
2. Roch A, Bach-Gansmo T, Muller RN (1993) In vitro relaxometric characterization of superparamagnetic contrast agents. *MAGMA* **1**: 83.
3. Fahlvik AK, Holtz E, Leander P, Schroder U, Klaveness J (1990) Magnetic starch microspheres, efficacy and elimination. A new organ-specific contrast agent for magnetic resonance imaging. *Invest Radiol* **25**: 113.
4. Colet JM, Van Haverbeke Y, Muller RN (1994) Evidences for attachment of magnetic starch microspheres to Kupffer cells receptors in excised and perfused rat liver. *Invest Radiol.* **29**: S223.
5. Harashima H, Ohnishi Y, Kiwada H (1992) In vivo evaluation of the effect of the size and the opsonization on the hepatic extraction of liposomes in rats: an application of Oldendorf method. *Biopharm Drug Disp* **13**: 549.
6. Harashima H, Sakata K, Kiwada H (1993) Distinction between the depletion of opsonins and the saturation of uptake in the dose-dependent hepatic uptake of liposomes. *Pharma Res* **10**: 606.
7. Artursson P, Sjöholm I (1986) Effect of opsonins on the macrophage uptake of polyacrylstarch microparticles. *Int J Pharm* **32**: 165.
8. Artursson P, Johansson D, Sjöholm I (1988) Receptor-mediated uptake of starch and mannan microparticles by macrophages: Relative contribution of receptors for complement, immunoglobulins and carbohydrates. *Biomaterials* **9**: 241.

A new MRI formulation for flow and motion applications

P.R. Moran

Wake Forest University, The Bowman Gray School of Medicine, Winston-Salem, NC 27157-1022, USA

A rigorous reformulation of the magnetic resonance (MR) image formulation model (IFM) can use the integrally cumulative nature of MRI phase shifts for encoding and of time-of-flight travel corrections for magnitude. This approach characterizes each independent gradient element by its cumulant waveforms, $K_N(t)$, instead of by particular time expansion in gradient moments. The lowest-order cumulant gradient that gives a simple monopolar waveform governs all resulting phase-encoding properties. Each gradient element specifically encodes one and only one motion-order variable. Phase sensitizations to "higher order" do not exist; they are mathematical psuedophasings. Magnetization isochromats may have arbitrarily complicated velocity history, $V(t)$, appearing in both time-of-flight and motion phase-shift formulas. The subject's intravoxel motion subdistributions each automatically reference the correct mean time of encoding action and its encoding duration. This formulation yields very simple and generalizable IFM expressions for MRI acquired data, with no theoretical confusion regarding higher-order phase shifts and nonphased time-of-flight effects.

Keywords: flow-imaging, MR motion artifacts, MR phase shifts.

INTRODUCTION

Magnetic resonance (MR) flow imaging is an obvious case in which time-of-flight (TOF) effects for moving magnetization generate one kind of MR contrast, whereas velocity phase-shift sensitization provides a different contrast (or artifact) phenomenon [1, 2]. But TOF and phase-shift effects are two aspects of the very same physical events in the subject imaging and should be treated together. As internal motions become more complex, theoretical interpretation of MR currently becomes impossibly difficult. Signal attenuation properties due to fluctuative motions (e.g., perfusive flow, stenotic jets) are one example. Publications by van Tyen et al. [3] and by Urchuk and Plewes [4] provide especially complete and pertinent bibliographies relating to these kinds of problems.

Much recent literature indicates how confusion arises from traditional MR treatment of TOF and phase shift as if they were separate, independent effects. When TOF travel actually occurs over some MR interval prior to the true time of signal detection,

Address for correspondence: Department of Radiology, Bowman Gray School of Medicine, Medical Center Boulevard, Winston-Salem, NC 27157-1022, USA.

then normal position-encoded phase-shift "correction" obviously must physically occur. Otherwise, the measured MR echo signal would not give the correct phase to reconstruct location of precessing magnetization, as it truly existed at encoding time. With the conventional gradient moments model of MRI, however, this adjustment for actual encoding time appears mathematically as if it were a phase-encoding specific for velocity. Some consequences have been explored by Simonetti, et al. [5]. Such unphased TOF image corrections may be called "psuedophasings." Similar confusions can occur for all higher-order MR motion as well; e.g., acceleration gives TOF to velocity.

This article outlines a reformulated MR Image formation model, to include possibly very complex internal motions. Natural MR relations between motion quantities, TOF travel, and imaged position then develop simultaneously. We have found this formulation eliminates automatically much of the theory confusion and mathematical intractability. A gratifyingly simple MR image formation model results with excellent generality and evident usefulness. However, one must carefully review the MR subject's magnetization functions that are encoded by an MR sequence, especially when complicated motion occurs, examine fundamental solutions to Bloch's equations when motion transport terms are added, and review how to describe a complicated MR gradient sequence. This short article outlines only the basic concepts and expressions for the new MR cumulative transport image formation model (IFM), leaving particular applications to later publication.

CUMULATIVE TRANSPORT MR QUANTITIES

The gradient field sequence

For a specific MR cycle and a specific TE reference for echo data acquisition in that cycle, the magnetic gradient field, $\mathbf{G}(t)\cdot\mathbf{r}$, can be written uniquely by a sum of independent "phase-gradient" modulation elements, $\Sigma_n \mathbf{F}_n(t)\cdot\mathbf{r}$. The action of each elemental F waveform varies with MRI cycle/sample, and each F element has an independent amplitude (or sampling time) incrementation, in nested-loop fashion, which identifies it as an element separate from all others. The F modulation includes phase inversion or creation from RF pulses and is zero prior to the effective time of initial excitation, T_A, for the magnetic moments detected at TE. We define a local time zero origin at the run time T_A point for that cycle, for example as shown in Fig. 1. We shall also consider that any data sampling time, $t_s - \text{TE}$), within the detection datagate, is a subinterval of (0, TE) whether $t_s - \text{TE}$ is positive or negative. We take $F(t)$ in imaging units, e.g., H/cm. As each F element is independent of all others, the associated phase shift is additive to and independent of all others. Phase modulation produced by an F element in one single uniquely moving, magnetically precessing spin group can then be expressed as an integral cumulative effect:

$$\phi_n(\mathbf{r}|\text{TE}) = 2\pi \int_0^{\text{TE}} \mathbf{F}_n(t) \cdot \mathbf{R}(t)\, dt \tag{1}$$

Bloch's equations require a specific meaning for position variables on the left side, namely, that (r| TE) means the voxel location of this magnetic moment isochromat group, conditioned on the specific detection TE time. We henceforth reserve $\mathbf{r}$ to denote position at TE detection time, making its conditional notation implicit unless needed. Under those conditions, the "time of flight (TOF) travel," $\mathbf{R}(t)$ in Eq. (1) refers to just one isochromat and is most usefully written as

$$\mathbf{R}(t) = \mathbf{r} - \int_t^{\text{TE}} \mathbf{V}(t')\, dt' \tag{2}$$

so that $\mathbf{r}$ is the correct voxel location of detection, i.e., for t equal to the TE time. The velocity integral is the isochromat's TOF travel over the TE $- t$ interval; we

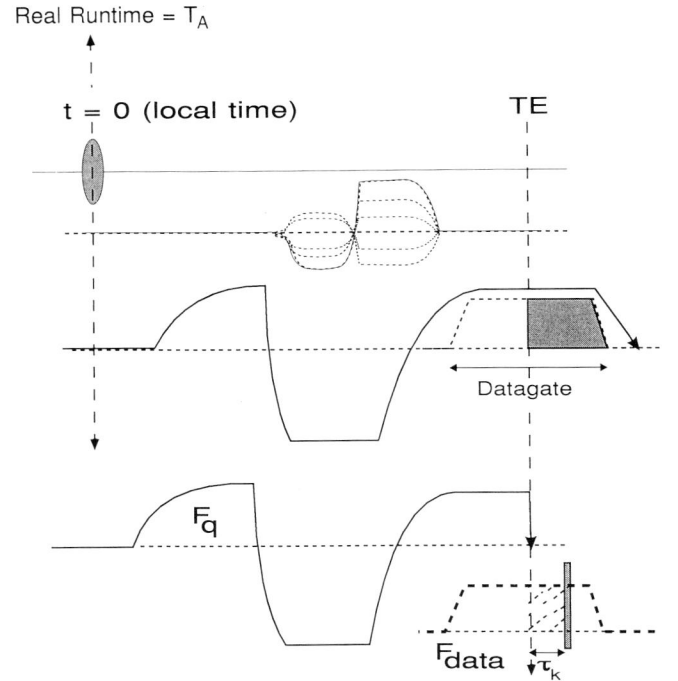

Fig. 1. The MR sequence timing diagram shows an example of initial RF pulse, two gradient directions, and three independent gradient elements. They are the pulsed-encoding (PE) elemental waveform, which is compensated for velocity, and the two independent elements along the "readout" direction. The latter are the second-echo quadrupolar waveform and the monopolar data aquisition waveform.

assume that MR acquisition gating methods synchronize pulsatile velocity to each scan cycle.

Transport solutions and motion orders

Equations (1) and (2) refer to a single "isochromat," a spin group with identical velocity histories, and all arriving in the voxel at $\mathbf{r}$ at the specified TE time. The final MR result, of course, will be an integral over a distribution of all possible positions and velocity histories, modulated by a product of phase factors, $\exp(i\phi_n)$. The TOF travel formula in Eq. (2) is a solution for Boltzman's transport equation not only for a transporting phase bolus [shown in Eq. (1)] but also for magnitude of precessing magnetization, M, as found in the TOF solution:

$$M(\mathbf{R}|T) = M((\mathbf{R} + \delta\mathbf{R})|\text{TE}); \quad \delta\mathbf{R} = \int_T^{\text{TE}} \mathbf{V}(t')\, dt' \tag{3}$$

for each isochromat whose $\mathbf{V}(t)$ contributes. We see that Eq. (3) is just the usual MR time-of-flight equation by which a bolus of magnetization is displaced downstream by $\delta\mathbf{R}$ between two time conditions of determination. Conditional time dependence, as used in Eqs.

F(quad.) GRADIENT

readout gradient
"velocity" compensated

sequence element: " K_0 "

t = 0
t = TE

first running integral;
the cumulant waveform: " K_1 "

second running integral;
the cumulant waveform: " K_2 "

This "eigencumulant" waveform
has a monopolar profile on (0,TE)

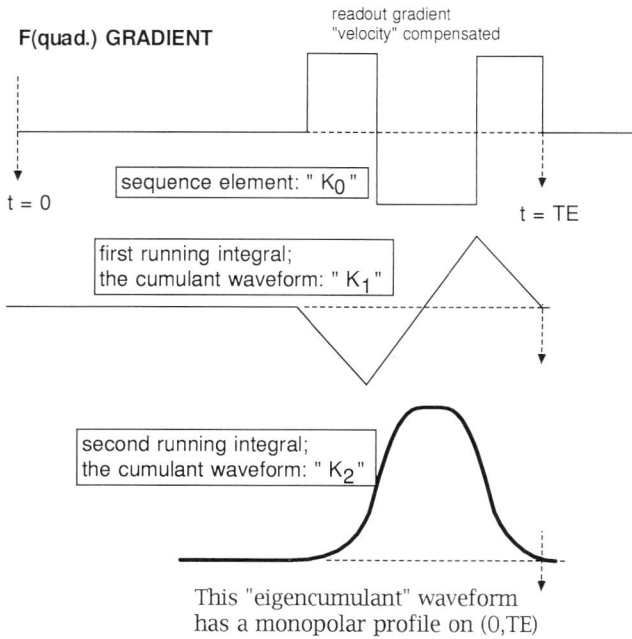

Fig. 2. The quadrupolar F gradient evolves to its cumulant descriptor as shown by the original $F(t)$ waveform, its first running integral $K_1(t)$, and its second running integral $K_2(t)$. As $K_2(t)$ has the first-occurring nonzero definite integral on (0, TE), it is the eigencumulant for a quadrupolar F element and sensitizes specifically only to second-order motion, $v_2(t)$, the acceleration quantity [$v_2 = a(t)$] for a particular isochromat group in the subject.

(1)–(3), at first seems to be confusing notation, but it is needed to distinguish actual signal detection reference time (i.e., a TE time) from the sequence run time, t, and/or different encoding action times. The natural definition of higher-order isochromat motions (denoted by v_n) is then given by derivatives of the TOF travel, $R(t)$,

$$v_n(t) \equiv d\{v_{n-1}\}/dt = (v_n|TE) - \int_t^{TE} v_{n+1}(t')\, dt'$$

$$v_0(t) \equiv R(t) = (r|TE) - \int_t^{TE} v_{n+1}(t')\, dt' \qquad (4)$$

$$v_1(t) \equiv V(t) = (V|TE) - \int_t^{TE} a(t')\, dt'$$

Note that every v_n has its own time-of-flight relation, all in the same form as Eq. (2).

The phase expression in Eq. (1) is an integral (cumulative) function, and all TOF relations in Eqs. (4) are cumulative. This suggests that a basic integrally cumulant waveform also should characterize each independent F waveform. Waveform "cumulants", $K_N(t)$, are related to moment polynomials but do not depend on specific choice of time origin. We may define the $K_N(t)$ by the inverse of that for the motion-

order quantities in Eq. (4)

$$K_N(t) = (-1)^N \int_0^t K_{N-1}(t')\, dt'$$

$$K_0(t) \equiv F(t)$$

with the special "eigencumulant" case, $K_n(t)$, whose full integral value is nonzero f_n,

$$f_n \equiv \int_0^{TE} K_n(t')\, dt',$$

$$\text{iff } \int_0^{TE} K_N(t')\, dt' \text{ is zero for all } N < n \qquad (5)$$

The eigencumulant order, n, will equal the characteristic multipolarity of that particular elemental F-gradient modulation. The $K_n(t)$ eigencumulant is always the first occurring *monopolar* waveform that derives from a specific $F(t)$, as illustrated in Fig. 2 for the sequence "second-echo" F(quadrupolar) used in the example of Fig. 1. This formulation greatly simplifies complex-motion MR theory because, when Eqs. (4) and (5) are substituted into Eq. (1), only v_n and K_n alone survive after integrations by parts. The result is

$$\phi_n(r|TE) = 2\pi \int_0^{TE} K_n(t) \cdot v_n(t)\, dt \equiv 2\pi f_n \cdot u_n \qquad (6)$$

where u_n is an averaged value of the specific $v_n(t)$ motion. To a good approximation in all realistic cases, a u_n component can be evaluated from the equivalent-square version of $K_n(t)$, as sketched in Fig. 3. The phase in Eq. (6) is now identical in form to position

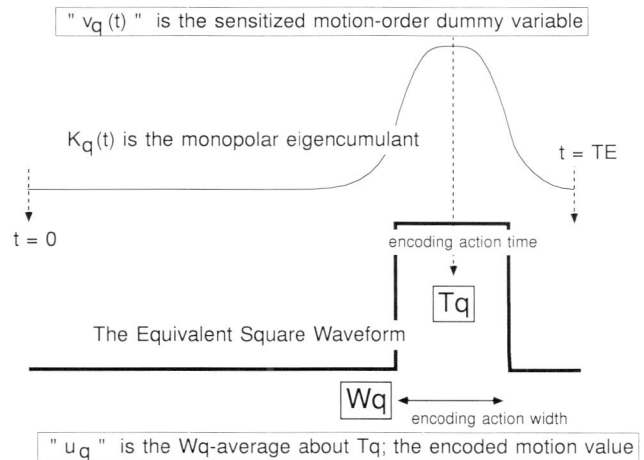

" $v_q(t)$ " is the sensitized motion-order dummy variable

$K_q(t)$ is the monopolar eigencumulant

t = TE

t = 0

encoding action time

Tq

The Equivalent Square Waveform

Wq
encoding action width

" u_q " is the Wq-average about Tq; the encoded motion value

Fig. 3. The encoded variable u_2, is the sensitized motion, equal to $v_2(t)$ averaged over an encoding action width, W_n, centered at the mean time of encoding action, T_n. These are given to good approximation by the correlation width and the mean time of the $K_2(t)$ monopolar waveform, as indicated by the "effective-square" shape in the figure.

encoding (zero order) of a MRI pulsed-encoding PE-gradient monopolar F_0 waveform [1, 2], and this is true for any sensitized order of motion. The phase-encoded variable, $\mathbf{u}_n$, is given by an average of $\mathbf{v}_n(t)$ over an encoding timewidth, W_n,

$$\mathbf{u}_n = (1/W_n) \int_{-W_n/2}^{/+W_n/2} \mathbf{v}_n(T_n + t') \, dt' \qquad (7)$$

The encodings of Eqs. (6) and (7) involve two time parameters, the encoding action meantime, T_n, and the active encoding timewidth, W_n. These are parameters determined only by $\mathbf{K}_n(t)$, the eigencumlant waveform for the F modulation and *not* by the time dependence of $\mathbf{V}(t)$. This result greatly simplifies the MR image model.

The cumulative transport formulation has shown that each elemental gradient F waveform sensitizes specifically to one and only to one motion-derivative quantity. The encoding time parameters, T_n and W_n, appear as arguments in the subject's magnetization functions that are encoded, as the encoding variables themselves will all be dummy variables of integration in evaluating the final detected MR signal. This formulation can give a wholly new perspective for theoretically describing motion effects in MR.

Magnetization distributions with complex motion

Moving magnetization generally must be expressed as a precessing jointly distributed magnetization, $S(\mathbf{V}, t; \mathbf{r}|\text{TE})$, which represents the (excited) magnetic moment (per dR^3) found in the voxel at $\mathbf{r}$, given detection at TE, and which has a velocity $\mathbf{V}$ any time (t)—an entire velocity history $\mathbf{V}(t)$ within range dV^3. Using Bayes' expansion, this multivariate distribution may be expressed in various forms, as conditional products of motion-order subdistributions. An example is

$$S(\mathbf{V}, t; \mathbf{r}|\text{TE}) \, d^3V \, d^3r = M(\mathbf{r}|\text{TE}) \, d^3r \, P(\mathbf{V}, t|\mathbf{r}) \, d^3V(t)$$
$$= M(\mathbf{R}|T_0)$$
$$\cdot (\Pi_{n=1}^{(N-1)} \, p_n(\mathbf{u}_n, T_n|\mathbf{r}) \, d^3\mathbf{u}_n) \qquad (8)$$
$$\cdot p_N(\mathbf{v}_N, t|r) \, d^3\mathbf{v}_{N_1}.$$

The general distribution of all isochromats in the subject is the total magnetization in the voxel multiplied by the time-dependent velocity history voxel dispersion, $P(V, t|r)$. But this isocromat fraction itself expands as a product of motion-derivative subdistributions, terminating in some highest-order time-dependent subdistribution not sensitized via Eqs. (6) and (7). Any nonsensitized subdistribution integrates to unity in the detected signal expression. Each independent gradient element of the MR sequence selects either $M(\mathbf{R})$ for position encoding or else selects one of the

intravoxel $p_n(\mathbf{v}_n(t)$ subdistributions for motion encoding. Each encoded variable value, $\mathbf{u}_n$, will be the motion average as in Eq. (7), taken about the eigencumulant mean time, T_n, consequently, all complexity formerly encountered as an infinite series of higher moment values collapses simply into how and which different motion-derivative quantities are present in voxels when $\mathbf{K}_n(t)$-encoding action actually occurs. Each motion subdistribution may have TOF correction over the interval (TE $- T_n$). Zero-order variables, ($\mathbf{u}_0$, $\mathbf{f}_0$) are conventionally called ($\mathbf{R}$, $\mathbf{k}$).

SIGNAL-FORMATION MODEL

The acquired MR signal, $A^\sim(f. .)$ for a given encoding cycle and echo-signal sample, will given by the image formation model as the product integral,

$$A \sim (k, f_1, f_2, \ldots) = \int\int\int \cdots M(\mathbf{R} + \delta\mathbf{R}|\text{TE})$$
$$\cdot \exp\{-2\pi\mathbf{k} \cdot \mathbf{R})$$
$$\cdot d^3R(\, p_1(\mathbf{u}_1, T_v|r)$$
$$\times \exp\{-2\pi\mathbf{f}_1 \cdot \mathbf{u}_1) \, d^3\mathbf{u}_1) \qquad (9a)$$
$$\times (\ldots \ldots) \times (\, p_n(\mathbf{u}_n, T_n|r)$$
$$\cdot \exp\{-2\pi\mathbf{f}_n \cdot \mathbf{u}_n) \, d^3\mathbf{u}_n)$$

the $M(\mathbf{R}|\mathbf{T})$ time of flight is special because M is the detected signal quantity;

$$\delta\mathbf{R} \approx \int_{T_0}^{\text{TE}} \mathbf{V}(t') \, dt' = \mathbf{u}_1 \times (\text{TE} - T_0) \qquad (9b)$$

Boldface vector quantities are treated component by component. Higher-order-motion TOF corrections between T_n and TE are not physically critical in MRI for the p_n subdistributions. However, positional TOF for M described by Eqs. (9a) and (9b) generates several kinds of MR motion artifacts, e.g., oblique flow image misregistration. An elaboration of the TOF results from Eq. (9b), in terms of the position-encoding F_0 waveform shape, is straightforward but outside the scope of this short article. The conditional dependences for magnetization functions also extend easily, describing scans with many echoes acquired for each excitation. The TE reference for ($\mathbf{r}|\text{TE}$) also has an implicit TE-cycle dependence which may be correlated with the series of k spatial encoding values. Intravoxel velocity distributions may flucutuate with TE-cycle numbers, the result directly describing erratic motion artifacts. The cumulative transport formulation is extremely general, and the product of individual sensitized motion functions of Eq. (9a) shows that the ultimate result also is remarkably simple.

For each independent gradient element in the MRI sequence only one motion quantity is senisitized; no further series of higher-order motion phase shifts appears, as in method-of-moments approaches. The new formulation shows that all such apparent higher-order predictions arise spuriously as pseudophasing that admixed TOF travel with specific motion phase shift. When one accounts immediately for TOF, these pseudophases do not appear, because then each encoded motion function, $p_n(\mathbf{u}_n, T_n | r, TE)$, references the actual gradient encoding time, T_n, and not some other arbitrarily specified time. Although $M(r)$ is the actually detected quantity, its TOF adjustments do have a critical role in possible motion artifacts effects. All such possibilities are given in a rigorous and relatively simple way by the MR signal formation in Eqs. (9a) and (9b), where the MR reconstructed image, $A(r, \ldots)$ is the Inverse Fourier transform of $A\tilde{}(k, f_1, f_2, \ldots)$. The results, for example, predict directly the form of oblique flow artifacts and PE gradient-element compensations addressed in Refs. 1 and 2, without requiring any special ad hoc arguments used in earlier works.

An application example

The averaging of a motion variable over W_n shown in Fig. 3 illustrates how average acceleration, $\langle \mathbf{a} \rangle = \mathbf{u}_2$, is phase sensitized by a second echo sequence via $\mathbf{F}_q$ [see Eq. (7)]. This new IFM has proven particularly useful for analyzing motion fluctuation effects. By writing the time-dependent isochromat accelerative quantity, $\mathbf{v}_2(t)$, as the sum of a coherent acceleration, $\mathbf{a}(t)$, and an incoherent fluctuating term, $\delta\mathbf{a}(t)$, the phase-modula-

tion result becomes

$$
\begin{aligned}
\boldsymbol{\phi}_q(\mathbf{r} | TE) &= 2\pi \int_0^{TE} \mathbf{v}_2(t) \mathbf{K}_2(t)\, dt \\
&= 2\pi (\mathbf{f}_2 \cdot \langle \mathbf{a} \rangle) + 2\pi \{\mathbf{f}_2 / W_2\} \cdot \Delta\mathbf{V}
\end{aligned}
\tag{10}
$$

where $\Delta\mathbf{V}$ is the random variable of velocity deviation in the encoding time W-width. Equation (10) shows one example where the new formulation can resolve formerly perplexing issues: We note that motion-fluctuation phasing depends on a random variable at one order lower than the motion derivative that is specifically sensitized by an F gradient. By inspection of the $\Delta\mathbf{V}$ deviation quantity of Eq. (10), one also notes that *intracycle* fluctuations (within W_n), as well as much longer correlation time *intercycle* fluctuations, enter through the dependence on $[p(\mathbf{u}, T | r, TE(k))]$ conditional variables. Both kinds of fluctuations can contribute strongly to attenuation artifacts in the reconstructed image.

REFERENCES

1. Moran PR (1991) Experiments for two MR imaging theories of motion phase sensitivity. *Radiology* **180**: 115–119.
2. Frank LR, Adrian PC, Buxton RB (1992) Elimination of oblique flow artrifacts in MRI. *MRM* **25**: 299–307.
3. van Tyen R, Saloner D, Jou LD, Berger S (1993) MR imaging of flow through Tortous vessels: a numerical simulation. *MRM* **31**: 184–195.
4. Urchuk SN, Plewes DB (1992) Mechanisms of flow-induced signal loss in MR angiography. *J Magn Reson Imaging* **2**: 453–462.
5. Simonetti OP, Wendt RE III, Duerk JL (1991) Significance of the point of expansion in interpretation of gradient moments and motion sensitivity. *J Magn Reson Imaging* **1**: 569–578.

Role of imaging parameters in phase mapping flow measurement

P.E. Summers,* M.G. Taylor and T.S. Padayachee

United Medical and Dental Schools of Guy's and St. Thomas's Hospitals, London, UK

The influences of several primary imaging parameters on flow measurements made by the magnetic resonance phase mapping technique have been studied. In cine phase mapping, the echo time and flip angle had minimal effect on the flow measurement. Velocity sensitivity, slice thickness, and slice position were found to have well-behaved effects on the flow measurements. Angulation of either the slice or the tube away from normal intersection significantly affected the flow measurement. Further, the effect differs with the axis of rotation of the slice. Compensation for tube angulation by slice angulation improves flow measurements. Phase mapping is, thus, most heavily affected by gradient-related parameters. Hard limits on the choice of imaging parameters are few, but appropriate choices can compensate for or prevent some systematic errors.

Keywords: MR flowmetry, phase mapping.

INTRODUCTION

In magnetic resonance (MR), velocity-induced phase mapping uses a calibrated bipolar magnetic field gradient to establish a linear relationship between the mean velocity in the gradient direction of material in a source voxel and the phase of the related image pixel [1, 2]. Although velocity encoding may be implemented along any combination of axes, the slice selection direction is most often used. Local velocity and vessel area can then be determined in a single scan, allowing flow to be calculated. The reproducibility and correlation of MR phase mapping with other modalities have been studied [3, 4]. In this study, we have examined the influence of imaging parameters on *in vitro* MR flow measurements.

MATERIALS AND METHODS

Measurements were performed on a 1.5-T Philips S15 Gyroscan scanner using the flow-adjusted gradients (FLAG) imaging sequence. Calibration was initially tested using a rotating gel-filled disc phantom. The

flow phantom for the current study consisted of a water-filled perspex box with a perspex tube crossing horizontally (2.54 cm inside diameter). To reduce entrance effects, 50 diameters of tube separated the entrance connector from the imaging region. Steady and pulsatile pumps were available to provide a flow of a tap water–methyl cellulose (5 g L^{-1}) suspension doped with sodium chloride (19 g L^{-1}). Timed collection (TC) provided reference flow values to which MR measurements are referred herein by the ratio MR : TC.

The baseline imaging parameters used through this series of experiments were 200 mm field of view, 5 mm slice width, 256^2 acquisition and reconstruction, 16.5 ms echo time, with 33 frames 30 ms apart for ECG-gated studies, and 180 ms repetition time for ungated studies. A pulsatile pump (60 bpm, 2–4 L min^{-1}, 50% systolic fraction) was used in most studies. Studies of the effect of rotating the slice away from transverse or rotating the tube in a coronal plane used a steady pump (2 L min^{-1}). The flow rate was kept within 2% for any individual study. During each experiment, a particular imaging parameter (TE, FOV, flip angle, acquisition matrix, velocity sensitivity, slice position, or slice–tube angle) was varied. The frame interval was not varied in order to maintain temporal resolution of the pulsatile flow. After interleaved acquisition of a flow sensitive and insensitive image pair, phase

* Address for correspondence: MR Physics Group, Radiological Sciences, UMDS—Guy's Hospital, London SE1 9RT, UK.

subtraction of the data was performed, and the resultant phase maps calculated. Images were analyzed on a SUN workstation using in-house software.

RESULTS

The fixed frame rate restricted the range of echo times studied to 16–25 ms. The echo time and similarly, flip angles of 10–90° influenced the modulus image appearance but had negligible effect on the ratio of MR flow measurements to timed collection, MR : TC.

Choice of a velocity-encoding range (VENC) insufficient for the peak pulsatile velocities caused phase wrapping in the relevant image(s) of an ECG-gated image set. Reducing velocity sensitivity (VS = 0.5/ VENC) eliminated the presence of phase wrapping. Below the cutoff for phase wrapping, choice of VS had minimal effect on flow measurement, except at the lowest value available on our scanner.

Slice thickness influenced the variability of MR : TC. The deviation in measurements was most pronounced for thin slices (< 5 mm). The signal-to-noise ratio (S/N) of the modulus images was seen to increase with slice thickness.

Increasing the in-plane pixel size increased the MR : TC ratio. This effect was present while increasing the FOV or decreasing the scan acquisition resolution. The relationship appeared monotonic but not linear.

A linear dependence (δMR : TC $\approx$ 2% cm^{-1}) of MR : TC upon position along the magnet bore was found. There was a concomitant variation in the background phase. A correction algorithm using samples from neighboring positions in the frequency-encoding direction appeared to partially correct the MR flow measurements.

MR : TC was seen to vary with axis and extent of tube–slice angulation. For rotation of the slice around the frequency encoding axis, a linear decrease in MR : TC was seen. This was coupled with an increasingly severe phase banding of the background phase. For rotation of the slice about the phase-encoding direction, a decrease in MR : TC occurred only for angulations >25°. Conversely, rotating the tube about the phase-encoding axis caused an increase in MR : TC, particularly for angles >25°. Reorienting the slice to match the tube largely corrected the MR flow measurements. The background correction described above was effective for slices angled about the phase-encoding direction, but the severity of background variation made the technique ineffective for angles >20° about the frequency-encoding direction. Tube area measurements increased with slice–tube angle more rapidly than 1/cos θ.

DISCUSSION

The relative insensitivity of phase mapping to echo time and flip angle are in keeping with their independence from the gradient evolution of the pulse sequence. They can, therefore, be used to manipulate the contrast between vessel and static tissue. Thus, TE should be minimized to reduce turbulent effects, and maximize the possible temporal resolution—provided gradient compromises are not made. The tissue–flow contrast can be expected to influence the flow measurements as the intrapixel velocity averaging depends on the relative magnitudes of the signals from the static and moving populations of spins.

The velocity sensitivity should be chosen for a peak velocity greater than that expected in the studied vessel. The lower limit to VS is determined by the ability to accurately define a gradient with small first moment in the presence of eddy currents. It should be noted that temporal averaging in ungated imaging of pulsatile flow may mask the wrap-around effect.

The relative stability of flow measurements for the thicker slices studied suggests that thick slices should be used. Two drawbacks to this approach are the need to avoid branches and bends in *in vivo* flow mapping and the mixing of excitation populations across the slice. The latter has been described as a mechanism influencing phase mapping measurements [5, 6]. The slice thickness may also influence the flow measurement through the demand for balancing increasing gradient strength as thinner slices are used. Hence, slice thickness should be chosen based on the available straight length of vessel and with consideration of the expected velocities.

In the absence of a signal from surrounding material, the increase in MR : TC with increased in-plane pixel dimensions agrees with a simple model of phase contributions in boundary pixels [7, 8]. Signal-generating static tissue should reduce this effect but will be dependent on flip angle and repetition time. That the effect is small for practicable imaging resolutions suggests phase mapping may be performed with the minimum number of phase-encoding steps required to identify the vessels of interest. As this will reduce the accuracy of the area measurement, it is essential that the intensity of static and flowing spins be manipulated suitably to allow velocity averaging within the pixels to occur. Otherwise, a high-resolution scan should be performed to reduce this form of partial volume effect.

The positional dependence of phase-mapping measurements may arise from eddy current patterns in the unshielded magnet used herein. A background correction technique should be applied if slice offsets are greater than a few centimeters. It may be possible to create a look-up table from phantom data for use if the surrounding tissue is itself likely to move or generate insufficient signal for a coherent local phase to be measured (e.g., lung).

The change in flow measurement for an angled tube illustrates an often overlooked aspect of MR imaging. Based on plane geometry, the increase in area intersected by the slice should be offset by a decrease in the projected component of velocity in the slice select direction. For slices having non-negligible thickness relative to their in-plane pixel dimensions, solid geometry applies. Thus, the number of pixels in the intersection between a tube and a slab increases more rapidly than $1/\cos\theta$. This is problematic for phase mapping in phantoms, as the negligible signal from the tube wall in the edge voxels is dominated by the large signal from moving fluid. Thus, the velocity-induced phase is unrealistically high in the resultant pixels and the flow lumen is overestimated. Furthermore, if the tube–slice rotation is about the frequency encoding axis, a phase displacement artifact will arise which may influence the flow measurement [9].

When angled slices are requested, effective velocity encoding demands that the relative contributions of the cooperating imaging and velocity-encoding gradients be properly calculated and that the positional and velocity encoding procedures keep their independence. The first of these will increase in importance with the angle of obliquity. The second will be particularly susceptible to eddy currents and mistiming of gradient lobes. This may account for the difference in effect of rotating the slice or tube about the phase-encoding direction as the moment of the readout gradients will be opposite for our experimental design. Phase misregistration will preferentially occur for rotation about the frequency-encoding axis. Finally, in phantoms, the above-mentioned solid-geometry-based partial-volume effects are to be expected.

CONCLUSIONS

It appears that pixel dimensions, echo time, and obliquity of flow to the imaging plane should be minimized for localized flow measurement by phase mapping. Slice thickness and flip angle should be chosen to allow vessel delineation and to minimize the effects of partial voluming. Where possible, a form of background correction for slice position and possibly angulation may be necessary.

ACKNOWLEDGMENTS

We thank Dr. M. Tarnawski and Mr. M. Graves for their time and support, and the Wellcome Trust for their financial support of this study.

REFERENCES

1. Moran PR (1982) A flow velocity zeugmatographic interlace for NMR imaging in humans. *Magn Reson Imaging* **1:** 197–203.
2. Van Dijk P (1984) Direct cardiac NMR imaging of heart wall and blood flow velocity. *J Comput Assist Tomogr* **8**(3): 429.
3. Firmin D, Nayler G, Kilner P, Longmore D (1990) The application of phase shifts in NMR for flow measurement. *Magn Reson Med* **14:** 230–241.
4. Buonocore M, Bogren H (1992) Factors affecting the accuracy and precision of velocity-encoded phase imaging. *Magn Reson Med* **26:** 141–154.
5. Gao J, Gore J (1991) A numerical investigation of the dependence of NMR signal from pulsatile blood flow in cine pulse sequences. *Med Phys* **18**(3): 342–349.
6. Yuan C, Gullberg G, Parker D (1989) Flow-induced phase effects and compensation technique for slice-selective pulses. *Magn Reson Med* **9:** 161–176.
7. Tarnawski M, Porter D, Graves MJ, Taylor MG, Smith MA (1989) Flow determination in small vessels by magnetic resonance imaging. *8th SMRM Meeting*, Amsterdam, Vol. 2, p. 896.
8. Tang C, Blatter D, Parker D (1993) Accuracy of phase-contrast flow measurement in the presence of partial volume effects. *J Magn Reson Imaging* **3:** 377–385.
9. Schulthess G, Higgins C (1985) Blood flow imaging with MR: Spin-phase phenomena. *Radiology* **157**(3): 687–695.

Velocity mapping of coronary artery blood flow

Jennifer Keegan*, David Firmin, Peter Gatehouse and Donald Longmore

Royal Brompton National Heart and Lung Hospital, London SW3 6NP, UK

A segmented *k*-space gradient-echo phase velocity mapping sequence has been developed for the measurement of through-plane and in-plane coronary artery blood flow velocity in a single breath-hold. The sequence was validated in phantom models representing stenosed and unstenosed coronary arteries and also in the descending aortas of several normal volunteers. In-plane and through-plane *in vivo* velocity maps of coronary arteries in normal subjects have been obtained and the problems associated with their acquisition are discussed.

Keywords: flow MRI, velocity mapping, coronary flow.

INTRODUCTION

Over the last 5 years, cardiologists have increasingly emphasized the need to quantify moderate coronary stenoses, the regression or progression of which has been shown to be a strong predictor of clinically important end points including myocardial infarction and cardiac death [1]. The use of segmented *k*-space breath-hold coronary angiography for the detection of severe (flow-limiting) coronary stenoses by the detection of signal loss due to turbulence at or beyond the site of stenosis has already been described [2], but such an approach is qualitative. A means of quantifying stenosis severity is desirable and we suggest that one possible approach may be to use the continuity equation in conjunction with breath-hold phase velocity mapping of coronary artery blood flow velocity.

METHOD

A segmented *k*-space breath-hold phase velocity mapping sequence with fat presaturation for in-plane and through-plane velocity mapping of coronary arteries was implemented on a Picker International 1.5-T scanner [3]. Two velocity sensitized images are acquired in a single breath-hold, the phase map subtrac-

Address for correspondence: MR Unit, Royal Brompton National Heart and Lung Hospital, Sydney Street, London SW3 6NP, UK.

tion of which results in a velocity map sensitized to flow velocities of ±25 cm s^{-1}. The acquisition of two sensitised images, rather than of a reference and more highly sensitized image, minimizes artifacts due to beat to beat variations in flow over the breath-hold period. The slice thickness used was 5 mm and the field of view was 150–200 mm $\times$ 200 mm, resulting in an in-plane pixel size of 1.6 mm $\times$ 1.6 mm. Four phase-encoding steps were performed per cardiac cycle resulting in a breath-hold period of 24–32 heartbeats, depending on the phase-encode direction field of view. The sequence was validated against a standard nonsegmented phase velocity mapping sequence in a pulsatile flow phantom where the peak flow velocity and the peak rate of change of flow velocity were similar to those found in normal coronary arteries, and, with a higher velocity window, in the descending aortas of several normal volunteers where much higher velocities and accelerations are found. *In vitro* through-plane velocity maps were also obtained in phantoms consisting of 5-mm diameter tubes with asymmetric area reducing stenoses of 34% and 57% through which copper sulphate solution flowed at approximately 10 cm s^{-1}.

Both through-plane and in-plane *in vivo* velocity maps of coronary arteries in several normal subjects were obtained in early diastole when coronary flow is at its highest and the heart is relatively stationary.

Diaphragm and chest wall position variations were studied in consecutive breath-hold periods, both at end expiration and at end inspiration.

RESULTS AND DISCUSSION

The velocities measured by the segmented sequence with four phase-encoding steps per segment agreed well those measured by the standard nonsegmented sequence in both the pulsatile flow phantom and in the descending aortas of the normal volunteers, as shown in Fig. 1. The through-plane stenosis phantom velocity maps showed mean velocity increases of 1.41 and 2.30 at the sites of the 34% and 57% stenoses,

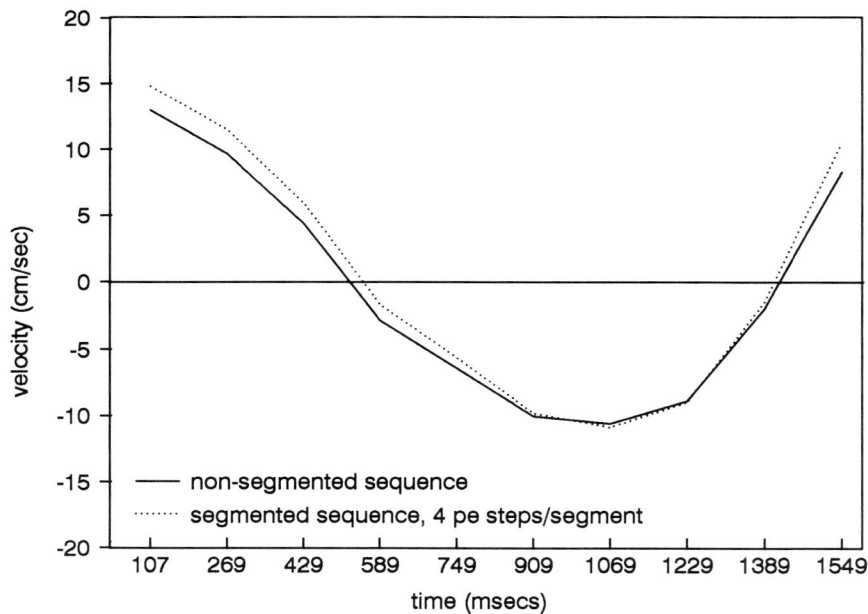

(a)

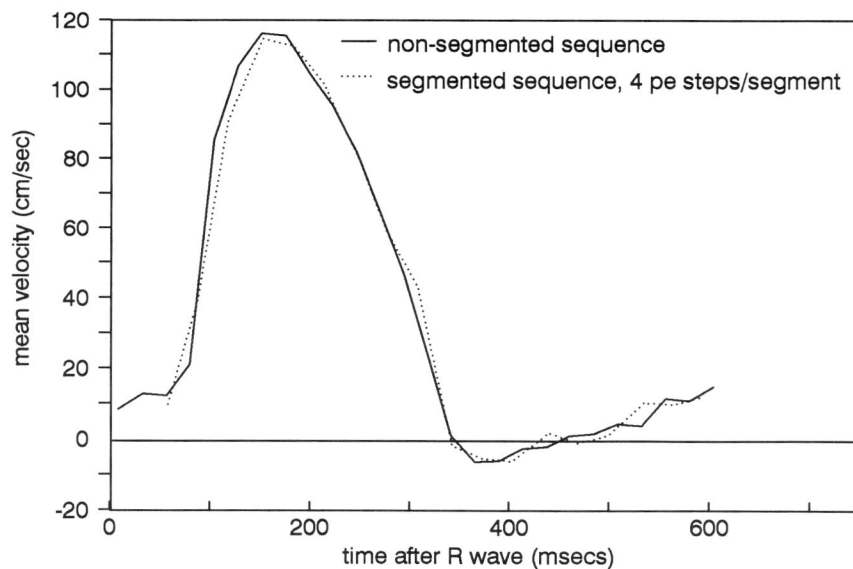

(b)

Fig. 1. Velocity–time curves measured by a standard nonsegmented phase velocity mapping sequence and by the segmented sequence with four phase-encoding steps per segment in (a), the coronary artery model, and (b) the descending aorta of a normal volunteer.

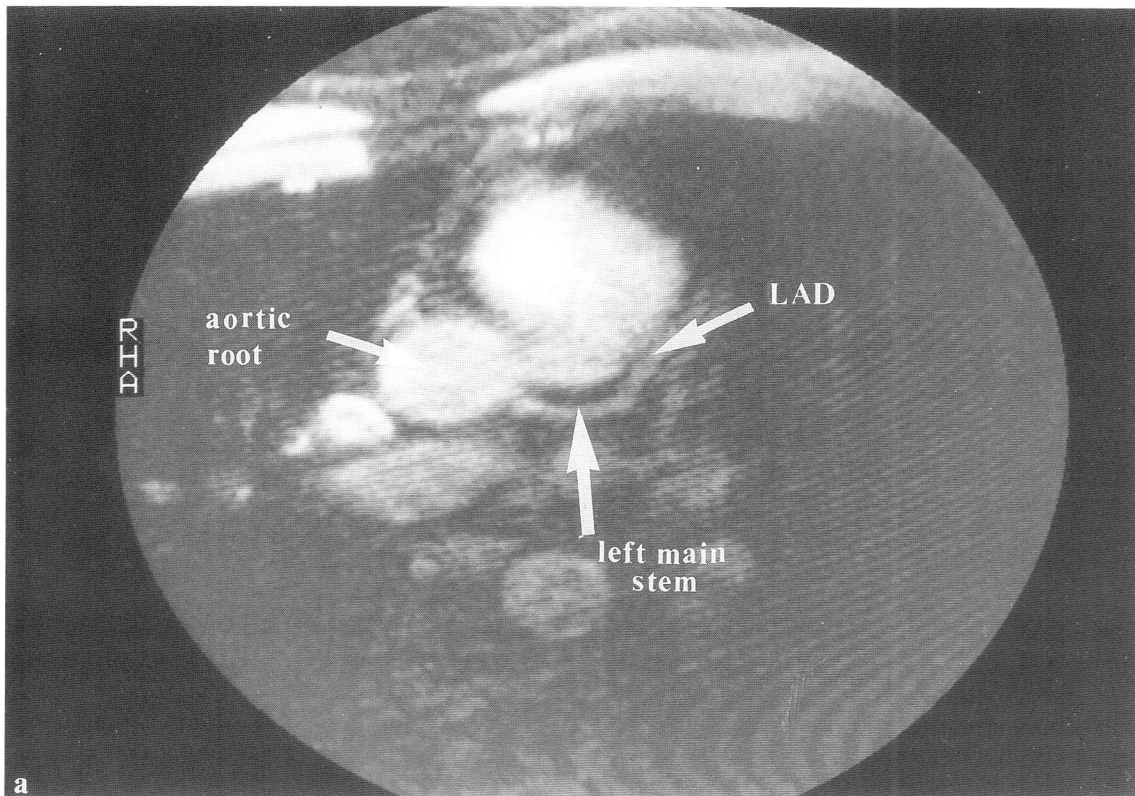

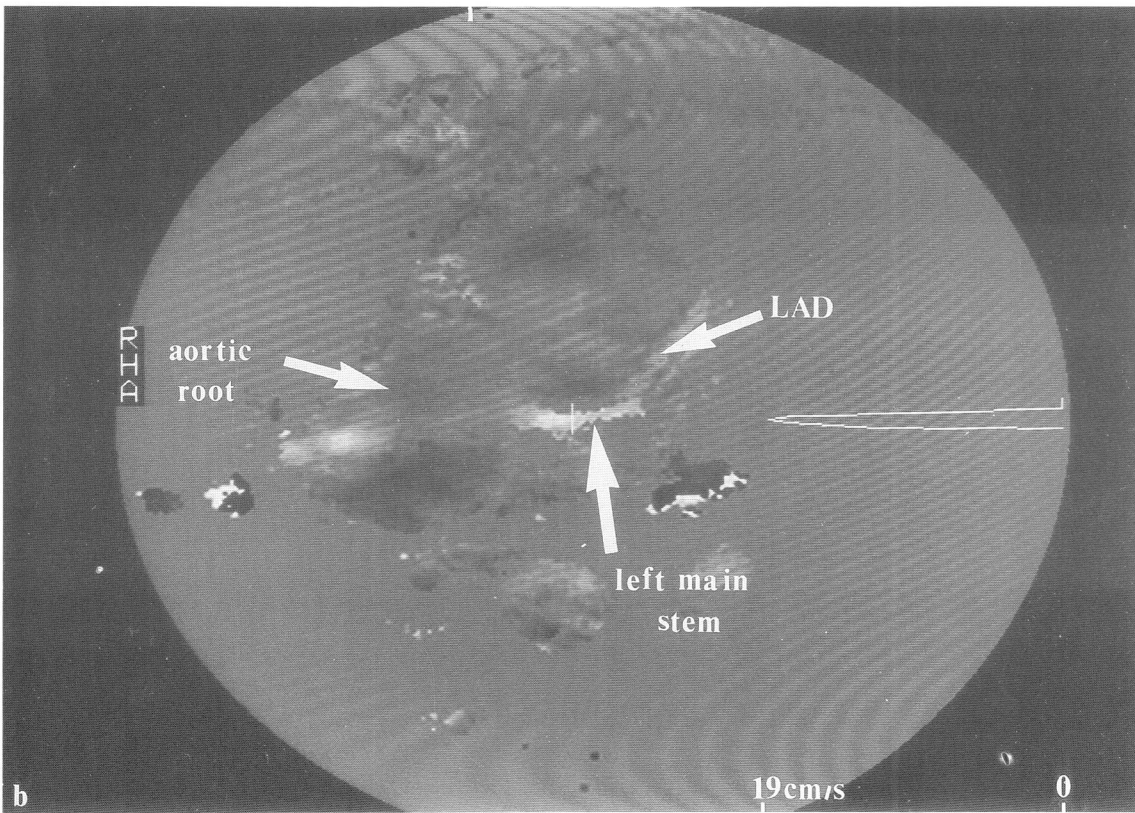

Fig. 2. In-plane early diastolic magnitude image (a) and corresponding velocity map (b) of the left main stem artery in a normal subject.

respectively, compared with increases of 1.52 and 2.33 expected from the application of the continuity equation, thereby demonstrating the feasibility of using such an approach for stenosis quantification *in vitro.*

Figure 2 is an example of a fat-suppressed in-plane magnitude image and velocity map in the left main stem and left anterior descending (LAD) arteries of a normal subject in early diastole. The imaging plane has been orientated so that the left main stem artery is in the direction of velocity encoding. A profile through the left main stem artery shows a peak velocity of 19 cm s^{-1} at this timing in the cardiac cycle. In 15 subjects studied, the arterial velocity ranged from 3 to 29 cm s^{-1}, depending largely on the exact timing in the cardiac cycle, with relatively small changes in the gating delay resulting in considerable velocity changes. Because of vessel tortuosity and problems of misregistration of the vessel due to uneven breath-holding, through-plane velocity maps were easier to achieve than those in-plane. However, for stenosis assessment, we feel that in-plane velocity mapping may provide the best approach, as flow velocities prestenosis, postenosis and at stenosis can be measured in a single breath-hold rather than the three individual breath-holds required for through-plane assessment, thereby eliminating problems with uneven breath-holding and any physiological changes in flow from breath-hold to breath-hold.

Repeat breath-holding at end inspiration and at end expiration showed that there was greater variation in both diaphragm and chest wall positions at end inspiration than end expiration. At both end inspiration and end expiration, the diapragm position was more variable than the chest wall position (by approximately a factor of 4), but a linear relationship between the two suggested that only one of the positions need be monitored for improving breath-hold consistency.

CONCLUSIONS

We have developed a sequence for the in-plane and through-plane phase velocity mapping of coronary artery blood flow and have demonstrated its use *in vivo* in normal subjects. We have also demonstrated *in vitro* the application of the continuity equation to stenosis assessment in several phantoms. Although a considerable number of *in vitro* and *in vivo* studies need to be performed in order to fully assess the applicability of this technique *in vivo,* we believe that the use of such an approach for the assessment of stenoses may be feasible.

REFERENCES

1. Waters D, Craven T, Lesperance J (1993) Prognostic significance of progression of coronary atherosclerosis. *Circulation* **87**(4): 1067–1075.
2. Manning WJ, Li W, Edelman R (1993) A preliminary report comparing magnetic resonance coronary angiography with conventional angiography. *N Engl J Med* **328:** 828–832.
3. Keegan J, Firmin DN, Gatehouse PD, Longmore DB (1994) The application of breath-hold phase velocity mapping techniques to the measurement of coronary artery blood flow velocity: Phantom data and initial in vivo results. *Magn Reson Med.* **31**:526–36.

MR high-resolution imaging of arterial intimal hyperplasia at 1.5 T

C. Sampson,[1,]* R. Edmondson,[2] J. Keegan,[1] S. Humphreys,[2] R. Hughes,[1]
D. Talbot,[1] P. Andrews,[1] D. Firmin[1] and D. Longmore[1]

[1]*The MRI Unit, Royal Brompton Hospital, London SW3 6NP, UK*
[2]*The Thrombosis Research Unit, Kings College Hospital London UK*

Intimal hyperplasia is the earliest microscopic change detectable in the arterial wall in the development of arteriosclerosis and atherosclerosis. To enable high-resolution imaging of this, a standard 1.5-T machine was modified using inserted gradient coils of 30 cm internal diameter and surface radio-frequency coils. Six rabbit aorta specimens with injury-induced intimal hyperplasia and two normal rabbit aorta specimens were imaged using a spin-echo sequence of TE 40. Pixel sizes as small as 20 μ × 20 μ could be obtained and the area of intimal hyperplasia could be measured at 80 μ × 40 μ. The results were compared with those made by a computer-linked microscope. In the injured aortas, there was a low-signal region on magnetic resonance imaging which corresponded to the media of the vessel wall when compared with the histology. T_1 and T_2 constants for the media were determined and compared with those of a normal specimen. The T_1 constant was shorter for the media of the injured aorta than in the normal. This could be related to the disruption of the internal elastic lamina and migration of muscle cells to the intima which occurs following injury. The popliteal artery of four normal volunteers was imaged and the area of the wall could be measured at a pixel size of 312 μ × 160 μ. This suggests that *in vivo* studies of intimal hyperplasia arteriosclerosis and atherosclerosis could be made.

Keywords: high-resolution MRI, intimal hyperplasia.

INTRODUCTION

The complications of arteriosclerosis and atherosclerosis are common and affect both the coronary arteries and the peripheral vascular system. Following treatment of stenotic lesions by percutaneous angioplasty, 30–40% recur [1], and following surgical reconstruction using bypass grafts, failure can occur due to the development of lesions which appear similar to arteriosclerosis at the distal end of the graft [2]. Thickening of the intima has been demonstrated to be the earliest histological change following injury and is also seen in spontaneous atherosclerosis, particularly distal to the bifurcation of a vessel [3]. At present, animal models are used for the study of the prevention and regression of the pathology, in particular the effect of diet and drugs. Magnetic resonance imaging (MRI) is potentially a noninvasive method of studying the disease *in vivo*. At present, high-resolution imaging of atheromatous vessels has been limited to that of cadaver arteries using a small-bore 9-T magnet which is unsuitable for human *in vivo* studies [4]. We have modified a 1.5-T machine by the use of a set of small gradient coil inserts which increase the magnetic gradient but which are large enough to allow imaging of the vessels of the lower limb. We have assessed the system by imaging specimens of rabbit aorta and normal human popliteal arteries.

MATERIALS AND METHODS

The gradient coil inserts were of a three-arc design and the internal diameter was 30 cm. This increased the gradient strength from 10 to 60 mT-m^{-1}. The gradients were rescaled using a phantom. For imaging of the rabbit aortas, a 2-cm-diameter solenoid radio-

* Address for correspondence: The Cardiovascular Magnetic Resonance Research Unit, St. Lukes Hospital, Milwaukee, WI 53215, USA.

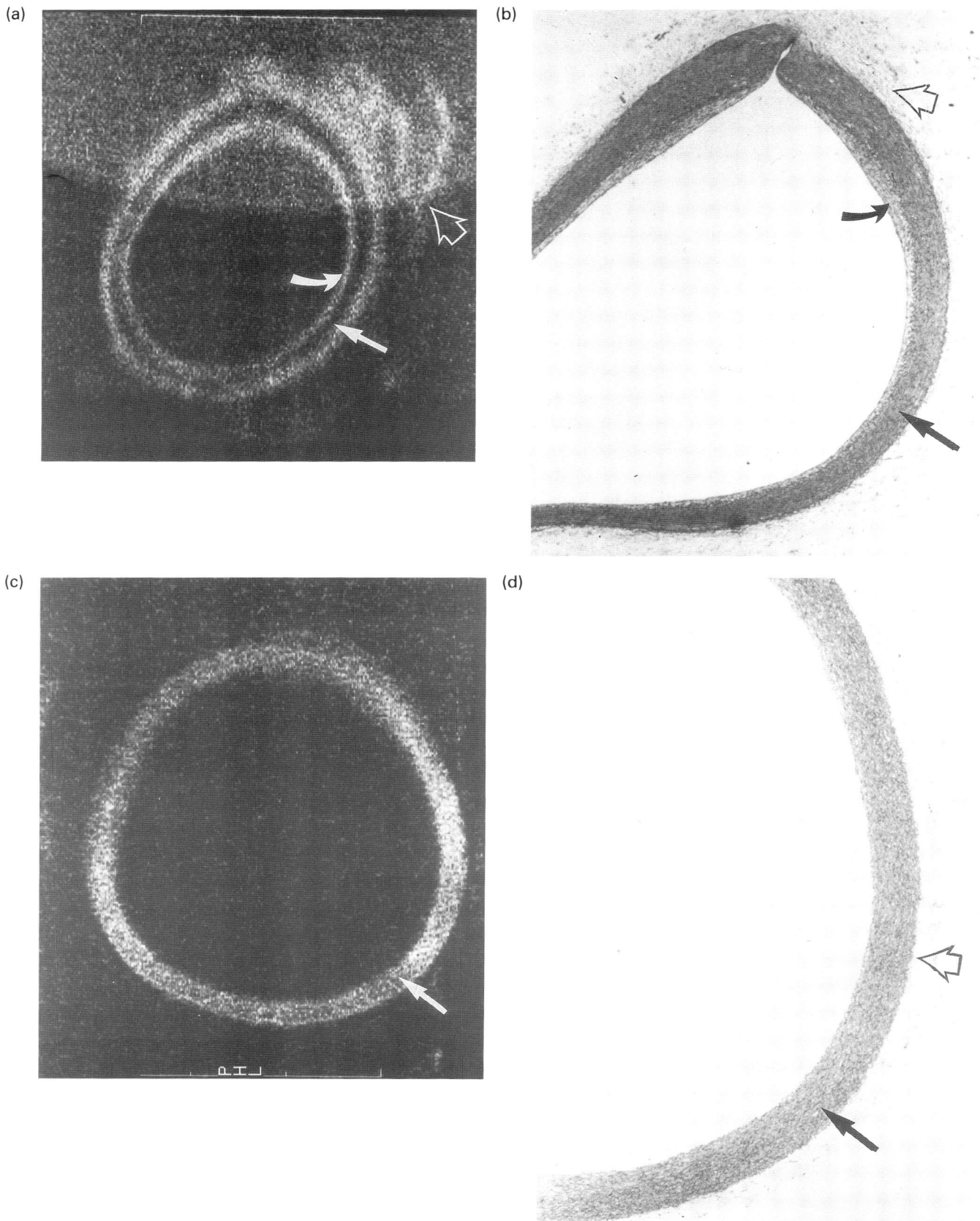

Fig. 1. (a) MRI and (b) histology of an injured rabbit aorta which has intimal hyperplasia, and (c) MRI and (d) histology of a noninjured rabbit aorta which has no intimal thickening. Curved arrow = intima; straight arrow = media; open arrow = adventitia.

frequency (RF) coil was used. A 12-cm-diameter quadrature coil was used for imaging the popliteal artery.

Six rabbit aorta specimens were obtained from animals used in a study of the effect of a thrombin inhibitor given at the time of injury of the aorta by an intravascular balloon catheter. Three animals were given the antithrombin agent (specimens 3–6). The animals were sacrificed 2 weeks postinjury and the aortas stored in 10% formalin. Each end of the aorta was examined histologically after staining. The areas of the lumen, intima, and media were measured using a computer-linked microscope. The middle portion of the aorta was attached to a perspex plate placed in a tube of normal saline and scanned using a spin-echo sequence with TE 40 and TR 500. A slice thickness of 3 mm was imaged and a field of view of 1 cm and a 512 × 512 matrix were used. This gave a pixel size of 20 μ × 20 μ. To improve the signal-to-noise ratio (S/N) 12 signal averages were acquired. Areas of the lumen and intima were measured by hand using a cursor. Two normal rabbit aortas were scanned for comparison. Histological examination was repeated after MR imaging on one normal and one abnormal specimen at approximately the position of the MR image.

The popliteal artery of four normal volunteers were scanned. The artery and its branches were located using a 3D time of flight MR angiography sequence. An ECG gated spin echo sequence TE40 and TR 500 was used to obtain a transaxial image of the artery. The FOV was 4 cms slice thickness 5 mm and a 128 × 256 matrix used. This gave a pixel size of 312u × 156u. Four signal averages were obtained.

Table 1. Microscopy and MRI transaxial area measurements of rabbit aorta.

	Area [10^{-7} m^2]				I/L [%][a]	
	Microscopy		MRI			
Specimen	Lumen	Intima	Lumen	Intima	Microscopy	MRI
1	0.24	0.30	0.39	0.47	20	17
	0.19	0.21	0.32	0.44	11	27
2	0.24	0.30	0.39	0.46	20	15
	0.26	0.29			10	
3	0.18	0.23	0.32	0.45	22	29
	0.09	0.13			30	
4	0.28	0.30	0.18	0.29	6	38
	0.34	0.36	0.19	0.25	6	24
			0.20	0.26		23
5	0.19	0.20	0.39	0.47	5	17
			0.40	0.47		15
			0.35	0.42		17
6	0.16	0.17	0.23	0.26	6	12
	0.25	0.26			4	

[a]I/L = ratio of intimal area to true lumen area as percentage.

RESULTS

All of the injured aorta specimens had intimal hyperplasia on histological examination. This was greater in the nontreated animals (specimens 1–3). On MRI, all of the injured specimens showed high signal from the

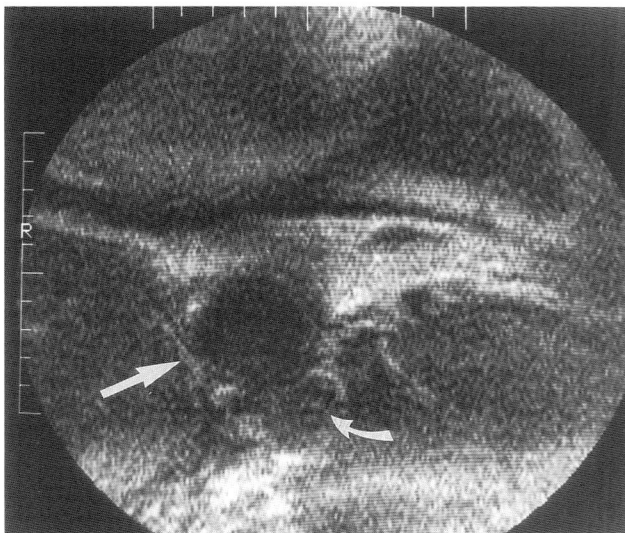

(a)

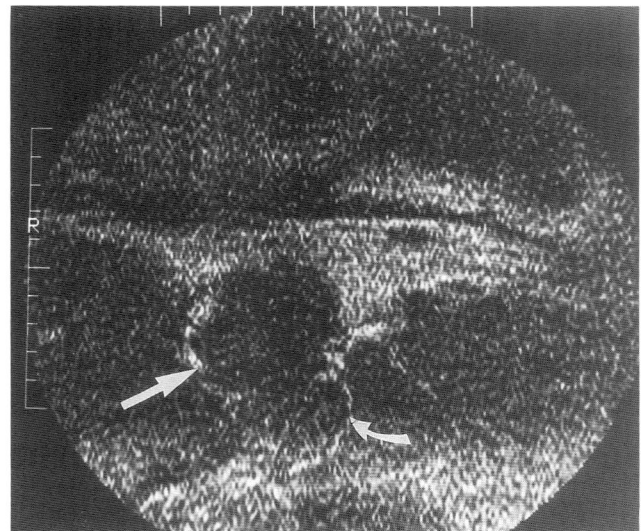

(b)

Fig. 2. Popliteal artery of normal subject. Pixel size 312 μ × 156 μ. (a) Four signal averages; (b) one signal average. Straight arrow = popliteal artery; curved arrow = popliteal vein.

intima and low signal from the adjacent media (Fig. 1a). The two noninjured specimens did not show any region of low signal (Fig. 1c) in the region of the media on MRI or any intimal hyperplasia on histological examination (Fig. 1d). The T_1 and T_2 constants were calculated from experiments using an inversion recovery sequence with varying recovery time for T_1 and a spin-echo sequence with varying echo times for T_2. In the region of the media, T_1 was shorter for the injured specimen (110 m) than for the noninjured specimen (248 m). Although T_2 was also shorter, this was within the error of the method (24 and 30 m).

A comparison of the measurements of the area of the lumen and of the area of the intima plus lumen are shown in Table 1. The ratio of the intimal area to the true lumen is also shown. Microscopy found less intimal hyperplasia in the three treated animals, but MRI did not find a difference in the two groups. The imaging time was 50 min.

The scanning time for the normal popliteal artery was 18 min, but the scanning time could be reduced to 4 min by using a single acquisition. Although the S/N was poorer, the arterial wall could still be seen (Fig. 2).

DISCUSSION

The results show that there is a difference in the appearance on MRI of an artery which has intimal hyperplasia compared with a normal vessel which, to some extent, corresponds to the histological findings. The shortening of T_1 in the media of vessels with postinjury intimal hyperplasia may be related to the disruption of the internal elastic lamina or to the migration of muscle cells from the media into the intima. Possible mechanisms include molecular diffusion and magnetization transfer. Further experiments

are necessary using fresh specimens. The comparison between microscopy and MRI measurements is limited because different sites in the aorta were used by the two modalities and the degree of intimal hyperplasia can vary within the same specimen. There are also errors for both methods. However, the results are encouraging and suggest that information of clinical relevance could be obtained. The time required for imaging at present limits the use of high-resolution work in patients. However, improvement in RF coil design to enable a better S/N may overcome this.

CONCLUSION

The use of small-diameter gradient insert coils enables high-resolution imaging at 1.5 T. This may have future use in the imaging *in vivo* of the development and treatment of arteriosclerosis and atheroma of the vessels of the leg.

ACKNOWLEDGMENTS

We thank Alistair Hall and David Gilderdale for their invaluable assistance in the design of the RF coils.

REFERENCES

1. Popma JJ, Califf RM, Topal EJ (1991) *Circulation* **84:** 1426–1436.
2. Imparato AM, Bracco A, Kim GE, Zeff R (1972) *Surgery* **72:** 1007–1017.
3. Badimon L, Badimon JJ, Gold HK, Fuster V (1992) *Am J Cardiac Imaging* **6:** 278–288.
4. Pearlman JD, Badimon JJ (1992) *Am J Cardiac Imaging* **6:** 325–332.

Clinical applications and techniques of echo-planar imaging

Franz Schmitt,[1]* S. Warach,[2] P. Wielopolski[2] and R.R. Edelman[2]

[1]*Siemens Medical Systems, Erlangen, Germany*
[2]*Beth Isreal Hospital, Boston, MA, USA*

The ultrafast magnetic resonance imaging technique known as echo-planar imaging has undergone considerable technical improvements in recent years. It is currently being evaluated at only a few institutions worldwide. Although EPI, invented by P. Mansfield in 1977, is the oldest fast MRI technique, it is still not widely available on clinical scanners. Only 20–30 EPI scanners exist worldwide, compared to about 7000 conventional MRI scanners. The main reason why EPI has not emerged from the scientific prototype niche is its high demands on hardware and software. However, the time is now coming when EPI is entering the clinical stage. We describe the common EPI sequence types, show clinical results, and describe the contrast in the measured images.

Keywords: ultrafast MRI, echo-planar imaging, EPI.

EPI GENERAL

Echo-planar imaging (EPI), invented by Peter Mansfield [1], is currently the fastest magnetic resonance imaging (MRI) technique available. It has been shown that EPI can provide head and body images of biomedically useful quality in 30–120 ms. These images are completely free of motion artifacts and provide almost unlimited proton density, T_1- and T_2-weighted contrast. EPI can also be used to measure a variety of physiological parameters such as diffusion, perfusion, and brain functions.

EPI is characterized by a train of gradient echoes, where in a single excitation a complete data set is acquired. A major advantage of EPI is its speed. EPI can acquire a complete set of slices in the time conventional MRI takes to acquire a single slice. When comparing EPI and other MRI techniques, this speed advantage has to be kept in mind.

Below we will describe the common EPI sequence types, show clinical results, and describe the contrast in the measured images.

*Address for correspondence: Siemens Medical Systems, Dept. MRE 5, Henkestrasse 127, 91052 Erlangen, Germany.

EPI PULSE SEQUENCES

With EPI, the data are acquired using a train of bipolar gradient pulses. Therefore, EPI is basically a gradient-echo technique. The length of the gradient pulse train is limited by the T_2^* decay:

$$1/T_2^* = 1/T_2 + \gamma \Delta B \qquad (1)$$

T_2^* characterizes the T_2 decay in the presence of field inhomogeneities, ΔB. In this case we speak only about the susceptibility induced local field inhomogeneities. Figure 1 shows some typical T_2^* decays. Large inhomogeneities cause fast T_2^* decay and small inhomogeneities cause slow T_2^* decay. Therefore, the data-acquisition window is limited to times less than 120 ms. For cardiac EPI this is still not fast enough. To achieve artifact-free images, the data have to be acquired in a time frame of less than 50 ms.

EPI can be combined with any kind of spin preparation technique, such as inversion recovery (IR), magnetization transfer contrast (MTC), and fat saturation (FATSAT). Fat saturation is essential for EPI due to the very weak phase-encoding (PC) gradient amplitude. A typical value for the PC gradient is 0.1 mT m^{-1}. This is about 250 times less than the readout (RO) gradient. An incomplete FATSAT causes a shift of the fat signal, which causes the fat to appear several centimeters

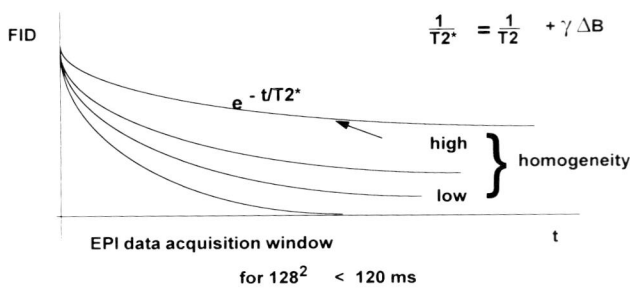

$$\frac{1}{T2^*} = \frac{1}{T2} + \gamma \Delta B$$

Fig. 1. EPI data acquisition window and its relation to the T_2^* decay.

from the water in the resulting image. This shift, Δx_{FW} can be described by

$$\Delta x_{FW} = 3.5 \times 10^{-6} B_0 / G_{PC} \qquad (2)$$

where B_0 represents the main magnetic field strength and G_{PC} is the PC gradient amplitude.

Spin-density-weighted contrast

Figure 2 shows the simplest EPI sequence possible. After the FATSAT pulse, a single-slice selective 90° pulse is applied. The data are sampled under an free-induction decay (FID). The contrast is typically spin density weighted (Fig. 3) if the echo time TE is short.

Susceptibility-weighted contrast (T_2^*)

If a long TE is used, the resulting images are called susceptibility or T_2^* weighted. This type of sequence is typically used for perfusion studies in the brain, the heart, and for functional MRI. Figure 4 shows four images from a cardiac perfusion study with a Gd-DTPA contrast bolus infusion. The myocardial signal is reduced due to the uptake of Gd-DTPA.

T_2 contrast

To minimize susceptibility effects in EPI, a 180° pulse can be used to refocus field inhomogeneities as in a conventional spin-echo (SE) excitation scheme (Fig. 5). The images show the typical T_2 contrast, due to the increase in effective TE time. An abdominal application is shown in Fig. 6. T_1-weighted fast low-angle shot images are shown in the upper row. T_2-weighted images (TE: 53/120 ms) of the same patient with multiple lesions (hemangioma in liver and two cysts in kidney) are shown in the lower row.

T_1 contrast

T_1 contrast can be achieved by applying an IR pulse prior to of the EPI pulse sequence (FID or SE excitation, Fig. 7). The FATSAT pulse has to be closest to the SE-excitation radio frequency pulses. The inversion time (TI) is typically set to null a specific tissue signal. In abdominal liver imaging, TI is adjusted to minimize the liver signal. This achieves best liver/lesion contrast. Figure 8 shows a series of images out of a T_1-weighted cardiac perfusion study. T_1 is adjusted to null the blood signal. Therefore, the selected myocardial ROI signal is reduced before the Gd-DTPA bolus and increased after the passage. The signal difference can be up to a factor of 3.

DIFFUSION IMAGING

Diffusion effects in MRI [2] are very sensitive to any kind of motion. Motion in MRI can be, for example, patient motion or brain pulsation. To avoid motion effects, a fast MRI technique must be used. EPI is especially suitable for that purpose [3]. It has been shown in animals [4] and patients [5, 6] that EPI

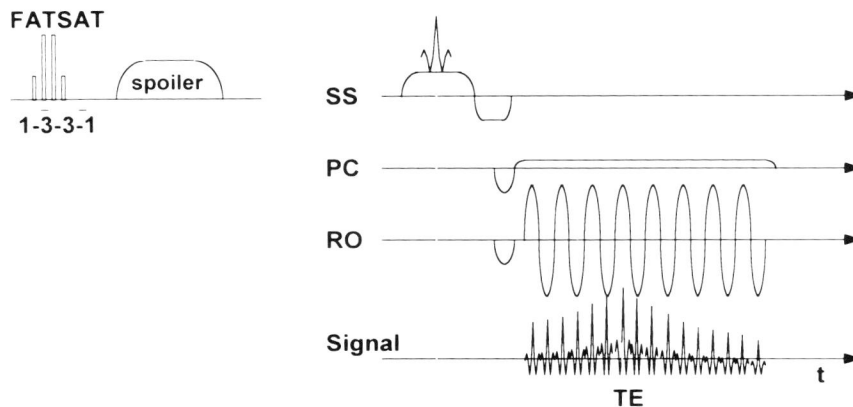

Fig. 2. T_2^*-weighted EPI–FID sequence.

- TE 26 ms

- Δz 6 mm

- FOV 250x187 mm

- N 160x256

- $\delta x < 1$mm

- T_{acq} 130 ms

- CP-spine coil

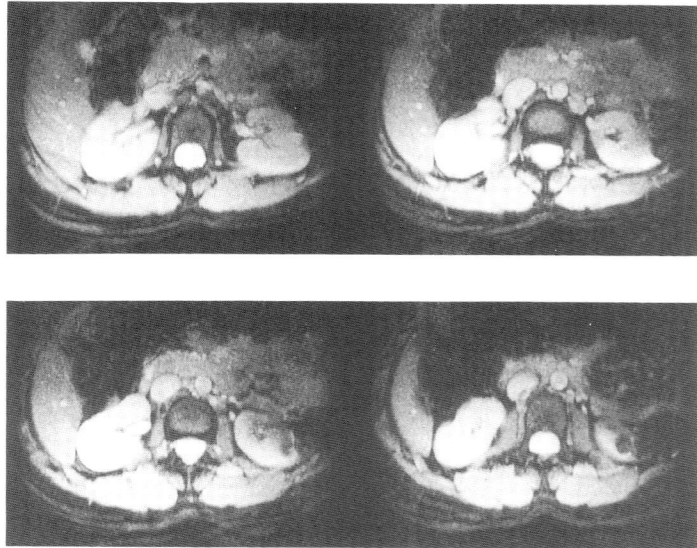

Fig. 3. Single-shot, multislice, high-resolution EPI of the kidneys. The total measurement time per slice was approximately 140 ms.

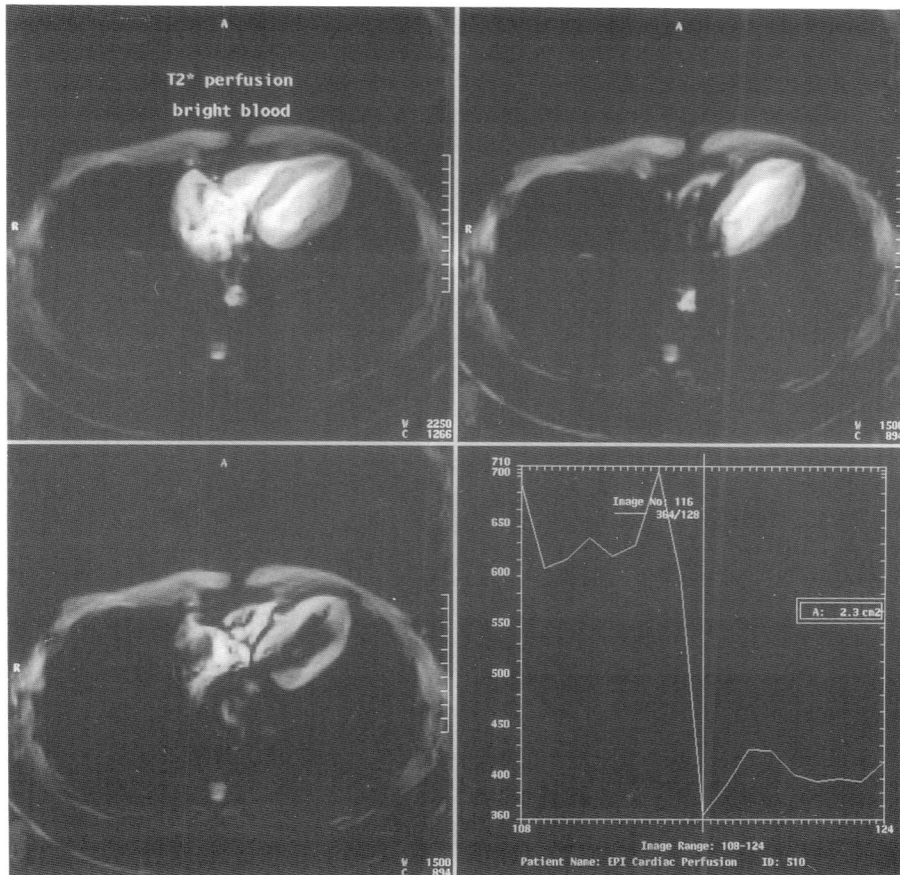

Fig. 4. T_2^*-weighted cardiac perfusion study using Gd-DTPA as contrast agent.

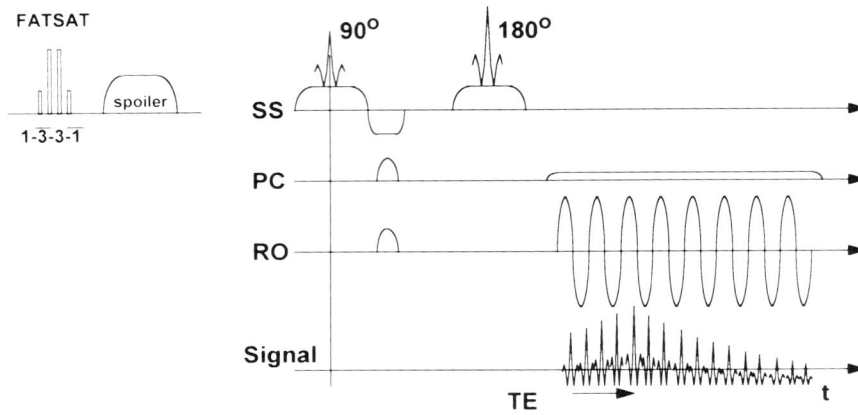

Fig. 5. T_2-weighted EPI–SE sequence.

diffusion can depict clearly ischemic lesions in stroke patients, even shortly after the onset of the stroke. Diffusion-weighted imaging will change the management of stroke patients because it allows unique

detection, follow-up, and treatment. Figure 9 shows the Stejskal–Tanner [7] version of the EPI–SE diffusion sequence. This sequence is basically an SE–EPI sequence with large dephasing gradients before and

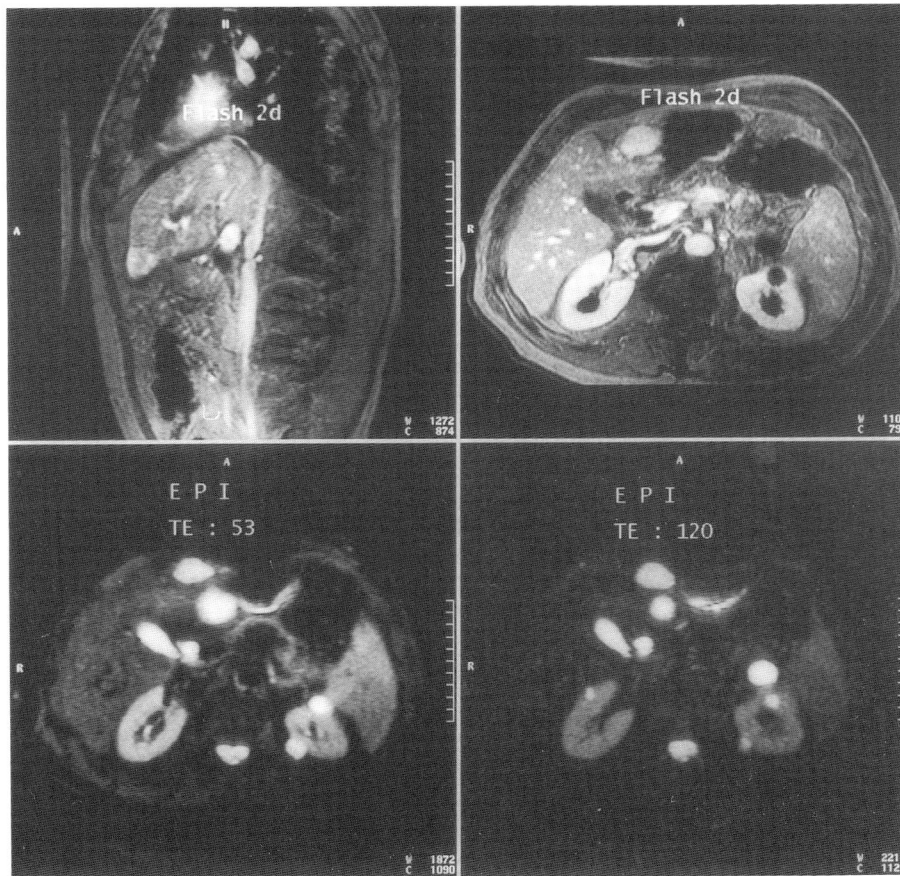

Fig. 6. EPI–T_2-weighted abdominal images of a patient with an hemangioma in the liver and two kidney cysts. Upper row: sagital and axial FLASH 2D T_1-weighted; lower row: EPI–SE with TE 53/120 ms.

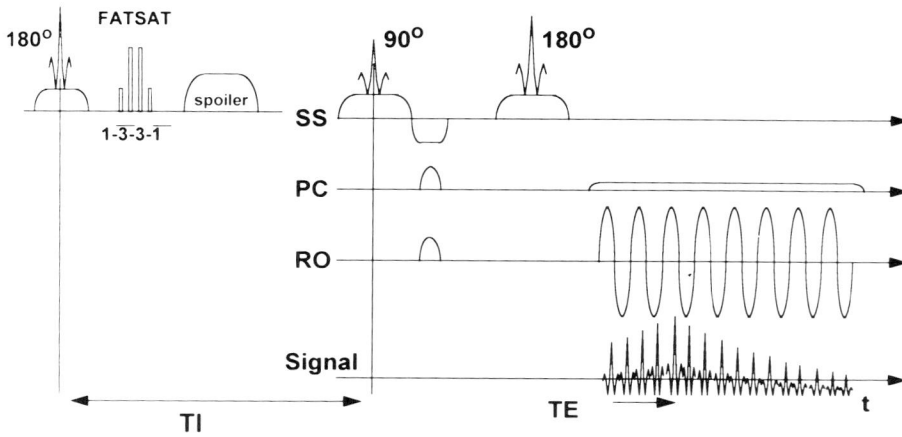

Fig. 7. IR–EPI–SE sequence for T_1 weighting.

after the 180° pulse. Typical diffusion gradients have a length of 20 ms and an amplitude of 20–30 mT m^{-1}. With diffusion gradient lobes, the signal from spins is dephased when they move a small distance compared to the free diffusion length. The signal decay is described as

$$S_D(t) = S_0(t)e^{-b/D} \tag{3}$$

where b is the diffusion-weighting b factor in units of seconds per square millimeter. For the pulse sequence

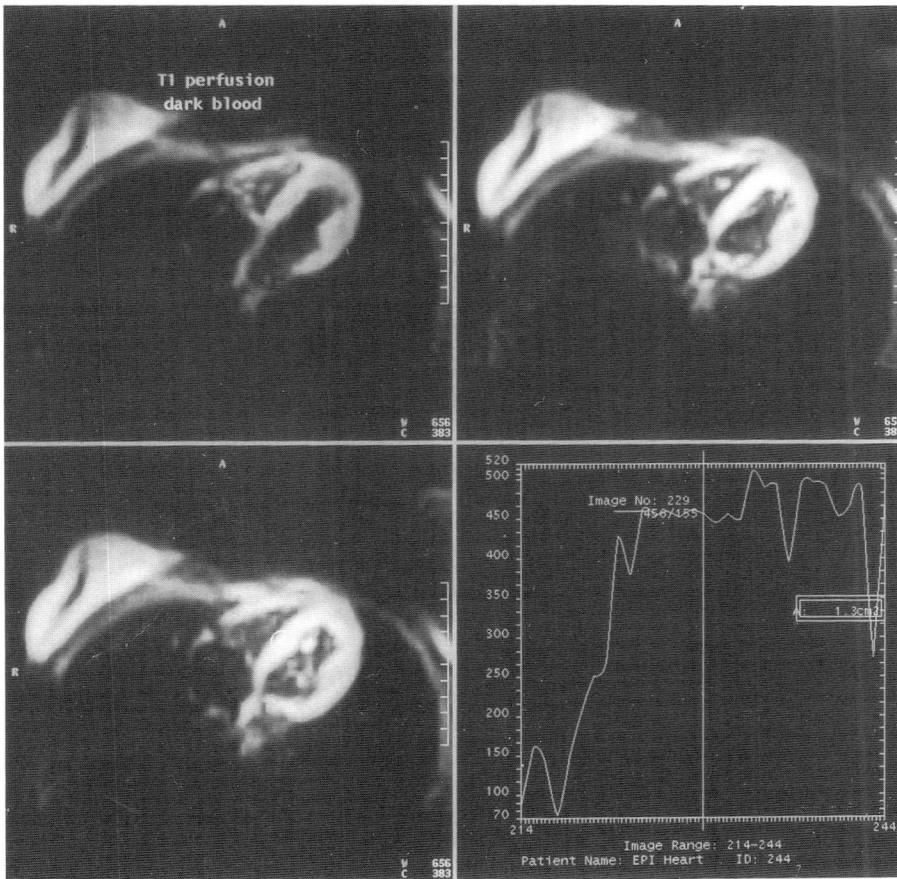

Fig. 8. T_1-weighted cardiac perfusion study. TI is adjusted to null the blood signal.

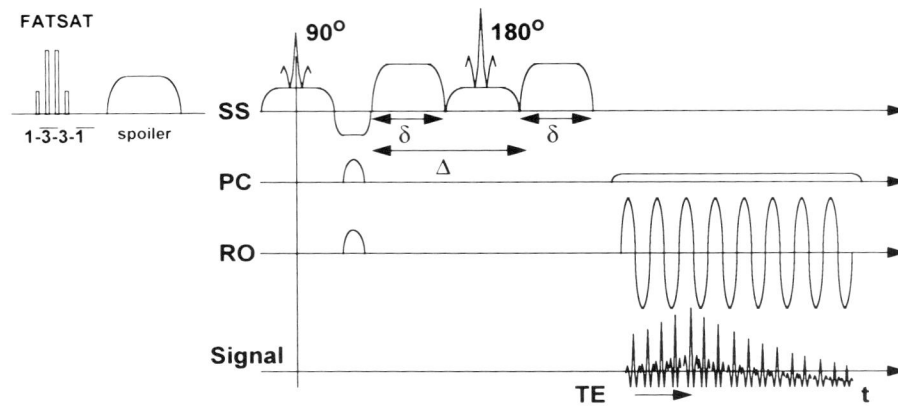

Fig. 9. Stejskal–Tanner EPI–SE diffusion-weighted sequence.

shown in Fig. 9, b is given by

$$b = \gamma^2\delta^2 G^2(\Delta - \delta/3) \qquad (4)$$

Here the gradient ramp time is neglected, i.e., it is short compared to the pulse duration. D describes the tissue-dependent diffusion constant measured in units of square millimeters per second. In diffusion-weighted EPI images of stroke (Fig. 10b), the ischemic lesion appears bright. This means the diffusion constant D is reduced compared to normal tissue (Fig. 10c). A T_2-weighted EPI image of the same patient (Fig. 10a)

does not show any signal change in the ischemic area. Another lesion shown in this image was diagnosed as a chronic stroke.

Diffusion weighting in the abdomen and chest is also possible in combination with EPI. However, a different sequence type has to be used. Best results for cardiac diffusion are gained with variations of STEAM sequences [8–10]. Figure 11 shows an EPI–STEAM sequence used to acquire images from a healthy volunteer shown in Fig. 12. From the top left to the bottom right, the b value was increased. The signal is reduced corresponding to the increase of the b value.

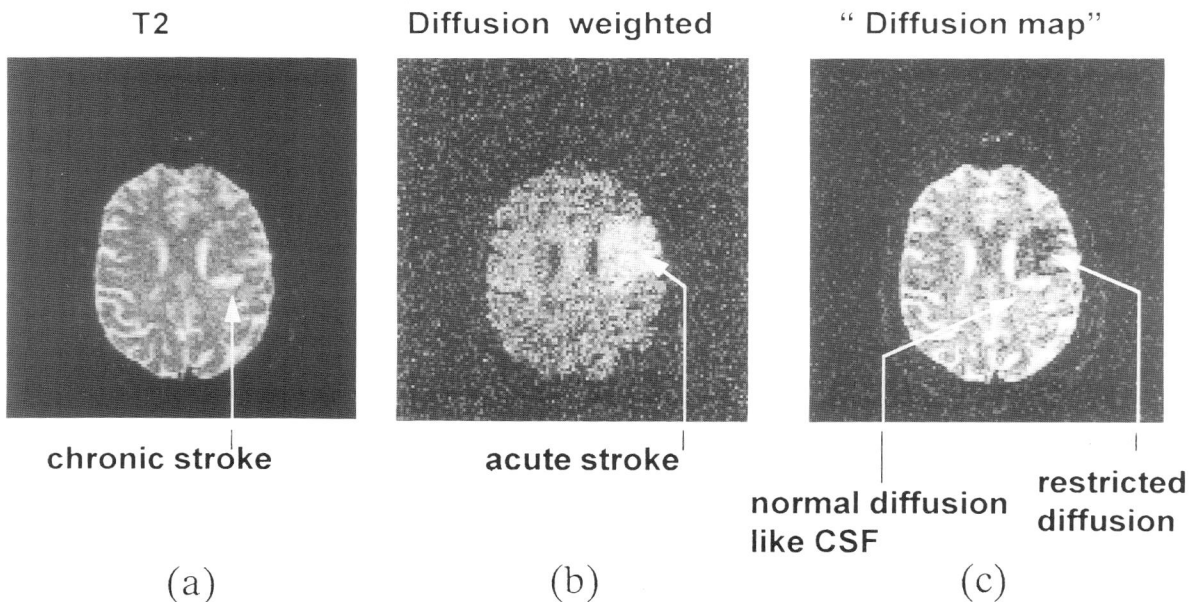

Fig. 10. Diffusion weighting in stroke: (a) EPI–T_2-weighted image shows only chronic stroke lesions; (b) EPI–diffusion-weighted image shows high signal in ischemic lesions and low signal in chronic stroke lesions; (c) EPI–diffusion map shows low diffusion constant in lesion.

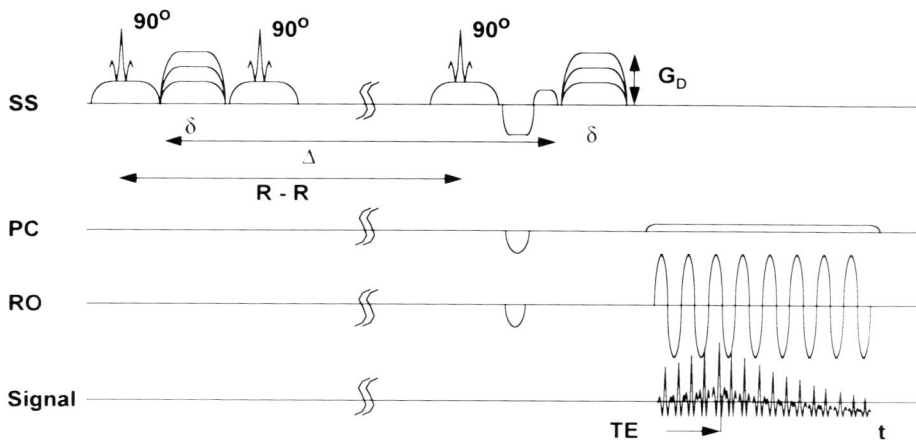

Fig. 11. EPI–STEAM sequence for cardiac and abdominal diffusion-weighted imaging.

CONCLUSION

Echo-planar imaging shows a clear advantage for dynamic and motion-sensitive imaging. The main advantage of EPI is its ability to scan a whole volume in a short time compared to the body's inherent motion and the clinical time constraints. The increased availability of EPI hardware will also have an impor-

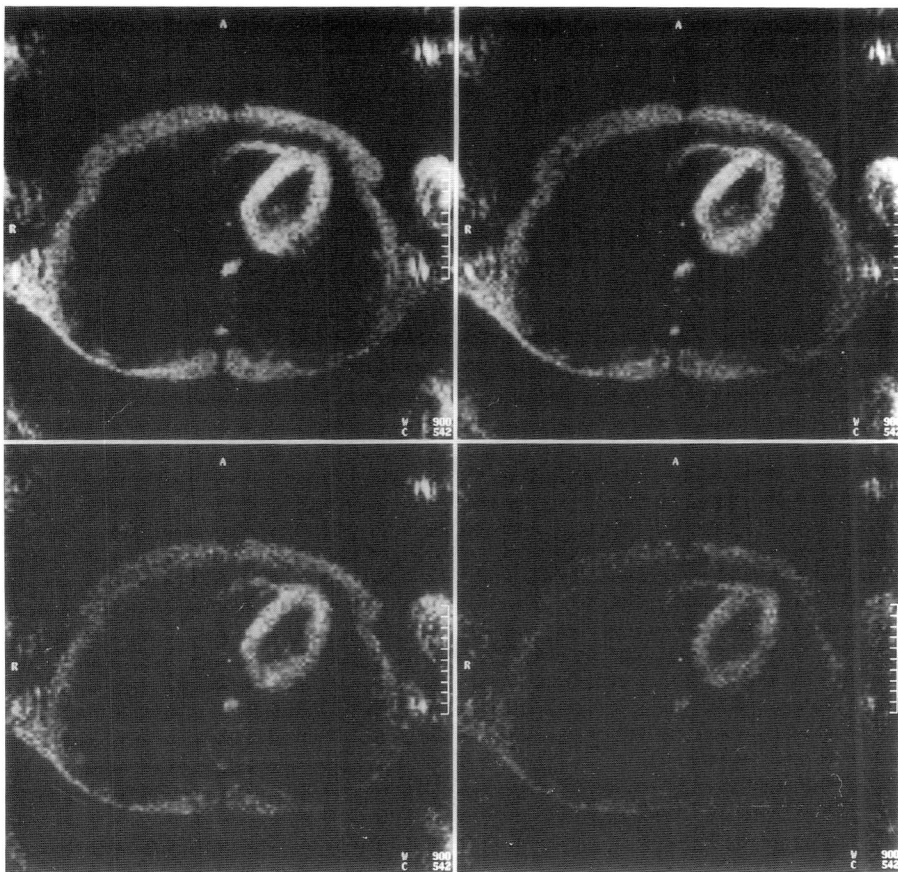

Fig. 12. EPI–diffusion-weighted imaging of the myocardium. From top left to bottom right the b value was increased ($b = 3/12/20/42$ s mm^{-2}) to achieve signal attenuation in the myocardium caused by diffusion.

tant impact on other fast-imaging techniques like RARE [11] and GRASE (gradient and spin echo) [12].

REFERENCES

1. Mansfield P (1977) Multi-planar image formation using NMR spin echoes. *J Phys C* L55–L58.
2. Le Bihan D (1991) Molecular diffusion nuclear magnetic resonance imaging. *Magn Reson Quart* **7:** 1–30.
3. Turner R, Le Bihan D, Chesnick AS (1991) Echo-planar imaging of diffusion and perfusion. *Magn Reson Med* **19:** 247–253.
4. Moseley ME, Mintorovitch J, Asgari H, Vexler Z, Kucharczyk J (1991) Diffusion/perfusion MR characterization of hyperacute cerebral ischemia. SMRM Book of Abstracts, p. 330.
5. Warach S, Chen D, Li W, Ronthal M, Edelman RR (1992) Fast magnetic resonance diffusion weighted imaging of acute human stroke. *Neurology* **42:** 1717–1723.
6. Warach S, Wielopolski P, Edelman RR (1993) Identification of the ischemic penumbra of acute human stroke using echo planar diffusion and perfusion imaging. SMRM Book of Abstracts; p. 249.
7. Stejskal EO, Tanner JE (1965) Spin diffusion measurements: spin-echo in the presence of a time-dependent field-gradient. *J Chem Phys* **42:** 288–292.
8. Merbold KD, Hanicke W, Bruhn H, Gyngell ML, Frahm J (1992) Diffusion imaging of the human brain in vivo using high speed STEAM MRI. *Magn Reson Med* **23:** 179–192.
9. Edelman RR, Gaa J, Prasad PV, Pearlman JD (1993) Diffusion imaging of the human heart. SMRM Book of Abstracts, p. 286.
10. Müller MF, Prasad PV, Siewert B, Raptopoulus V, Nissenbaum MA, Lewis WD, Edelman RR (1993) Abdominal diffusion mapping using a whole body echo planar system. SMRM Book of Abstracts, p. 45.
11. Hennig J, Friedburg H (1988) Clinical applications and methodological developments of the RARE technique. *Magn Reson Imaging* **6:** 391–395.
12. Oshio K, Feinberg DA (1991) GRASE (gradient- and spin-echo) imaging: a novel fast MRI technique. *Magn Reson Imaging* **20:** 344–349.

High-resolution echo-planar imaging at 3.0 T

R. Bowtell,* P. Mansfield, R.J. Coxon, P.R. Harvey and P.M. Glover

Magnetic Resonance Centre, University of Nottingham, University Park, Nottingham, UK

Echo-planar imaging (EPI) is a snapshot technique, which is useful in a wide range of clinical applications, including the study of physiological function. Over recent years, EPI has found a major new use in functional imaging of the brain. Many EPI experiments can benefit from the increased signal-to-noise ratio (S/N) which results from imaging at high magnetic field. Recently, we have built a 3.0-T EPI scanner at Nottingham University. The low-level radiofrequency and control electronics have been constructed in-house. This, coupled with software written specifically for the system, results in a performance and flexibility exceeding that of a commercial system. A quiet head gradient set produces gradients of up to 30 mT m^{-1}. It is driven using a series multiresonant filter circuit, which allows the production of high-strength, trapezoidal- or sinusoidal-switched gradients.

Using this scanner it has been possible to obtain images comprising 256 × 256 pixels, with a 2.5-mm slice and 0.75 mm in-plane resolution, in 140 ms. Multislicing allows a volume set of 16, 128 × 128 images to be obtained in 1.6 s. A comparison of tests performed at fields of 0.5 T and 3.0 T on the same phantom indicates a better than linear increase in S/N with field strength. EPI images obtained at 3.0 T have been used in studies of brain activation during visual stimulation and execution of a simple motor task.

Keywords: echo-planar imaging, high magnetic field, image distortion.

INTRODUCTION

The application of conventional magnetic resonance imaging techniques in medicine is limited by relatively long data acquisition times, which can lead to the production of motion artifacts in images and to slow patient throughput. Echo-planar imaging (EPI) [1, 2] obviates these problems, as it allows the generation of two- or even three-dimensional images in times of the order of 20–150 ms. Such acquisition times mean that by using EPI it is possible to follow rapid dynamic processes in the body and also to interactively optimize image appearance. Recently, EPI has found widespread application in functional brain imaging [3, 4], where its high speed allows investigation of the rapid signal changes that occur during brain activation.

The high speed of EPI is achieved at a cost of a reduction in S/N which results from acquisition of a full set of echoes from a single free-induction decay.

Any loss in S/N can to some extent be recovered by operating with a higher static magnetic field strength, B_0, as this leads to higher equilibrium magnetization and resonant frequency. A gain in S/N achieved by using a high magnetic field strength can be traded against improved resolution, reduced acquisition time, or a combination of both these parameters. In the functional imaging method based on the elevation of T_2^*, which occurs in activated brain regions as a result of a reduced concentration of deoxyhemoglobin in the capillaries and venules [5], further increases in the sensitivity of the technique can be achieved by raising B_0, because the extra magnetic fields introduced by susceptibility differences are magnified by the increase in field strength. There are, thus, potentially significant gains to be made by adopting a higher static magnetic field strength in EPI, particularly in functional imaging [6]. Unfortunately, there are also a number of drawbacks to imaging at high field: some which affect all imaging techniques, such as the increased difficulty of constructing efficient volume radiofrequency (RF) coils, and some which effect EPI particularly strongly, such as the increased image distortion resulting from spatially varying magnetic

* Address for correspondence: Magnetic Resonance Centre, University of Nottingham, University Park, Nottingham NG7 2RD, UK.

fields induced by magnetic susceptibility differences in the sample, as well as increased Lorentz forces on the gradient coils leading to greater acoustic noise in the magnet bore. These effects have to be overcome if high-field EPI is to fulfill its full potential. In this article we describe an EPI scanner which operates at a static magnetic field of 3.0 T [2]. Initial results from the system are presented and methods of overcoming the above problems are discussed.

METHODS

Apparatus

The system is based around a 3.0-T, 100-cm-bore magnet that was constructed by Oxford Magnet Technology. The low-level RF electronics and the waveform controller were constructed in-house [7]. These are interfaced to a Sun SPARC Station 370 computer and an AT&T Pixel Machine, which together allow the acquisition and processing of 128×128 EP images at a rate of up to 10 frames per second.

EPI requires the use of strong, oscillating magnetic field gradients. At high static magnetic field strengths the resulting large oscillating forces on the gradient coil wires can generate significant sound intensity in the magnet bore, thus leading to potential patient discomfort. To overcome this effect, the gradient coil set in use in the 3.0-T system was designed to be force and torque balanced [8] and, thus, relatively quiet. The x, y, and z gradient coils of this set [9], which has an inner bore 40 cm in diameter, have efficiencies of 0.059, 0.037, and 0.16 mT m^{-1} A^{-1} and inductances of 269, 269, and 192 μH.

Resonant gradient coil driving systems offer significant advantages in the generation of the large oscillating currents needed in EPI. Simple series or parallel resonant circuits can be used to generate sinusoidally varying field gradients. However, the use of trapezoidal gradient waveforms is often desirable, as they allow higher image resolution at a given peak current, and at a given resolution they are less likely to cause peripheral nerve stimulation [10]. Such gradients can be generated using multimode resonant gradient coil drivers [11]. The 3.0-T system uses a fifth-order circuit with a fundamental frequency of 520 Hz, in conjunction with a bank of eight, Series 7700 Techron amplifiers. This combination can produce trapezoidal waveforms with a rise time of 150 μs and a peak gradient strength of 30 mT m^{-1}.

A linear bird-cage coil was used in RF reception and transmission. This incorporates a patchwork RF screen, composed of a mosaic of small sections of copper sheet, which overlap one another but which are separated by a thin layer of insulator. The screen forms a continuous path for RF currents, thus screening the bird-cage coil but does not sustain eddy currents at the gradient switching frequency. Such eddy currents are best eliminated because they can cause ghosting in EP images.

S/N comparison

In order to investigate the performance of the 3.0-T system, a comparison of EP images obtained at low and high static magnetic fields was made [12]. A 15-cm-diameter cylindrical phantom was imaged using the 3.0-T system and then using a 0.5-T imaging system, which was built in house. In both cases the same EPI sequence was employed and a similar diameter (27 cm) linear RF bird-cage coil was used. Analysis of the resulting images indicates that the S/N is approximately a factor of 7 greater in the images obtained at 3.0 T. The S/N has obviously not increased as $\omega^{7/4}$, as predicted by simple theory [13]. This is because of the increased coil loading by the saline phantom at high frequency, which meant that the Q of the RF coil operating at 128 MHz is actually less than that of the coil used at 22 MHz. However, the seven-fold gain in S/N, achieved by moving from 0.5 to 3.0 T, is highly advantageous and can, for example, be translated into a factor of 1.9 improvement in resolution in all three dimensions.

RESULTS

128 × 128 images

Figure 1 shows four 128×128-pixel, gradient-echo, EP images, taken from a multislice set of 16 images which was acquired in 1.6 s. The effective echo time was 10 ms and each image was generated by acquiring 72 echoes. The first 16 echoes, which span the center of k-space, were used to produce a phase map. This was then used to phase correct the image generated from the full set of 72 echoes [14]. The in-plane resolution of these images is 1.2×1.5 mm^2 and the slice thickness is 5 mm. Figure 2 shows four 128×128, spin-echo images of the same volunteer. The image parameters are the same as in the images of Fig. 1, except here the echo time, TE, is 60 ms. The increased TE yields the strong T_2 contrast which is evident in these images.

256 × 256 images

The increased intrinsic S/N at 3.0 T has allowed the matrix size to be increased to 256×256. This was accomplished by keeping the time per echo constant and simply doubling the number of echoes acquired and the sampling rate. Figure 3 shows two of the

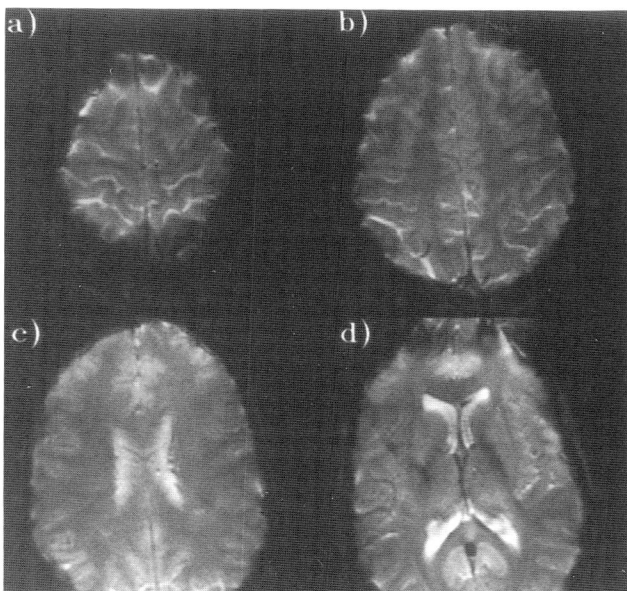

Fig. 1. 128 × 128 gradient echo, EP images obtained at 3.0 T. The resolution is 1.2 × 1.5 mm² and the slice thickness is 5 mm. These four images were taken from a multislice set of 16 which was acquired in 1.6 s. (TE = 10 ms.)

resulting images. Figure 3a is a gradient echo image (TE = 10 ms), whereas Fig. 3b is a spin-echo image (TE = 60 ms). In both images, the in-plane resolution is 0.75 mm and the slice thickness is 2.5 mm. Comparison of Fig. 3 with Figs. 1 and 2 indicates that there is

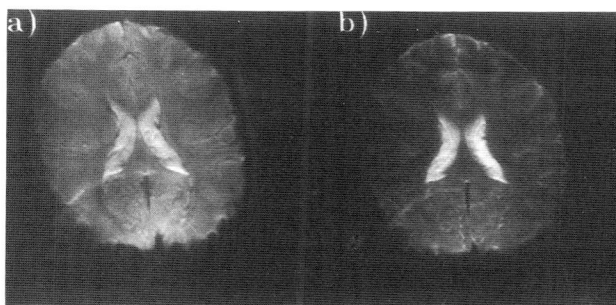

Fig. 2. 128 × 128 spin-echo, EP images acquired with the same resolution and slice thickness as in Fig. 1. (TE = 60 ms.)

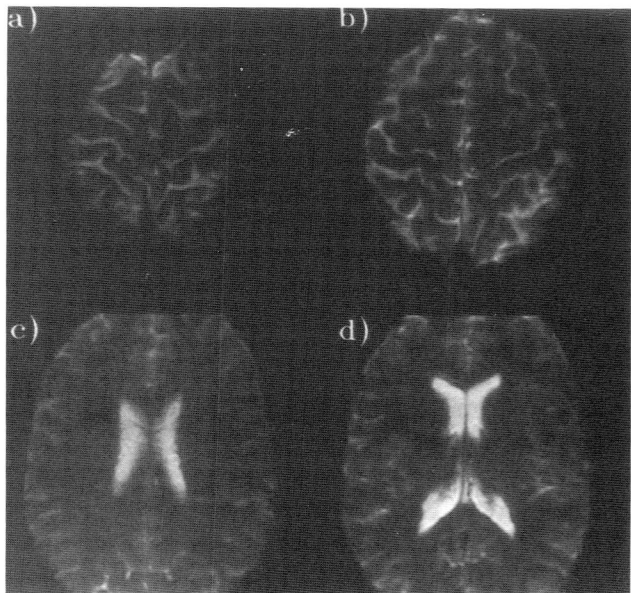

Fig. 3. 256 × 256 (a) gradient-echo (TE = 10 ms) and (b) spin-echo (TE = 60 ms) images. In both cases, the in-plane resolution is 0.75 mm and the slice thickness 2.5 mm.

increased detail in the 256 × 256 matrix image, implying a true increase in resolution. Images such as those shown in Figs. 1–3 have been used to investigate brain activation during visual stimulation and execution of a simple motor task [15].

Image distortion

Although the image quality is high in Figs. 1–3, there is some evidence of distortion close to the interfaces between skull and brain. This results from the spatially varying magnetic field that is induced at a boundary between media of different magnetic susceptibilities. In EPI the distortion due to such a field occurs in the direction of the blipped gradient, in which the frequency separation of pixels is smallest. In an experiment in which N echoes are acquired with each echo lasting a time τ, it can be shown that a susceptibility induced field B_e will cause a distortion of n_e pixels, where

$$n_e = \frac{\gamma B_e N \tau}{2\pi} \tag{1}$$

With $\tau = 1$ ms and $N = 128$, substitution into Eq. (1) indicates that a susceptibility difference of just 1 ppm at 3.0 T can cause a distortion of 16 pixels. Susceptibility-induced distortion can clearly be a problem in EP images obtained at a high magnetic field. There are several possible routes to reduction of this effect. Equation (1) indicates that reduction of τ or N will reduce n_e. However, both of these changes can be problematic. If the resolution is to be maintained, reducing the value of τ necessitates an increase in switched gradient strength, which may be difficult to achieve and which will inevitably lead to increased rate of change of flux in the patient's body when the gradient is switched and, hence, possible peripheral nerve stimulation. Reduction of N leads to a reduced field of view in the blipped gradient direction.

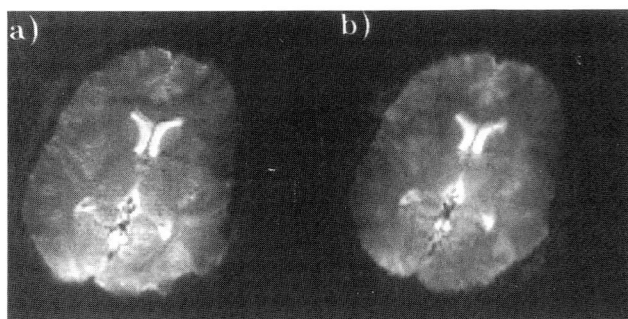

Fig. 4. (a) 128 × 128 head image acquired with a positive blipped gradient. (b) Corrected image which was generated by postprocessing using (a) and a similar image acquired with a negative blipped gradient.

An alternative way of reducing image distortion is through image postprocessing. We have recently evaluated a method based on a technique for correcting distortion in 2D Fourier transform (FT) images [16]. In one-dimensional form the technique involves gathering two profiles: the first with a positive read gradient and the second with a negative read gradient. Reversing the read gradient polarity effectively causes the distortion to occur in the opposite sense in the profile. By evaluating a running integral of each profile intensity and comparing the two integrals it is possible to generate an undistorted profile [16]. In the application to EPI [17], images are gathered with a positive and then negative polarity blipped gradient. By breaking down the image into a set of one-dimensional profiles and then correcting each profile in the manner described above, a corrected image can be generated. Figure 4 shows the result of applying this method to a 128 × 128-pixel head image obtained at 3.0 T. Figure 4a is an image acquired with a positive blipped gradient, whereas Fig. 4b shows the corrected image. In Fig. 4a there is noticeable distortion at the back of the head, which has been removed by the postprocessing algorithm in Fig. 4b. However, there is some evidence of blurring in the corrected image. This may have resulted from movement but is most likely to have been caused by slight mismatches in the intensities in the two images. Further effort is currently being applied to refining the algorithm so as to overcome this problem.

CONCLUSION

A specially constructed 3.0-T, echo-planar imaging system has been described and some of the first results from this system have been presented. The latter include 256 × 256-pixel images of the head, with submillimeter resolution. A new method of correcting susceptibility distortion in EP images by postprocessing has also been reported.

ACKNOWLEDGMENTS

We would like to thank the British Technology Group, the Department of Health and the University of Nottingham, for funding the construction of the 3.0-T imaging system. We thank the MRC for current support of this project. The RF coil used for this work was constructed by A. Howseman of Surrey Medical Imaging Systems. We would also like to acknowledge the help of B. Chapman, M-J. Commandre, D.J.O. McIntyre, and I. Thexton.

REFERENCES

1. Mansfield P (1977) Multi-planar image formation using NMR spin echoes. *J Phys [E]* **10:** 55–62.
2. Mansfield P, Coxon R, Glover P (1994) Echo-planar imaging of the brain at 3.0 T: first normal volunteer results. *Journal of Computer Assisted Tomography* **18:** 339–343.
3. Belliveau JW, Kennedy DN, McKinstry RC, Buchbinder BR, Weisskoff RM, Cohen MS, Vevea JM, Brady TJ, Rosen BR (1991) Functional mapping of the human visual cortex by Magnetic Resonance Imaging. *Science* **254:** 716–719.
4. Bandettini PA, Wong EC, Hinks RS, Tikofsky RS, Hyde JS (1992) Time course EPI of human brain function during task activation. *Magn Reson Med* **25:** 390–397.
5. Ogawa S, Lee TM, Nayak AS, Glynn P (1990) Oxygenation-sensitive contrast in magnetic resonance images of rodent brain at high fields. *Magn Reson Med* **14:** 68–78.
6. Turner R, Jezzard P, Wen H, Kwong KK, Le Bihan D, Zeffiro T, Balaban RS (1993) Functional mapping of the human visual cortex at 4 and 1.5 Tesla using deoxygenation contrast EPI. *Magn Reson Med* **29:** 277–279.
7. Glover PM (1993) High field magnetic resonance imaging. *Ph.D. Thesis, University of Nottingham.*
8. Mansfield P, Glover PM, Bowtell R (1994) Active acoustic screening: design principles for quiet gradient coils in MRI. *Meas Sci Technol* **5:** 1021–1025.
9. Mansfield P, Chapman BLW, Bowtell R, Glover PM, Harvey P (1994) Active acoustic screening: reduction of noise in gradient coils by net Lorentz force balancing. *Magn Reson Med* (in press).
10. Mansfield P, Harvey PR (1993) Limits to neural stimulation in echo-planar imaging. *Magn Reson Med* **29:** 746–758.

11. Mansfield P, Harvey PR, Coxon R (1991) Multi-mode resonant gradient coil circuit for ultra high speed NMR imaging. *Meas Sci Technol* **2**: 1051–1058.

12. Glover P, Coxon R, Mansfield P (1993) Echo-planar imaging at 3.0 T. *Book of Abstracts of the 10th Annual Meeting of the European Society for Magnetic Resonance in Medicine and Biology, Rome.* p. 46.

13. Mansfield P, Morris PG (1982) *NMR Imaging in Biomedicine.* New York: Academic Press.

14. Cohen MS, Weisskoff RM (1991) Ultra-fast imaging. *Magn Reson Imag* **9**: 1–37.

15. Hykin J, Bowtell R, Glover P, Coxon R, Gowland P, Worthington B, Blumhardt, Mansfield P (1994) Functional brain imaging using EPI at 3.0 T. *MAGMA* **2** (this issue).

16. Chang H, Fitzpatrick JM (1992) A technique for accurate magnetic resonance imaging in the presence of field inhomogeneities. *IEEE Trans Med Imaging* **MI-11**: 319–329.

17. Bowtell R, McIntyre DJO, Commandre MJ, Glover PM, Mansfield P (1994) *Proceedings of the 2nd Annual Meeting of the Society of Magnetic Resonance, San Francisco* (p 411).

Intracranial functional MR angiography in humans

Valérie Belle,[1] Chantal Delon-Martin,[1] Raphaël Massarelli,[1] Jean Decety,[3]
Jean-François Le Bas,[1,4] Alim Louis Benabid[1,4] and Christoph Segebarth[1,2]*

[1]INSERM U318, Unité de Recherche en Neurobiologie Préclinique, Université Joseph Fourier, 38043 Grenoble Cedex, France
[2]Hôpital Erasme, Université Libre de Bruxelles, B1070 Bruxelles, Belgium
[3]INSERM U94, 69500 Bron, France
[4]Centre Hospitalier Universitaire, Université Joseph Fourier, 38043 Grenoble Cedex, France

Functional MR angiography (fMRA) images have been generated from the brain of healthy volunteers, in response to a hand motor task. Two sets of 3D phase-contrast MR images were, therefore, acquired, one during a resting and one during a task activation period. The MR images measured during rest were subtracted from those measured during task performance. The fMRA images were eventually obtained by calculating maximum intensity projections from the set of subtraction images. The results confirm earlier observations that there is a significant functional response from pial veins to motor activity.

Keywords: functional magnetic resonance imaging, fMRI, functional magnetic resonance angiography, fMRA, motor systems, vessels.

INTRODUCTION

The potential of MRI for detecting functional changes in cortical activity has triggered widespread interest within the scientific and medical community. This interest is reflected by the large number of functional MRI (fMRI) studies already published. The fMRI studies have been concerned mainly by the primary visual [1] and the somatic sensory and motor cortices [2], but the frontal cortex has also been the subject of fMRI investigation [3].

The precise origin of the signals detected in fMRI is the subject of debate. Initially, it was commonly accepted that the fMRI signals originated from the cortex. Recently, however, it has been suggested that extracerebral vessels may contribute significantly to signal contrast in fMRI [4, 5].

In a recent study [6], we have demonstrated that the predominating signals in gradient-echo fMRI of motor activity are due to extracerebral veins tributary to the sagittal sinus. The demonstration was obtained by exploring the upper part of the brain in a slice-per-slice mode, in MR conditions which matched those usually applied in gradient-echo fMRI. The fMR images thus obtained were stacked, and maximum intensity projections (MIPs) derived from the set of fMR images were compared with regular MR angiograms obtained from the same volume. The fMR MIPs constituted the first examples of functional MR angiography (fMRA) images.

While particularly demonstrative, the fMRA images thus obtained presented a suboptimal signal-to-noise ratio (S/N), as they had been derived from a large set of 2D MR images acquired in a multiple single-slice mode. In the present study, we have, therefore, used a 3D MR acquisition technique in order to optimize the S/N of the fMRA images. In order to detect selectively the fMR signals from flowing spins only, we have applied a phase-contrast (PC) MR approach [7].

MATERIALS AND METHODS

Six healthy volunteers were examined on a 1.5-T clinical MR imager (Philips ACS II). The regular head coil was used for signal detection, whereas the body coil was used for excitation. The examinations were performed with the informed consent from each subject.

* Address for correspondence: INSERM U 318/GARN, Pavillon B, Centre Hospitalier Universitaire, BP 217 X, 38043 Grenoble Cedex, France.

The examination protocol included two pilot and four 3D PC fMRA scans.

In the first pilot scan, the brain was imaged in the sagittal orientation by means of a T_1-weighted 3D gradient-echo MR sequence. In the second pilot scan, a 3D PC MR sequence was applied in the axial direction. The image planes covered the upper part of the brain. They were angulated around the left–right axis so that their intersection with the sagittal plane was parallel with the bicommissural axis, as assessed on the mid-sagittal image obtained from the first pilot scan. An axially and a sagitally oriented MR angiogram (MIP) were calculated from the latter pilot scan, in view of the determination of geometrical parameters of the ensuing 3D PC fMRA scans. A reduced field of view (FOV) in the phase-encoding (left–right) direction of the fMRA images was determined on the basis of the axial MIP, whereas two regional saturation slabs, aimed at saturating the MR signals from the sagittal sinus, were positioned on the basis of the sagittal MIP.

Each one of the four 3D PC fMRA scans was built up from two identical 3D PC MR scans, the first of which was run during a resting period and the second of which was run either during a second resting period or during performance of a motor task. Functional MRA images were obtained by subtracting the PC MR images measured during rest from the corresponding images measured during performance of the motor task and by eventually calculating MIPs from the difference MR images. Regular MRA images were obtained by calculating MIPs from the PC MR images acquired during the resting period. A number of dummy scans ensured that the measurements were performed in steady-state conditions, during rest as well as during task performance. The major sequence parameters of the 3D PC MR scans are the following: TR = 67 ms, TE = 30 ms, α = 30°, FOV = 132 × 220 mm², number of slices = 35 (reconstruction onto 70 slices by means of Fourier interpolation), slice thickness at acquisition = 2 mm, scan matrix = 38 × 128, reconstruction matrix = 154 × 256, pixel bandwidth = 35 Hz. Total acquisition time was 7.5 min. The motor tasks consisted of a finger-to-thumb opposition in a self-paced, deliberate order, either unilaterally or bilaterally.

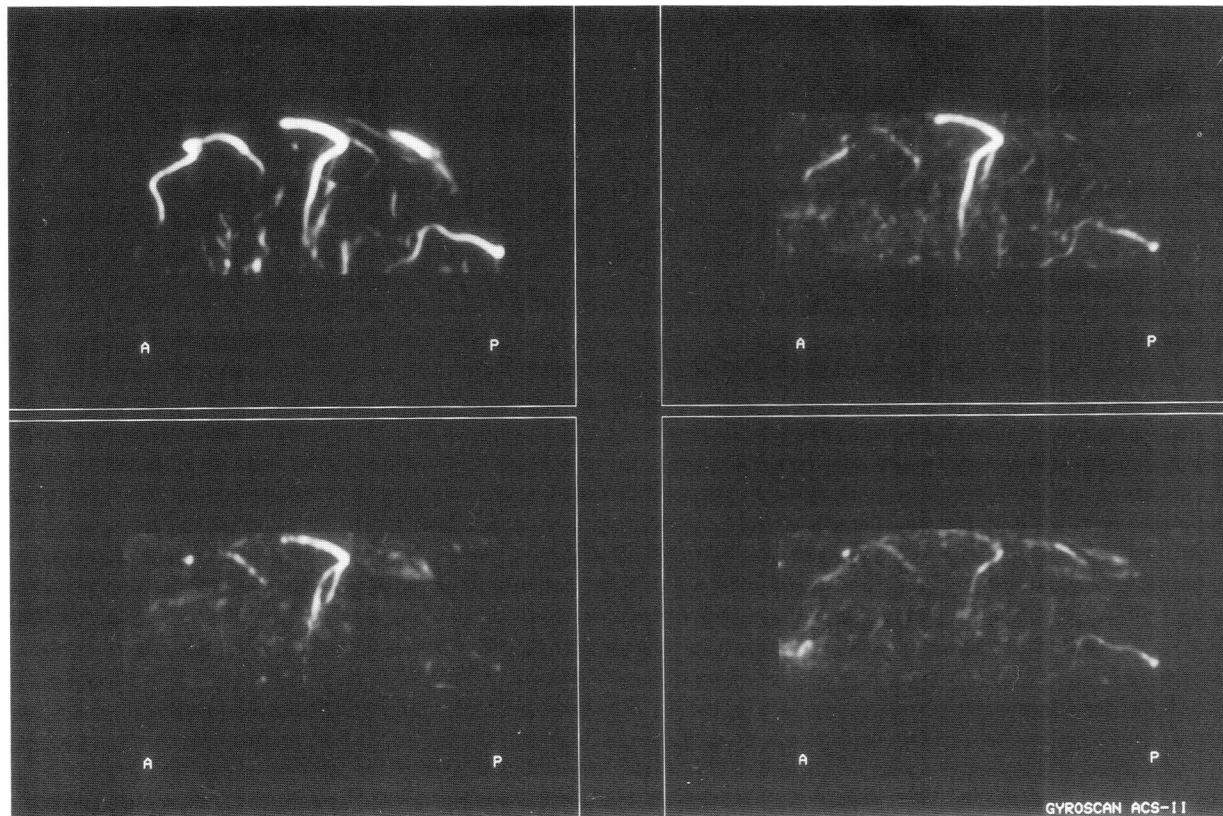

Fig. 1. Four sagittal MR angiograms from the right hemisphere of a volunteer. Upper left quadrant: regular MR angiogram. Upper right and lower two quadrants: functional MR angiograms obtained, clockwise, in response to a bilateral, a right- and a left-hand motor task.

RESULTS

The results presented here constitute a typical example of those obtained on the different volunteers. The four quadrants of Fig. 1 represent sagittal MIPs from the right hemisphere of a volunteer. Clockwise, and starting from the upper left quadrant, one regular and three functional MR angiograms are shown. The functional MR angiograms have been obtained in response to a bilateral, a right- and a left-hand motor task, respectively.

DISCUSSION

This study demonstrates that an extracerebral vascular response to motor activity can be visualized by means of 3D PC MR techniques. Although these techniques are sensitive to moving spins only, the signal intensities in the PC fMRA images may originate from task-induced changes in T_2^* (Blood Oxygenation Level Dependent, BOLD effect) [8] as well as in flow velocity. Further study is needed in order to assess both contributions. Comparison of the regular and the functional MR angiograms confirms previous findings that the extracerebral vascular response to motor activity is due to pial veins [4, 6]. Comparison of the results obtained in this study with those reported earlier [6] shows that these veins are also those which contribute predominantly to signal contrast in gradient-echo fMRI. Also, in agreement with earlier observations in fMRI, the vascular response is mainly contralateral with respect to the motor task, in accordance with earlier observations reported in fMRI of the human motor cortex [9].

REFERENCES

1. Belliveau JW, Kennedy DN, McKinstry RC, Buchbinder BR, Weiskoff RM, Cohen MS, Vevea JM, Brady TJ, Rosen BR (1991) Functional mapping of the human visual cortex by magnetic resonance imaging. *Science* **254**: 716–719.
2. Bandettini PA, Wong EC, Hinks RS, Tikofsky RS, Hyde JS (1992) Time course EPI of human brain function during task activation. *Magn Reson Med* **25**: 390–397.
3. McCarthy G, Blamire AM, Rothman DL, Gruetter R, Shulman RG (1993) Echo-planar magnetic resonance imaging studies of frontal cortex activation during word generation in humans *Proc Natl Acad Sci USA* **90**: 4952–4956.
4. Lai S, Hopkins AL, Haacke EM, Li D, Wasserman BA, Buckley P, Friedman L, Meltzer H, Hedera P, Friedland R (1993) Identification of vascular structures as a major source of signal contrast in high resolution 2D and 3D functional activation imaging of the motor cortex at 1.5 T: Preliminary results. *Magn Reson Med* **30**: 387–392.
5. Hajnal JV, Oatridge A, Schwieso J, Young IR, Bidder GM (1993) Cautionary remarks on the role of veins in the variability of functional imaging experiments (Abstract). *Twelfth Annual Meeting of the Society of Magnetic Resonance in Medicine (1993)*, p. 166.
6. Segebarth C, Belle V, Delon C, Massarelli R, Decety J, Le Bas JF, Décorps M, Benabid AL (1994) Functional MRI of the human brain. Predominance of signals from extracerebral veins. *NeuroReport* **5**: 813–816.
7. Dumoulin CL, Souza SP, Walker MF, Wagle W (1989) Three dimensional phase contrast angiography. *Magn. Reson. Med.* **9**: 139–149.
8. Ogawa S, Lee TM, Kay AR, Tank DW (1990) Brain magnetic resonance imaging with contrast dependent on blood oxygenation. *Proc Natl Acad Sci USA* **87**: 9867–9872.
9. Kim SG, Ashe J, Georgopopoulos AP, Merkle H, Ellermann JM, Menon RS, Ogawa S, Ugurbil K (1993) Functional imaging of human motor cortex at high magnetic field. *J Neurophysiol* **69**: 297–302.

Functional brain imaging using EPI at 3 T

J. Hykin,[1]* R. Bowtell,[1] P. Mansfield,[1] P. Glover,[1] R. Coxon,[1]
B. Worthington,[2] and L. Blumhardt[3]

[1] *Magnetic Resonance Centre and Departments of* [2]*Radiology and* [3]*Neurology, University of Nottingham,
Nottingham NG7 2RD, UK*

Functional magnetic resonance imaging (fMRI) is becoming an important tool in the mapping of
brain activation. However there are two main concerns that need to be answered before functional
imaging can be considered truly useful as a neurophysiological tool. The first is that the detected
activation may be derived from large veins and, thus, be spatially separate from the underlying
brain activity. The second is the incomplete understanding of the brain transfer function and its
relation to brain activity, blood flow, and metabolism. This work contains initial results that will help
address these points. Models of the brain vasculature predict that signal changes on SE (spin-echo)
images are expected to be much smaller in magnitude but very accurate in localizing true areas of
activation than on GE (gradient-echo) images which are susceptable to large veins. By comparing
activation from SE and GE EPI at 3 T, we have shown that the regions of activation are spatially very
similar, suggesting that GE activation is closely linked to the underlying brain activity. We have
identified an experimental impulse response of the brain following 8-s visual stimulation. This
impulse response can be used to successfully predict the frequency response obtained experimentally and its shape suggests a resonance phenomenon. This suggests the brain transfer function can
be modeled from linear response theory corresponding to the inherent feedback control mechanisms of the brain homeostasis. Continuation of this early work will help to identify the links
between fMRI signal change and underlying brain physiology.

Keywords: functional imaging, EPI, brain transfer function.

INTRODUCTION

Functional brain imaging using MRI is rapidly becoming a very important technique in classifying functional brain anatomy [1]. Although many such studies
have already been published, there is still some concern over what the activation truly represents. There
are two main areas of concern: first, that activation
may be derived from large veins which are removed
spatially from the underlying brain activity and, second, that the actual form of the signal change following activation is not fully described or explained. It is
essential that these areas be investigated if we are to
successfully explain and identify true areas of brain
activity.

This article presents the results from initial experiments that examine these two concerns. We have

*investigated the brain transfer function by determin-
ing the brain impulse response. By comparing spin-
echo (SE) and gradient-echo (GE) echo-planar imaging (EPI) functional activation we have been able to
identify whether a significant amount of the activation
seen during GE experiments is from veins distant from
the capillary level activation seen on SE experiments.

METHOD

Imaging

All scans were performed at 3 T on a dedicated EPI
scanner. The imaging sequence was a half-Fourier
technique with the signal obtained under a gradient
or spin echo. The imaging pixel matrix was either 128^2
or 256^2, with single slices obtained in 70 ms and a
16-slice whole brain set in 1 s. The in-plane resolution
was typically 1.5×1.5 mm with a 5-mm slice thickness
[2]. The very high quality of these images allows the
activation to be superimposed on the images from

---

* *Address for correspondence: Magnetic Resonance Centre, University of Nottingham, Nottingham NG7 2RD, UK.*

which it was obtained, thus obviating the need for image registration. Head movement was reduced by packing the head into the radio-frequency (RF) coil with polystyrene foam.

Impulse response

The impulse response of the brain was assessed experimentally by using short bursts (8 s) of visual activation [provided by light proof LED (light-emitting diode) goggles manufactured by Grass Instruments with an 8-Hz flash rate), followed by 2 min of no activation. This process was repeated six times. Imaging was performed as above with TR = 2 s. The results of six experiments were averaged to provide one set of images representing the impulse response.

Although still in the scanner and in the same position, the volunteer was then visually stimulated using different frequencies of stimulation and a frequency response for the activation obtained. The impulse response was then used to predict this frequency response using linear system theory, and, thus, the linearity of the brain transfer function was assessed.

Pulse sequence experiments

The EPI module can be used under a spin echo or a gradient echo. Visual activation was applied subsequently to the same volunteer using GE and SE EPI. Even at 3 T the percentage change seen for a SE experiment is only a few percent; thus, to accurately determine its amplitude, 16 cycles of 64-s periods with visual stimulation on and off were used. In this way, the magnitude, phase, and spatial location of the signal changes for a GE and a SE were compared.

RESULTS

The activation was extracted from the images by using the Fourier filtering technique [3]. In this way, the image data is Fourier transformed in time, creating coefficient images reflecting the frequency spectrum of the signal change in pixels with time. Following a particular frequency of stimulation, the activation seen occurs in the corresponding Fourier coefficient image. The phase of this activation will describe the time delay of signal change with respect to the stimulation; this was seen to be approximately 3–5 s.

The impulse response obtained as described above is shown in Fig. 1. The regions of activation for SE and GE activation superimposed on the images from which they were obtained are shown in Fig. 2.

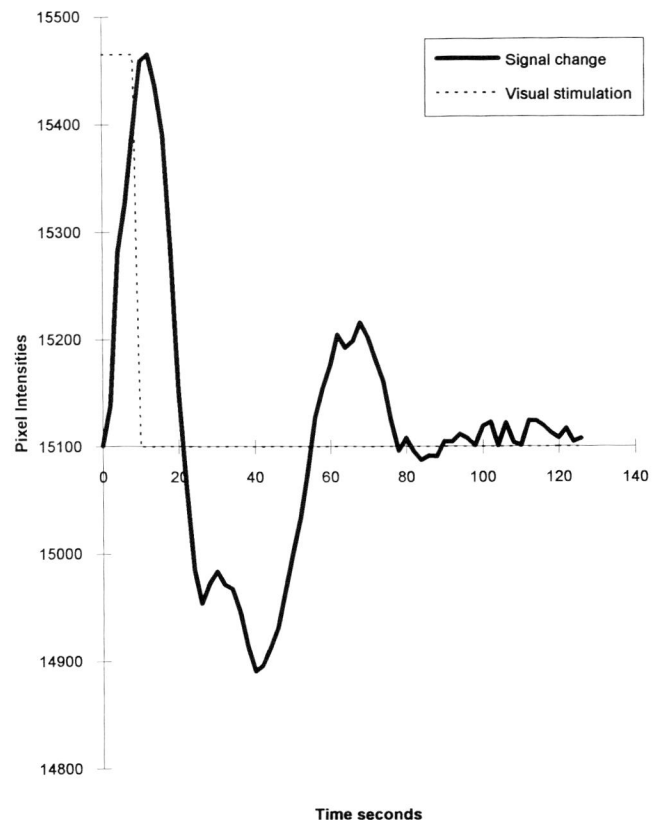

Fig. 1. EPI signal change with time in the visual cortex following a 8-s burst of visual stimulation, or impulse response.

DISCUSSION AND CONCLUSION

The shape and form of the impulse response is very revealing. It shows a slow delayed rise followed by a long undershoot and a further small rise. This appearance is similar to a damped resonant system and, thus, suggests a complex feedback controlled hemodynamic response. The impulse response accurately predicted the frequency response of the brain transfer function, suggesting that it is a linear system. Images obtained using the spin-echo experiment show a much smaller percentage change than a gradient-echo experiment (5% versus 20% for SE; TE = 80 ms GE; TE = 35 ms). It is known from our and other models [4] of the signal change based on the diffusion of protons around vessels containing blood with differing levels of hemoglobin saturation that a spin echo refocuses spin dephasing around large vessels, whereas a gradient echo is prone to producing large changes in signal from large vessels. Our results, therefore, confirm that the large percentage of changes seen for gradient echoes are from large vessels. If, however, the regions

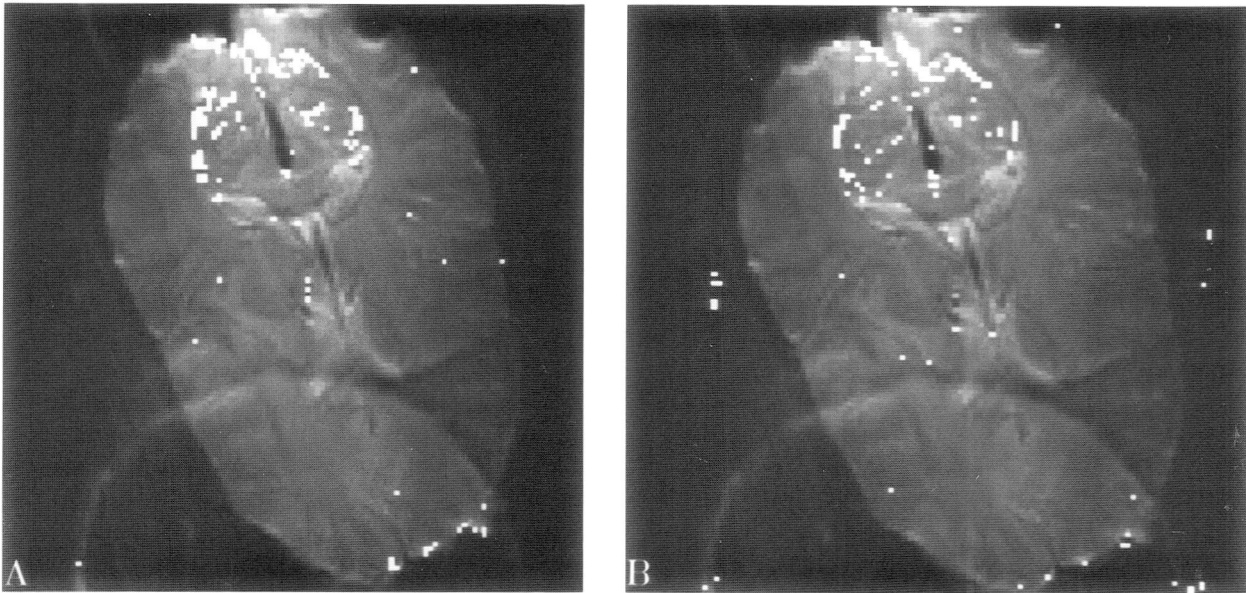

Fig. 2. Visual activation for a (a) SE and (b) GE EPI sequence with activation superimposed on the SE images from which the SE activation was obtained.

of activation are compared after a spin echo and gradient echo, then there is little difference. This suggests that the large vessels seen on gradient echo results are located very close to the small vessels and, thus, the true site of activation.

This preliminary work suggests two important results: first, that the signal change seen on gradient-echo experiments is predominantly derived close to capillary level activity and not from distal veins and, second, that the brain transfer function contains resonance and feedback phenomena and arises from a linear response process.

ACKNOWLEDGMENTS

We thank the British Technology Group, the Department of Health, the University of Nottingham, and the Medical Research Council for the major support of the 3-T EPI program.

REFERENCES

1. Ogawa S, Lee T, Nayak A, Glynn P (1990) Oxygenation-sensitive contrast in magnetic resonance image of rodent brain at high magnetic fields. *Magn Reson Med* **14:** 68–78.
2. Mansfield P, Coxon R, Glover P (1994) Echo-planar imaging of the brain at 3.0 T: First normal volunteer results. JCAT **18**(3): 339–343.
3. Doyle M, Mansfield P (1986) Real-time movie image enhancement in NMR. *J Phys E* **19:** 439–444.
4. Fisel C, Ackerman R, Buxton R, Garrido J, Belliveau J, Roseb B, Brady T (1992) MR contrast due microscopically heterogeneous magnetic susceptability: numerical simulations and applications to cerebral physiology. *Magn Reson Med* **17:** 348–356.

Perfusion and diffusion imaging

J. V. Hajnal and I. R. Young*

Robert Steiner MR Unit, Hammersmith Hospital, London W12 OHS, UK

This article reviews the measurement of perfusion and diffusion and discusses the implications of the observed anisotropy of diffusion of water molecules in some tissues. An experiment is described which shows how observations of diffusion anisotropy can be used to obtain structural information for a model system and to estimate tissue properties *in vivo*. Differences between perfusion and diffusion are highlighted, and the impact of the former on temperature measurements *in vivo* based on MRI is discussed. The article concludes that the observation of these phenomena are worth very substantial effort in order to elucidate a number of quite significant problems in the practice of magnetic resonance imaging today.

Keywords: perfusion, diffusion, anisotropy, measurement in MRI.

INTRODUCTION

Although commonly discussed together, and frequency regarded as being phenomena that can be observed by similar techniques, perfusion and diffusion in tissue are really quite different. The former refers to flow through the fine (capillary) section of the vasculature. The capillaries have diameters which are too small to be resolved by conventional magnetic resonance imaging (MRI) and have been modeled as being quasirandom in orientation [1] although there is a tendency for those bringing in arterial blood to roughly parallel those removing venous blood. Flow in any one capillary is, however, coherent, with typical flow rates of the order of millimeters per second.

Diffusion is a microscopic phenomenon associated with thermally driven random motion. In the context of *in vivo* MRI it relates to the movement of free water molecules inside tissues. Molecules in a free fluid move with equal probability in any direction at a rate that is determined by the diffusion coefficient, D, which has dimensions of length squared per unit time. The mean distance traveled by molecules in a time t is proportional to $\sqrt{Dt}$ and amounts to around 20 μm in 80 ms for water at body temperature. Thus, on the time scale of a typical T_2-weighted spin echo, molecules diffuse mean distances that are comparable to cellular dimensions. As a consequence, tissue structure has a profound impact on the apparent diffusion of water *in vivo* as observed by MRI. Perhaps the most notable manifestation of this is the apparent anisotropy of diffusion observed in both white matter and muscle.

This article discusses the measurement of perfusion and diffusion *in vivo* and the impact on the latter of anisotropy. An example is given of how diffusion anisotropy may be exploited to estimate the mean diameter of cylindrical barriers that may be associated with myelinated axons. Some observations of diffusion and perfusion *in vivo* are described, and some of the problems of understanding what is happening in the microcirculation are discussed.

CONVENTIONAL OBSERVATION OF DIFFUSION

Measurement of diffusion *in vivo* has conventionally relied on the pulsed gradient spin-echo (PGSE) method of Stejskal and Tanner [2]. Although standard for early diffusion work [1, 3, 4], this technique has also been used for accurate flow measurement [5]. The form of this pulse sequence is illustrated in Fig. 1, in which sensitization to movement is created by extra gradient pulses (shown shaded), which in this case are in the direction normal to the plane of the slice.

For coherent motion, this sequence results in a

* Address for correspondence: Robert Steiner Magnetic Resonance Unit, The Royal Postgraduate Medical School, Hammersmith Hospital, Du Cane Road, London W12 ONN, UK.

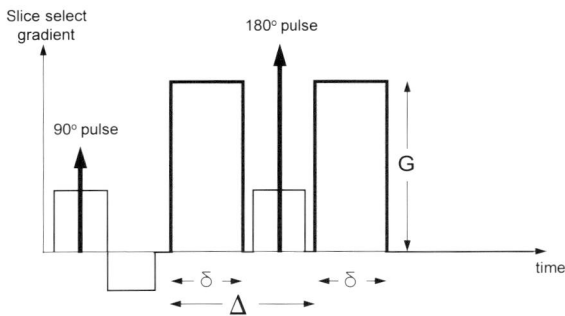

Fig. 1. Diagram of the PGSE sequence, with motion sensitization (shaded regions) along the slice selection direction.

phase shift of the received signal rather than a change in amplitude. When the motion is random (as with molecular diffusion) the relationship established in Ref. 2 for signal acquisition after an echo time TE is applicable:

$$S = S_0 \left(1 - \exp\left(-\frac{TR}{T_1} \right) \right) \exp\left(-\frac{TE}{T_2} - \gamma^2 D G^2 \delta^2 \left(\Delta - \frac{\delta}{3} \right) \right)$$

$$(1)$$

In this equation, S is the observed signal, S_0 is the signal available after full recovery, TR is the repetition time, γ is the gyro magnetic ratio, G is the gradient pulse amplitude, and δ and Δ are times defined in Fig. 1.

Equation (1) is generally written in compressed form

$$S = S_R \exp(-bD) \qquad (2)$$

where S_R is the available signal taking T_1 and T_2 relaxation into account and b is a diffusion sensitivity parameter [1] defined by

$$b = \gamma^2 G^2 \delta^2 (D - \delta/3) \qquad (3)$$

The value of the diffusion coefficient D can be calculated in principle by measuring the signal for a range of values of b and fitting the data using Eq. (2). A minimum of two different b values is required for this, in which case

$$D = \frac{1}{b_B - b_A} \ln \frac{S_A}{S_B} \qquad (4)$$

where S_A and S_B are signals obtained with diffusion sensitivities b_A and b_B.

Pixel intensities in images produced by the sequence in Fig. 1 are weighted by the local degree of diffusion of spins as specified by Eq. (2). In view of the extreme sensitivity of the PGSE sequence to subject motion, satisfactory images can only be obtained by careful attention to motion control, including cardiac gating, or the use of single-shot techniques such as echo-planar imaging (EPI). The latter provides an attractive combination of ease of use and capability for rapid data acquisition but has generally not achieved the resolution available from more conventional approaches.

For a simple fluid phantom the logarithm of the signal is found to decrease linearly with increasing b according to Eq. (2). However, *in vivo* it was observed that although this relationship appears to hold for moderate b values, it tends to fail both at high and low b values. The high b value behavior, in which the signal decays more slowly than expected, remains to be fully explained. For small b values, the signal rises above the straight log-linear curve and this is often attributed to perfusing blood, the signal from which is completely destroyed at larger values of b because it is undergoing relatively very fast motion.

A further complication arises in some tissues as Moseley et al. were the first to point out [6] with their observation of anisotropy in the diffusion coefficient in white matter in cat brain. This remarkable phenomenon can be explained by supposing that molecules could diffuse freely along tubular structures such as axons but are prevented by largely impermeable walls from more than very restricted movement in a radial direction across them. Then, if b is held constant, but the time between the gradient pulses (Δ) is varied, initially, when Δ is small, signals tend not to display strong dependencies on the direction of sensitization. As Δ is extended, however, signals after sensitization transverse to the axons are generally much greater than those after sensitization along them.

USE OF DIFFUSION ANISOTROPY TO OBTAIN STRUCTURAL INFORMATION

Diffusion anisotropy provides a means of studying microscopic tissue structure. Several theoretical models have been developed to describe the effect of restricting barriers of varying geometries. Tanner [7] considered arrays of parallel partially permeable planes, and Neuman calculated the signal from a PGSE for spherical and cylindrical impermeable barriers [8]. We have verified the applicability of Neuman's relationships using a microchannel plate. This is made of glass 0.5 mm thick, drilled with an array of nominally identical circular holes, 12.5 μ in diameter, with a center-to-center distance of 15 μ. The pores in the plate were filled with water, and excess water was

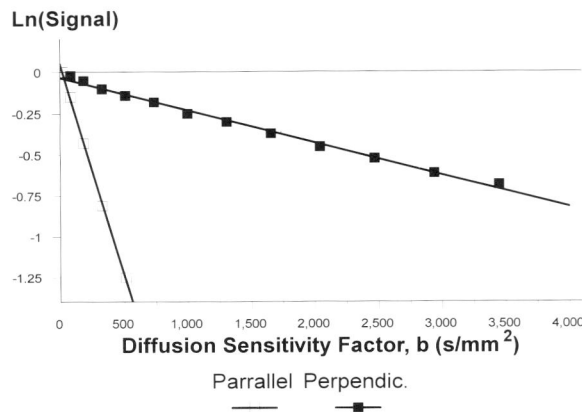

Fig. 2. Results from a microchannel plate experiment showing the logarithm of signal from a PGSE sequence at 0.15 T plotted against diffusion sensitivity (b). The two regression lines are for sensitization along the length of the pores (parallel) and transverse to them (perpendicular). The pore diameter was 12.5 μm.

removed carefully from the faces of the plate. Results of PGSE measurements at 0.15 T are shown in Fig. 2, in which the logarithm of the signals obtained with sensitization normal to and in the plane of the microchannel plate are plotted against the diffusion sensitivity of the sequence.

From this data the mean diameter of the pores was calculated using Neuman's formula to be 14 μ, which agrees quite well with the actual value. In a study performed on the corpus callosum of a normal volunteer, the measurements were obtained under normal conditions at 0.15 T (Fig. 3). The apparent mean axonal diameter was calculated to be about 22 μ [9]—again

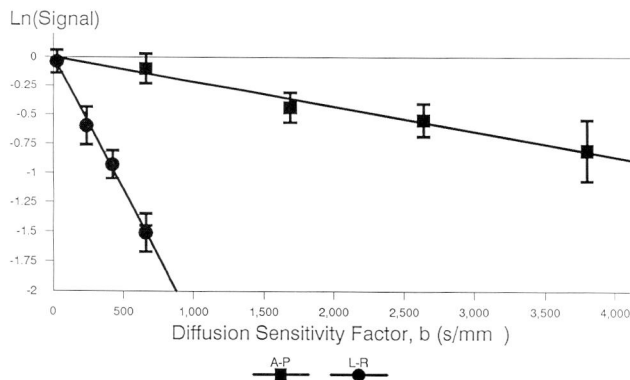

Fig. 3. Results comparable to those in Fig. 2 but for the corpus callosum of a normal adult volunteer. Points labeled L-R are for sensitization parallel to axons, those labelled A-P are for perpendicular sensitivities. On the basis of the results, the mean diameter of the mix of restricted intracellular and extracellular volumes of water was calculated to be 22 μm.

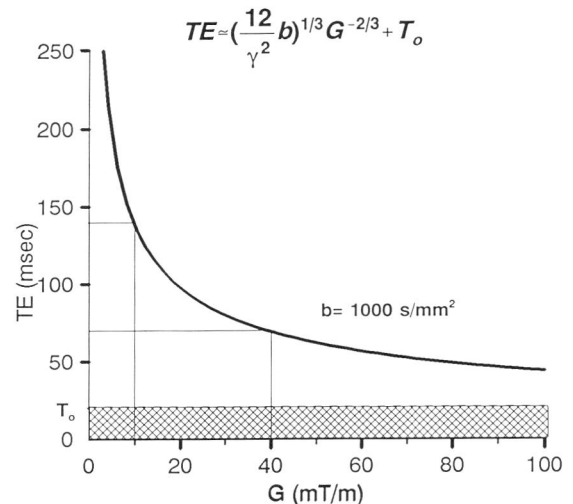

Fig. 4. Illustration to show the desirability of larger gradients for diffusion-weighted experiments. The curve is plotted for a b of 1000 s mm^{-2} to show the reduction in TE with increasing gradient strength. There is a minimum time overhead needed for RF pulses, spatial localization, and data acquisition (shown hatched), so that above around 40–50 mT m^{-1}, increases in gradient strength become much less useful.

generally in accord with expected values if it is assumed that signals may derive from both intraaxonal and extraaxonal water.

EQUIPMENT ISSUES

Diffusion-weighted sequences can be implemented on conventional machines and frequently are. Where measurement is needed, however, and large values of b (1000 s mm^{-2} or so) are required, gradient coils with strengths similar to, or greater than, those required for echo-planar imaging [10] are desirable. This is because although the diffusion weighting achieved for a given gradient strength can always be increased by extending δ and Δ, this is at the expense of increased TE—and results in substantial signal loss through transverse relaxation as well as diffusion weighting. Increasing peak gradient strength (for example, to 40 mT m^{-1}) allows large diffusion sensitivities to be achieved at relatively short echo times. Figure 4 is a plot of minimum echo time for a constant b of 1000 s mm^{-2} versus available gradient strength. It is noticeable that, with the sequence parameters employed, TE is markedly reduced in changing from 10 to 40 mT m^{-1} with more marginal reductions achieved beyond this value.

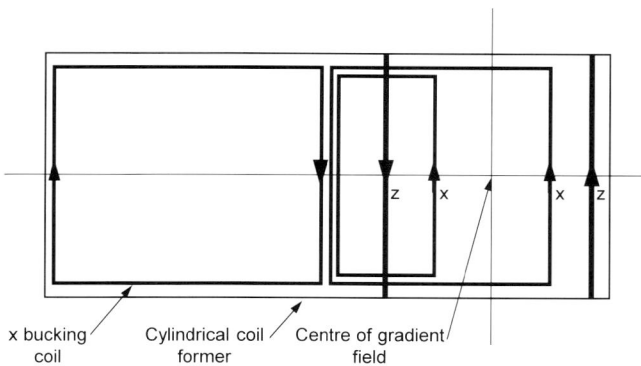

Fig. 5. Schematic diagram of an asymmetric gradient coil set, with attached bucking coils. *Z* is a conventional arrangement, but both *X* and *Y* (not shown) are folded back, and the unbalanced torques arising from this are compensated by the series-wound bucking windings.

Large gradients can conveniently be created by small insert gradient coils as most studies of interest are of the brain. However, the subject's shoulders restrict access to all except the top part of the brain with conventional gradient coil designs. One option is to use an asymmetrical system in which the Z-gradient is developed conventionally using a Maxwell pair, so defining the extent of the coil from its central plane toward one end. The return conductors for *X* and *Y* are folded back on themselves, so that both returns are on the same side of the coil central plane. This is effective in allowing excellent patient access to limited diameter coils but results in a very substantial torque on the coil assembly when the gradients are pulsed, making it hard to anchor them and stop mechanical vibration of the whole structure. A solution is the use of additional "bucking" coils wound in series with the field generating windings and an opposing balancing torque [11]. This is illustrated in Fig. 5, which shows such a coil assembly.

A general problem with insert coil systems arises because the gradient fields may terminate within the region of sensitivity of the RF coils used for transmission and reception. This may result in unwanted signals being aliased back into the desired image data. Care in the design of the RF coils and careful choice of slice selection arrangements can obviate these problems to a satisfactory extent.

CLINICAL RESULTS FROM DIFFUSION STUDIES

The main initial clinical application of diffusion-weighted imaging was in the study of stroke, where changes in the apparent diffusion coefficient have been observed before any other indications on conventional MR images [12]. The significance of diffusion-weighted imaging as an early indicator of acute injury is now also being explored in cases of perinatal hypoxic ischemic injury [13].

Reliable measurement of the apparent diffusion coefficient *in vivo* has proved to be difficult and has not added greatly to a clinical assessment of diffusion-weighted images. This is largely because of problems with motion artifact, partial volume effects, and the markedly anisotropic properties of white matter of the brain, in particular, and in peripheral muscle tissue [14]. Figure 6 illustrates the appearance of diffusion anisotropy *in vivo* (in this case in a volunteer study).

THE APPEARANCE OF PERFUSION IN NORMAL IMAGING AND ITS APPLICATIONS

Although perfusion and diffusion are often treated together as though they were synonyms for each other, their mechanisms and means of observation are very different. Because perfusion relates to the movement of blood through the microvasculature (venules) of parenchymal tissue, its observation is of significance in assessing the continuing viability of tissue. The study of perfused flow is currently of interest in connection with attempts to observe functional changes in the brain [15–17]. Signal changes associated with perfusion mediated variations in blood oxygenation states (the BOLD mechanism [18]) are attracting substantial attention at present. However, the ultimate efficacy of this model remains to be evaluated fully [19]. The use of bolus injections of Gd-DTPA to highlight changes due to perfusion is much more secure, although there is much work to be done to achieve the sort of quantitation performance that can be obtained with X-ray contrast agents. Work is however progressing on brain [20], heart [21], and kidney [22] using this approach.

The impact of perfusion changes is destined to play an increasing role in MRI as interventional procedures involving any sort of hyperthermia are studied more extensively. The body's thermoregulatory mechanism responds, with some degree of lag, to thermal stresses that persist for more than a short time. The ensuing changes in perfusion can compromise measurements of temperature through the observation of tissue parameters [23]. Because of the problems found with the measurement of T_1 (in particular as outlined in Ref. 23), the approach suggested by Le Bihan et al. [24]

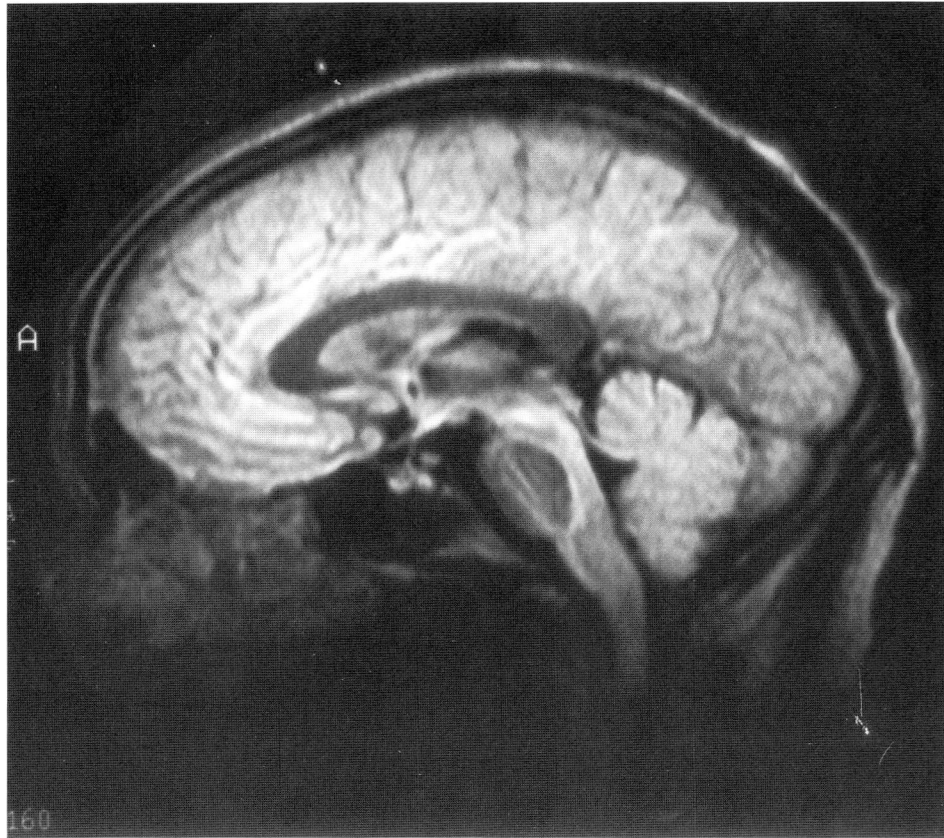

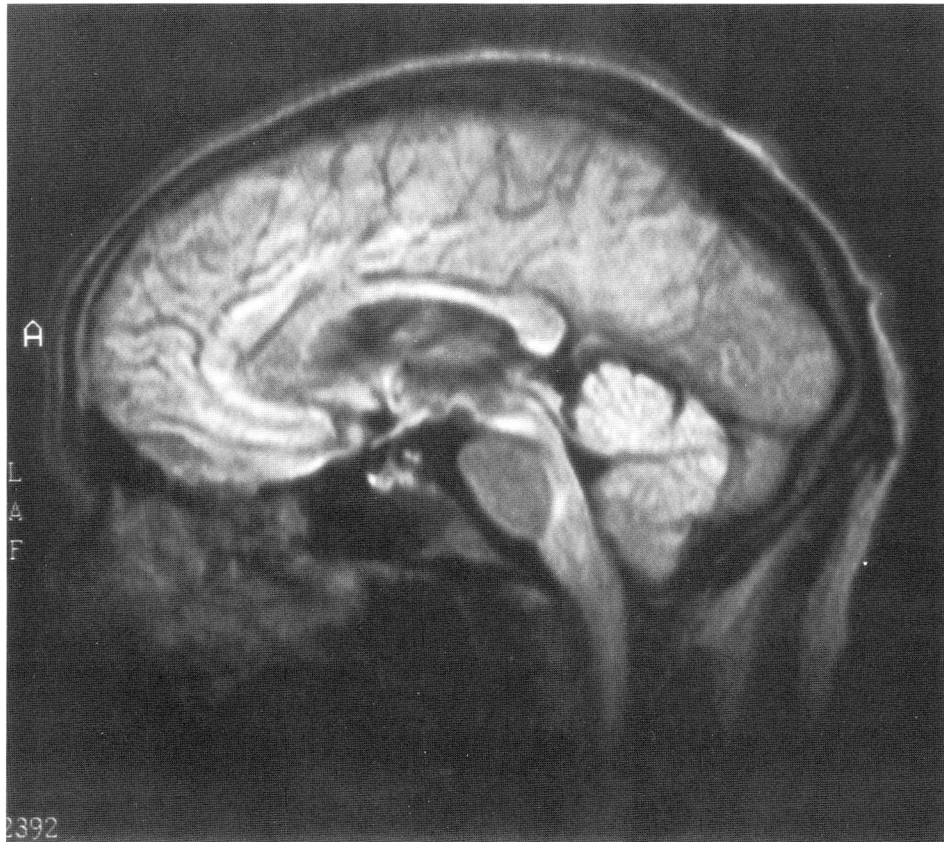

Fig. 6. Pair of sagittal images of a normal adult volunteer to illustrate the appearance of anisotropically restricted diffusion. In both cases the images were acquired at 1 T, with TR = 1500 ms (determined by cardiac gating), TE = 130 ms and b was 550 s mm^{-2}. (a) Sensitization in the L-R direction (perpendicular to the plane of the image). Note the loss of signal in the corpus callosum and parts of the pons. Fibers running head to foot in the pons are clearly seen against a low-signal background. (b) Sensitization in the A-P direction. The corpus callosum now has high signal and the ascending/descending tracts no longer stand out in the anterior of the pons.

using the diffusion coefficient may be better, even if more technically difficult [25]. Studies of both approaches are continuing *in vivo* [26, 27], with the hope that one or other method will provide a satisfactory means of local tissue temperature measurement *in vivo*.

CONCLUSION

The study of diffusion and perfusion *in vivo* is of increasing importance, and new applications are emerging for the quantitative investigation of both. It may take some time for these to become established, but they are likely to be central to the study of the functional performance of the body.

ACKNOWLEDGMENTS

We are grateful to the Medical Research Council and Picker International Inc. for their continuing support and to our colleagues at the Robert Steiner MR Unit at Hammersmith Hospital. It is a pleasure to acknowledge the assistance of Dr. Martin King in performing calculations for the diffusion studies.

REFERENCES

1. Le Bihan D, Breton E, Lallelmand D, Grenier P, Cabanis E, Laval-Jeantet M (1986) Imaging of intravoxel incoherent motions: application to diffusion and perfusion in neurological disorders. *Radiology* **161**: 401–407.
2. Stejskal EO, Tanner JE (1965) Spin diffusion measurements. Spin-echoes in the presence of a time-dependent field gradient. *J Chem Phys* **42**: 288–292.
3. Wesbey GE, Moseley ME, Ehman RL (1984) Translational molecular self-diffusion in magnetic resonance imaging. I. Effects on observed spin-echo relaxation. *Invest Radiol* **19**: 484–490.
4. Taylor DG, Bushell MC (1985) Spatial mapping of translational diffusion coefficients by the NMR imaging technique. *Phys Med Biol* **30**(4): 345–349.
5. Bryant DJ, Payne JA, Firmin DN, Longmore DB (1984) Measurement of flow with NMR imaging using a gradient pulse and phase difference technique. *J Comput Assist Tomogr* **8**(4): 588–593.
6. Moseley ME, Kucharczyk J, Asgari HS, Norman D (1991) Anisotropy in diffusion-weighted MR. *Magn Reson Med* **19**(2): 321–326.
7. Tanner JE (1974) Spin echo of spins diffusing in a bounded medium. *J Chem Phys* **60**: 4508.
8. Neuman CH (1978) Transient diffusion in a system partitioned by permeable barriers. Application to NMR measurements with a pulsed field gradient. *J Chem Phys* **69**: 1748–1754.
9. Hajnal JV, King M, Oatridge A (1992) Measurement of Diffusion Coefficients and Barrier Spacings in the Corpus Callosum. *Soc. Magn. Reson. Med., Proc. 11th Ann. Mtg.*, Berlin p. 1204.
10. Mansfield P (1977) Multi-planar image formation using NMR spin echoes. *J Phys C Solid State Phys* **10**: L55–L58.
11. Hajnal JV, Hall AS (1991) UK Patent Application No. 2,253,903.
12. Moseley ME, Cohen Y, Mintorvitch J, Chieluitt L, Shimizu H, Hucharczyk J, Wendland MF, Weinstein PR (1990) Early detection of regional cerebral ischemia in cats; comparison of diffusion and T2-weighted MRI and spectroscopy. *Magn Reson Med* **14**(2): 330–346.
13. Rutherford MA, Cowan FM, Manzur AY, Dubowitz LMS, Pennock JM, Hajnal JV, Young IR, Bydder GM (1991) MR imaging of anisotropically restricted diffusion in the brain of neonates and infants. *J Comput Assist Tomogr* **15**(2): 188–198.
14. Howe FA, Filler AG, Bell BA, Griffiths JR (1992) Magnetic resonance ueurography. *Magn Reson Med* **28**(2): 328–338.
15. Belliveau JW, Rosen BR, Kantor HL, Rzedzian RR, Kennedy DN, McKinstry RC, Vevea JM, Cohen MS, Pykett IL, Brady TJ (1990) Functional cerebral imaging by susceptibility-contrast NMR. *Magn Reson Med* **14**(3): 538–546.
16. Ogawa S, Tank DW, Menon R, Ellerman JM, Kim S-G, Merkle HH, Ugurbil K (1992) Intrinsic signal changes accompanying sensory stimulation: functional brain mapping with magnetic resonance imaging. *Proc Natl Acad Sci (USA)* **89**: 5951–5955.
17. Bandettini PA, Wong EC, Hinks RS, Tikofsky RS, Hyde JS (1992) Time course EPI of human brain function during task activation. *Magn Reson Med* **25**: 390–389.
18. Ogawa S, Lee T-M, Nayak AS, Glynn (1990) Oxygenation-sensitive contrast in magnetic resonance image of rodent brain at high magnetic fields. *Magn Reson Med* **14**(1): 68–78.
19. Hajnal JV, Myers R, Oatridge A, Schwieso JE, Young IR, Bydder GM (1994) Artifacts due to stimulus correlated motion in functional imaging of the brain. *Magn Reson Med* **31**(3): 283–291.
20. Haase A, Matthaei D, Hänicke W, Frahm J (1986) *Radiology* **160**: 537.
21. Wilke N, Simm C, Zhang J, Ellermann J, Ya X, Merkle H, Path G, Lüdemann H, Bache RJ, Ugurbil K (1993) Contrast-enhanced first pass myocardial perfusion imaging: correlation between myocardial blood flow in dogs at rest and during hyperemia. *Magn Reson Med* **29**(4): 485–497.
22. Choyke PL, Frank JA, Girton ME, Inscoe SW, Carvlin MJ, Black JL, Austin HA, Dwyer AJ (1989) *Radiology* **170**: 713.
23. Young IR, Hand JW, Oatridge A, Prior MV, Forse GR (1994) Further observations on the measurement of tissue T_1 to monitor temperature *in vivo* by MRI. *Magn Reson Med* **31**(3): 342–345.
24. Le Bihan D, Delannoy J, Levin RL (1989) Temperature

mapping with MR imaging of molecular diffusion: application to hyperthermia. *Radiology* **171**: 853–857.

25. Hall AS, Prior MV, Hand JW, Young IR, Dickinson RJ (1990) Observation of MR imaging of *in vivo* temperature changes induced by radio frequency hyperthermia. *J Comput Assist Tomogr* **14**(3): 430–436.

26. Morvan D, Leroy-Willig A, Malgouyres A, Cuenod CA, Jehenson P, Syrota A (1993) Simultaneous temperature and regional blood volume measurement in human muscle using an MRI fast diffusion technique. *Magn Reson Med* **29**(3): 371–377.

27. Young IR, Hand JW, Oatridge A, Prior MV (1994) Modelling and observation of temperature changes in vivo using MRI. *Magn Reson Med* (in press).

MRI of ischemic lesions in gerbil brain

P. D. Hockings,[1]* D. A. Middleton,[2] D. G. Reid,[2] S. Patel,[3] N. Milkowski[3] and D. M. Doddrell[1]

[1]*Center for Magnetic Resonance, University of Queensland, 4072 Australia*
[2]*SB Pharmaceuticals, The Frythe, Welwyn, Hertshire AL6 9AR, UK*
[3]*SB Pharmaceuticals, Harlow, Essex CM19 5AD, UK*

Brain temperature was varied during global forebrain ischemia in adult male Mongolian gerbils to produce a graded response to the ischemic insult. The severity of damage in the dorsal hippocampus was then quantified 4 days after the event with T_2-weighted 2DFT images and with histology. Statistically significant correlation was observed between magnetic resonance imaging (MRI) score and brain temperature and between MRI score and the area of the CA region in the dorsal hippocampus measured by histology.

Keywords: global forebrain ischemia, MRI, histology, gerbil.

INTRODUCTION

The pharmaceutical industry is working to develop effective medication to reduce the extent of neurodegeneration after a stroke. At the same time, it is trying to reduce the numbers of laboratory animals involved in drug trials both for cost reasons and to comply with the spirit of legislation like the UK Animal (Scientific Procedures) Act 1986. In this respect, MRI is useful because its noninvasive nature means that animals may be prescreened and those with anatomical abnormalities culled, thus allowing fewer animals to produce a statistically significant result. In addition, images obtained prior to a procedure allow the normal biological variation in any population to be taken into account when the effect of the procedure is being quantified.

A common animal model in stroke research involves global forebrain ischemia in the Mongolian gerbil. The present study was undertaken to determine whether T_2-weighted images could be used to quantitate neuronal damage at the level of the dorsal hippocampus using this model. Brain temperature was varied during bilateral carotid artery occlusion to produce a graded response to the ischemic insult [1].

---

* *Address for correspondence: SB Pharmaceuticals, The Frythe, Welwyn, Hertshire AL6 9AR, UK.*

MATERIALS AND METHODS

Images of the gerbil brain were obtained on a Bruker AMX300 spectrometer interfaced to a 89-mm vertical magnet with the Bruker Image Directed Spectroscopy probe. A gradient strength of 5 G cm^{-1} was available by pulsing the room-temperature shims. Images (2 cm field of view and 1.5 mm slice thickness) were collected with a multislice spin-echo sequence using a 60-ms TE and 2-s TR. Ischemic damage at the level of the dorsal hippocampus was quantified on a scale of 0 to 5 with 0 representing no damage and 5 maximal damage by comparison to a series of reference images.

Gerbils were prescreened by magnetic resonance imaging (MRI) and those showing abnormal hyperintensity in the hippocampus were rejected (4 out of 26). The remaining animals were anesthetized with 4.5% halothane and maintained on a heating blanket controlled by a Harvard Homeothermic Control Unit. Brain temperature was monitored by a thermocouple placed in the temporalis muscle and adjusted to 32°C, 36°C, or 40°C by moving a heat lamp an appropriate distance from the animal. When brain temperature had stabilized, both common carotid arteries were occluded for 6 min. Animals were reexamined by MRI 4 days postischemia.

Animals were removed from the magnet and anesthetized with a lethal dose of pentabarbitone. Brains were then removed for histology. Sections were stained with a Nissl stain to show neuronal damage and the

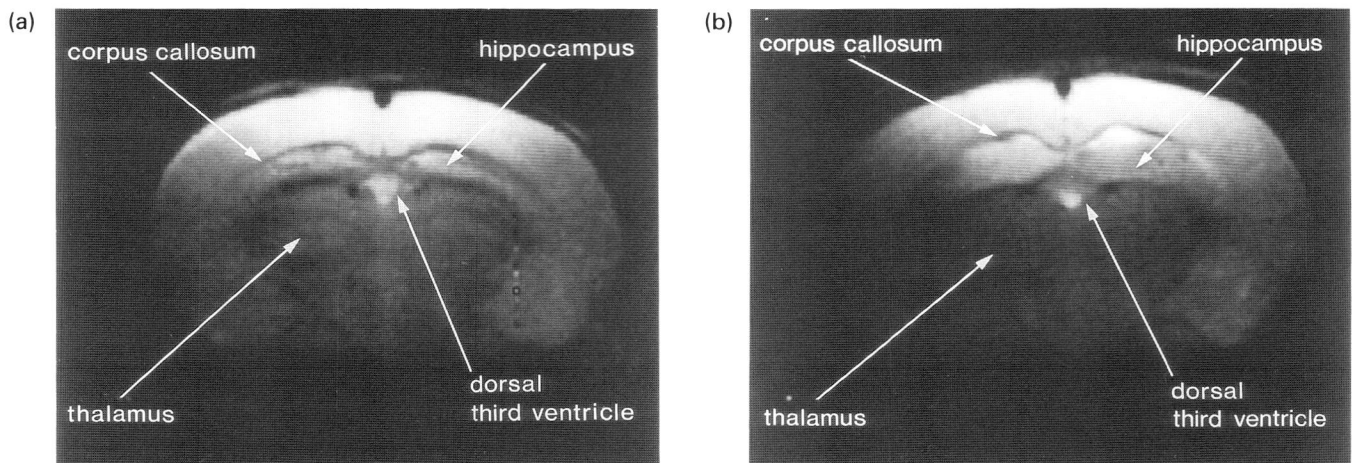

Fig. 1. Transverse spin-echo images of an adult male Mongolian gerbil obtained (a) prior to and (b) 4 days after 6 min bilateral carotid artery occlusion with a 2-cm field of view and 1.5 mm slice thickness. Acquisition parameters were 60 ms TE and 2 s TR with one average per phase increment. Images were acquired as a 256 × 256 matrix and zero filled to 512 × 512.

area of the CA hippocampal region mapped using a Quantimet 920 image analysis system.

RESULTS

Figure 1(a) shows an image through the level of the dorsal hippocampus prior to ischemia. The same animal 4 days postischemia is shown in Fig. 1(b). The hippocampus was swollen and hyperintense relative to the preischemic image. MRI scoring of hippocampal damage showed a statistically significant correlation ($p < 0.05$) to brain temperature during ischemia. The histology score at the same level showed no statistically significant correlation to brain temperature during ischemia. However, the correlation between MRI and histology results was significant (Fig. 2). The apparent discrepancy in these findings may simply reflect the fact that some of the animals used in the MRI study could not be scored in the histology study because the sections were damaged.

Severely damaged animals sometimes developed lesions in the thalamus and occasionally in the cortex.

CONCLUSION

We have shown that MRI can produce a graded scale of damage in the global ischemia model and is, therefore, suitable for use in drug studies. The good correlation with histology enables us to build on the database of results available through this technique.

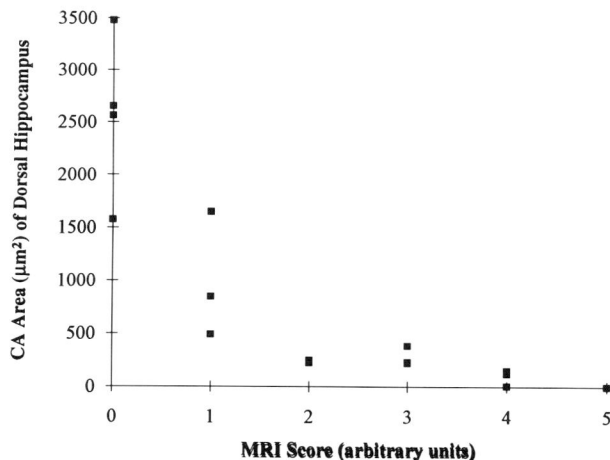

Fig. 2. Correlation between MRI score and CA area measured by histology in the dorsal hippocampus 4 days after 6 min bilateral carotid artery occlusion.

REFERENCES

1. Churn SB, Taft WC, Billingsley MS, Blair RE, DeLorenzo RJ (1990) Temperature modulation of ischemic neuronal death and inhibition of calcium/calmodulin-dependent protein kinase II in gerbils. *Stroke* **21**: 1715–1721.

Focal ischemia in cat brain as studied by diffusion-weighted and dynamic susceptibility-contrast magnetic resonance imaging

H.B. Verheul,[1] K.S. Tamminga,[2] R.M. Dijkhuizen,[1,2] J.-W. Berkelbach van der Sprenkel,[1] C.A.F. Tulleken[1] and K. Nicolay[2]*

[1]Department of Neurosurgery and [2]Bijvoet Center, Utrecht University, Utrecht NL-3584 CJ The Netherlands

Diffusion-weighted and susceptibility-contrast-enhanced magnetic resonance imaging were used to monitor the development of focal ischemia in cat brain. Diffusion-sensitized imaging was used to assess early ischemic tissue damage which was confirmed for the latest time point (~ 12 h) with postmortem histological analysis. T_2^*-sensitized FLASH was used to measure the first passage of a bolus of FeO particles. Gamma function fitting of ΔR_2^*–time curves resulted in 2D maps of relative hemodynamic parameters, including cerebral blood volume and flow. The present data provide indications for cerebral blood flow thresholds for acute as well as for delayed ischemic tissue damage.

Keywords: diffusion-weighted MRI, susceptibility contrast MRI, ischemia, brain, blood flow, cat.

INTRODUCTION

In the acute stage, a focal ischemic area in the brain encompasses regions with varying degrees of cerebral blood flow (CBF) reduction. Tissue near the occlusion site usually has a low residual CBF and will rapidly become irreversibly damaged. By contrast, more distant tissue may show more graded levels of hypoperfusion due to collateral flow. The latter tissue has collectively been termed the ischemic "penumbra" and can be salvaged by timely intervention [1]. The temporal evolution of tissue injury in penumbra regions and its relation to the level and duration of a perfusion deficit are still poorly understood [2].

Magnetic resonance (MR) techniques can noninvasively monitor the developing ischemic lesion with a favorable spatial and time resolution. First, diffusion-weighted (DW) magnetic resonance imaging (MRI), in which the signal intensity is sensitized to (intravoxel) incoherent microscopic motion (i.e., the apparent self-diffusion) of tissue water [3], detects the formation of ischemic tissue damage within minutes after the onset

of ischemia [4]. In early ischemia DW-MR images show an increased signal intensity which is caused by a decrease in the apparent diffusion coefficient (ADC) of brain tissue water. The decreased ADC has been associated with cytotoxic cell swelling [4], i.e., an increased water content of the intracellular compartment where self-diffusion of water possibly is more limited than in the extracellular space [5]. Interestingly, DW-MRI has shown great potential in the detection of a wide variety of morphologically silent brain pathologies, including acute excitotoxic lesions [6, 7] and experimental status epilepticus [8]. Second, dynamic susceptibility contrast MRI techniques, based on the measurement of the first passage of a (super)-paramagnetic T_2^*-contrast agent through the brain parenchyma, have been shown to give cerebrovascular hemodynamic information [9, 10] and, thus, may provide a powerful means to assess ischemia-related hypoperfusion.

The primary aim of this study was to assess the time course of ischemic damage as measured by DW-MRI in relation to the reduction in cerebral perfusion as deduced from susceptibility contrast MRI. Both techniques were combined to monitor regional ischemia in cat brain during the first 8–12 h after unilateral middle cerebral artery (MCA) occlusion.

* Address for correspondence: Department of in vivo NMR, Utrecht University, Bolognalaan 50, NL-3584 CJ Utrecht, The Netherlands.

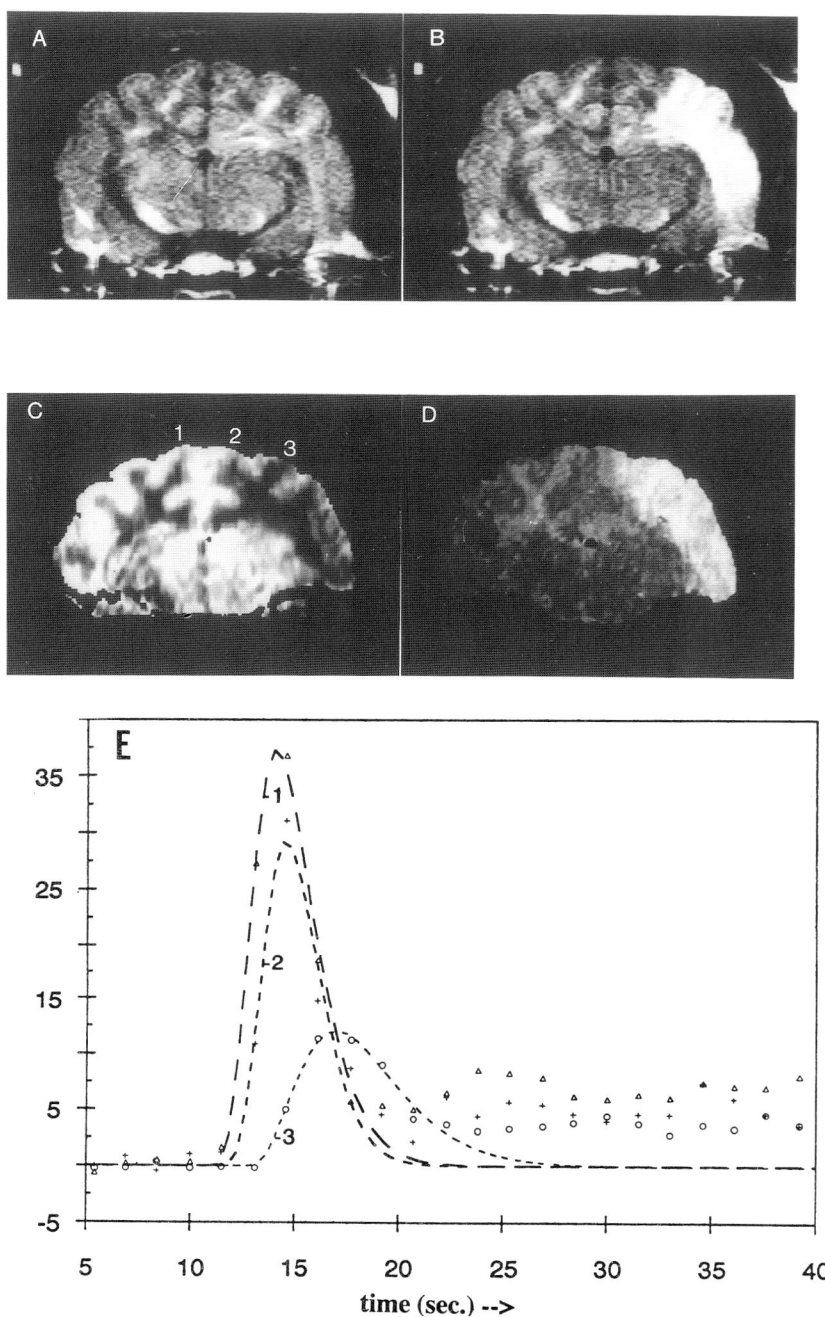

Fig. 1. Slowly developing tissue damage in focal brain ischemia in the cat. (A, B) DW-MR images collected at 1 and 8 h after MCA occlusion, respectively; (C, D) relative cerebral blood flow (CBF) index and time-to-peak maps calculated from a series of FLASH images collected during FeO bolus passage, 1 h after occlusion; bottom: examples of ΔR_2^*-time curves corresponding to pixels numbered in (C).

MATERIALS AND METHODS

Animal model

Focal ischemia was induced in 10 cats essentially as described previously [11]. A ligature was placed around the MCA at least 10 days prior to the NMR experiment. During the NMR experiment, the cat was ventilated on $O_2 : N_2O$ (30 : 70) and 1.5–2.5% isoflurane. Then, the ligature was exposed and connected to a thread so as to allow traction from outside the magnet. The animal's temperature, arterial blood pressure, and expired CO_2 were continuously monitored and maintained constant.

Magnetic resonance imaging

MRI was done on a SISCO 200/400 *in vivo* NMR spectrometer. Multislice coronal DW-MR images were acquired with spin-echo imaging [TR, 2.2 s; TE, 74 ms; NEX, 4; field of view (FOV), 8×8 cm²; nine contiguous slices]. Diffusion sensitization was done in *x, y,* and *z* directions simultaneously (*b* value 1211 s mm^{-2}). Slice thickness was 3.1 mm. Thirty single-slice, dynamic T_2^*-weighted FLASH images (TR, 12 ms; TE, 7 ms; tip angle, 15°; matrix size 128×128) were measured at 1.5-s intervals after an I.V. bolus injection of FeO particles (0.07 mmol Fe kg^{-1}; donated by Schering, Berlin). Separate bolus injections were spaced by at least 30 min. Other parameters used were as for the DW-MRI.

Data processing and analysis

FeO-induced changes in signal intensity were converted to ΔR_2^*–time curves [10] which reflect FeO concentration–time curves. These curves were then fitted on a pixel-by-pixel basis to a gamma-variate function [12] to correct for recirculation of the contrast agent. A relative assessment of the cerebral blood volume (CBV) was obtained by integrating the gamma curve. Absolute CBV determinations are not possible with this method as yet (see Ref. 13). The same holds for absolute data on cerebral blood flow (CBF). Importantly, however, Weisskoff et al. [13] have provided evidence that relative CBF estimates can be obtained from the dynamic MR data, especially when the same region is compared in two different situations (e.g., prior to and immediately after an intervention) or when comparing two regions with similar vascular topology. This condition applies to the present study which, therefore, provided acceptable relative estimates of the cerebral hemodynamic parameters, including a relative CBF index, mean transit time, and the time-to-peak [12]. Correlations between intensities in the DW-MR images and in the calculated hemodynamic parameter images were typically made in 40 regions-of-interest (ROI), regularly distributed throughout the ipsilateral and contralateral cortex.

RESULTS AND DISCUSSION

Figure 1 shows typical data on a cat in which a moderate degree of ischemia was observed. During the first 4 h postocclusion, the DW-MR images re-

mained largely unchanged (Fig. 1A), whereas a pronounced hyperintensity was seen at the 8 hr timepoint (Fig. 1B). Interestingly, the FeO-bolus passage experiments provided evidence that considerable hypoperfusion had already developed 1 h after the occlusion. Thus, Figs. 1C and D show maps of the relative CBF index and the time-to-peak, respectively. The ipsilateral part of the relative CBF index map (Fig. 1C) gave indications for an early hypoperfusion (1 h postocclusion), whereas ischemic cell damage still was absent on the DW images (Fig. 1A). The ipsilateral perfusion deficit was most evident from the time-to-peak map (Fig. 1D), especially because this parameter showed less differentiation between gray and white matter. Small alterations in bolus passage were, therefore, more sensitively visualized in the latter representation.

A detailed analysis of the correlation between time-dependent changes in DW-MR images and hemodynamic parameter maps in the 10 cats studied led to the following major findings. First, a relative CBF index below 20–25% of its (normal) contralateral value represents a threshold for immediate ischemic tissue damage (Fig. 2). Second, relative CBF indices between ~25–55% of control led to delayed ischemic tissue damage (Fig. 3). Relative CBF indices above 55% of

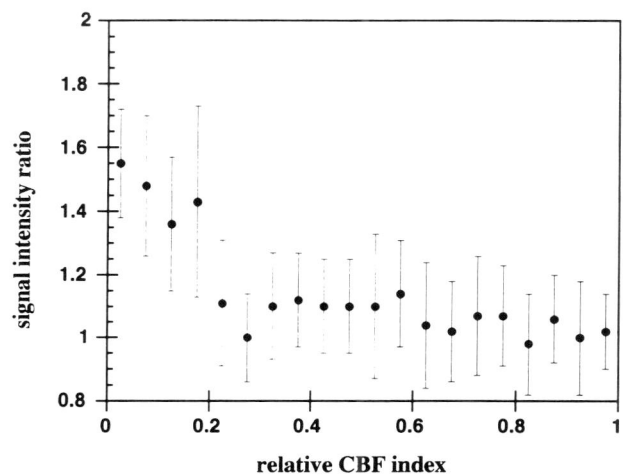

Fig. 2. Relationship between rCBF index and relative signal intensities in DW-MR images acquired directly before the relative flow evaluation. Relative CBF index values between 0 and 1 were clustered into 20 groups. Each group represents data from at least 10 ROIs. rCBF indices in individual ROIs in the ipsilateral hemisphere were scaled relative to the mean rCBF index of all ROIs in the contralateral hemisphere. Signal intensities in DW-MR images are expressed relative to the preischemic values in the same ROI. Data given are mean ± S.D.

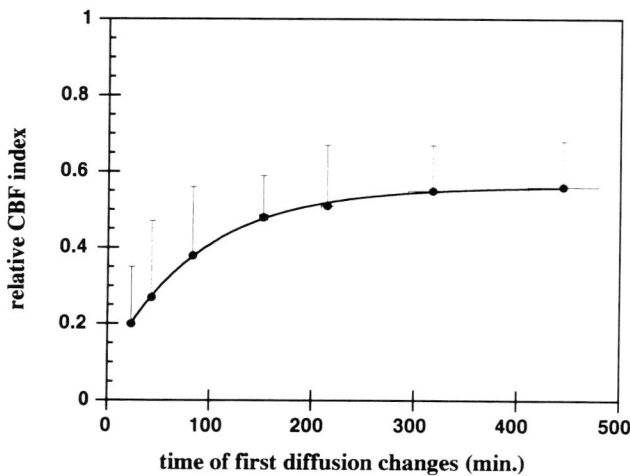

Fig. 3. Relationship between rCBF index as measured 1 h postocclusion and the time of the first significant signal intensity increase in DW-MRI. The latter was considered significant when amounting more than twice the standard deviation (evaluated from the contralateral ROIs). Details in text.

normal did not lead to altered signal intensity in DW-MRI up to 12 h postocclusion. Therefore, this degree of flow reduction might represent the threshold for the final morphological damage.

Histology confirmed that DW-MRI reported on the development of ischemia-induced tissue damage in the present model of experimental cerebral ischemia (not shown).

CONCLUSIONS

We have shown that *in vivo* MRI techniques offer unique possibilities for assessing the relationship between the development of tissue damage and tissue perfusion status in experimental brain ischemia. Now that we have established flow indices for acute and delayed ischemic tissue damage, our future research will address the issue of MR-based perfusion quantitation.

REFERENCES

1. Siesjö B (1992) Pathophysiology and treatment of focal cerebral ischemia. *J Neurosurg* **77:** 169.
2. Heiss W-D (1992) Experimental evidence of ischemic thresholds and functional recovery. *Stroke* **23:** 1668.
3. LeBihan D, Breton E, Lallemand D, Grenier P, Cabanis E, Laval-Jeantet M (1986) MR imaging of intravoxel incoherent motions: application to diffusion and perfusion in neurologic disorders. *Radiology* **161:** 401.
4. Moseley ME, Cohen Y, Mintorovitch J, Chileuitt L, Shimizu H, Kucharczyk J, Wendland MF, Weinstein PR (1990) Early detection of cerebral ischemia in cats: comparison of diffusion- and T_2-weighted MRI and spectroscopy. *Magn Reson Med* **14:** 330.
5. Van Gelderen P, De Vleeschouwer MHM, DesPres D, Pekar J, Van Zijl PCM, Moonen CTW (1994) Water diffusion and acute stroke. *Magn Reson Med* **31:** 154.
6. Verheul HB, Balázs R, Berkelbach van der Sprenkel J-W, Tulleken CAF, Nicolay K, Van Lookeren Campagne M (1993) Temporal evolution of NMDA induced excitotoxicity in the neonatal rat grain measured with ^{1}H nuclear magnetic resonance imaging. *Brain Res* **618:** 203.
7. Verheul HB, Balázs R, Berkelbach van der Sprenkel J-W, Tulleken CAF, Nicolay K, Tamminga KS, Van Lookeren Campagne M (1994) Comparison of diffusion-weighted MRI with changes in cell volume in rat model of brain injury. *NMR Biomed* **7:** 96–100.
8. Zhong J, Petroff OAC, Prichard JW, Gore JC (1993) Changes in water diffusion and relaxation in rat cerebrum during status epilepticus. *Magn Reson Med* **30:** 241.
9. Villringer A, Rosen BR, Belliveau JW, Ackerman JL, Lauffer RB, Buxton RB, Chao Y-S, Wedeen VJ, Brady TJ (1988) Dynamic imaging with Lanthanine chelates in normal brain: Contrast due to magnetic susceptibility effects. *Magn Reson Med* **6:** 164.
10. Rosen BR, Belliveau JW, Vevea JM, Brady TJ (1989) Perfusion imaging with NMR contrast agents. *Magn Reson Med* **14:** 249.
11. O'Brien MD, Waltz AG (1973) Transorbital approach for occluding the middle cerebral artery without craniectomy. *Stroke* **4:** 201.
12. Berninger WH, Axel L, Norman D, Napel S, Redington RW (1981) Functional imaging of the brain using computed tomography. *Radiology* **138:** 711.
13. Weisskoff RM, Chesler D, Boxerman JL, Rosen BR (1993) Pitfalls in MR measurement of tissue blood flow with intravascular tracers: which mean transit time? *Magn Reson Med* **29:** 553.

Fat suppression by echo interference

F. Hennel,* J.F. Nédélec and J.P. Macher

FORENAP Foundation, 68250 Rouffach, France

Two spectral components of a binary system, like water and fat in proton magnetic resonance imaging (MRI) can be separated by adding two signals acquired with a different delay (the Dixon method). The same effect can be obtained in a single acquisition by interference of two shifted echoes. The standard multiecho imaging technique based on the Carr–Purcell–Meiboom–Gill (CPMG) sequence has been modified by adding a time shift of $\tau/2$ after excitation. As a result, in the second and further periods of the sequence, the signal is a sum of two echoes which have opposite phases for this spectral component, which is off-resonance by $1/2\tau$. A magnitude image based on the first period of such nonsymmetric CPMG shows both components, whereas the second period gives an image of the on-resonance component only. The flip angle of the refocusing pulses must be adjusted to give equal amplitudes of the interfering echoes. A similar effect is obtained with the RARE sequence based on nonsymmetric CPMG with low-angle refocusing pulses.

Keywords: chemical shift imaging, fat suppression, signal interference.

INTRODUCTION

Separation of two spectral components of a binary system, like water and lipids in proton magnetic resonance imaging (MRI), can be achieved either by frequency-selective excitation or by comparison of the phases acquired by the two components in a certain evolution time. The latter approach, first proposed by Dixon [1], usually involves two acquisitions which differ by their time shifts from the center of the spin echo. Summation of the two complex images or raw data sets [2] cancels the contribution from this spectral component, which is off-resonance by $1/2\tau$, where τ is the shift between acquisitions. It will be demonstrated that the same effect can be obtained in a single acquisition by interference of two shifted signals.

METHODS

The Carr–Purcell–Meiboom–Gill (CPMG) sequence is known to generate a number of signals in addition to the train of direct spin echoes [3]. The simplest example is the stimulated echo emerging after the

second refocusing pulse as a result of freezing a part of magnetization on the z-axis in the previous period of the sequence. The stimulated echo and the second spin-echo can be shifted apart by moving the excitation pulse away from its original position (Fig. 1). The shift of the excitation pulse by $\tau/2$ gives a separation of the two echoes in time by τ. This situation corresponds to the summation of two shifted acquisitions in the Dixon method when the two interfering echoes have

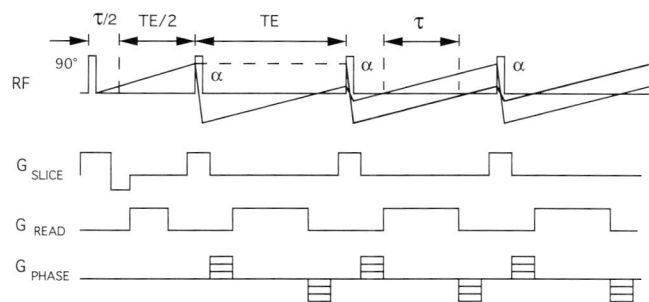

Fig. 1. Diagram of the nonsymmetric CPMG sequence for multiecho imaging. Evolution of the magnetization phase due to chemical shift is superimposed on the RF plot (for clarity, only two coherence pathways were selected). After the second refocusing pulse, the phase plot is split to two lines, corresponding to the spin echo and the stimulated echo, due to the shift of the excitation pulse by $\tau/2$. The signal is suppressed when the vertical distance between the two lines is 180°.

* Address for correspondence: FORENAP Foundation, Hospital Centre, 68250 Rouffach, France.

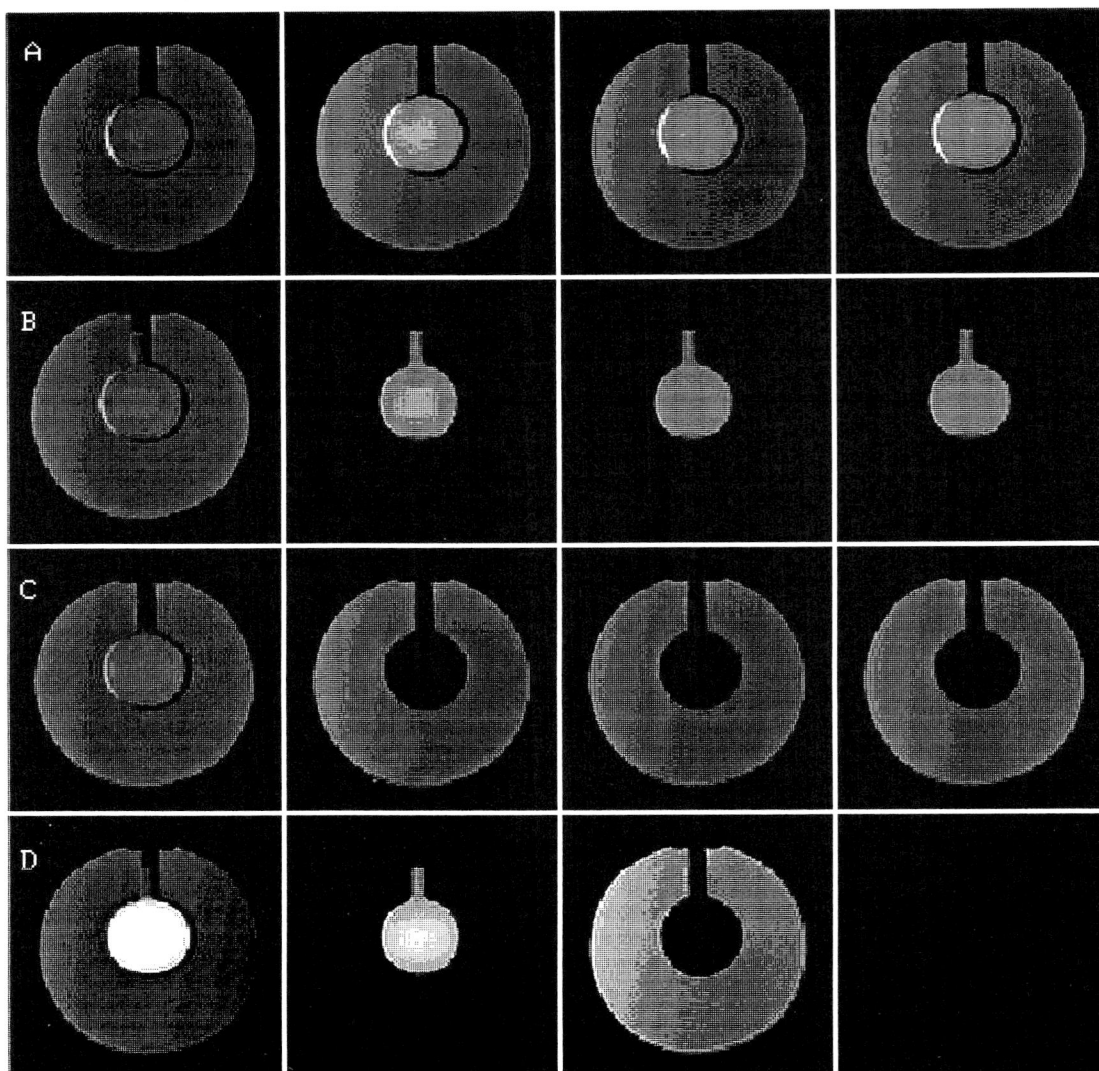

Fig. 2. Images of a phantom containing water (inner sphere) and oil (outer sphere). (A) Four echo images using symmetric CPMG; (B) four echo images using nonsymmetric CPMG; water on-resonance; (C) the same as (B), oil on resonance; (D) low-angle (110°) RARE images corresponding to (A–C).

equal amplitudes and when both follow the same trajectory in the k-space [4]. In such a case, the gradient echo generated at point **r** by the component which is off-resonance by v can be represented (in rotating frame) as

$$e^{2\pi i[\mathbf{k}\cdot\mathbf{r}+(t+\tau/2)v]} + e^{2\pi i[\mathbf{k}\cdot\mathbf{r}+(t-\tau/2)v]} = 2e^{2\pi i(\mathbf{k}\cdot\mathbf{r}+tv)}\cos(\pi\tau v),$$

where **k** is the time integral of the frequency gradient. The signal is maximal for the on-resonance component ($v = 0$) and zero for the one which has a chemical shift of $v = 1/2\tau$.

Equal amplitudes of the second spin echo and the stimulated echo can be obtained by adjusting the flip angle of the refocusing pulses. Using the transition matrix formalism [3], assuming $T_1 = T_2$, one finds the theoretical value of $\alpha = \arctan\sqrt{2} \approx 109.47°$. Manual adjustment can be done by looking at the two echoes separated using the readout gradient (gradient pulse after excitation different than one-half of the readout pulse). In order to keep the same k-space dependence of the two interfering echoes, each period of the CPMG sequence should be separately phase encoded as in the RARE method [5].

As can be seen from Fig. 1, the interference of two echoes shifted by τ takes place in all periods of the sequence starting from number two. As a result, the first period of the nonsymmetric CPMG sequence gives an image of both spectral components and following periods show only the on-resonance one. As the relative amplitudes of the pairs of echoes are different, the level of suppression in different periods is variant. Our computer simulations show that in the range of the flip angles from 80° to 120° the amplitude difference between interfering echoes is small and randomly oscillating, in agreement with Refs. 3 and 6. This leads to a strong suppression of the off-resonance component in the RARE method in which each period of CPMG yields a different line in *k*-space. Amplitude oscillations for the off-resonance component result in a scattered-point spread function in the phase-encoding direction and, thus, cause a reduced pixel intensity. This is a different mechanism to the one previously described in nonsymmetric RARE with refocusing pulses close to 180° [7], where the fat suppression was related to accumulation of the longitudinal magnetization for the off-resonance component.

RESULTS AND DISCUSSION

The nonsymmetric CPMG sequence has been used to obtain separate images of water and silicon oil contained in two concentric spheres (Fig. 2). The chemical shift between these components in the field of 3 T was 600 Hz and the corresponding shift of the excitation pulse ($\tau/2$) was 416 µs. Images based on the first echo show both components (displaced in the readout direction by the chemical shift). In the second and higher echo images, only water or only oil are visible, depending on which component is on resonance. A similar effect has been obtained using the RARE sequence with the refocusing flip angle of about 110°. The advantage of the described method with respect to the Dixon technique is a reduction of the acquisition time by half. The main difficulty in using the interference method is the sensitivity to the refocusing flip angle and, thus, to the homogeneity of the radio-frequency (RF) field. This should be reduced by use of adiabatic RF pulses.

REFERENCES

1. Dixon WT (1984) *Radiology* **153**: 189.
2. Szumowski J, Plewes DB (1987) *Radiology* **165**: 247.
3. Hennig J (1988) *J Magn Reson* **78**: 397.
4. Liunggren S (1983) *J Magn Reson* **54**: 338.
5. Hennig J, Friedburg H, Ströbel B (1986) *J Comput Assist Tomogr* **10**: 375.
6. Norris DG, Börnertt P, Reese T, Leibfritz D (1992) *Magn Reson Med* **27**: 142.
7. Higuchi H, Hiramatsu K, Mulkern RV (1992) *Magn Reson Med* **27**: 107.

Stereological estimation of the total volume of MR visible brain lesions in patients with multiple sclerosis

Neil Roberts,[1]* Silas Barbosa,[1] Lance D. Blumhardt,[2]
Ron A. Kawoski[3] and Richard H.T. Edwards[1]

[1]*Magnetic Resonance Research Centre, University of Liverpool, P.O. Box 147, Liverpool L69 3BX, UK*
[2]*Division of Clinical Neurology, Faculty of Medicine, Queens Medical Centre, Nottingham, NG7 2UH UK*
[3]*Biomedical Imaging Resource, Department of Physiology and Biophysics,
Mayo Foundation, Rochester, Minnesota 55905, USA*

Point counting represents a convenient and efficient technique for estimating the area of transects through multiple sclerosis (MS) lesions on magnetic resonance (MR) images obtained for sections through the brain. When sectioning has been performed according to the Cavalieri method, unbiased estimates of the total volume of MR-visible MS plaques can be obtained with a precision of 3–5% in 5–10 min.

Keywords: MRI, Matheron formula, multiple sclerosis, nugget effect, point counting, stereology volume.

INTRODUCTION

Quantification of the total volume of magnetic resonance (MR) visible lesions in the brain of patients with multiple sclerosis (MS) is of interest as a means of monitoring disease progress [1, 2]. Acute MS lesions are readily visualized as high-signal-intensity regions on T_2-weighted MR images. But, how should the MR images be obtained and analyzed in order to achieve predefined levels of precision in estimating the total lesion volume? Answers to these questions are provided by a topic in applied mathematics known as stereology.

Stereology is all about sampling. Sampling should be efficient so that the workload is optimized. It should also follow a design such that the geometric quantities obtained (e.g., volume) are free from systematic error, i.e., bias. The Cavalieri method describes how an unbiased estimate of the volume of an object may be estimated from the measurement of transect areas on an appropriate series of sections through the object. However, automatic segmentation of MS le-

sions using image analysis techniques is not straightforward [3]. Problems arise, for example, in instructing the image analyzer how to extract a complete boundary for periventricular lesions. Point counting represents an alternative convenient and efficient method for analyzing the images.

METHOD

Irrespective of their shape, an unbiased estimate of the total volume, V, of a collection of objects can be obtained by the Cavalieri method, which involves simultaneously cutting the objects with a series of parallel planes a distance T apart. If noninvasive scanning techniques such as magnetic resonance imaging (MRI) are employed, the images obtained refer to slabs of tissue of certain thickness rather than true planes, and T may be defined as the distance between the mid-planes of consecutive slices. To avoid bias, the first section must be placed at a uniform random position in an interval of length T. If the area of the object transects on the images can be measured exactly (e.g., by automatic image analysis techniques), then

$$\text{est}_1 V = T(A_1 + A_2 + \cdots + A_m) \quad [\text{cm}^3] \quad (1)$$

* Address for correspondence: Magnetic Resonance Research Centre, University of Liverpool, P.O. Box 147, Liverpool L69 3BX, UK.

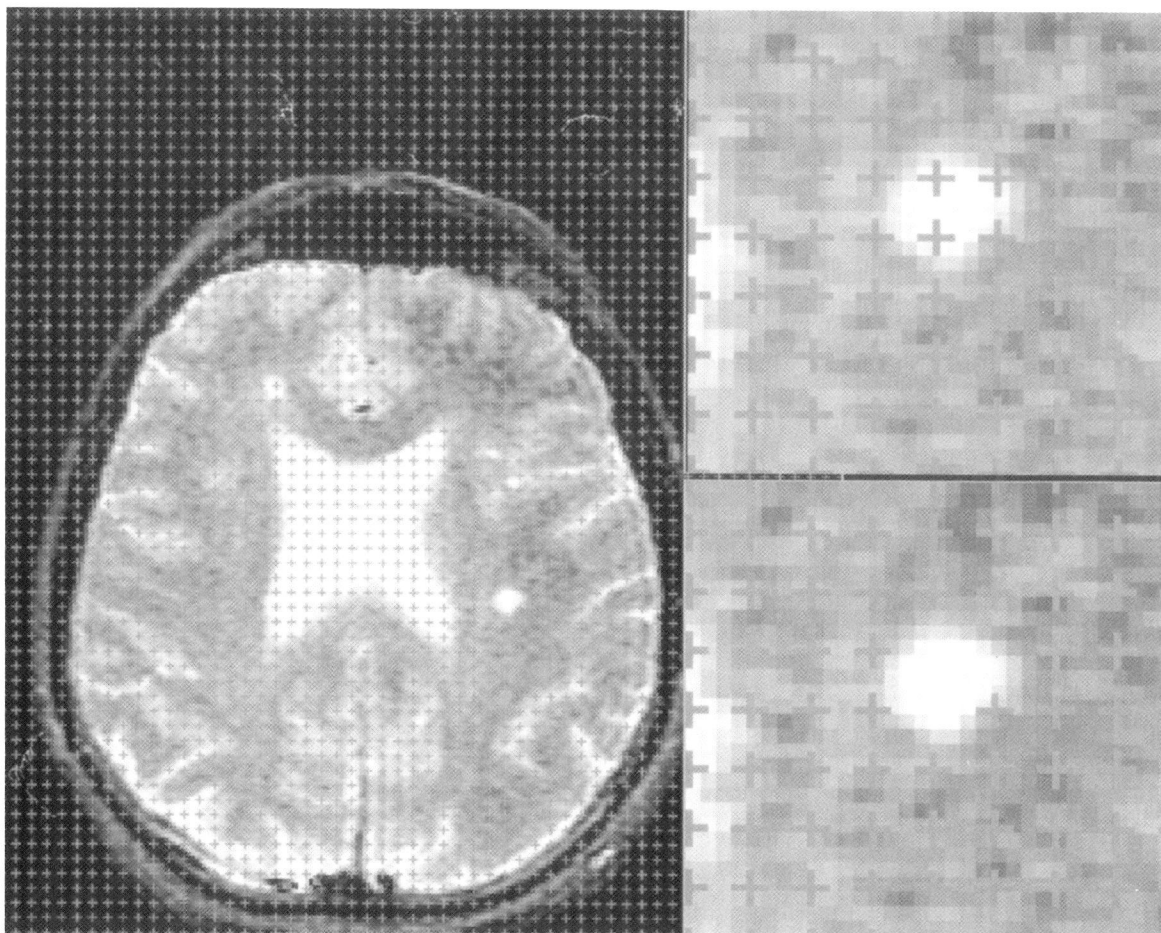

Fig. 1. A square grid of test points of separation four pixels is overlain with uniform random position on each MR image on the computer screen, and a record kept of the number of points which lie within the boundaries of the transects through the MS plaques. The two small panels show enlargements of a transect through an MS plaque before (top) and after (bottom) an operator has selected those points lying within the boundary of the transect. A transect through a second MS plaque (more anteriorly placed in the opposite hemisphere) remains to be analyzed.

is an unbiased estimator of V, where m is the number of sections and $A_1, A_2, \ldots, A_m$ are the corresponding total transect areas on the m sections. The precision of the estimator $\mathrm{est}_1 V$ may be measured by its coefficient of error or "relative standard error," namely, $\mathrm{CE}(\mathrm{est}_1 V) = \mathrm{SE}(\mathrm{est}_1 V)/V$. To predict $\mathrm{CE}(\mathrm{est}_2 V)$ is not straightforward because the transect areas $A_1, A_2, \ldots, A_m$ are not independent quantities. The special formula

$$\widehat{\mathrm{CE}}(\mathrm{est}_2 V) = \left(\sum_{i=1}^{m} A_i \right)^{-1}$$

$$\cdot \left\{ \frac{1}{12} \left(3 \sum_{i=1}^{m} A_i^2 + \sum_{i=1}^{m-2} A_i A_{i+2} - 4 \sum_{i=1}^{m-1} A_i A_{i+1} \right) \right\} \tag{2}$$

was developed by Gundersen and Jensen [4], based on

models of the correlation structure of the data, as suggested by Matheron [5].

If the section areas cannot be properly segmented and measured automatically, then the semiautomatic approach based on manual contour tracing of the digital section images should never be adopted. Instead, the method of point counting should be employed. Each image is overlayed with a regular grid of test points (called a test system in stereology; see Fig. 1) and an operator counts the number of points hitting the object transects on the corresponding sections. The unbiased volume estimator becomes

$$\mathrm{est}_2 V = T \frac{a}{p} (P_1 + P_2 + \cdots + P_m) \quad [\mathrm{cm}^3], \tag{3}$$

where $P_1, P_2, \ldots, P_m$ denote the point counts and a/p

represents the area associated with each test point: If a square grid is used with distance d between test points, then $a/p = d^2$. Note that each section area A_i is now estimated by $(a/p)P_i$. The subscript 2 in $\text{est}_2 V$ indicates that the volume is estimated by a two-stage sampling, namely, sectioning and point counting. In the present study, point counting has been facilitated via a stereology interface added to the ANALYZE software [6] (MAYO Foundation, USA) (see Fig. 1).

When transect areas are estimated by point counting rather than measured exactly, strictly it is not sufficient just to replace the P's with A's in Eq. (2). Cruz-Orive [7] has, instead, developed the formula

$$\widehat{CE}(\text{est}_2 V) = \left(\sum_{i=1}^{m} P_i \right)^{-1} \left\{ \frac{1}{12} \left(3 \sum_{i=1}^{m} P_i^2 \right. \right.$$
$$\left. + \sum_{i=1}^{m-2} P_i P_{i+2} - 4 \sum_{i=1}^{m-1} P_i P_{i+1} \right) \qquad (4)$$
$$\left. + 0.0543 \frac{\overline{B}}{\sqrt{\overline{A}}} \left(m \sum_{i=1}^{m} P_i \right)^{1/2} \right\}^{1/2} .$$

The new term on the third line of the equation is called the "nugget effect" term. It involves the dimensionless shape coefficient $B/\sqrt{\overline{A}}$, where $\overline{A}$, and $\overline{B}$ represent the mean area and the boundary length of the object transects per section, respectively. $\overline{A}$ may be estimated by point counting and $\overline{B}$ by counting intersections I between the transect boundaries and an isotropically positioned square grid of test lines [8]. Pilot studies have shown that the value of $\overline{B}/\sqrt{\overline{A}}$ for a collection of MS lesions typically ranges between 4.0 and 8.0. The size of the "nugget effect" term decreases as the grid size is decreased and more and more points are counted on the lesion transects.

DISCUSSION

As a prerequisite for point counting being a sound approach to estimating MS lesion volume, it is essential that the sizes and positions of the objects of interest are accurately reproduced and can be defined on the MR images. Accordingly, at the outset, all those involved in obtaining the point counts must agree on the precise rules that they will use for defining a test point as being within the transect of an MS lesion on the MR images.

The grid spacing shown in Fig. 1 was chosen so that a total of about 100 to 200 points will be counted within the MS lesion transects on a series of MR images obtained through the human brain. To obtain a similar number of point counts with respect to obtaining the reference volume of the white matter containing the lesions, a much wider spacing of grid points may be used. Further discussion relevant to determining how many section images should be obtained and how many points counted on these images in order that predefined levels of precision can be achieved in estimating the volume of a variety of structures are to be found in Mayhew and Olsen [9], Roberts et al. [10], Pache et al. [8] and Roberts et al [11].

ACKNOWLEDGMENTS

We gratefully acknowledge support from the North West Cancer Research Fund, the Marilyn Houlton Trust for Motor Neurone Disease and the Cancer and Polio Research Fund Limited. N. R. received a Fellowship from the European Science Exchange Programme of the Royal Society and the Swiss National Science Foundation to visit the University of Berne; he and L.M.C-O. acknowledge support from the Swiss National Science Foundation grant No. 3-28610.90.

REFERENCES

1. Ormerod IEC, Miller DH, McDonald WI, du Boulay EPGH, Rudge P, Kendall BE, Moseley IF, Johnson G, Tofts PS, Halliday AM, Bronstein AM, Scaravilli F, Harding AE, Barnes D, Zikha KJ (1987) The role of NMR imaging in the assessment of multiple sclerosis and isolated neurological lesions: A quantitative study. *Brain* **110:** 1579–1616.

2. Isaac C, Genton M, Grochowski E, Palner M, Kastrukoff LF, Oger J, Paty DW (1988) Multiple sclerosis: A serial study using MRI in relapsing patients. *Neurology* **38:** 1511–1515.

3. Wicks DAG, Tofts PS, Miller DH, du Boulay GH, Feinstein A, Sacares RP, Harvey I, Brenner R, McDonald WI (1992) Volume measurement of multiple sclerosis lesions with magnetic resonance images. A preliminary study. *Neuroradiology* **34:** 475–479.

4. Gundersen HJG, Jensen EB (1987) The efficiency of systematic sampling in stereology and its prediction. *J Microsc* **121:** 65–73.

5. Matheron G (1971) *The Theory of Regionalized Variables and its Applications,* Les Cahiers du Centre de Morphologie Mathematique de Fontainebleau, No 5. Fontainebleu: Ecole National Superieure des Mines de Paris.

6. Cruz-Orive LM (1993) Systematic sampling in stereology. *Bull Int. Statist Inst* **55**(2): 451–468.

7. Robb RA (1990) A software system for interactive and quantitative analysis of biomedical images. In *3D Imaging in Medicine*, (Hohne KH, Fuchs H, Pizer SM, eds) pp. 333–361. NATO ASI Series. Geneva: NATO.

8. Pache JC, Roberts N, Zimmermann A, Vock P, Cruz-Orive LM (1993) Vertical LM sectioning and parallel CT scanning designs for stereology: Application to human lung. *J Microsc* **170:** 3–24.

9. Mayhew TM, Olsen DR (1991) Magnetic resonance imaging (MRI) and model-free estimates of brain volume determined using the Cavalieri principle. *J Anat* **178:** 133–144.

10. Roberts N, Cruz-Orive LM, Reid N, Brodie D, Bourne M, Edwards RHT (1993) Unbiased estimation of human body composition by the Cavalieri method using magnetic resonance imaging. *J Microsc* **171:** 239–253.

11. Roberts, N, Garden, AS, Cruz-Orive, LN, Whitehouse, GM, Edwards, RMT (1994) Estimation of fetal volume by magnetic resonance imaging and stereology. *British Journal of Radiology,* **67:** 1067–1077.

New approaches to selective pulse design

Peter G. Morris,[1]* David E. Rourke,[2] Dominick J.O. McIntyre[3] and Abdullah Al-Beshr[1]

[1]*Magnetic Resonance Center, Department of Physics, University of Nottingham, University Park, Nottingham NG7 2RD, UK*
[2]*Institute for Biodiagnostics, National Research Council of Canada, Winnipeg, Manitoba R3B 1Y6, Canada*
[3]*Division of Biochemistry, Department of Cellular and Molecular Sciences, St. George's Hospital Medical School, London SW17 0RE, UK*

Selective pulse design for noninteracting spins is equivalent to inversion of the Bloch equations. Until recently, few analytical solutions to this problem were known. However, approaches based on inverse-scattering theory have now led to general solutions that offer ever higher precision in meeting target responses. The concept of soliton pulses (pulses that leave the spin system unaffected) turns out to be a particularly valuable one because half-solitons (both $\pi/2$ and π pulses) are inherently phase compensated. Such pulses are important for observation of short T_2 species, where substantial signal loss could occur in any refocusing period. Multiply-selective pulses, suitable for simultaneous suppression of several "solvent" lines have been generated by inverse-scattering theory and have considerable potential in both *in vivo* magnetic resonance spectroscopy and in routine high-resolution NMR. Although analytical solutions show great promise, it is likely that optimization methods will continue to be of value for the foreseeable future. The use of the SPINCALC scheme that operates in a switched stationary reference frame is illustrated through its use to design adiabatic refocusing pulses that do not lead to cumulative errors when used in multiple-echo trains.

Keywords: selective pulse, inverse scattering theory, SPINCALC, soliton pulse, refocusing pulse, self-focusing pulse.

INTRODUCTION

Since the first paper on the subject of selective pulses by Garroway, Grannell, and Mansfield in 1974 [1], the guiding principle for their design has remained Fourier transform theory. Thus, to excite a slice with a perfect square profile, the radiofrequency (RF) carrier is modulated by a sinc function. However, the spin system behaves in an approximately linear fashion (as required by Fourier transform theory) only for small flip angles, and the response departs substantially from the linear prediction for π pulses [2].

Pulse design (for noninteracting spins), amounts to the inversion of the Bloch equations: We know the response we would like to have and must calculate the radiofrequency envelope required to achieve it. No completely general solution to this problem exists, although, as discussed below, some analytical and optimization schemes come close to this ideal. Improvements in the performance of selective pulses have resulted from the use of standard numerical optimization schemes such as optimal control theory [3, 4]. However, these and other gradient descent methods are prone to terminate prematurely in local minima. This difficulty is avoided in simulated annealing, which permits positive excursions during the minimization of the error functional [5]. Simulated annealing has enjoyed particular success in the generation of self-focusing pulses [2, 6, 7]. It has also been used for optimization of multidimensional pulses [8].

Many other optimization schemes have been proposed, including some quite novel ones; for example, one inspired by the natural processes of genetic evolution [9] and a second, neural network approach, by a synaptic model of brain function. All these optimization schemes involve evaluating the effects of random variations in parameters and incorporating

---

* Address for correspondence: Magnetic Resonance Centre, Department of Physics, University of Nottingham, University Park, Nottingham NG7 2RD, UK.

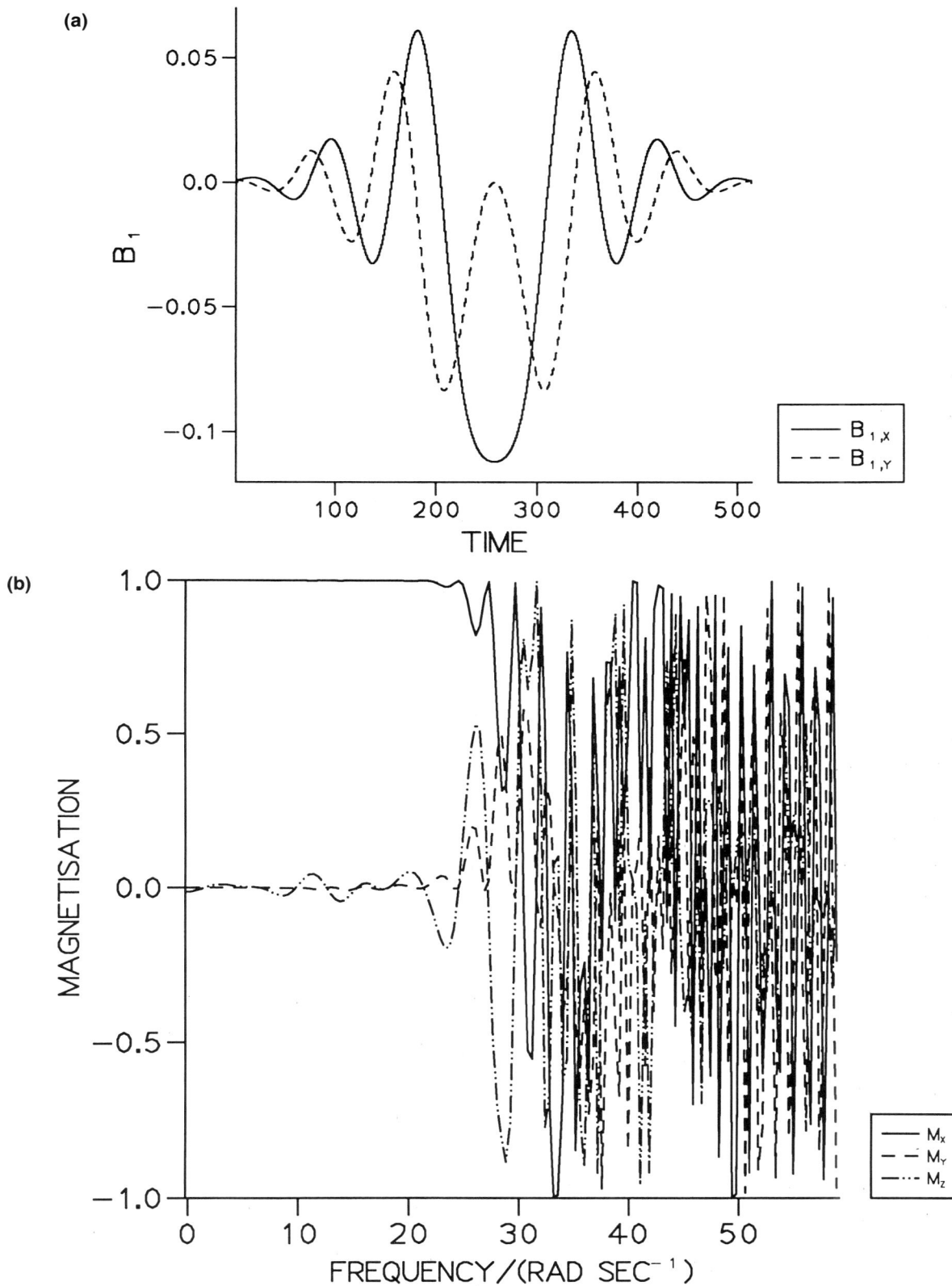

Fig. 1. (a) Complex amplitudes of adiabatic refocusing pulse, optimized using SPINCALC. (b) Response after a train of 4 phase cycled (XYXY) optimized π pulses with the magnetization originally along the x-direction.

(c)

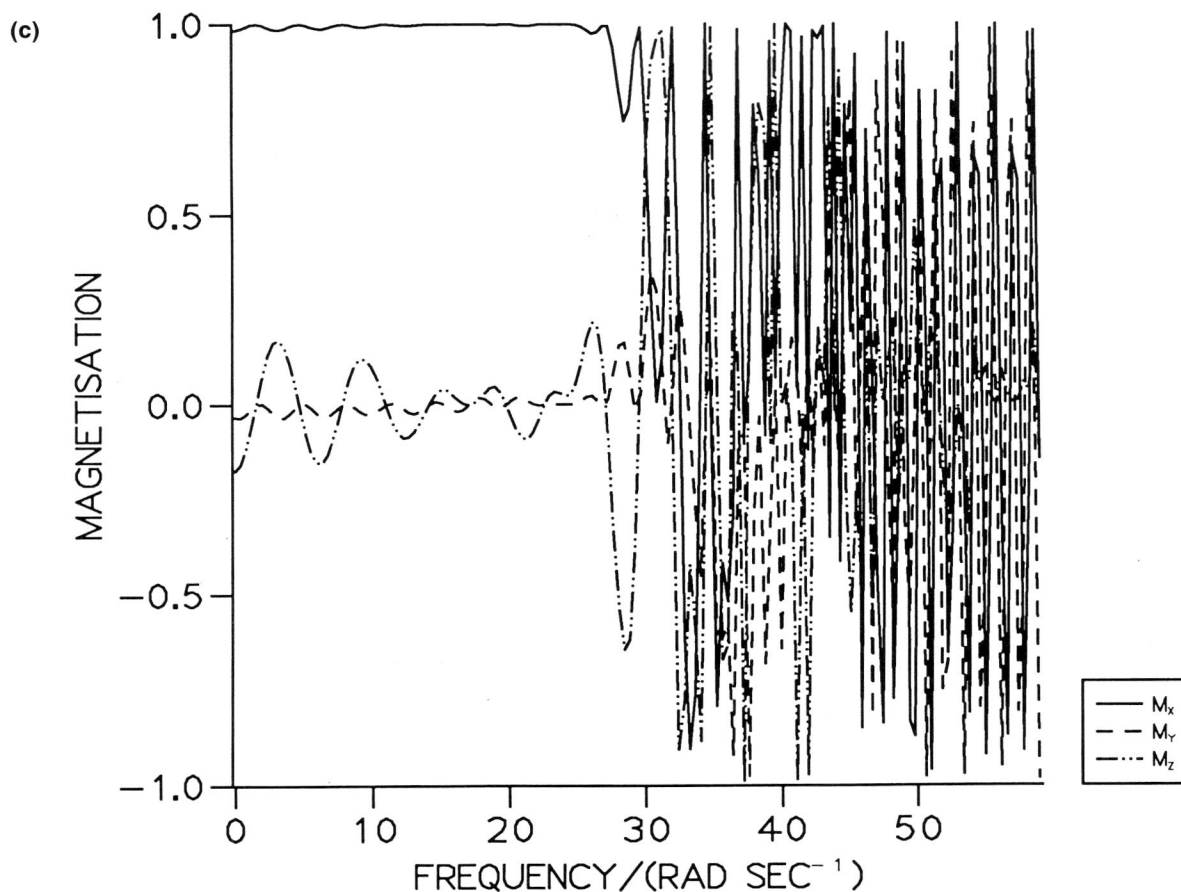

Fig. 1. (Continued) (c) Response after a train of 4 phase-cycled (XYXY) hyperbolic secant pulses, with the magnetization originally along the x-direction.

those that lead to favorable outcomes. Inherently, such methods are computationally intensive. This article reviews two approaches to the rational design of selective pulses (i.e., not involving random changes): an optimization method, SPINCALC, and an analytical approach based on inverse-scattering theory.

SPINCALC

SPINCALC was introduced by Ngo and Morris in 1986 [10–12]. It is a numerical optimization scheme that relies on a transformation to a stationary reference frame to effectively linearize the Bloch equations and enable their inversion. In the absence of relaxation, the Bloch equation describing the magnetization $\mathbf{M}(t, q)$ of a single isochromat q is

$$\frac{d}{dt}\mathbf{M}(t, q) = -\gamma\mathbf{B}(t, q) \times \mathbf{M}(t, q) \qquad (1)$$

This corresponds to rotation of $\mathbf{M}(t, q)$ about the

(time-varying) effective field. At the end of the pulse (time T), the magnetization will have undergone a total rotation $R_{tot}(q)$, such that

$$\mathbf{M}(T, q) = R_{tot}(q)\mathbf{M}(0, q) \qquad (2)$$

where the total rotation matrix, $R_{tot}(q)$, is given by the product $R_n(q) \cdots R_2(q) R_1(q)$, corresponding to the n discrete time intervals of the pulse envelope. For each q, a new rotation matrix is sought that rotates the magnetization to a position closer to the desired response:

$$R_{tot,new}(q) = \delta R_n(q)R_{n(q)} \cdots \delta R_1(q)R_1(q) \qquad (3)$$

This product cannot be reordered because the rotation matrices do not commute. (A small change made near the start of the pulse does not usually achieve the same effect as a similar change made near the end of the pulse.) Transformation to a switched frame of reference defined by

$$\delta R'_m(q) = U_m(q)\delta R_m(q)U_m(q)^{-1} \qquad (4)$$

where

$$U_m(q) = R_n(q)R_{n-1}(q) \cdots R_{m+1}(q)$$
$$= 1$$

$$\text{for} \quad m = n - 1, n - 2, \cdots, 0$$
$$m = n$$

solves the problem, for then

$$R_{\text{tot,new}}(q) = \delta R'_n(q) \cdots \delta R'_1(q)R_{\text{tot}}(q) \quad (5)$$

and, for small changes, the product of these matrices can be replaced with a sum of small vectors:

$$\delta \mathbf{R}_{\text{tot}}(q) = \Sigma_m \, \delta \mathbf{R}'_m(q) \quad (6)$$

Values for $\delta \mathbf{R}'_m(q)$ are determined for each degree of freedom (e.g., RF amplitude and phase), and least squares fitting is used to assemble the desired response from them. Additional constraints can be imposed at this stage, to minimize peak or mean radiofrequency power, for example.

SPINCALC can be used to design virtually any type of selective pulse. It has been used to generate "pancake flip" pulses and a number of phase-compensated pulses (self-refocused or prefocused). Some of the latter were derived using a selective $\pi/2$–selective π pair as an initial guess, and the optimized solution retains many of the features of its progenitor [11], whereas others were derived *ab initio* [12].

The hyperbolic secant is a near-perfect adiabatic inversion pulse [13, 14], but it fails as a refocusing (pancake flip) pulse. It is well known that refocusing does occur after each pair of such pulses. However, because the hyperbolic secant function must be curtailed in practice, the magnetization precesses around the B_1 direction, instead of being perfectly spin-locked. This leads to an error which, though negligible for a single echo, accumulates through a multiple-echo sequence. The SPINCALC technique has been used to generate a complex adiabatic pulse of finite duration that avoids this problem. The complex amplitudes (B_{1x}, B_{1y}) of this optimized pulse are shown in Fig. 1a. The responses after four consecutive refocusing pulses are compared for optimized and hyperbolic secant pulses in Figs. 1b and c, respectively.

ANALYTICAL SOLUTIONS: THE INVERSE-SCATTERING TRANSFORM

Until recently, the only familiar example of an analytical solution of the Bloch equations was the hyperbolic secant pulse. However, interest has grown in general methods for obtaining exact solutions. The Shinnar–Le Roux (SLR) algorithm [15], originally developed for generating specific M_z responses, without regard for the effects on the transverse magnetization, has been developed to produce selective pulses of controlled phase, including self-refocusing pulses. It can be shown that the SLR algorithm is actually a special case of the inverse-scattering transform [16], which relates the potential function to the measured scattering coefficients of a one-dimensional wave function. The potential corresponds to the radiofrequency pulse envelope, and the scattering matrix is simply related to the desired magnetization profile. We have shown how to obtain general solutions, provided the desired magnetization profile is described by a rational function [17]. As the number of poles is increased, the response becomes ever closer to a perfect top hat function. However, a price is paid in the increasingly high radiofrequency amplitude needed. In practice, a compromise is sought between these conflicting requirements. Doubly-selective pulses have also been designed by this method that lend themselves to multiple "solvent" suppression, for example, water and lipid in ^{1}H *in vivo* spectra. Although in principle this can be achieved by simple cosine modulation of a single selective pulse, this fails as the separation becomes comparable to the width of the excited regions (another manifestation of the nonlinearity of the NMR spin system).

A "soliton lattice algorithm" has been developed that allows the inversion problem for rational reflection coefficients to be reduced to one for zero reflection coefficient [18]. The solutions to the zero reflection coefficient problem are "solitons"—pulses that leave the spin system undisturbed. Although at first sight this does not appear to be particularly helpful, such pulses have been advocated for suppression of motional artifacts. More importantly, whereas a soliton pulse achieves nothing, half-solitons turn out to be almost perfect refocusing pulses (both $\pi/2$ and π pulses). The reduction in time that can be achieved through the use of a prefocused $\pi/2$ pulse is particularly valuable in studies of short T_2 species, such as the ^{31}P resonances of ATP. An extremely efficient way of determining soliton pulses has been found. The computation time for this "soliton–lattice algorithm" is proportional to the number of time points defining the pulse, and for a typical pulse it would usually be much less than 1 CPU minute. A more general algorithm, using a conventional stereographic projection method, has been described [19] that does not require the magnetization response to be defined as a rational function. Although it is much less efficient than the soliton lattice algorithm, it is conceptually simple and easy to implement.

CONCLUSION

The inverse-scattering transform is a powerful new analytical approach to selective pulse design, permitting target responses to be approached with arbitrarily high precision. The soliton–lattice algorithm is a particularly efficient and elegant solution to the general design of self-focused pulses. However, a role still remains for nonanalytical approaches, such as SPIN-CALC, in optimizing for novel target responses, or subject to some constraint such as peak or mean radiofrequency power. They also have a role in the design of pulse sequences that compensate for known field (B_0 and B_1) inhomogeneities.

REFERENCES

1. Garroway AN, Grannell PK, Mansfield P (1974) Image formation in NMR by a selective irradiative process. *J Phys C* **7**: L457–L462.
2. Morris PG, McIntyre DJO, Rourke DE, Ngo JT (1986) Rational approaches to the design of NMR selective pulses. *NMR Biomed* **5/6**: 257–266.
3. Conolly S, Macovski A (1985) Selective pulse design via optimal control theory. Proceedings of the 4th Annual Meeting, Society of Magnetic Resonance in Medicare p. 958.
4. Lent AH , Kritzer MR (1985) A new rf pulse shape for narrowband inversion: the WOW-180. *Proceedings of the 4th Annual Meeting, Society of Magnetic Resonance in Medicine* p. 1015.
5. Kirkpatrick S, Gelatt CD, Vecchi MP (1983) Optimization by simulated annealing. *Science* **220**: 671–680.
6. Rourke DE, McIntyre DJO, Morris PG (1989) A simulated annealing approach to the design of phase-compensated selective pulses. *Proceedings of the 8th Annual Meeting, Society of Magnetic Resonance in Medicine* p. 863.
7. Geen H, Wimperis S, Freeman R (1989) Band-selective pulses without phase distortion. A simulated annealing approach. *J Magn Reson* **85**: 620–627.
8. Hardy CJ, Bottomley PA, O'Donnell M, Roemer P (1988) Optimization of two-dimensional spatially selective NMR pulses by simulated annealing. *J Magn Reson* **77**: 233–250.
9. Wu X-L, Xu P, Freeman R (1991) Delayed-focus pulses for magnetic resonance imaging: an evolutionary approach. *Magn Reson Med* **20**: 165–170.
10. Ngo JT, Morris PG (1986) A new method for the optimization of NMR selective pulses. *Biochem Soc Trans* **14**: 1271–1272.
11. Ngo JT, Morris PG (1987) General solution to the NMR excitation problem for noninteracting spins. *Magn Reson Med* **5**: 217–237.
12. Ngo JT, Morris PG (1986) Selective excitation: something for nothing. *TAMU Newsletter* **337**: 38–39.
13. Baum J, Tycko R, Pines A (1983) Broadband population inversion by phase-modulated pulses. *J Chem Phys* **79**: 4643–4644.
14. Silver MS, Joseph RI, Chen C-N, Sank VJ, Hoult DI (1984) *Nature* **310**: 681–683.
15. Shinnar M, Eleff SM, Subramanian VH, Leigh JS (1989) The synthesis of pulse sequences yielding arbitrary magnetization vectors. *Magn Reson Med* **12**: 74–80.
16. Buonocore MH (1993) RF pulse design using the inverse scattering transform. *Magn Reson Med* **29**: 470–477.
17. Rourke DE, Morris PG (1992) The inverse scattering transform and its use in the exact inversion of the Bloch equation for non-interacting spins. *J Magn Reson* **99**: 118–138.
18. Rourke DE, Morris PG (1992) Half solitons as solutions to the Zakharov–Shabat eigenvalue problem for rational reflection coefficient with application in the design of selective pulses in nuclear magnetic resonance. *Phys Rev A* **46**: 3631–3636.
19. Rourke DE, Prior MJW, Morris PG, Lohman JAB (1994) Stereographic method of exactly calculating selective pulses. *J Magn Reson A* **107**: 203–214.

The soliton–lattice algorithm and selective pulses

David E. Rourke,* Piotr Kozlowski, Beatrice G. Winsborrow and John K. Saunders

Institute for Biodiagnostics, National Research Council of Canada, 435 Ellice Avenue, Winnipeg, Canada R3B 1Y6

The soliton–lattice algorithm, an exact algebraic method of inverting the Bloch equation to obtain frequency-selective radio-frequency pulses is described. Some general properties of pulses are described that were obtained with the help of this algorithm. It is used to obtain two new pulses. A highly prefocused pulse is shown that can be used in short-echo-time *in vivo* ^{31}P spectroscopic imaging, and an adiabatic selective inversion pulse is obtained.

Keywords: selective pulses, inverse scattering theory, solitons.

INTRODUCTION

A problem of some importance in NMR is to be able to exactly invert the equation of motion of the spin system (the Bloch equation) [1]. This would enable the design of radio-frequency (RF) pulses to control precisely the magnetization response of a sample. An algebraic method of inversion would also be expected to give some insight into the relationship between spin response and RF pulse. Hence, practical considerations such as pulse duration limits and B_1 inhomogeneity could be taken into account.

THE SOLITON–LATTICE ALGORITHM

The soliton–lattice algorithm [2, 3] is an algebraic method of inversion, applicable to the design of frequency-selective RF pulses (i.e., the main magnetic field and any gradients must be constant in time during the application of the pulse).

There are two key steps in its derivation. First, the Bloch equation, neglecting relaxation, can be reduced to an equation from scattering theory—the Zakharov–Shabat eigenvalue problem [4–6]. Hence, the RF pulse can be thought of as a scattering potential, from which the initial magnetization is scattered, producing final magnetization. The inverse-scattering problem (obtain-

ing the potential, given the response to the potential) is, therefore, equivalent to inverting the Bloch equation.

Second, all scattering systems can be reduced to one or two systems in which no scattering occurs— "reflectionless" systems. Reflectionless potentials, or solitons, can be calculated very efficiently using the Bäcklund transform [7, 8]. Given the soliton potentials, the required RF pulse may be obtained easily [2, 3]. The entire process of obtaining the RF pulse is called the soliton–lattice algorithm.

SOME GENERAL PROPERTIES OF THE INVERSION

Uniqueness

An important consideration in an inversion method is its uniqueness. It can be shown that the soliton–lattice algorithm is unique for pulses on semi-infinite support [3]. This includes self-refocused pulses. Consequences of uniqueness include the result that if a self-refocused pulse gives rise to the symmetries $m_x(\omega_3) = -m_x(-\omega_3)$, $m_y(\omega_3) = m_y(-\omega_3)$, and $m_z(\omega_3) = m_z(-\omega_3)$, where (m_x, m_y, m_z) are the components of the magnetization response at the end of the pulse, as a function of resonance offset ω_3, then that pulse is purely real.

Pulse duration

For small pulse amplitude (i.e., when the spin system response behaves in a linear fashion to the RF pulse), the duration of a selective pulse, δt, is related to the width of the slice's transition region, δf, by an "uncertainty" relation [9], $\delta t \delta f \sim 1$.

* Address for correspondence: Institute for Biodiagnostics, National Research Council of Canada, 435 Ellice Avenue, Winnipeg, Canada R3B 1Y6.

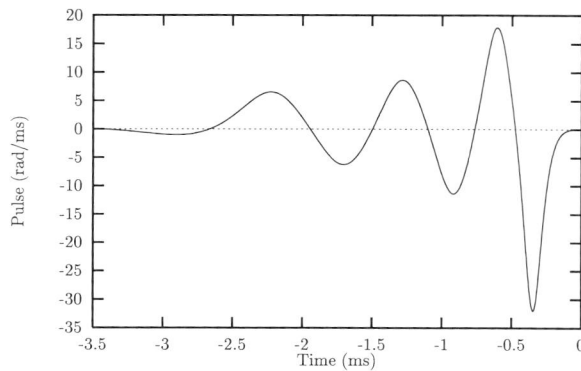

Fig. 1. Highly prefocused selective pulse, requiring an additional free-precession of 1 ms.

In the general case, where the system is nonlinear, the pulse amplitude dies away as $e^{-2K|t|}$. The quantity K is determined by $r(\xi)$, the "reflection coefficient" of the system, which is simply related to the desired final magnetization, and is a function of ξ, the "dimensionless resonance offset" [2, 6]. K is defined as the imaginary part of ξ_{min}, where ξ_{min} is the solution of $r(\xi)r^*(\xi^*) + 1 = 0$ that is in the upper half-complex ξ plane and is closest to the real axis (the asterisk denotes the complex conjugate).

Hence, the pulse duration can be taken to be when $e^{-2K|t|}$ goes below some critical value.

EXAMPLES

A highly prefocused selective pulse

Prefocused selective pulses selectively excite a pulse, with the magnetization within the slice not coming into focus until some time after the pulse has ended, with the slice-select gradient being held constant throughout the pulse and the subsequent free-precession [10].

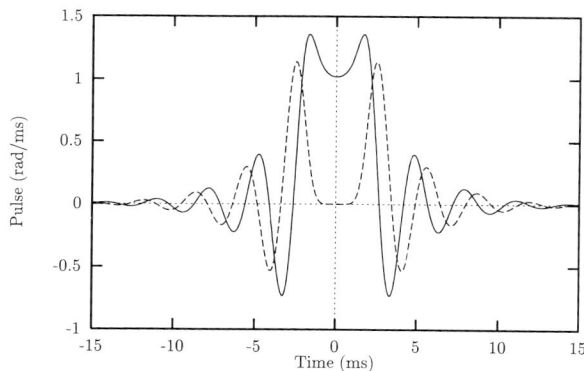

Fig. 2. Adiabatic selective inversion pulse. Solid line: real part; dashed line: imaginary part.

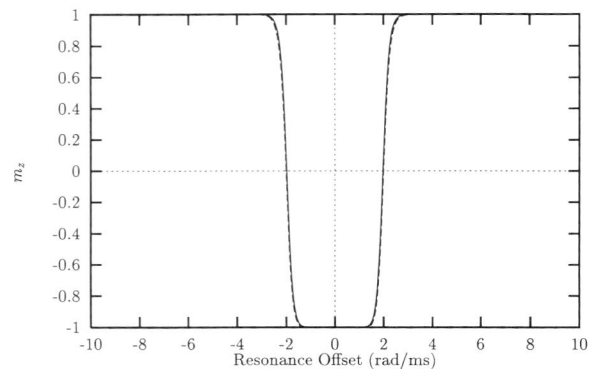

Fig. 3. Response to the adiabatic selective inversion pulse of Fig. 2 (dashed line) and to the same pulse but scaled in amplitude by a factor 2 (solid line). The two lines are almost indistinguishable due to the adiabatic nature of the pulse.

We have used the soliton–lattice algorithm to design a 3.5-ms prefocused pulse, requiring subsequent free-precession of 1 ms; this is shown in Fig. 1. We have demonstrated its utility in short-echo-time *in vivo* ^{31}P spectroscopic imaging [11]. By applying the phase encoding during the free-precession period, and because no refocusing pulse is needed, the signal may be collected immediately after the free-precession—i.e., the echo time is 1 ms.

An adiabatic selective inversion pulse

The soliton–lattice algorithm has been used [3] to calculate an adiabatic selective inversion pulse (shown in Fig. 2). Figure 3 shows the magnetization response, m_z, to this pulse and to the pulse after it has been scaled by a factor of 2. They are almost indistinguishable. It is hoped that the method used to obtain this pulse can be generalized to obtain adiabatic 90° selective excitation pulses, which would be very useful in, for example, surface coil magnetic resonance imaging.

CONCLUSION

The soliton–lattice algorithm is an extremely efficient, exact method of obtaining RF pulses, given the desired magnetization response. It typically can obtain an RF pulse evaluated at 1000 points in under 10 CPU seconds on a Unix workstation.

As it is an algebraic method, it offers some insight into the relationship between magnetization response and RF pulse. It is hoped, in particular, that this will enable the design of RF pulses which are insensitive to their amplitude.

REFERENCES

1. Mansfield P, Morris PG (1982) NMR imaging in biomedicine. In *Advances in Magnetic Resonance* (Suppl. 2). Orlando, FL: Academic Press.
2. Rourke DE, Morris PG (1992) Half-solitons as solutions to the Zakharov–Shabat eigenvalue problem for rational reflection coefficient, with application in the design of selective pulses in nmr. *Phys Rev A* **46**(7): 3631–3636.
3. Rourke DE, Saunders JK (1994) Half-solitons as solutions to the Zakharov–Shabat eigenvalue problem for rational reflection coefficient. II. Potentials on infinite support. *J Math Phys* **35**(2): 848–872.
4. Zakharov VE, Shabat AB (1972) Exact theory of two-dimensional self-focusing and one-dimensional self-modulation of waves in nonlinear media. *Sov Phys JETP* **34**(1): 62–69.
5. Ablowitz MJ, Kaup DJ, Newell AC, Segur H (1974) The inverse scattering transform—Fourier analysis for nonlinear problems. *Studies Appl Math* **53**(4): 249–315.
6. Rourke DE, Morris PG (1992) The inverse scattering transform and its use in the exact inversion of the Bloch equation for noninteracting spins. *J Magn Reson* **99**: 118–138.
7. Konopelchenko BG (1982) Elementary Bäcklund transformations, nonlinear superposition principle and solutions of the integrable equations. *Phys Lett A* **87**(9): 445–448.
8. Calogero F, Degasperis A (1984) Elementary Bäcklund transformations, nonlinear superposition formulae and algebraic constructions of solutions for the nonlinear evolution equations solvable by the Zakharov-Shabat spectral transform. *Physica D* **14**: 103–116.
9. Wang Z (1989) Theory of selective excitation by scaled frequency–amplitude sweep. *J Magn Reson* **81**: 617–622.
10. Ngo JT, Morris PG (1987) General solution to the nmr excitation problem for noninteracting spins. *Magn Reson Med* **5**: 217–237.
11. Kozlowski P, Rourke DE, Winsborrow BG, Saunders JK (1994) Highly prefocused selective pulses—a tool for in-vivo ^{31}P spectroscopic imaging. *J Magn Reson Ser B* **104**: 280–283.

Data sampling in MR relaxation

Christian Labadie,* Daniel Gounot, Yves Mauss and Barbu Dumitresco

Institut de Physique Biologique, Université Louis Pasteur, Strasbourg, France

Four time spacing methods for the sampling of magnetic resonance relaxation data are investigated: linear, logarithmic, geometric with time offset, and pure geometric spacing methods. They are compared with the respective normalized root-mean-square errors of the four parameters of biexponential inversion recoveries. Linear spacing was found to be inappropriate for NMR. Geometric spacing may be the method of choice to detect an unexpected exponent when sampling is performed from $1/28.7$ of the shortest time constant up to five times the longest one.

Keywords: MR relaxation, time spacing, T_1 and T_2 estimation, inverse Laplace transform.

INTRODUCTION

The multiexponential analysis of relaxation data has gained considerable interest in one-dimensional nuclear magnetic resonance (1D-NMR) [1], in 2D-NMR [2], in magnetic resonance imaging (MRI) [3], and in MR applications to porous media [4]. A recent review published in the field of dynamic light scattering has compared most numerical methods available to perform the relaxation data analysis, also called *general inverse Laplace transformation* (GILT) [5]. A simplified classification of the most popular numerical methods is as follows: (i) δ-function methods (e.g., DISCRETE) [6], (ii) analytical methods (e.g., stretched exponential) [4], (iii) regularized grid methods (e.g., CONTIN) [7], and (iv) nonregularized grid methods (e.g., MinPeak) [8]. Although much effort has gone into improving the solution to the GILT, the MR relaxation (MRR) data sampling procedure itself has not been investigated very much.

The spacing of the data points in time affects the information content of the data [5, p. 228]. The data acquisition should cover both the fast region of the decay and the return to the baseline [5, Fig. 4.27]. In this study, the effect that the time spacing method has on the estimation of the time constants and the amplitudes has been computed with the covariance matrix of biexponential inversion recoveries. The upper limit of five times the longest time constant is

* Address for correspondence: Institut de Physique Biologique, 43, rue Kirschléger, F-67085 Strasbourg Cedex, France.

widely adopted [9]; a lower limit for the fast region is suggested.

MATERIAL AND METHODS

Time spacing methods

Four kinds of time spacing methods were investigated. An example of each one is depicted in Fig. 1. The time axis represents an example of MRR experiments comprising a spoil gradient delay following the end of the preparation and acquisitions of non-negligible duration.

(i) The *linear spacing method* (or arithmetic progression) is the most commonly employed procedure in NMR (e.g., CPMG or Look-Locker [9, 10]). It produces equal time intervals on a linear scale:

$$t_n = t_1 + (n - 1)\alpha \quad (1)$$

where t_n is the time of the nth measurement, n is an integer value ranging from 1 to N, the number of data points, and α is a time increment.

(ii) The *logarithmic spacing method* (or geometric progression) is usually chosen to construct the time list of inversion recovery experiments [4], which produces t values equispaced logarithmically:

$$t_n = t_1 \alpha^{n-1} \quad (2)$$

where α is a constant time ratio.

(iii) The *geometric spacing method* produces geometrically progressing intervals between successive

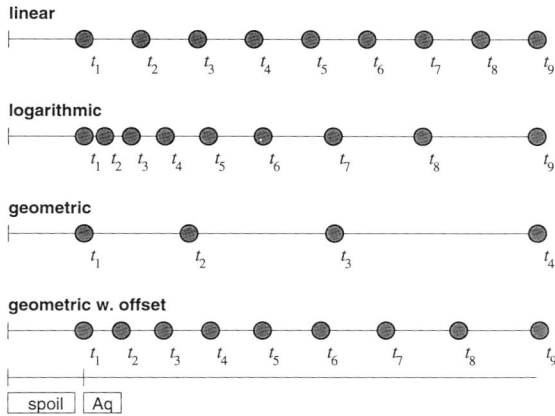

linear

t_1 t_2 t_3 t_4 t_5 t_6 t_7 t_8 t_9

logarithmic

t_1 t_2 t_3 t_4 t_5 t_6 t_7 t_8 t_9

geometric

t_1 t_2 t_3 t_4

geometric w. offset

t_1 t_2 t_3 t_4 t_5 t_6 t_7 t_8 t_9

spoil Aq

Fig. 1. Sketch of the following time spacing methods: linear [Eq. (1)], logarithmic [Eq. (2)], geometric [Eq. (3)], and geometric with time offset [Eq. (4)]. For certain applications, logarithmic spacing may not allow sufficient time for the acquisition (Aq). A relatively long initial delay, such as a spoil gradient (spoil), is incompatible with pure geometric spacing; the introduction of a time offset may help solving this aspect in part.

data points. Thus, t_n is the result of a geometric sum:

$$t_n = t_1 \frac{\alpha^n - 1}{\alpha - 1} \tag{3}$$

where α is the constant ratio between successive intervals.

(iv) The *geometric spacing method with time offset* may be of interest in MRI [3] because it allows an initial delay t_1 (e.g., spoil) which may exceed the smallest interval $t_2 - t_1$ (e.g., acquisition):

$$t_n = t_1 + (t_2 - t_1) \frac{\alpha^{n-1} - 1}{\alpha - 1} \tag{4}$$

Depending on the adjustment of the parameters, this method may approximate either linear, logarithmic, or geometric spacings.

Computation of the root-mean-square error

The effect of sampling was studied using the root-mean-square (rms) errors of the parameters (i.e., amplitudes and time constants). The rms errors were directly obtained from the square root of the diagonal elements of S^{-1}, the inverse of the covariance matrix, without data simulation, where S was constructed with the partial derivatives of the magnetization:

$$s_{ij} = \sum_{n=1}^{N} \frac{\partial M(t_n)}{\partial p_i} \times \frac{\partial M(t_n)}{\partial p_j} \tag{5}$$

where p is an array holding the parameters and $M(t_n)$ is the magnetization of a biexponential inversion-

recovery model:

$$M(t_n) = \sum_{m=1}^{2} a_m \left(-1 + 2 \exp\left(\frac{-t_n}{T_{1m}}\right) \right) \tag{6}$$

Each computation was performed with 64 sampling times and up to 5 times the longest time constant. Both amplitudes contributed equally, and the resulting rms errors, $\sigma_e(p)$, were normalized ($a_m = 0.5$). The rms error of a parameter p_i, $\sigma(p_i)$, is inversely proportional to the signal-to-noise ratio (S/N):

$$\sigma(p_i) = \frac{\sigma_e(p_i)}{\text{S/N}} \tag{8}$$

where the S/N ratio is the sum of the amplitudes a_m divided by the rms of the noise.

RESULTS AND DISCUSSION

A systematic search of the minimum rms error for each time spacing method was performed for r values, the ratio of the long-time over the short-time constants, ranging from 1.26 up to 1000. Figure 2 shows the rms errors of amplitudes (top) and time constants (bottom) as a function of $\log(r)$.

In dynamic light scattering, the resolution is usually of three or four δ-functions per decade (respectively $r = 2.1$ or 1.8) [5, p. 202]. Indeed, Fig. 2 shows that with 64 data points the rms errors tend to get extremely large for ratios smaller than 2.1. For example, with $r = 1.41$, the rms error of the time constant is ~ 16; thus, to resolve the two exponents one needs a S/N of at least 253 [$2\sigma_e(\log T_1) \sqrt{2 \ln 2}/\log(r)$], i.e., at half-height, the two components do not overlap; but in order to reduce the error of the amplitude to less than 10%, the S/N should be greater than 4600 [$\sigma_e(a_m)/a_m/10\%$], which is difficult to achieve in MRR (especially in MRI [3]). Although Fig. 2 is limited to a biexponential model with 64 data points, it gives an idea of the resolution to be expected for a given S/N and a given time spacing method.

For r values greater than 3, linear spacing influences the rms errors dramatically and is clearly inappropriate for MRR. Surprisingly, geometric spacing is as good or even slightly better than logarithmic.

However, the optimum initial waiting delay t_1 for geometric spacing is shorter than that for logarithmic spacing, respectively $1/33.4$ and $1/5.8$ of the shortest-time constant (not shown). The optimized value of t_1 depends on whether the time constant or the amplitude estimation is critical; in order to optimize the time constant, t_1 should be set to slightly earlier values. Furthermore, this depends on the relative fraction of each component. As a rule of thumb, we matched

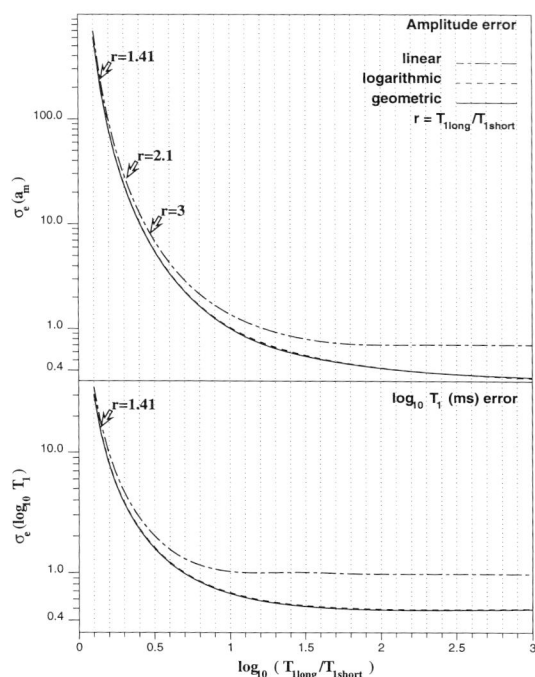

Fig. 2. Plot of the rms errors for the amplitude (top) and the time constant (bottom). Those rms errors were the average of the respective diagonal elements of the inverse of the covariance matrix [Eq. (5)] of a biexponential inversion recovery. They were computed with 64 data sampling times for 3 different spacing methods. Sampling was performed up to five times the long-time constant. The initial delay t_1 was optimized in order to produce the lowest rms error. A ratio r less than 2.1 may be considered as the limit of the resolution achievable with typical S/N.

$dM(t_n)/d\log(t_n)$, the derivative of the magnetization versus $\log(t_n)$, in both regions of the decay (not shown), which suggested an empirical limit for the beginning of sampling equal to $\frac{1}{28.7}$ of the shortest-time constant.

As shown in Fig. 1, logarithmic spacing places many points on the early part of the decay. If the lower limit of $\frac{1}{5.8}$ is not respected, logarithmic spacing may undersample the long component and the baseline. For geometric spacing, the plot of the minimum rms errors versus the optimum initial delay t_1 is more shallow than that for logarithmic spacing (not shown). Geometric spacing may help detecting an unexpected expo-

nent by spreading data points more uniformly along the decay.

ACKNOWLEDGMENTS

CL thanks Dr. S.W. Provencher for very kindly offering constant help and suggestions, Pr. C.S. Springer, Jr., Dr. J.-H. Lee, and Pr. G.S. Harbison for stimulating conversations, Dr. H. Ohlenbusch for corrections, and the U.S. National Institutes of Health for support (Grant No. GM 32125 to CSS).

REFERENCES

1. Kroeker RM, Henkelman RM (1986) Analysis of biological NMR relaxation data with continuous distributions of relaxation times. *J Magn Reson* **69**: 218–235.
2. Lee J-H, Labadie C, Springer CS, Harbison GS (1993) Two-dimensional inverse Laplace transform NMR: Altered relaxation times allow dectection of exchange correlation. *J Am Chem Soc* **115**: 7761–7764.
3. Labadie C, Lee J-H, Vetek G, Springer CS (1994) Relaxographic imaging. *J Magn Reson* **B 105**: 59–112.
4. Borgia GC, Brancolini A, Brown RJS, Fantazzini P, Ragazzini G (1994) Water–air saturation changes in restricted geometries studied by proton relaxation. *Magn Reson Imaging* **12**: 191–195.
5. Stepanek P (1993) Data analysis in dynamic light scattering. In *Dynamic Light Scattering,* (Brown W, ed.) pp. 177–241. Oxford: Clarendon Press.
6. Provencher SW, Vogel RH (1980) Information loss with transform methods in system identification—A new set of transforms with high information-content. *Math Biosci* **50**: 251–262.
7. Provencher SW (1982) CONTIN: A general purpose constrained regularization program for inverting noisy linear algebraic and integral equations. *Comput Phys Commun* **27**: 229–242.
8. Provencher SW (1992) Low-bias macroscopic analysis of polydispersity. In *Laser Light Scattering in Biochemistry* (Harding SE, Sattelle DB, Bloomfield VA, eds.) pp. 92–111. Cambridge: Royal Society of Chemistry.
9. Kaptein R, Dijkstra K, Tarr CE (1976) A single-scan Fourier transform method for measuring spin-lattice relaxation times. *J Magn Reson* **24**: 295–300.
10. Look DC, Locker DR (1970) Time saving in measurement of NMR and EPR relaxation times. *Rev Sci Instrum* **41**: 250–251.

Biplanar gradient coil design by simulated annealing

A. M. Peters and R. W. Bowtell*

Magnetic Resonance Centre, Department of Physics, University of Nottingham, Nottingham NG7 2RD, UK

Simulated annealing has been applied to the design of biplanar gradient coils for use in NMR microscopy. This method allows a variety of coil parameters to be considered, such as homogeneity over a specified region of interest (ROI), power dissipation, and efficiency. Chosen parameters are represented in an overall figure of merit which is then minimized by the simulated annealing approach. Unlike most analytical techniques which rely on the use of the stream function, with this technique the coil properties are calculated directly from the wire positions, so there is no stage of approximation between current density and the actual coil design. Using this technique, we have designed biplanar x and z gradient coils for use in an 11.7-T NMR microscope. In each case, the coils were composed of straight wire units. The plane spacing was set at 10 mm and the ROI was a central cube of side 6 mm. Starting from a design generated using the target field approach, simulated annealing was applied with the aim of minimizing the ratio of power dissipation per unit current to the square root of coil efficiency while maintaining adequate gradient homogeneity. The efficiency and power dissipation per unit current of the resulting x and z coils were 117 mT m^{-1} A^{-1} and 0.1 W A^{-2}, and 99 mT m^{-1} A^{-1} and 0.4 W A^{-2}, respectively.

Keywords: gradient coils, MRI gradients, coil design, NMR microscopy, simulated annealing.

INTRODUCTION

The characteristics of the gradient set are central to the performance of any magnetic resonance imaging (MRI) system. In general, we require a gradient set with high efficiency, good homogeneity over the sample volume, a low resistance to minimize power dissipation, and a low inductance to minimize the switching time. Obviously, some of these parameters are in direct conflict with each other and so the coil design must represent some compromise between the above requirements. The exact compromise reached will depend on the particular application for which the coil is intended.

During the last 30 years, a number of methods for the design of gradient coils have been developed. An important step in coil design was the introduction of the stream function, which is the integral of current density. By placing discrete wires on equally spaced contours of a stream function, wire paths can be generated which approximate the current density. This idea is used in the target field approach [1], which

involves the inversion of Ampere's law to derive a current density on the coil surface directly from a specified target field function. Once the current density is known, the stream function can be calculated and the wire paths generated as described above. This method is capable of producing designs rapidly; however, the field variation is constrained to follow an analytic function which may not always be appropriate. Coil properties such as efficiency also depend on the target field function in a manner which is not always obvious. In addition, when the coil is built, the current distribution must be approximated by discrete wire paths. This approximation can lead to a discrepancy between designed and achieved coil behavior, particularly when the number of discrete wires is small. Because this approach does not work in real space, it can also be difficult to limit the spatial extent of the coil.

Design methods involving the minimization of a function based on the coil properties have also been applied. Wong [2] addressed the problem of approximation to a continuous current distribution. He defined an error function for the coil which contained terms for the efficiency, homogeneity, and inductance of the coil. This function was then minimized by conjugate gradient descent. Instead of a continuous

* Address for correspondence: Magnetic Resonance Centre University of Nottingham, University Park, Nottingham, NG7 2RD, UK.

current distribution, the field was calculated directly from the wire paths using the Biot–Savart law. The drawback with this approach is that in the minimization of the error function, although conjugate gradient descent will always find a minimum in the function, this minimum may not be the global minimum, and so may not represent the best possible arrangement of wires. This problem arises because during the minimization a change in the wire positions is only accepted if it results in a decrease in the error function. Because of this, once the system has entered a local minimum, there is no mechanism for escape. Simulated annealing [3, 4] is a minimization technique which offers such a possibility. It has already been used successfully by Crozier et al to design cylindrical z gradient coils [5].

METHOD

A figure of merit which again may contain many parameters is defined for the coil. This is then minimized by the simulated annealing approach. If during the minimization a change in the wire positions results in a decrease in the figure of merit, the change is always accepted. However, unlike conjugate gradient descent, a change resulting in an increase in the figure of merit also has a probability of being accepted. This probability, p, is related to the Boltzmann distribution,

$$p \propto \exp\left(\frac{-|dE|}{KT}\right) \tag{1}$$

where dE is the increase in the figure of merit, k is Boltzmann's constant, and T is an effective temperature. If T is high, then the probability of accepting an increase in the figure of merit is high, and the system is essentially free. As the minimization proceeds, T is reduced, which reduces the probability of accepting an increase in the figure of merit. Both the initial value and the rate of decrease of T are important. If T is too low or reduced too quickly, then the system will quench into a local minimum. If T is initially too high or reduced too slowly, then the computational time required increases with no benefit.

Using this method, we have designed biplanar x and z gradient coils based on straight wire units for use in an 11.7-T, 89-mm-bore microscope system. The efficiency of a coil varies as the inverse square of the coil size, making the production of small coils highly advantageous. The biplanar design allows the coil to be as small as is consistent with adequate gradient homogeneity over the sample volume while still allowing access to the sample. This geometry also allows the

orientation of the sample with respect to the gradients to be accurately determined. The design requirements for both coils were that they should have a high efficiency and low resistance and be linear over a cube of side 6 mm to within 5%. Further restrictions on the gradient coils were that they should fit inside a cylinder of 33 mm diameter. These requirements dictated that the coil consist of two y-z planes separated by a distance of 10 mm, with a plane width of 28 mm in the y direction. It was decided that there should be 40 straight wire units for the x gradient and 24 for the z gradient on each plane.

The figure of merit used for this design was of the form

$$\text{Figure of merit} = a\left(\frac{1}{|E|}\right) + bH + c\sqrt{R} \tag{2}$$

where E is the efficiency, H represents the homogeneity, and R is the resistance of the coil. a, b, and c are weighting coefficients for each of the elements. By adjusting the relative values of these, the effect of each element can be changed. This leads to an intuitive method of design, as each coefficient relates to one single coil characteristic. For each arrangement of wires investigated by the minimization algorithm, the field is calculated at a number of points in the region of interest. From this, the efficiency can be calculated directly. The homogeneity term used was the sum of the squares of the deviations from a linear gradient at each point in the region of interest. A wire diameter was calculated such that the closest two wires just touched. This was then used with the total wire length to calculate the resistance of the coil.

RESULTS AND DISCUSSION

Initial designs were obtained without the resistance term in the figure of merit ($c = 0$). These produced x and z gradients of the required homogeneity with efficiencies of 150 mT m^1 A^{-1} and 116 mT m^{-1} A^{-1}, respectively. However, such high efficiency was only achieved with a coil resistance of several kilohms, which would result in unacceptable power dissipation in the coil. The large resistance resulted from very small wire separations which lead to a small wire diameter. When the weighting term for the resistance was increased, it had the effect of increasing the wire separations and, therefore, the wire diameter. Final coil designs were obtained with efficiencies of 117 mT m^{-1} A^{-1} and 99 mT m^{-1} A^{-1} for the x and z coils, respectively. The resistances were 0.1 Ω and 0.4 Ω. The wire positions for these coils are shown in Figs. 1 and 2.

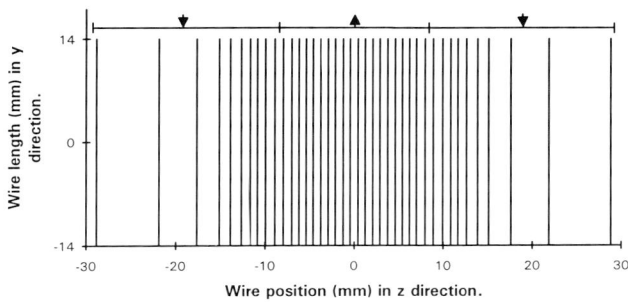

Fig. 1. Wire positions for one plane of the *x* gradient coil. The current direction, shown by the arrows, is the same in the opposite plane.

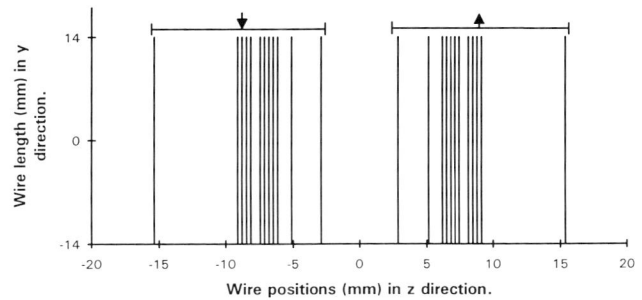

Fig. 2. Wire positions for one plane of the *z* gradient coil. The current direction, shown by the arrows, is reversed in the opposite plane.

The time required to perform the minimization increases rapidly with the number of wires in the coil, as each wire position is an independent variable. Computational time is also dependent on the number of parameters in the figure of merit and the number of points in the region of interest at which the field is calculated. Even using the symmetry of the coil to reduce the number of calculations required, the designs took approximately 3 h for the *z* coil and 10 h for the *x*, running on an IBM RS6000. It is the computational time required to perform the minimization, which limits the range of application of this method. When the number of wires in the coil is small, the approximation from a current distribution to discrete wires which is used in other methods is poor, whereas this method can give good results in a reasonable time. As the number of wires increases, the advantage of this method is diminished. This method is, therefore, particularly suitable for the design of coils with few wires, or with a geometry not easily handled by other methods.

REFERENCES

1. Turner R (1986) A target field approach to optimal coil design. *J Phys D* **19:** L147–151.
2. Wong EC, Jesmanowicz A, Hyde JS (1991) Coil optimisation for MRI by conjugate gradient descent. *Magn Reson Med* **21:** 39–48.
3. Metropolis N, Rosenbluth AW, Rosenbluth MN, Teller AH, Teller E (1953) Equation of state calculations by fast computing machines. *J Chem Phys* **6:** 1087–1092.
4. Kirkpatrick S, Gelatt CD, Vecchi MP (1983) Optimisation by simulated annealing. *Science* **220:** 671–680.
5. Crozier S, Doddrell DM (1993) Gradient coil design by simulated annealing. *J Mag Reson A* **103:** 354–357.

Active screening in RF coil design

P. Mansfield,* A. Freeman and R. Bowtell

Magnetic Resonance Centre, University of Nottingham, Nottingham NG7 2RD, UK

Active magnetic screening can be made to operate satisfactorily at RF frequencies up to approximately 8 MHz for small diameter short solenoids. The principles can be used to construct magnetically orthogonal coils which are geometrically coaxial. Such coils have a wide range of uses in NMR.

Keywords: radio-frequency coils, active screening.

INTRODUCTION

Active magnetic screening was originally introduced by Mansfield and Chapman [1, 2] to circumvent the problem of magnetic interaction of gradient coils when rapidly switched within the close confines of a superconductive magnet. The typical operating frequency in this application is around 1 kHz. Radio-frequency (RF) applications were proposed by them but not implemented. This article is, therefore, concerned with the first practical realization of the concept.

MATERIALS AND METHODS

A small 74-mm-diameter solenoid with a length of 48 mm was actively screened with a screen of 108 mm diameter. The whole assembly was screened with a Faraday screen over which was wound a 120-mm-diameter secondary coil. To avoid proximity effects, the gap between the screen and secondary coil should ideally be ≥ 7 mm. The coil arrangement is shown in Fig. 1.

The primary solenoid has six turns, the screen three turns suitably distributed, and the secondary coil six turns. A further small search coil of diameter 35 mm and one turn was placed coaxially inside the coil assembly. The purpose of this coil is to simulate an NMR signal from a sample placed within the primary solenoid.

* Address all correspondence to Sir Peter Mansfield, Magnetic Resonance Centre, University of Nottingham, Nottingham N97 2RD, UK.

The physical arrangement of this coil assembly constrained the RF operating frequency to 8 MHz. Lack of a suitable magnetic field prevented us from performing NMR experiments with the coil. All results have, therefore, been obtained by injecting a simulated NMR signal into the assembly via the search coil.

THEORY

In order to make the electrical measurements under matched conditions, the coil formed part of the test circuit shown in Fig. 2. Here $M_{1,2}$ and M_3 are 50-Ω matching circuits, the latter, not shown, being for the unscreened primary coil, and Q_1, Q_2, and Q_3 are the quality factors of the outer secondary, screened primary, and unscreened primary coils, respectively. The capacitors C_n are chosen to make all coils resonant at a frequency $f = 8.0$ MHz. The search coil is untuned and driven by a constant voltage V. The measured signals on each output are V_1 and V_2. The output from the unscreened primary is V_3.

The signal enhancement factor, Γ, for the arrangement described above is given by

$$\Gamma = \frac{V_1 + V_2}{V_3\sqrt{2}} = \frac{1 + \sqrt{(Q_2/Q_1)}\, K\sqrt{F}}{\sqrt{(Q_3/Q_1)}\, K\sqrt{2}} \qquad (1)$$

where F is the field factor for the screened solenoid and K is a coil geometry factor given by

$$K = \left(\frac{a_1}{a_3}\right)^{3/2} \left(\frac{1 + (l_1/a_1)^2}{1 + (l_3/a_3)^2}\right)^{1/4}. \qquad (2)$$

In this expression, a_1 and a_3 are the radii of the outer secondary coil and screened primary coil and l_1 and l_3

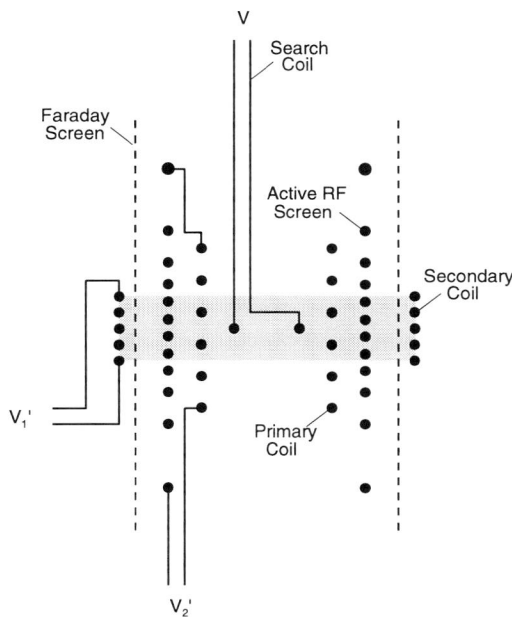

Fig. 1. Diagram showing the coil arrangement comprising an actively screened primary coil, a Faraday screen, and a secondary coil coaxial with the primary coil axis.

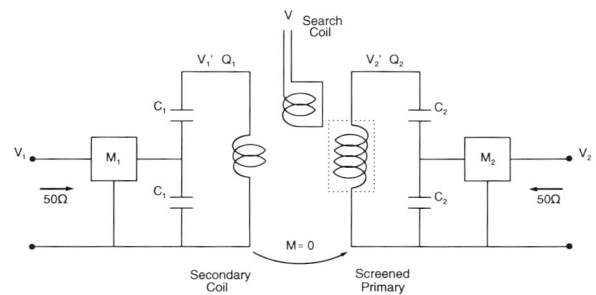

Fig. 2. Diagram of the test circuit. The dotted line around the primary coil is intended to indicate that it is magnetically screened, thereby making the mutual inductance $M = 0$ between the screened primary and secondary coils.

are the coil half-lengths, respectively. Equation (1) is valid only if the noise from the two ports is uncorrelated. This is the case if the mutual inductance $M \simeq 0$.

For the experimental coil, the values of the coil parameters were $a_1/a_3 = 1.58$, $l_1/a_1 = 0.40$, $l_3/a_3 = 0.63$, and $F = 0.65$. The RF screen radius $a_2 = 1.42a_3$.

RESULTS

Measurements were made by sweeping the frequency of the input V and simultaneously measuring V_1 and V_2 on a network analyzer. From the frequency response data, we have measured the Q values and corresponding peak voltage outputs as follows: $Q_1 = 43$, $V_1 = 2.5V$; $Q_2 = 38$, $V_2 = 3.1$ V. For the unscreened primary, we have $Q_3 = 47$, $V_3 = 5.1$ V.

From Eqs. (1) and (2) together with the coil parameters we evaluate a theoretical signal enhancement factor $\Gamma_{THEOR} = 0.87$. The experimental value using the above-stated measurements is $\Gamma_{EXP} = 0.78$. We empha-

size that Eqs. (1) and (2) hold for $M = 0$. When $M \neq 0$, as in our case, a small correction can be applied which reduces the theoretical signal enhancement factor by $\Delta\Gamma$, thus bringing it closer to the observed value.

CONCLUSIONS

With the particular coil parameters chosen, an improvement in signal-to-noise ratio (S/N), i.e., $\Gamma > 1$, is not predicted. However, the agreement between the theoretical and experimental values supports the essential correctness of our approach. By varying the parameters, it should be possible to design synchronously tuned magnetically orthogonal coils which produce an improvement in S/N over that obtainable by a single unscreened coil.

This is one particular application of active RF screening. Others include the possibility of transmitting on one coil and receiving from the second, useful in pulsed NMR and in double resonance experiments.

REFERENCES

1. Mansfield P, Chapman B (1986) Active magnetic screening of gradient coils in NMR imaging. *J Magn Reson* **66:** 573–576.
2. Mansfield P, Chapman B (1986) Active magnetic screening of coils for static and time-dependent magnetic field generation in NMR imaging. *J Phys E* **19:** 540–545.

NMR microscopy of single neurons at 500 MHz

Stephen J. Blackband,[3,6]* Richard W. Bowtell,[1] Andrew Peters,[1] Jonathan C. Sharp,[4]
Peter Mansfield,[1] Edward W. Hsu,[2] Nanci Aiken[5] and Anthony Horsman[6]

[1]MR Centre, Nottingham University, Nottingham NG7 2RD, UK Departments of [2]Biomedical Engineering and [3]Radiology,
Johns Hopkins University Hospital, Baltimore, USA
[4]Institute of Biodiagnostics, Winnipeg, Canada
[5]NMR Department, Fox Chase Cancer Centre, Philadelphia, USA
[6]MR Centre, Hull Royal Infirmary, Hull, UK

Previous NMR microimaging studies at 360 MHz have demonstrated a clear differentiation between the nucleus and cytoplasm in isolated single neurons. In particular, the T_2 of the cell nucleus is ~ 2.5 times larger than that of the cytoplasm. In order to determine the magnitude of possible T_2^* influences on these observations, images of single cells have been obtained at 500 MHz using spin-echo and line-narrowing sequences. Comparison of the images acquired by the two sequences, and of the spin-echo images at 360 and 500 MHz, imply that any T_2^* contributions are relatively small. Consequently, the measured T_2 differences in spin-echo imaging represent a true difference in the T_2 relaxation in the two cellular compartments.

Keywords: NMR microscopy, single neurons, T_2 measurements, T_2^* measurements.

INTRODUCTION

Previous studies of isolated aplysia neurons at 8.5 T highlight differences in the NMR characteristics of the nuclear and cytoplasmic compartments, even though spin density images appear homogeneous [1, 2]. The T_2 of the cell cytoplasm (29.0 ± 1.4 ms) is ~ 2.5 times shorter than that of the nucleus (78 ± 14 ms). Figure 1 shows a T_2-weighted image of a neuron where the contrast between the cell nucleus and cytoplasm is evident. Of concern is the significance of T_2^* contributions to the measured T_2 (and the image contrast) in microimaging studies at high magnetic field strengths, to the extent that susceptibility effects arising from differences in the subcellular composition and organization, and not true T_2 relaxation, may be the major cause of the observed differences in T_2.

Sharp et al. [3] have recently demonstrated the application of Carr-Purcell-Meiboom-Gill (CPMG) based, or 'line-narrowing,' imaging technique for eliminating T_2^* effects in imaging sequences. In this article, we present the first images of single neurons at 500 MHz. Further, line-narrowed and spin-echo imaging are quantitatively compared in order to determine the T_2^* contribution to the calculated T_2 relaxation times.

METHODS

Aplysia californica were obtained from Alacrity Biological Supply Inc., or Marinus Inc., California, USA, and shipped to Nottingham University, UK. Single L7 neurons were isolated as described previously [2]. Imaging experiments were performed on an 11.7-T, 89-mm-bore Oxford magnet interfaced to a home-built imaging console [4]. A series of T_2-weighted spin-echo images at a resolution of 20 × 20 × 160 μm were obtained in 13:48 min each on seven cells. Using a CPMG-based line-narrowing sequence [3], a series of correspondingly T_2-weighted images at a resolution of 20 × 20 × 160 μm on three of the cells and 27 × 27 × 160 μm on four of the cells were obtained.

Image data sets were analyzed as previously described [2]. Limitations in the cell viability time resulted in data being acquired with differing numbers of echoes in the T_2 fits. Consequently, data were averaged using standard weighted means and vari-

* Address for correspondence: MR Centre, Hull Royal Infirmary, Anlaby Road, Hull, HU3 2JZ, UK.

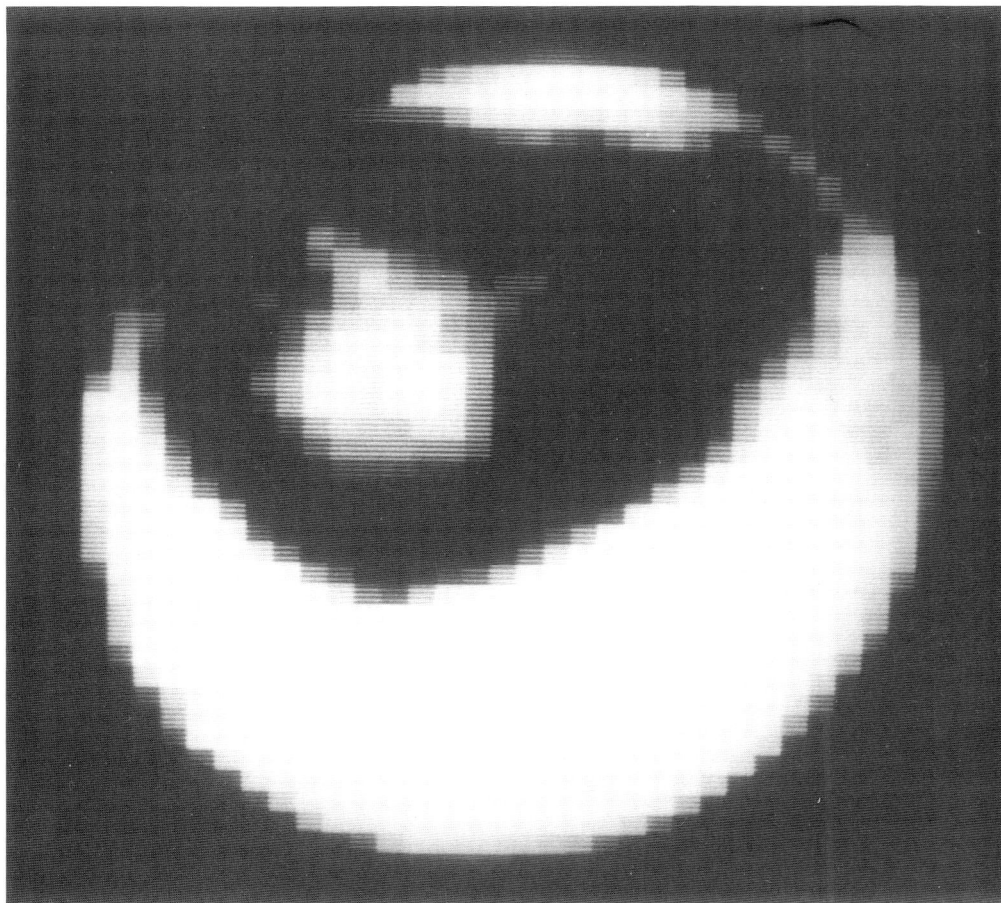

Fig. 1. T_2 weighted image of an isolated Aplysia neuron at 360 MHz. Images resolution is $20 \times 20 \times 100 \ \mu$m, $TR = 3$ s, $TE = 50$ ms. The central bright nucleus is surrounded by a dark cytoplasm which in turn is surrounded by artificial sea water.

ances, and data were compared using a weighted paired t-test.

RESULTS

Figure 2 shows example images from the same cell at two echo times using spin-echo and line-narrowed imaging sequences. All seven cells showed similar contrast. The nucleus and cytoplasm are clearly distinguished and the images appear qualitatively similar to those obtained previously [2] at 360 MHz. Further, the image contrast appears similar in the spin-echo and line-narrowed images, which immediately implies that any T_2^* contributions must be small or negligible.

The data were then analyzed to obtain quantitative T_2 measurements in the two cell compartments as described previously [2]. Two cells did not contain adequate nuclear areas for fitting and, consequently, seven cytoplasmic and five nuclear T_2 fits were ob-

tained. The mean values for the spin-echo determined T_2 relaxation rates were 41.9 ± 5.2 s^{-1} and 15.8 ± 2.6 s^{-1} for the cytoplasm and nucleus, respectively, whereas similar rates determined using the line narrowed sequence were 32.3 ± 3.6 s^{-1} and 11.8 ± 3.1 s^{-1}. In both cases, the nuclear T_2 relaxation time is again ~ 2.5 times that of the cytoplasm.

A weighted paired t-test indicates that the differences between the nuclear relaxation rates obtained by the two imaging techniques at 500 MHz is statistically insignificant ($P > 0.4$), whereas a similar comparison for the cytoplasm is marginally statistically significant ($P < 0.04$). We also note that both the cytoplasmic and nuclear relaxation rates obtained by the line-narrowed technique are approximately 25% lower than that of the spin-echo technique and conclude that any T_2^* contribution to the measured T_2 using spin-echo techniques will be $\sim 25\%$ or less.

A comparison of the spin-echo data obtained in this study at 500 MHz and a previous study at 360 MHz

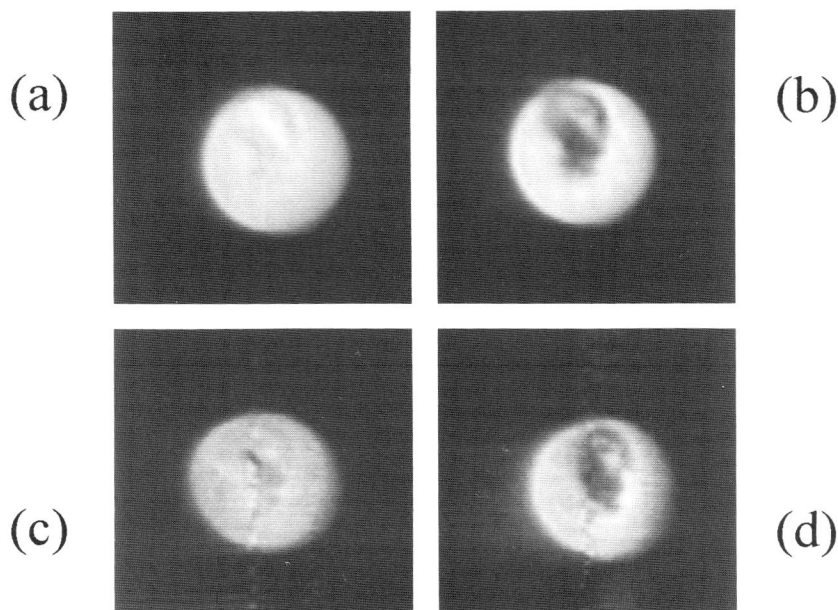

Fig. 2. Example spin echo (a,b) and line narrowed (c,d) images of a single neuron. $TR = 3$ s, image matrix $= 128 \times 128$, 2 averages. The echo times are 10 (a,c) and 50 (b,d) ms.

(33.5 ± 1.8 s^{-1} for the cytoplasm and 7.1 ± 1.2 s^{-1} for the nucleus) shows no significant difference ($P > 0.1$ for the nucleus and $P > 0.07$ for the cytoplasm). Again, this observation implies that any T_2^* contribution to the observed relaxation rates must, therefore, be small, as we would expect any T_2^* contribution to increase with field strength.

CONCLUSIONS

We conclude that any T_2^* contribution to the observed T_2 relaxation rate from the two compartments is similar in proportion, and set an upper limit of approximately 25% at 500 MHz. The data imply that the T_2 generated contrast between the cell nucleus and cytoplasm reflects primarily a true difference in the T$_2$ relaxation of the water in those two compartments and is not an "artifact" associated with microsusceptibility effects at high field strengths and spatial resolutions. The images presented also represent the first images of single neurons at 500 MHz and are comparable to similar studies performed at 360 MHz. Improved experiments are required to determine more accurately the possible T_2^* contribution.

ACKNOWLEDGMENTS

This work was supported in part by the Yorkshire Cancer Research Campaign. Collaborative studies between Hull, Nottingham, and Baltimore was supported by NATO grant (CRG 930244). Additional support was provided by SERC (A.P.), NIH grant CA09630 (N.A.), a Howard Hughes Fellowship (E.H.), and an institutional ICNMR grant from Johns Hopkins.

REFERENCES

1. Schoeniger JS, Aiken NR, Blackband SJ (1991) NMR Microscopy of Single Neurons. Society of Magnetic Resonance in Medicine, Tenth Annual Meeting, San Francisco.
2. Schoeniger JS, Aiken NR, Hsu EW, Blackband SJ (1994) Relaxation time and diffusion NMR microscopy of single neurons. *J. Magn. Reson.* B, **103**: 261–273.
3. Sharp JC, Bowtell RW, Mansfield P (1993) Elimination of susceptibility distortions and reduction of diffusion attenuation in NMR microscopy by line narrowed 2DFT. *Magn Reson Med* **29**: 407.
4. Bowtell RW, Brown GD, Glover PM, McJury M, Mansfield P (1990) Resolution of cellular structures by NMR microscopy at 11-7T *Philos. Trans. Roy. Soc.* **A333**: 457.

Relative assessment of brain iron levels using MRI at 3 tesla

R.J. Ordidge,[1]* J.M. Gorell,[2] J.C. Deniau,[2,3] R.A. Knight[2,3] and J.A. Helpern[2,3]

[1]*Department of Medical Physics and Bioengineering, University College of London, UK*
[2]*Department of Neurology, Henry Ford Hospital & Health Sciences Center, Detroit, USA*
[3]*Department of Physics, Oakland University, Rochester, MI, USA*

High field MR (magnetic resonance) images can be made sensitive to the relative concentration of tissue iron through the use of T_2^*-weighted contrast. This has enabled tissue iron levels to be assessed noninvasively by quantification of transverse relaxation rates. High field MRI may provide a new method to investigate neurological diseases which result in alteration of brain iron levels in specific areas of the human brain. Parkinson's disease (PD) results in an increase in iron concentration within the lateral region of the substantia nigra (SN), and provides one potential application of this methodology. Preliminary results of our findings are that there is a significant difference in SN iron levels in PD patients compared with age-matched controls, assessed by quantification of the reversible line-broadening component of transverse relaxation rate, R_2'.

Keywords: T_2^*-weighted MRI, brain iron, Parkinson's disease.

INTRODUCTION

Non-heme iron within brain tissue is stored mainly in the form of ferritin. Total iron levels are particularly high in the extrapyramidal brain regions (globus pallidus, substantia nigra, putamen, and caudate nucleus). Furthermore, these levels are known to be changed in specific regions in various neurological diseases. In Parkinson's disease (PD), the level of iron concentration measured postmortem has been shown to be increased by approximately 35% in the substantia nigra (SN) [1].

High field magnetic resonance imaging (MRI) is highly sensitive to the local magnetic field perturbations produced by tissue iron and deoxygenated blood. The transverse relaxation rate (R_2^*) is composed of two contributions which are responsible for reversible signal decay (at rate R_2') and irreversible decay (at rate R_2), using

$$R_2^* = R_2 + R_2'$$

where $R_2^* = 1/T_2^*$, $R2 = 1/T_2$, and $R_2' = 1/T_2'$.

Previous work has concentrated on the use of heavily T_2-weighted MRIs to provide a relative assessment of brain iron levels [2, 3]. However, T_2 relaxation is sensitive to a variety of relaxation mechanisms and, hence, may not provide contrast which is specific to changes in tissue iron levels. T_2^* is strongly dependent on T_2, causing similar difficulties in interpretation. Therefore, in this study we have concentrated on the evaluation of R_2' ($1/T_2'$), which we believe will more faithfully reflect the line-broadening effects from microscopically distributed paramagnetic material within biological tissue.

In order to assess the feasibility and utility of our methods, we have performed a preliminary study of transverse relaxation rates in the SN region of PD patients using a 3-T MRI system.

METHOD AND RESULTS

Measurements were made using a 3-T, 80-cm-bore magnet (Magnex Scientific, Abingdon, UK) linked to a Bruker Biospec 1 spectrometer (Bruker Medical Instruments, Billerica, USA). Following patient positioning, the subject was scanned to obtain axial images through the mid-brain in a section which clearly depicted the SN. A multiple-echo sequence was used and involved application of a modulated readout gradient to produce one spin-echo image (from the first echo with

* *Address for correspondence: Department of Medical Physics and Bioengineering, 11–20, Capper Street, University College of London, London, WC1E 6JA, UK.*

Table 1.

Parameters	Normal ($n = 9$)	PD ($n = 9$)	P- and F-values
R_2 (in s^{-1})	29.2 ± 3.9	26.8 ± 7.7	$P = 0.12, F = 2.65$
R_2^* (in s^{-1})	37.4 ± 3.1	54.4 ± 10.0	$P < 0.001, F = 26.7$
R_2' (in s^{-1})	8.2 ± 4.1	30.1 ± 7.7	$P < 0.001, F = 56.7$

TE = 29 ms, TR = 2 s, slice thickness = 5 mm, 128×128 image matrix), followed by a series of seven gradient-echo images with a sequentially incremented level of T_2^* contrast as defined by the period between echoes (8 ms). A second imaging experiment was then performed as before, but with a 24-ms increment in the delay between 90° and 180° excitation pulses, making the fourth echo a spin echo with TE = 77 ms. This provided a series of images with different relative weighting of T_2/T_2^* contrast. R_2 and R_2^* were then obtained by exponential fitting of data obtained from a region within the SN, using the image intensities from both sequences of eight images.

Measurements were performed on a small group of PD patients ($n = 9$, aged 47–72) and an equal number of age-matched controls. Diagnosis of PD was made if patients showed two or more of the cardinal signs of the condition. R_2, R_2^*, and R'_2 values for these groups are shown in Table 1. R_2 values do not discriminate between PD and control subjects ($P = 0.12$, F factor = 2.7); however, R_2^* and R'_2 values indicate that both parameters can be used to distinguish between the patient groups ($P < 0.001$). Furthermore, R'_2 values seem to be more effective than R_2^* in distinguishing between the patient groups (F factors of 56.7 and

26.7, respectively), suggesting that this parameter is more representative of the concentration of brain iron.

CONCLUSION

Previous studies of PD using heavily T_2-weighted MRI have provided inconclusive evidence of an increase of iron content in the SN [2–5]. In this study, measurements of R'_2 using a 3-T MRI system shows clear discrimination between PD and control subjects. Therefore, we believe that measurements of T_2 and T_2^*, in order to calculate T'_2 and R'_2, represents an effective approach to the study of brain iron levels.

REFERENCES

1. Dexter DT, Wells FR, Lees AJ, Agid F, Agid Y, Jenner P, Marsden CD (1989) Increased nigral iron content and alterations in other metal ions occuring in brain in Parkinson's disease. *J Neurochem.* **52:** 1830–1836.
2. Drayer B, Burger P, Darwin R, Riederer S, Herfkins R, Johnson GA (1986) Magnetic resonance imaging of brain iron. *Am J Nuclear Reson* **7:** 373–380.
3. Antonini A, Leenders KL, Meier D, Oertel WH, Boesiger P, Anliker M (1993) T2 relaxation time in patients with Parkinson's disease. *Neurology* **43:** 697–700.
4. Rutledge JN, Hilal SK, Silver AJ, Defendini R, Fahn S (1987) Study of movement disorders and brain iron by MR. *Am J Nuclear Reson* **8:** 397–411.
5. Braffman BH, Grossman RI, Goldberg HI, Stern MB, Hurtig HI, Hackney DB, Bilaniuk LT, Zimmerman RA (1989) MR imaging of Parkinson's disease with spin-echo and gradient-echo sequences. *Am J Nuclear Reson* **152:** 159–165.

Imaging gray brain matter with a double-inversion pulse sequence to suppress CSF and white matter signals

Thomas W. Redpath and Francis W. Smith

MRI Centre, Aberdeen Royal Infirmary, Foresterhill, Aberdeen AB9 2ZB, UK

The design of a double-inversion recovery (DIR) sequence, to selectively image gray brain matter, is described. A suitable choice of inversion times allows the cerebrospinal fluid (CSF) and white matter to be suppressed, to image the cortex alone. Consistently good results were achieved in a group of normal volunteers using the same inversion times throughout. The DIR sequence was found give clear delineation of the complex folds of the cerebral cortex.

Keywords: double-inversion recovery, brain cortex, segmentation.

INTRODUCTION

Inversion recovery (IR) sequences can be used to null the signal of a single tissue by appropriate choice of the inversion interval TI. For the case where the z-magnetization is fully recovered this is

$$TI = (\ln 2)T_1$$

where T_1 is the tissue's longitudinal relaxation time. The most common example of this is the STIR sequence [1], where TI is chosen to suppress fat.

The use of an additional inversion pulse allows two tissues (e.g., fat and fluid) to be nulled simultaneously and is termed a double-inversion recovery (DIR) sequence [1]. Figure 1 outlines a simple explanation of the DIR sequence applied to nulling cerebrospinal fluid (CSF) and white-matter signals. In the interval TI_1 between the inverting pulses, brain tissue magnetization recovers almost fully, whereas CSF, with its substantially longer T_1, recovers to only a small fraction of M_0, the equilibrium magnetization. The second inversion interval TI_2 is chosen to null white-matter magnetization. Gray matter, with a longer T_1, remains negative and generates a signal. CSF magnetization recovers slowly to pass through the null point at the same time as white matter.

Address for correspondence: MRI Centre, Aberdeen Royal Infirmary, Foresterhill, Aberdeen AB9 2ZB, UK.

THEORY

The sequence consists of two inverting pulses preceding a conventional spin-echo sequence. The inversion times TI_1 and TI_2 are defined in Fig. 1. The interval between the 90° and the refocusing 180° radio-frequency (RF) pulses is τ and equals TE/2 for the sequence used.

The value of the available z-magnetization M_A present immediately prior to the 90° imaging pulse can be calculated from the Bloch equations, assuming dynamic equilibrium from one TR interval to the next, and that all transverse magnetization decays or is spoiled after signal observation, before the sequence repeats. The method is described by Redpath [2] and gives

$$M_A = M_0[1 - 2E_2 + 2E_1E_2 - E_C(2E_\tau^{-1} - 1)]$$

where

$$E_1 = \exp(-TI_1/T_1)$$

$$E_2 = \exp(-TI_2/T_1)$$

$$E_C = \exp(-TR/T_1)$$

and

$$E_\tau = \exp(-\tau/T_1)$$

For a 90° imaging pulse, the NMR signal is, therefore,

$$S = kM_A E_\tau^2 \Delta V$$

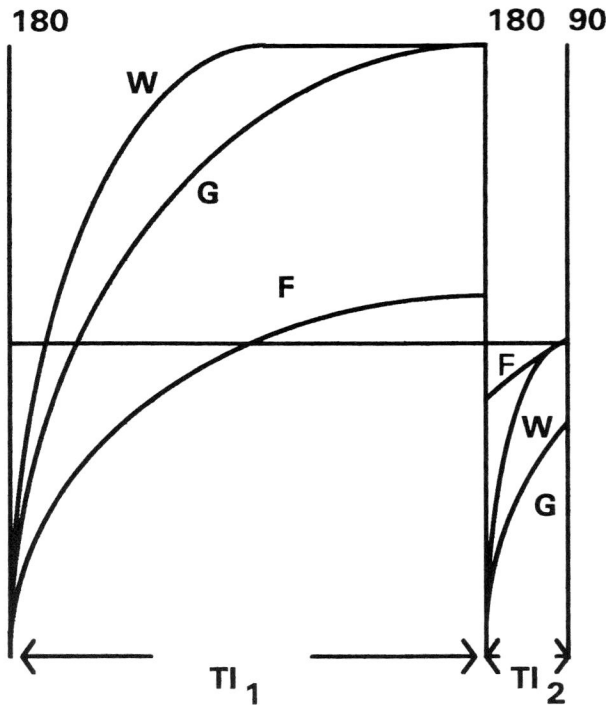

Fig. 1. The evolution of M_z through the inverting intervals TI_1 and TI_2 is sketched for cerebrospinal fluid (F), gray (G), and white (W) matter.

where ΔV is the volume of the voxel and k is a measure of the overall system gain.

In order to null the signals from two tissues, it is necessary to choose TI_1 and TI_2 to satisfy

$$1 - 2E_2 + 2E_1E_2 - E_C(2E_\tau^{-1} - 1) = 0$$

at both T_1 values. This can be done graphically as follows. Rewrite the above equation to give

$$E_2 = \frac{E_C(2E_\tau^{-1} - 1) - 1}{2(E_1 - 1)}$$

TI_2 can then be plotted as a function of TI_1 for the particular T_1 to be nulled, because

$$TI_2 = -T_1 \ln E_2$$

A second curve is produced for the second tissue to be nulled, and the intercept of the two curves gives the TI_1 and TI_2 required to null both tissues simultaneously.

In order to calculate sequence timings, knowledge of the expected T_1 values of gray and white matter and CSF is required. Henriksen et al. [3] conducted a multicenter trial to measure human T_1 values *in vivo* using normal volunteers. The conclusion was that the empirical fit of T_1 versus frequency proposed by Fischer gave a good description of the T_1 values of

gray and white matter obtained at the various field strengths used. The expected T_1 values for gray and white matter are 920 ms and 530 ms, respectively, at 0.95 T (40.5 MHz). The variation of Henriksen's measurements from this fit is sometimes large, by as much as 10% for gray matter and 20% for white matter. Condon et al. [4] concluded that the T_1 of CSF exceeded 3 s at 6 MHz. Hopkins et al. [5] measured the T_1 of CSF *in vivo* at 6.2, 25, and 60 MHz and found it to equal 4.3 s, with no evidence of field dependence.

Assuming T_1 values of 530 ms for white matter and 4.3 s for CSF, graphs of TI_2 versus TI_1 were produced for TR = 8 s and τ = 10 ms in order to find inversion timings to null CSF and white matter simultaneously, as described above. Table 1 summarizes the findings.

METHODS

The study was performed on a 0.95-T Siemens Impact scanner (Siemens AG, Erlangen, Germany), using the system's circularly polarized transmit–receive head coil.

The inversion timings required in practice were estimated by scanning a normal 31-year-old male volunteer. First, a multislice T_2-weighted transaxial multislice scan (TR = 4000 ms, TE = 128 ms) was acquired parallel to the radiological baseline, with the central slice through the anterior horns of the lateral ventricles. This scan effectively acted as an anatomical reference, allowing the structures seen in the DIR scans to be identified. White-TI_2 was varied to null frontal white matter adjacent anterior to the lateral horns of the ventricles, and then TI_1 was varied to null the CSF within the horns. All the DIR scans used TR = 8 s and τ = 10 ms. Other TR values were not investigated.

Once the inversion timings needed to selectively image gray brain matter had been determined, normal volunteers were scanned to measure the degree of suppression which could be routinely achieved. The T_2-weighted reference scan was obtained as before [field of view (FOV) = 230 mm, slice width = 5 mm,

Table 1. Estimated inversion times.

TR [ms]	TI_1 [ms]	TI_2 [ms]
4000	1700	350
6000	2250	360
8000	2650	360

Note: The estimated inversion times required to null white matter and CSF are given for various TR values. The T_1 values of white matter and CSF are assumed to be 530 ms and 4.3 s, respectively.

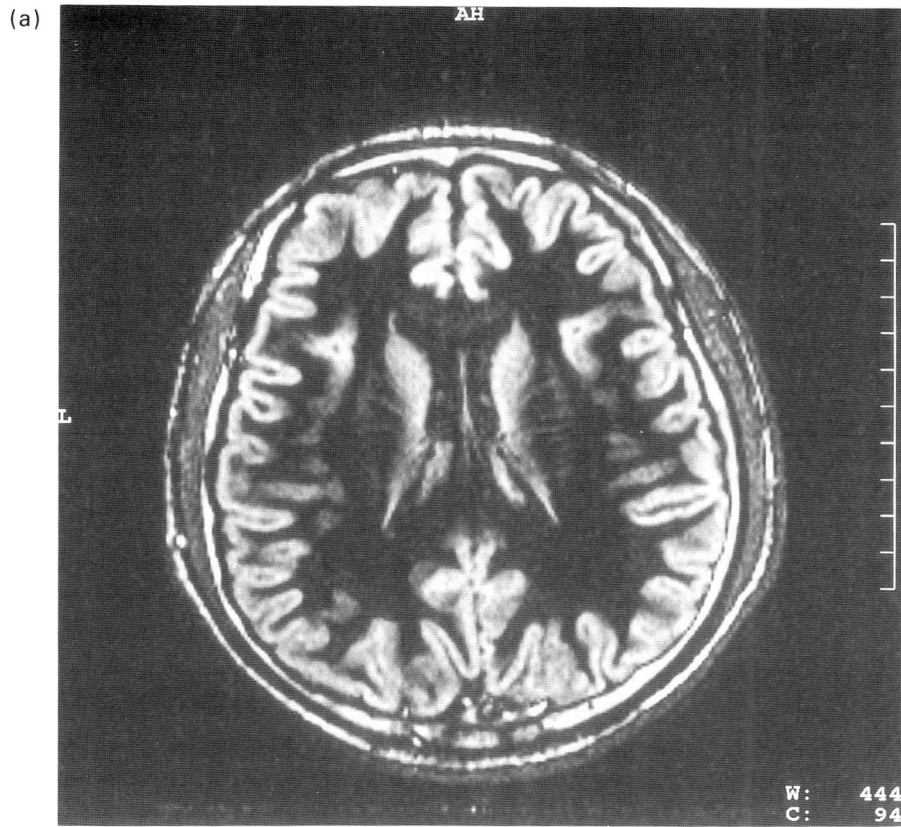

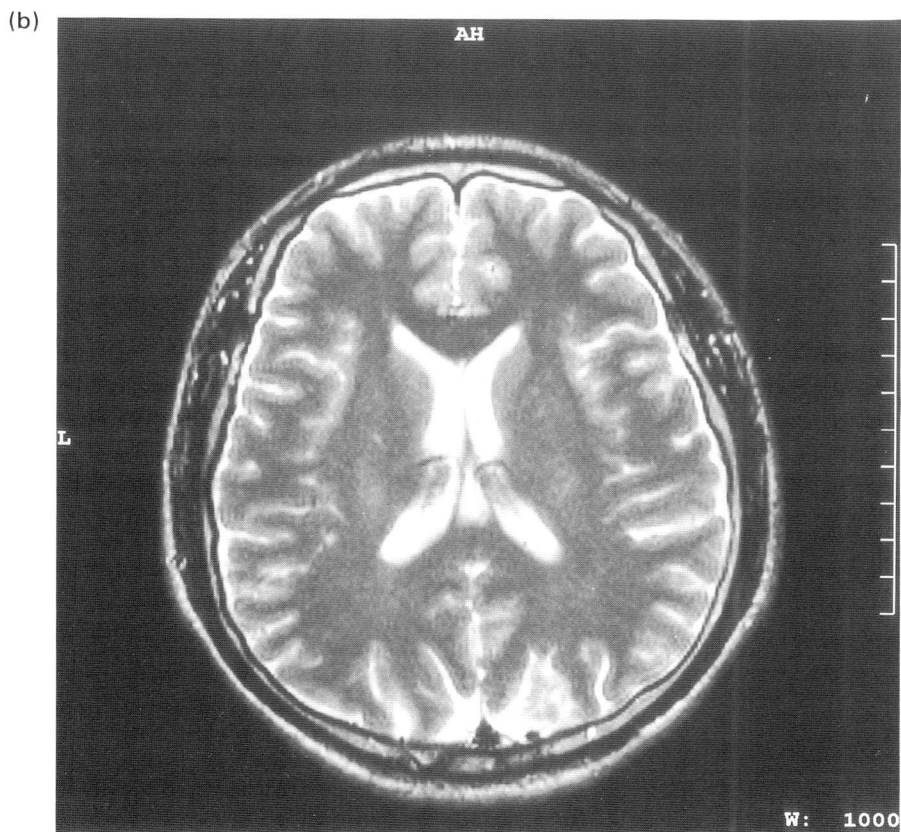

Fig. 2. (a) Gray-matter selective DIR (TR/TI$_1$/TI$_2$/TE = 8000/2300/300/20 ms); (b) T_2-weighted reference (TR/TE = 4000/128 ms) images of a normal volunteer at identical levels.

gap = 2.5 mm]. The DIR scan set was then acquired at matching slice positions with the same FOV and slice parameters. The matrix used was 192 × 256, resulting in an acquisition time of 25.6 min for the DIR image set, using a single acquisition (NSA = 1). Seven volunteers (five male, two female), ranging in age from 25 to 42 years (average age 30 years, sample standard deviation 6 years), were scanned.

The degree of suppression achieved was estimated by measuring the signal difference to sum ratio

$$D = (S_1 - S_2)/(S_1 + S_2)$$

for pairs of tissues, where S_1 and S_2 are the means of their respective signals, taken from region-of-interest (ROI) measurements. D is independent of the system gain k and is, therefore, a useful figure for comparing contrast between different types of scan and between different subjects. Ideally, D should equal $\pm$ 1.0, for complete suppression of the signal from one of the pair of tissues. The average signal in air is not zero, as might be expected, but it is a small positive number, reflecting the intrinsic white noise level in the magnitude image [6]. Therefore, even for tissue and air, the magnitude of D is less than 1.0. Only for an infinite signal-to-noise ratio would the ideal value be achieved.

For each volunteer's white-matter suppressed scan, a single D value was calculated for (i) gray and white matter, (ii) gray matter and CSF, and (iii) gray matter and air. The air region was taken outside the head, in an area unaffected by image artefacts. The CSF measurement was taken within the anterior horns of the lateral ventricles, the white-matter measurement anterior and lateral to this, from within the frontal hemispheres. The cortex ROI was chosen from the thickest and most uniform area possible, adjacent to the longitudinal fissure.

RESULTS

The optimum inversion times for DIR scans with TR/TE = 8000/20 ms were found to be TI_1 = 2300 ms and TI_2 = 300 ms for the white-matter and CSF suppressed scan, compared to the predicted values of 2650 ms and 360 ms, respectively. Figure 2a shows a selective DIR transverse scan of the cortex of a normal, male, 27-year-old volunteer, at the level of the lateral ventricles. Figure 2b shows the T_2-weighted spin-echo reference image for comparison.

Table 2 shows the degree of suppression which was achieved as measured by the signal difference to sum ratio D, given as the mean and sample standard deviation of the group. A negative value of D means that the second tissue of the pair has a higher signal

Table 2. Measured D ratios.

Sequence	Tissue pair	D
Cortex selective	GM/WM	0.80 ± 0.08
	GM/CSF	0.78 ± 0.08
	GM/air	0.88 ± 0.02
T_2-weighted SE	GM/WM	0.24 ± 0.04
	GM/CSF	−0.38 ± 0.01
	WM/CSF	−0.57 ± 0.03
	GM/air	0.92 ± 0.01
	WM/air	0.87 ± 0.02

Note: The range of D values obtained for the normal volunteers are given for the cortex-selective DIR sequence. Values for the T_2-weighted spin-echo (SE) reference scan are given for comparison.

than the first. The results of the T_2-weighted sequence are shown for comparison.

DISCUSSION AND CONCLUSIONS

The long TR necessitates a very long acquisition time, which probably precludes the routine clinical use of the DIR sequence for selective imaging of the cerebral cortex. However, rapid spin-echo acquisition methods may allow acquisition times to be reduced to more acceptable levels.

Good degrees of unwanted signal suppression were achieved for the group of normal volunteers with the gray-matter selective sequence. This indicates that the T_1 values of white matter and CSF did not vary sufficiently within the group to invalidate the use of fixed TI_1 and TI_2 settings. Specifically designed pulse sequences can be used to assess CSF volumes by MRI [7]. Computerized image segmentation methods, applied to MR images, can also be used to produce separate maps of brain tissue and CSF [8]. The DIR sequence offers a method of further segmenting brain tissue by using the T_1 differences between tissues to null unwanted signals.

ACKNOWLEDGMENTS

This work was supported by a grant from Tenovus (Scotland).

REFERENCES

1. Bydder GM, Young IR (1985) MR imaging: clinical use of the inversion recovery sequence. *J Comput Assist Tomogr* **9:** 659–675.

2. Redpath TW (1982) Calibration of the Aberdeen NMR imager for proton spin-lattice relaxation time measurements in vivo. *Phys Med Biol* **27**: 1057–1065.

3. Henriksen O, De Certaines JD, Spisni A et al. (1993) V. In vivo field dependence of proton relaxation times in human brain, liver and skeletal muscle: a multicenter study. *Magn Reson Imaging* **11**: 851–856.

4. Condon B, Patterson J, Jenkins A et al. (1987) MR Relaxation times of cerebrospinal fluid. *J Comput Assist Tomogr* **11**: 203–207.

5. Hopkins AL, Yeung HN, Bratton CB (1986) Multiple field strength in vivo T_1 and T_2 for cerebrospinal fluid protons. *Magn Reson Med* **3**: 303–311.

6. Edelstein WA, Bottomley PA, Pfeifer LM (1984) A signal-to-noise calibration procedure for NMR imaging systems. *Med Phys* **11**: 180–185.

7. Condon BR, Patterson J, Wyper D et al. (1986) A quantitative index of ventricular and extraventricular intracranial CSF volumes using MR imaging. *J Comput Assist Tomogr* **10**: 784–792.

8. Kohn MI, Tanna NK, Herman GT et al. (1991) Analysis of brain and cerebrospinal fluid volumes with MR imaging. Part I. Methods, reliability, and validation. *Radiology* **178**: 115–122.

Hybrid sequences for rapid T_1 imaging

Simon J. Doran

INSERM Unité 318, Group d'Application de la RMN à la Neurobiologie, Grenoble, France

This article generalizes the concept of the Look-Locker T_1-measurement sequence to include both EPI-like and Snapshot FLASH-like elements and it provides a bridge between a number of previously demonstrated methods of quantitative T_1 imaging. It is shown that a segmented k-space acquisition provides numerous advantages if sufficient time is available.

Keywords: T_1 measurement, Look–Locker, hybrid sequence, segmented k-space, point-spread function.

Because of the long-recognized potential in both clinic and laboratory of calculated T_1 images, much effort has been expended in trying to optimize experiments for obtaining quantitative T_1 data in a manageable time. The two sequences currently vying for the title of fastest are Inversion-Recovery Snapshot FLASH (IR-SnF) [1] and Inversion-Recovery Look–Locker EPI (echo-planar imaging) (IR-LL-EPI) [2], both of which are based on the original concept of Look and Locker [3] and acquire their entire data set in the minimum time theoretically possible (i.e., ~ $5T_1$). Although there are applications for which such ultrafast methods are indispensible, it is shown here that if the available imaging time is of the order of *minutes* and not seconds, then there are good reasons to use a "hybrid" or "segmented k-space" acquisition.

Hybrid sequences (e.g., Ref. 4), which acquire between 2 and 32 lines of k-space per "shot," represent a compromise between the high speed of the SnF and EPI imaging modules and the ease of implementation of the standard spin echo or gradient echo. Hybrids have the following general advantages over SnF and EPI:

(i) the ability to make measurements with standard, nonspecialist imagers;

Address for correspondence: INSERM Unité 318 (GARN), Pavillon B, CHU Albert Michallon, BP 217 X, 38043 Grenoble Cedex, France.

(ii) per experiment (though not necessarily per unit time), a higher signal-to-noise ratio (S/N) than SnF and possibly EPI, too—in the first case, because there are fewer excitation pulses to "use up" longitudinal magnetization (pulses may also have a larger flip angle, "gaining" transverse magnetization), and in the second case because of reduced $T_2{}^*$ decay during acquisition and a lower receiver bandwidth;

(iii) the ability to make measurement in shorter $T_2{}^*$ conditions than is possible for EPI;

(iv) the possibility of higher-resolution images (there is a direct trade-off between imaging time and resolution).

Look–Locker hybrids [see explanation in Fig. 1a] form a bridge between a number of previously described sequences, each of which represents one of the limiting cases (IR-SnF: $m = 1$, $n = n_\phi$, $q = 1$; IR-LL-EPI: $m = n_\phi$, $n = 1$, $q = 1$; TOMROP [5]: $m = 1$, $n = 1$, $q = n_\phi$, where n_ϕ is the number of phase-encode (PE) steps). As well as the advantages above, these hybrids offer the following: (i) the ability to measure shorter T_1 values than is possible by either IR-SnF or IR-LL-EPI and (ii) freedom from T_1 artifacts due to the image point-spread function (PSF) in systems with interfaces between high and low T_1's.

The hybrid initially chosen for testing has $m = 1$ and $n = 4$, with the phase-encoding scheme shown in Fig. 1b. It can be shown that magnetization recovery in the $[(\alpha - \tau)_4 - T]_p$ experiment can be described in a way

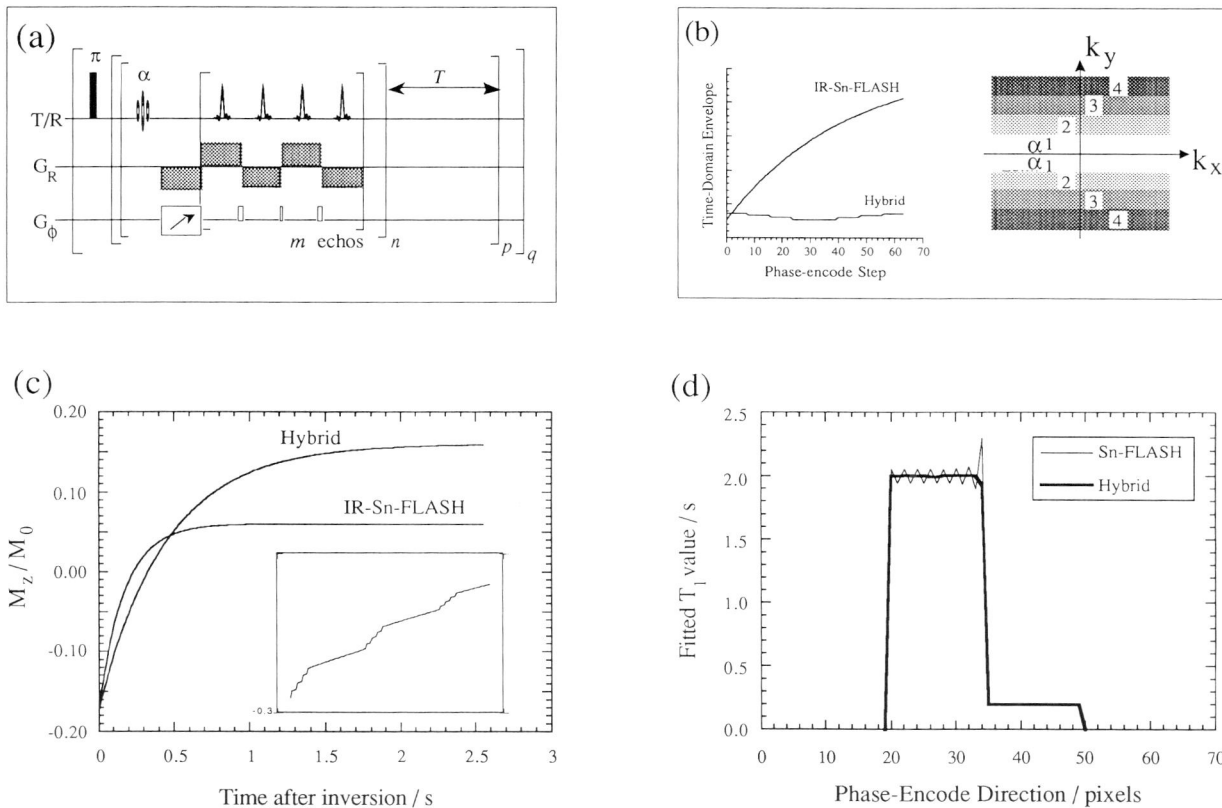

Fig. 1. (a) General hybrid Look–Locker imaging sequence. q inversions of the spin system are performed, each followed by a period of approximately $5T_{1max}$ (where T_{1max} is the longest T_1 of the sample), in which p groups of n low flip-angle excitations occur. Each group corresponds to a differently T_1-weighted image and is followed by a delay T. From each excitation, m echoes are acquired during a time τ, so that there are mn acquisitions per group, each of which can be phase-encoded differently. Note that the mnq is equal to the number of phase-encode steps and that the total imaging time is $5qT_{1max}$. (b) Sampling of k-space for an $m = 1$, $n = 4$ hybrid sequence. Left: Time-domain "envelope" function (i.e., the value of M_z immediately before the sampling pulse) by which the acquired data are multiplied, for the first image of an IR-Sn-FLASH and an $m = 1$, $n = 4$ hybrid sequence. The PSF (i.e., the FT of this envelope function) is convolved with the image. It causes a serious ringing artifact which carries through into the fitted T_1 values. Right: For a 64-PE-step experiment, steps 24–39 are acquired from excitation 1, steps 16–23 and 40–47 from excitation 2, steps 8–15 and 48–55 from excitation 3 and steps 0–7 and 56–63 from excitation 4. (c) Simulation of evolution of

very similar to that proposed [1] for the $[(\alpha - \tau)_{128}]_p$ original IR-SnF experiment: $M_z = \beta [1 - \gamma \exp(-t/T_1^*)]$, with $T_1^* = (4\tau + T)/[(4\tau + T)/T_1 + \ln(\cos^4 \alpha)]$, where τ is the gap between α pulses, i.e., the duration

longitudinal magnetization of a species with $T_1 = 0.5$ s under IR-Sn-FLASH ($\alpha = 10°$, 16 images, each of 64 PE steps, gap between PE-steps = 4 ms) and an $m = 1$, $n = 4$ hybrid sequence ($\alpha = 10°$, gap between α pulses = 4 ms, gap between groups $T = 256$ ms), with (inset) a zoom of the behavior of M_z during the first three pulse groups of such a hybrid sequence. Note how for the same flip angle, the magnetization recovers to a much larger value in the hybrid experiment. Although the hybrid sequence takes 16 times as long to obtain data for a complete T_1 image, the S/N advantage means that for this typical choice of values, it takes only *twice* as long to obtain data with the same S/N as by Sn-FLASH. Note also that T_1^* is longer for the hybrid experiment. This makes it easier to measure in cases where T_1 itself is short. (d) A typical plot of fitted T_1 values (fits made to simulated data) for an original sample containing short (0.2 s) and long (2 s) T_1 objects adjacent in the PE direction. Thin line: IR-Sn-FLASH ($\alpha = 5°$, gap between α pulses = 4 ms, 16 images of 64 PE steps, max. error in T_1 due to PSF 14.8%); thick line $m = 1$, $n = 4$ hybrid sequence ($\alpha = 5°$, gap between α pulses = 4 ms, gap between groups $T = 256$ ms, max. error in T_1 due to PSF 3.9%).

of the n loop in Fig. 1a. Although more complicated than Deichmann and Haase's original expressions, β and γ are still easily calculable functions of α, τ, T, and T_1. Figure 1c compares the recovery path of longitudinal magnetization in a standard IR-SnF experiment and the hybrid described. This hybrid is particularly advantageous in samples containing sharp interfaces between different T_1 values. Fig. 1d compares the theoretical performance of IR-SnF and the hybrid for measuring the T_1 of a sample which contains a T_1 component of 2 s immediately adjacent to a T_1 of 0.2 s.

REFERENCES

1. Deichmann R, Haase A (1992) Quantification of T1 values by SNAPSHOT FLASH NMR imaging. *J Magn Reson* **96:** 608–612.

2. Gowland P, Mansfield P (1993) Accurate measurement of T1 in vivo in less than 3 seconds using echo-planar imaging. *Magn Reson Med* **30:** 351–354.

3. Look DC, Locker DR (1970) Time saving in measurement of NMR and EPR relaxation times. *Rev Sci Instrum* **41:** 250–251.

4. McKinnon GC (1993) Ultrafast interleaved gradient-echo-planar imaging on a standard scanner. *Magn Reson Med* **30:** 609–616.

5. Gowland PA, Leach MO (1992) Fast and accurate measurements of T1 using a multi-readout single inversion-recovery sequence. *Magn Reson Med* **26:** 79-88.

3D MRI and angiography of human extremities using a local gradient coil

P. Gibbs,[1,*] S.J. Blackband,[1] B. O'Connor,[2] J.S. Schoeniger,[3]
I. Chakrabarti,[4] D.L. Buckley[1] and A. Horsman[1]

[1]Centre for MR Investigations, Hull Royal Infirmary Hull, UK
[2]Department of Applied Physics, University of Hull, Hull, UK
[3]Centre for Computational Engineering, Sandia National Laboratories, Livermore, California, USA
[4]University Department of Orthopaedics, Newcastle-upon-Tyne, UK

The limits of the spatial resolution achievable on a standard GE Signa 1.5-T imaging machine have been explored by interfacing a 12-cm-diameter local gradient set to such a system. Using a range of purpose-built radio-frequency (RF) coils, 3D gradient echo images with a spatial resolution of $100 \times 100 \times 500$ μ have been routinely obtained on the finger. Also produced were $100 \times 200 \times 500$ μ resolution angiograms of the finger detailing submillimeter vessels, with a velocity encoding of 6 cm s^{-1}. High-resolution fat/water suppressed images and isotropic data sets with a resolution of 170 μ are also demonstrated. With regard to the investigation of the mechanics of the human finger, isotropic data sets are desirable if accurate segmentation is to be implemented. A preliminary study illustrating the potential for producing a magnetic-resonance-based computer simulation of the mechanics of the human finger shows the distal interphalangeal joint extended and then in flexion.

Keywords: angiography, finger, high resolution.

INTRODUCTION

The available signal-to-noise ratio (S/N) determines the maximum achievable spatial resolution in a magnetic resonance imaging (MRI) system. At a given field strength, decreasing the size of the radio-frequency (RF) coil used is an efficient way of increasing S/N [1]. Relatively high spatial resolutions can, therefore, be achieved on clinical systems using surface coil technology. However, as the size of the RF coil is decreased, any further increases in spatial resolution are eventually limited by the characteristics of the gradient coil system. The maximum available gradient strength can be increased by reducing the dimensions of the gradient coils at the

expense of the size of the sample that may be examined.

Previous workers [2] have demonstrated the improvements in spatial resolution achievable with a small-diameter gradient set in order to produce images of the hand and wrist. However, this work reported single-slice acquisitions only. Thin contiguous slices are essential in high spatial resolution experiments because the important pathology may be very small. The full potential of the high resolution afforded by local gradient coil technology is only realized when the increase in S/N inherent in a 3D image acquisition is utilized.

Using a series of purpose-built RF coils and a 12-cm-diameter local gradient set, we demonstrate the image quality achievable in 3D imaging of the finger. The potential for angiographic studies of the extremities is also explored and possible clinical applications are discussed.

* Address for correspondence: Centre for MR Investigations, Hull Royal Infirmary, Hull, UK.

METHODS

An important consideration during the design of the local gradient coil set was the need for integration with the GE 1.5-T Signa in such a way that all the clinical sequences currently available could be utilized. This obviates the need for any pulse sequence programming and also enables the use of normal clinical protocols. The gradient set was constructed to a Helmholtz–Golay design [3] using wire wound on a plastic former.

Utilization of the reduced switching times, available with a smaller-sized gradient set, would have enabled the implementation of very short echo time sequences but would also have involved substantial software development and gradient amplifier modification. Con-sequently, standard clinical gradient rise times were employed. The gradient amplifiers used in normal clinical scanning are incorporated into the system, resulting in an increase of the maximum gradient strength from 10 to 60 mT m^{-1}. Hardware interfacing takes a maximum of 10 min.

A number of solenoid, saddle, and birdcage RF coils were constructed with lengths varying from 1.5 to 6.5 cm and internal diameters from 2.2 to 2.5 cm. The highest S/N images were obtained using the solenoid [4], although this requires the finger to be oriented vertically in the magnet bore. Patient comfort is improved using the birdcage or saddle RF coil geom-etries. In all situations, volunteers easily tolerated the 30 min required for a typical 3D imaging and angiogra-phy study. Gradient-echo and phase-contrast angio-grams were obtained, using standard clinical proto-

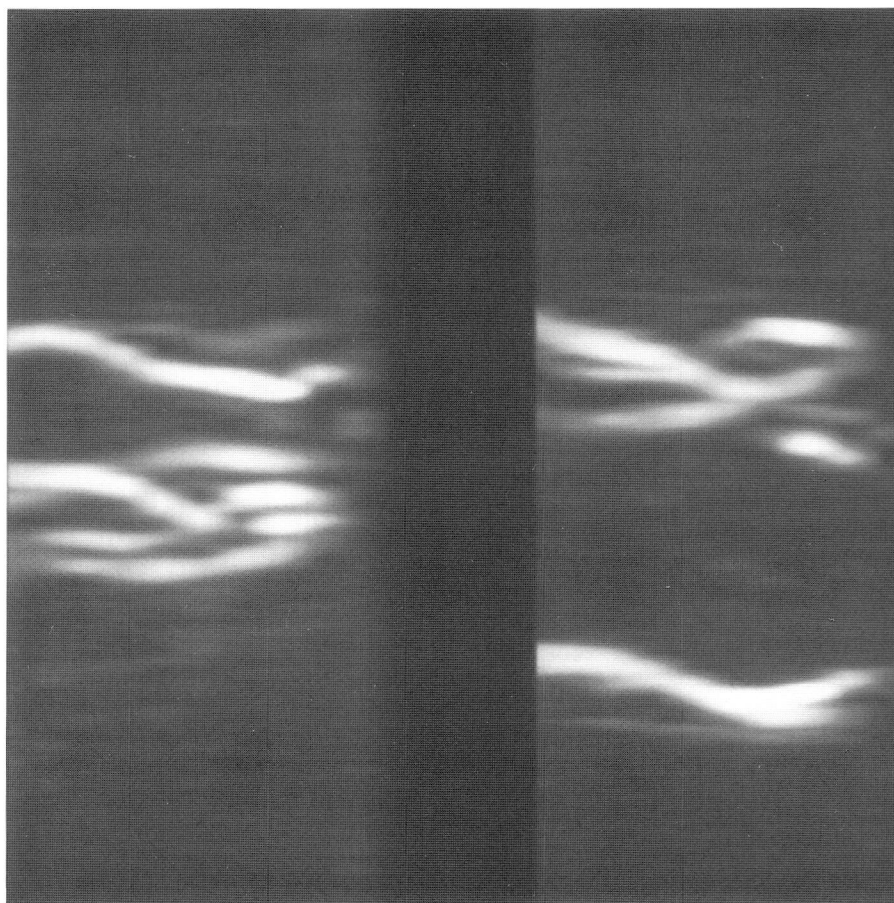

Fig. 1. Two projection angiograms of a finger illustrating the arterial and venous structure present. TE = 8.2 ms (frac-tional echo), TR = 50 ms, flip angle = 45°, field of view = 2.6 cm, matrix size = 256 × 128. Spatial resolution is 100 × 200 × 500 μ.

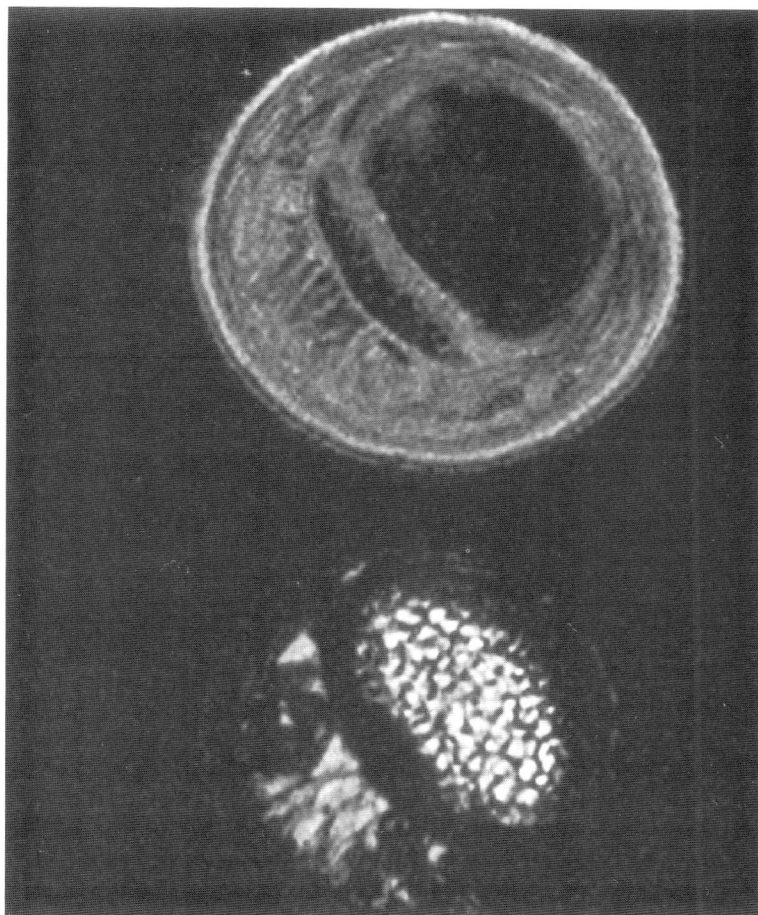

Fig. 2. (a) Axial image of distal interphalangeal joint obtained with fat suppression and (b) corresponding water-suppressed image. Acquisition parameters are TE = 5 ms (fractional echo), TR = 50 ms, flip angle = 30°, field of view = 2.6 cm, matrix size = 256 × 256. Spatial resolution is 100 × 100 × 500 μ.

cols, with three to six times the maximum spatial resolution previously achievable.

RESULTS

Three-dimensional gradient-echo images with in-plane resolutions of 100 × 100 μ and a slice thickness of 500 μ have previously been reported [5]. Angiographic studies have also been carried out on volunteers. The major arteries and veins within the finger are clearly visible in Fig. 1, with typically 10 pixels spanning a vessel diameter. Due to the increased gradient strength available, the angiography experiment is very sensitive to slow flow rates, thus enabling detailed observation of peripheral vessels.

Because the local gradient coil system is fully compatible with all clinically available software, high-resolution fat- or water-suppressed images can be easily produced using a chemical shift selective presaturation pulse. Figure 2 illustrates fat and water images of the finger with an in-plane resolution of 100 × 100 μ. In the fat image, the marrow within the bone is clearly seen along with characteristic globules of fat within the soft tissues.

Figure 3 illustrates alternate axial images of the distal interphalangeal joint obtained with an isotropic resolution of 170 μ. These images were taken from a 60-slice 3D data set obtained in just under 14 min. Such isotropic images are desirable if attempts are to be made to investigate the mechanics of human joints. Preliminary examples of images obtained using a saddle coil with the finger bending are shown in Fig. 4. Although a similar sized birdcage coil would give improved S/N, the open geometry of the saddle coil permits the finger end to bend out of the side of the

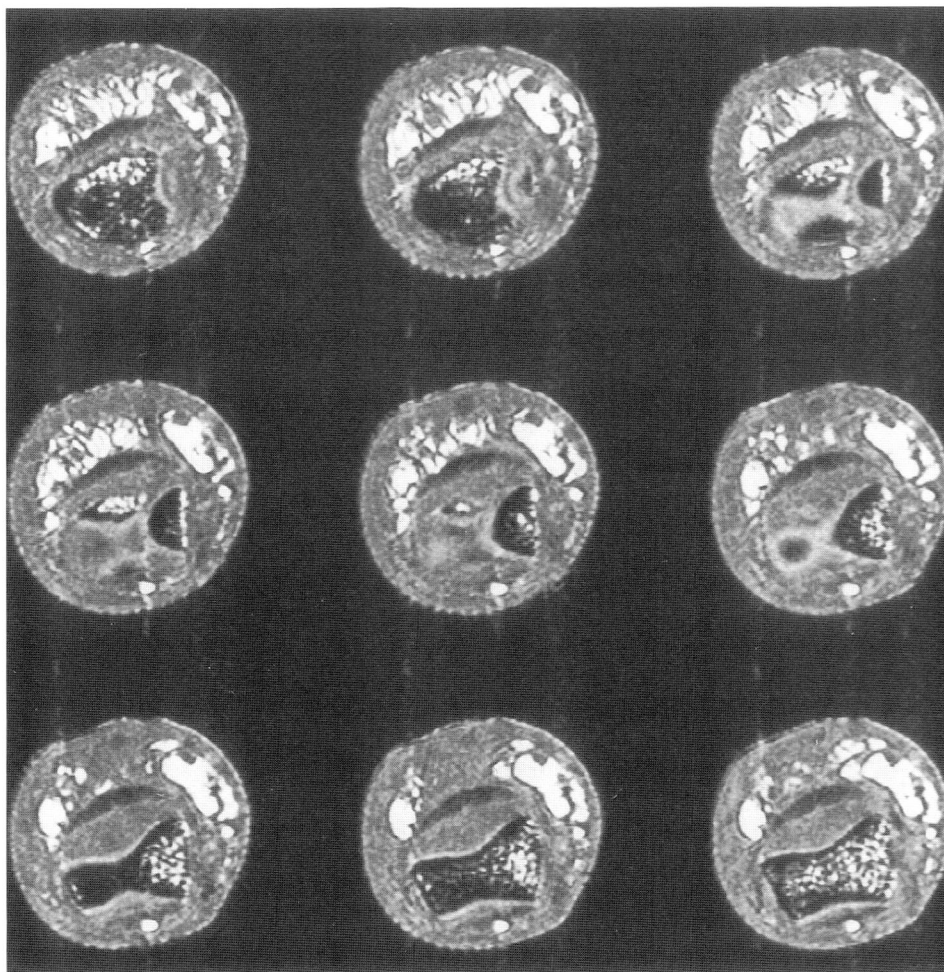

Fig. 3. Nine axial images of the finger taken from a set of 60 with an isotropic resolution of 170 μ. Acquisition parameters are TE = 5 ms (fractional echo), TR = 50 ms, flip angle = 45°, field of view = 4.33 cm, matrix size = 256 × 256.

coil. In Fig. 4a, the finger is extended; Fig. 4b shows the distal joint in flexion. Shortening and thickening of the flexor tendon are apparent. The distal interphalangeal joint is the simplest joint in the human body, and work is currently underway to investigate the potential of high-resolution MR data as a basis for the development of a computerised finite-element model of the human finger.

CONCLUSIONS

A local gradient coil system and various purpose-built RF coils have been used to obtain high-resolution images and angiograms of the human finger. The increased gradient strength available improves sensitivity to the lower flow rates found within the human extremities. Compatibility with all currently available commercial software allows the full range of protocols routinely used to be exploited to obtain the required contrast in the finger. Various RF coil designs have been utilized.

Finger-bending studies illustrate the potential of high-resolution imaging in the investigation of the mechanics of human joints. The possible use of diffusion-weighted and magnetization transfer sensitive pulse sequences as means of improving joint contrast are also currently under investigation.

Potential clinical applications include the use of angiographic studies in the assessment of peripheral vascular disease and diabetic microangiopathy, the examination of various joint disorders such as rheumatoid arthritis, and the design of prosthetic devices.

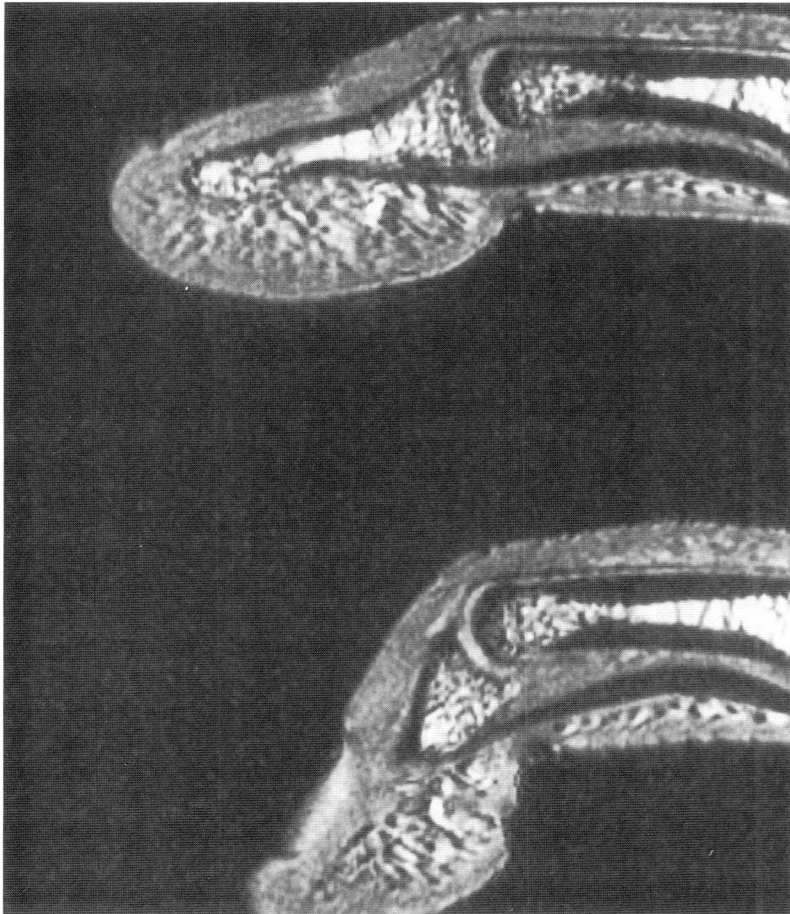

Fig. 4. Sagittal images of the finger obtained with a saddle coil. The finger is extended in the coil in the upper image and the distal joint is in flexion in the lower image. Acquisition parameters are TE = 5 ms (fractional echo), TR = 50 ms, flip angle = 45°, field of view = 5.33 cm, matrix size = 256 × 256. Spatial resolution is 200 × 200 × 670 μ.

ACKNOWLEDGMENTS

Many thanks to Dr. Elliot McVeigh for his involvement in preliminary studies at Johns Hopkins University Hospital, Baltimore. The Centre for MR Investigations is funded by the Yorkshire Cancer Research Campaign.

REFERENCES

1. Mansfield P, Morris PG (1982) *NMR Imaging in Biomedicine*, New York: Academic Press.

2. Wong EC, Jesmanowicz A, Hyde JS (1991) High resolution short echo-time MR imaging of the fingers and wrist with a local gradient coil. *Radiology* **181**: 393–397.

3. Bottomley PA (1981) A versatile magnetic field gradient control system for NMR imaging. *J Phys [E]* **14**: 1081–1087.

4. Hoult DI, Richards RE (1976) The signal-to-noise ratio of the nuclear magnetic resonance experiment. *J Magn Reson* **24**: 71–85.

5. Blackband SJ, Chakrabarti I, Gibbs P, Buckley DL, Horsman A (1994) Fingers: Three-dimensional MR imaging and angiography with a local gradient coil. *Radiology* **190**: 895–899.

Progress toward whole-body proton–electron double-resonance imaging of free radicals

David J. Lurie

Department of Bio-Medical Physics, University of Aberdeen, Aberdeen AB9 2ZD, UK

Proton–electron double-resonance imaging (PEDRI) has been developed recently for imaging free radicals in biological samples and small animals. This article summarizes the techniques of PEDRI and the related field-cycled method, FC-PEDRI, and discusses the difficulties in scaling the techniques up to whole-body size. Imaging free radicals with broad EPR lines in humans would require excessive radiofrequency (RF) power, but the use of magnetic field cycling alleviates this problem and improves the signal-to-noise ratio. The results of computer simulations of field-cycled PEDRI are presented, which show that optimum EPR irradiation frequencies exist, depending on the free radical's electron relaxation times and on the applied RF power.

Keywords: free radicals, imaging, double resonance, field cycling, DNP.

INTRODUCTION

Free radicals are defined as molecules with one or more unpaired electrons in their outer orbitals. Over recent years, the role of free radicals in the development of many diseases has become apparent to the medical community, but despite this fact the direct observation of naturally occurring free radicals in animals or humans remains an elusive goal, with the experimental evidence for free-radical involvement in disease being largely indirect. We, and others, have been working for a number of years on a technique called proton–electron double-resonance imaging (PEDRI), the ultimate aim of which is the imaging of endogenous and exogenous free radicals in animals and humans. This article discusses some of the difficulties encountered in applying this method on a large scale and suggests some ways in which the technique can be optimized.

PEDRI

PEDRI is a combination of proton NMR imaging with dynamic nuclear polarization (DNP). The latter (also known as the Overhauser effect) involves the observation of the NMR signal of a solvent while irradiating

Address for correspondence: *Department of Bio-Medical Physics, University of Aberdeen, Foresterhill, Aberdeen AB9 2ZD, UK.*

the EPR resonance of a free-radical solute. Provided the free radicals' unpaired electrons are causing relaxation of the nuclei under observation, the EPR irradiation can, under favorable conditions, result in a large increase in amplitude of the observed NMR signal. The enhanced NMR signal arises from an increase (and usually also a reversal) in the nuclear spin polarization, resulting in a nuclear magnetization which may be much greater than that predicted by the normal Boltzmann distribution.

In the simplest implementation of PEDRI, an NMR image is collected while irradiating an EPR resonance of the free radical of interest [1]. The NMR signal is enhanced in regions of the sample containing the free radical, and these parts are revealed by increased intensity in the final image. Subtraction of images obtained with and without EPR irradiation yields an image showing only those parts of the sample where free radicals are present.

The enhancement factor, E, in a DNP experiment is defined as the ratio of the NMR signal amplitudes A_z and A_0 obtained respectively with and without EPR irradiation. The well-known theory of DNP [2] predicts the following expression for E:

$$E = 1 - \rho f s \frac{|\gamma_S|}{\gamma_I} \qquad (1)$$

where ρ, f, and s are known as the coupling, leakage, and saturation factors, respectively; γ_S and γ_I are the electron and proton gyromagnetic ratios, with $|\gamma_S|/\gamma_I = 659$.

The coupling factor describes the nature of the interactions between the unpaired electrons and protons; with small free-radical molecules in aqueous solution, the interactions are predominantly dipolar, and ρ takes the value $\frac{1}{2}$.

The leakage factor takes account of the fraction of proton longitudinal relaxation that arises from the presence of the free radical in solution:

$$f = 1 - \frac{T_1}{T_1^0} \qquad (2)$$

where T_1 is the spin lattice relaxation time of the free-radical solution, and T_1^0 is the spin lattice relaxation time of the solution without free radical. The dependence of the enhancement on the free-radical concentration is described through the leakage factor.

Maximum enhancement is only observed when the EPR resonance is completely saturated; s gives the extent of saturation as a function of the applied radiofrequency (RF) magnetic field strength, B_2, and the electronic longitudinal and transverse relaxation times τ_1 and τ_2:

$$s = \frac{1}{n}\left[\frac{\gamma_S^2 B_2^2 \tau_1 \tau_2}{1 + \gamma_S^2 B_2^2 \tau_1 \tau_2}\right] \qquad (3)$$

Here, n is the number of hyperfine lines in the free radical's EPR spectrum ($n = 3$ for nitroxide free radicals).

It can be seen from the above equations that the maximum enhancement factor, obtained by complete saturation ($s = \frac{1}{3}$) of a concentrated solution ($f = 1$) is $E = -109$.

THE PROSPECTS FOR WHOLE-BODY PEDRI

In a given magnetic field B_0, the EPR frequency is approximately 659 times the proton NMR frequency. Just as EPR imaging of biological samples must be performed at frequencies below about 300 MHz, to minimize nonresonant absorption and to allow sufficient penetration into the sample, so PEDRI is restricted to this regime for the same reasons. Thus, PEDRI must be implemented at magnetic fields of 10 mT or less, well below the range of magnetic fields employed in clinical MRI. Because the signal-to-noise ratio (S/N) of the NMR experiment varies roughly as $B_0^{7/4}$, this brings into question the feasibility of whole-body PEDRI imaging.

If one could achieve enhancement factors close to the theoretical maximum, the inherent lack of S/N might be alleviated, but, in fact, enhancement factors $|E| > 5$ are not seen *in vivo* with nitroxide free radicals, which have EPR linewidths of the order of 0.2 mT, and require copious amounts of RF power to saturate the EPR resonance. For example, our initial *in vivo* PEDRI work at 10 mT achieved an enhancement factor of -3 in the kidneys of a rat injected with an intravenous dose of 0.4 mmol kg^{-1} of PCA nitroxide solution, with an applied RF power of 30 W at 238 MHz [3].

A free radical with a single, very narrow EPR resonance would undoubtedly allow enhancements of the order of 100 to be obtained *in vivo*, with a corresponding improvement in S/N and image quality, but the fact remains that currently available compounds suitable for use as PEDRI "contrast agents" do not possess these properties. Furthermore, if we hope to detect naturally occurring free radicals (with or without the "chemical amplification" technique of spin trapping), then it is important to concentrate on the detection and imaging of compounds such as the nitroxides, with their somewhat unfavorable EPR characteristics.

In fact, the power requirement of the EPR irradiation is the main limiting factor in applying PEDRI on a whole-body scale. The power P deposited in a spherical conducting sample of radius b can be written as

$$P = \pi\omega^2 B_2^2 b^5 / 15\eta \qquad (4)$$

where ω is the angular frequency, B_2 is the RF magnetic field in the rotating frame, and η is the solution's resistivity [4]. In our rat experiments, the instantaneous power absorbed by the animal was approximately 15 W (estimated by the ratio of loaded and unloaded resonator Q factors). (The animal was not cooked because the EPR irradiation was applied in bursts long enough to produce enhancement, separated sufficiently to reduce the average power.) Equations (1)–(3) show that with a particular free radical (giving ρ, τ_1, and τ_2) in a given environment (giving f) the enhancement depends on the degree of saturation, which is, in turn, a function of B_2, independent of sample size. Taking the "radius" of the rat to be 4 cm, the instantaneous power absorbed by a 16-cm "radius" human would be of the order of 15 kW to achieve the same enhancement under identical conditions! This figure equates to a specific absorption rate (SAR) of roughly 1 kW kg^{-1} and would require the use of a pulse sequence with an EPR irradiation duty cycle of 0.4% to bring the RF exposure within the limits of current guidelines (4 W kg^{-1} SAR). Bearing in mind that the EPR irradiation must last roughly three times T_1 (300–500 ms) to achieve enhancement, this suggests a sequence repetition time of more than 1 min, which is clearly impracticable.

The alternative is to irradiate the EPR at a lower frequency, because the power required to achieve a given B_2 depends quadratically on the frequency. Suppose one uses a pulse sequence where the EPR irradiation is applied in 300-ms bursts, with a repetition time of 2000 ms, giving a duty cycle of 15%. Then, one can afford to apply an instantaneous SAR of 27 W kg^{-1}, and the upper limit of the EPR frequency is found by appropriate scaling to b and ω to be 39 MHz. With nitroxide free radicals such as TEMPOL or PCA, this frequency implies a magnetic field B_0 of around 2.5 mT, with an NMR frequency of 106 kHz, and disastrous consequences for the S/N!

FIELD-CYCLED PEDRI

The above arguments suggest that the prospects for whole-body PEDRI are not good. For once, however, nature is on the side of the experimenter. The nuclear polarization, once increased by a sufficiently long and intense period of EPR irradiation, decays toward the Boltzmann distribution with a time constant equal to T_1. In other words, the nuclear spin system "stores" the enhanced magnetization and, even *in vivo*, the storage period is long enough to permit the applied magnetic field to be changed during the pulse sequence, using the techniques of magnetic field cycling [5]. We have dubbed the combination of techniques field-cycled PEDRI (FC-PEDRI) [6], and we will now demonstrate that the whole-body imaging of broadline free radicals by FC-PEDRI is a realistic proposition.

Like any field cycling pulse sequence, the FC-PEDRI sequence can be divided into polarization, evolution, and detection periods, at applied magnetic fields of B_0^P, B_0^E, and B_0^D, lasting for times t^P, t^E, and t^D, respectively. Initial nuclear polarization occurs at B_0^P, and the equilibrium magnetization is simply proportional to the magnetic field. The EPR irradiation is applied during the evolution period at a frequency determined by B_0^E and the nuclear magnetization increases with time constant T_1 toward an equilibrium value proportional to EB_0^E. Finally, the magnetic field is increased as rapidly as possible to B_0^D and the longitudinal magnetization is read by a 90° pulse, accompanied by the normal magnetic field gradients. It is convenient to use an interleaved pulse sequence, with EPR irradiation occurring before alternate 90° pulses, the final image being formed by subtraction of data collected with and without EPR irradiation. FC-PEDRI

provides two distinct benefits over the fixed-field PEDRI experiment:

1. By judicious choice of B_0^E the EPR irradiation frequency can be chosen to stay within power deposition requirements.
2. The major factor determining the NMR signal strength (and therefore the S/N) is the *detection* magnetic field B_0^D. This is because we are detecting the signal induced in the receiver coil (as in all NMR experiments), which is proportional to the detection frequency as well as the magnitude of the magnetization.

OPTIMIZATION OF FC-PEDRI PULSE SEQUENCE

If we assume that the applied EPR irradiation power is fixed at some nonhazardous value and that B_0^D is also fixed, then we can attempt to predict the optimum values of EPR frequency and B_0^E, as well as B_0^P and the timing of the pulse sequence. This is best accomplished by computer simulation, as it is necessary to include the effects of field switching times, which may be a significant fraction of the nuclear T_1.

A model of the interleaved pulse sequence was set up based on the specification of a whole-body FC-PEDRI system that we are currently constructing, with a detection magnetic field $B_0^D = 60$ mT. The change ΔM_z in the longitudinal magnetization M_z is calculated during time interval Δt ($\ll T_1$) by

$$\Delta M_z = (M_{eq} - M_z)[1 - \exp(-\Delta t/T_1)] \qquad (5)$$

where M_{eq} is the equilibrium magnetization at the time, proportional to the currently applied magnetic field (B_0^P, B_0^E, or B_0^D, or an intermediate value during field ramps), except during EPR irradiation, when M_{eq} is proportional to EB_0^E.

The final signal strength, which is to be maximized, is taken as the difference between the nuclear magnetization values just after the start of the detection period, obtained respectively with and without EPR irradiation. The results of the FC-PEDRI simulations are expressed relative to the signals from a simulated interleaved PEDRI experiment at a fixed field of 10 mT, with an EPR irradiation at 237 MHz at the same power as that used in the FC-PEDRI experiment. The equilibrium enhancement factor is calculated from Eqs. (1)–(4) by inserting values for τ_1, τ_2, and f. A particular value for B_2 at 237 MHz is assumed (which sets the power level), and this is scaled in inverse proportion to ω, via Eq. (4), to determine the value of E at lower values of B_0^E. Figure 1 shows the variation

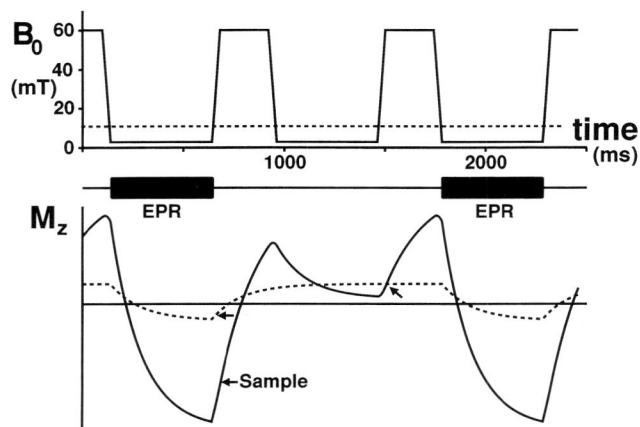

Fig. 1. Computer simulation of longitudinal proton magnetization M_z in a fixed-field PEDRI experiment at 10 mT (dashed lines) and an optimized FC-PEDRI experiment at the same applied RF power (sufficient to generate $B_2 = 12$ μT at 237 MHz). Sample parameters: τ_1, $\tau_2 = 0.1$ μs; $f = 0.4$; $T_1 = 200$ ms (60 mT), 150 ms (10 mT). FC-PEDRI parameters are $B_0^P = B_0^D = 60$ mT, $B_0^E = 2.5$ mT, EPR irradiation frequency 40 MHz, sequence timing $t^P = t^D = 100$ ms, $t^E = 500$ ms, ramp time between field levels 40 ms. Solid blocks indicate timing of EPR irradiation. Arrows indicate magnetization at time of NMR detection pulse.

with time of the longitudinal magnetization in an optimized FC-PEDRI experiment. For comparison, a similar plot is included for a fixed-field (10 mT) PEDRI experiment on the same sample, with the same applied RF power and the same overall sequence timing. The parameters used in the simulations are listed in the figure caption.

RESULTS AND CONCLUSIONS

Figure 2 summarizes the results of a number of FC-PEDRI simulations and shows a plot of the "FC advantage" (the ratio of the difference signals obtained from interleaved FC-PEDRI and PEDRI experiments) at three electron relaxation time values, as a function of EPR irradiation frequency. Different RF power levels yield families of curves with different maximum advantage values and optimum frequencies. However, the simulations indicate that the broader the line, or the lower the irradiation power, the lower is the irradiation frequency that must be used in order to optimize the experiment.

The fact that there *is* an optimum irradiation frequency can be explained qualitatively as follows: At high frequencies, the RF power limit dictates that only small B_2 values are generated, insufficient to cause significant saturation of the EPR line. As lower values

of ω are used, at correspondingly smaller values of B_0^E, the nonenhanced equilibrium magnetization decreases in proportion to the field, but the EPR saturation rises because of the larger B_2, increasing the enhancement, so that at some frequency $|EB_0^E|$ is maximized. At lower irradiation frequencies the decrease in B_0^E is no longer compensated by increased enhancement because the saturation is not linear with B_2 at high saturation levels, and the FC advantage drops once again.

Interactive use of the simulations allows one to reach the following general conclusions regarding the optimization and use of FC-PEDRI:

1. In contrast to conventional field-cycling experiments, there is no advantage to be gained from an increased polarization field ($B_0^P > B_0^D$). Because $E < 1$ (and usually <0), an increased B_0^P means that M_z has "further to go" to reach M_{eq} during the evolution period.
2. As far as possible, the evolution period should be made sufficiently long so that M_z reaches M_{eq}. In other words, $t^E \geq 3T_1$.
3. The larger the field-cycling apparatus, the more difficult it is to ramp rapidly the magnetic field between levels. Although field switching times

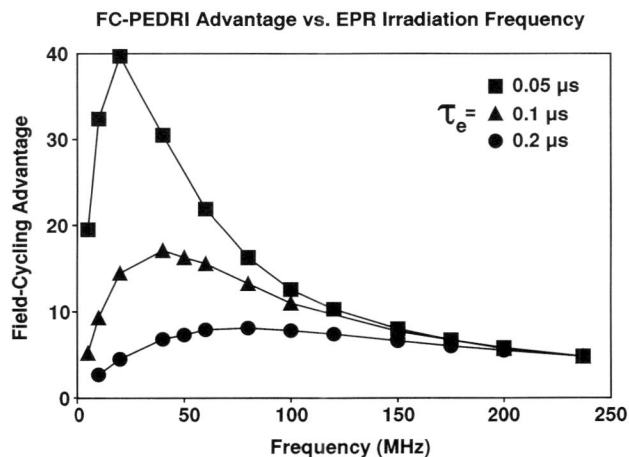

Fig. 2. Results of simulations of FC-PEDRI experiments with different electron relaxation times ($\tau_e = \tau_1 = \tau_2$) and the same RF power (sufficient to generate $B_2 = 12$ μT at 237 MHz), showing plots of FC advantage versus EPR irradiation frequency. FC advantage is defined as $(B_0^D(S - S_{EPR})_{FC})/(B_0^F(S - S_{EPR})_F)$, where S and S_{EPR} are respectively the NMR signals obtained without and with EPR irradiation. Subscripts FC and F indicate field-cycled and fixed-field experiments, while B_0^F is the field at which the latter are performed, namely, 10 mT. The ratio B_0^D/B_0^F gives the increase in signal due to NMR detection at the higher frequency. Sequence parameters are the same as those listed for Fig. 1.

should be kept as fast as possible (particularly between the evolution and detection periods), even with ramp times that are a significant fraction of T_1, FC-PEDRI offers a large S/N advantage over the fixed-field experiment at the same RF power.

This work indicates that whole-body field-cycled PEDRI will be capable of imaging free radicals with broad EPR lines without undue RF exposure. Work is underway to refine the FC-PEDRI model further and to confirm the predictions experimentally.

ACKNOWLEDGMENTS

The author thanks the Medical Research Council and the University of Aberdeen Research Committee for their continued support of this project.

REFERENCES

1. Lurie DJ, Bussell DM, Bell LH, Mallard JR (1988) Proton–electron double-resonance imaging of free radical solutions. *J Magn Reson* **76**: 366–370.
2. Dwek RA, Richards RE, Taylor D (1969) Nuclear electron double resonance in liquids. *Annu Rev NMR Spectrosc* **2**: 293–344.
3. Lurie DJ, Nicholson I, Foster MA, Mallard JR (1990) Free radicals imaged in-vivo in the rat by using proton–electron double-resonance imaging. *Phil Trans Roy Soc Lond* **A333**: 453–456.
4. Chen C-N, Hoult DI (1989) *Biomedical Magnetic Resonance Technology.* Bristol: IOP Publishing Ltd.
5. Noack F (1986) NMR Field-cycling spectroscopy: principles and applications. *Prog NMR Spectrosc* **18**: 171–276.
6. Lurie DJ, Hutchison JMS, Bell LH, Nicholson I, Bussell DM, Mallard JR (1989) Field-cycled proton–electron double resonance imaging of free radicals in large aqueous samples. *J Magn Reson* **84**: 431–437.

ABSTRACTS OF INVITED PAPERS

P07

Magnetization transfer contrast in MRI

R. S. BALABAN
NHLBI, Laboratory of Cardiac Energetics
Bethesda, Maryland 20892 USA

Magnetization transfer contrast (MTC) in magnetic resonance imaging (MRI) is generated via the dipolar interaction of bulk water protons (H_f) with the protons contained in macromolecules (H_r). The extent of the dipolar interaction of H_f and H_r is dependent on H_r molecular dynamics and surface chemistry results in the selectivity of MTC. MTC is generated by combining saturation transfer techniques with standard MR imaging procedures. Generally, MTC is produced by selectively saturating H_r with off-resonance RF energy. The specific practical and theoretical aspects of saturation transfer between H_r and H_f is an area of current debate. Of major practical importance is the specificity and power of the scheme used to saturate H_r. By the appropriate choice of frequency and power for H_r irradiation, the power deposition for generating MTC can be reduced by factors of > 10. In addition, the specific lineshapes of H_r and H_f is important in the interpretation of MTC. H_r has been shown to have a complex lineshape composed of both Gaussian and Lorentzian lines which can originate from different motional domains. Recent studies using selective ^2H labeling of macromolecular systems has revealed the topology of the spin coupling within the macromolecule and insights into the nature of the specific interaction site of water. The probing of the macromolecular structures via the magnetic interactions of water may provide a new tool in tissue characterization with MRI. In the last 3 years, MTC has been applied to the clinical studies with useful applications demonstrated the knee, eye, brain, breast, and heart. The application of MTC to accentuate MR angiography and contrast agent studies has also been demonstrated. Thus, MTC is quickly becoming another tool in maximizing the specificity and diagnostic potential of MRI.

S01

Advances in the study of brain function through rapid magnetic resonance imaging

M.S. COHEN
UCLA Departments of Neurology and Radiological Sciences, Los Angeles, USA

The human brain is on the one hand, characterized by substantial topographical localization of function in which fairly discrete regions subserve elements of cognitive processing. On the other hand, the brains of individuals differ greatly. The scientific task of *mapping* brain function is increasingly dependent on individual studies.

Through magnetic resonance imaging, the intrinsic contrast effects of blood flow and changes in blood oxygen content offer the neuroscientist a unique opportunity to assess changes in brain activity in human subjects without exposure to ionizing radiation. As a consequence, one can, in principle, ask subtle questions requiring multiple imaging sessions on single subjects, such as whether related neural processing (e.g., detection of motion or identification of objects) is subserved by the selfsame cortical regions. Such studies are clearly beyond the scope of present-day PET devices and can be asked to only a limited degree in invasive surgical procedures.

The degree to which functional MR activation studies (fMRI) may be used in individuals is an area of active and crucial research. Baseline fluctuations in signal intensity add noise to the functional studies that is not easily overcome with the usual imaging armamentarium such as increases in field strength or improvements in surface coils; much of this fluctuation is due to physiological factors in the subject. We will present data that attempt to characterize the fMRI signal and its variability within and across individuals and will show results demonstrating focal blood flow changes visible in response to a variety of cognitive and behavioral tasks.

C15

Functional magnetic resonance imaging of a spatial working memory task

A.M. BLAMIRE, G. MCCARTHY, A. PUCE,
A.C. NOBRE, F. HYDER, G. BLOCH, D. ROTHMAN,
P. GOLDMAN-RAKIC and R. G. SHULMAN

Yale University, New Haven, Connecticut, USA and VA Medical Center, West Haven, Connecticut, USA

Introduction: Working memory is the capacity to keep a running record of ongoing events. Measurements in primates implicate areas of prefrontal cortex (PFC) in performance of spatial working memory tasks [1]. Recent PET studies in humans support this finding [2]. We have used functional MRI to investigate human PFC during a spatial working memory task.

Methods: Eight subjects (four female) were studied at 2.1 T using an echo-planar imaging sequence. A single coronal slice was localized in PFC, 4 cm anterior to the anterior commissure. Images were acquired with a repetition time of 3 s and a gradient echo time of 50 ms. Stimuli were presented using an active matrix LCD display system and laptop computer and were viewed using prismatic glasses. Five subjects were studied twice. Activated areas were identified by *t*-test.

Tasks: In all tasks, subjects viewed the same stimuli. A random selection of 20 novel shapes were presented at different locations in the subjects field of view. In most cases, the shape was white, but occasionally a red shape appeared. In the "BASELINE" task, no stimuli were presented and no responses were made. In the "SENSORY" task, the subject responded when the object was red. In the "MEMORY" task, the subject monitored the objects and responded if any object appeared in the same location twice. In the "DOT" task, a small red dot appeared within the object and the subject was to respond when this occurred. Subjects performed the first three tasks only in their initial study and all four tasks at restudy.

Results: Focal activation was consistently observed in all subjects. The foci were in middle frontal gyri (areas 9 and 46). The "MEMORY" task gave the largest response in all subjects. In some subjects, activation was also observed in the "DOT" and "SENSORY" tasks.

Discussion: These results support the involvement of PFC in working memory tasks. Across-subject averaging suggested that the "SENSORY" and "DOT" tasks activated areas distinct from those involved in the "MEMORY" task.

1. Goldman-Rakic P et al. (1990) *Quart J Quant Biol* **55:** 1025–1038.
2. Petrides et al. (1993) *Proc Natl Acad Sci USA* **90:** 73–77.

C16

Localization of stimulus rate-dependent activation in the human auditory cortex using fMRI

A. DHANKHAR, B. D. WEXLER, A. M. BLAMIRE and
R. G. SHULMAN

Yale University School of Medicine, New Haven, Connecticut, USA

Introduction: PET studies have correlated regional cerebral blood flow (rCBF) in the human primary and secondary auditory cortices with the rate of stimulus presentation [1]. We investigated stimulus rate-specific responses in these regions using fMRI.

Methods: Six right-handed (two male), native English speakers were studied at 2.1 T using an echo-planar imaging sequence. Two or four axial-oblique slices were localized in the superior temporal gyrus. Images were acquired with a TR of 3.75 or 7.5 s and a gradient echo time of 50 ms. For stimulus presentation, subjects were padded headphones connected to an audio system.

Tasks: Stimuli were nouns presented at 0, 10, 50, 90, and 130 words per minute (wpm) in 1-min stimulation blocks repeated in counterbalanced and quasi-random-order. Sixteen images were acquired for each slice. Stimuli were presented during images 5–12. Repeated sets for each frequency were added together. Activated areas were identified by *t*-test as before [2] and quantified by a count of significant pixels.

Results: (1) Localized activation was consistently observed in all subjects in the transverse temporal and the superior temporal gyri as previously reported [1, 3]. (2) A significant increase in the volume of the activated region 10–50 wpm (113%), 10–90 wpm (194%), and 10–130 wpm (134%) was observed in all subjects. (3) Rate-dependent increases in the $\Delta S/S_0$ appeared to be less pronounced than increases in the activated volume. (4) Hemispherical asymmetry in activated volume was observed in all subjects. Five subjects showed left hemispherical dominance at all rates. One subject was right dominant.

Discussion: The results suggest the importance of dynamic neuronal recruitment, leading to a spread of the activated volume with increased processing demands. Lateral asymmetry in auditory processing parallels lateralized models of speech and cognitive processing.

1. Price C et al. (1992) *Neurosci Lett* **146**: 179–182.
2. McCarthy G et al. (1993) *Proc Natl Acad Sci USA* **90**: 4952–4956.
3. Binder JT et al. (1993) *Proc XIIth Annual Meeting SMRM*, Vol. 1, p. 5.

C17

A study of language production by functional MRI

A.M. BLAMIRE, A. BELGER, G. MCCARTHY and R.G. SHULMAN
VA Medical Center, West Haven, Connecticut, USA
Yale University School of Medicine, New Haven, Connecticut, USA

Introduction: Previous studies using PET [1] and functional MRI [2] have demonstrated frontal lobe activation during verb generation tasks. Our previous fMRI study showed totally overlapping activated areas for both verb generation and repetition in a single axial slice. The goal of this study was to investigate possible anatomical segregation of activated areas during an overt verb generation, a covert generation, and an overt noun repetition task using multislice imaging.

Methods: Data were collected using an asymmetric spin-echo, echo-planar imaging sequence on a 2.1-T MR system. Four coronal slices were imaged, ranging from the anterior commisure to 1 cm anterior to the end of the corpus callosum in the mid-sagittal plane. Slice thickness was 5 mm, repetition time was 6 s, and gradient echo time was 50 ms. Word stimuli were presented visually every 3 s at central field. Subject movement was minimized by a restraining head holder, and subsequent motion analysis indicated negligible movement. Activated regions were identified by t-tests [2].

Results: Bilateral activation was observed in all four slices. A spatial separation was observed between frontal lobe areas involved in the overt generation and repetition tasks. The more anterior regions were only activated during the generation task, whereas posterior frontal regions were equally activated by both the overt generation and the repeat tasks, both of which involved verbal output. Little or no activation was observed in these areas in the covert generation task.

Conclusions: These results are consistent with our previous observation of activity in area 47 using auditory stimulus presentation. They also show how the high spatial resolution of multislice fMRI has resolved areas involved in generation and repetition in this task.

1. Petersen SE et al. (1988) *Nature* **331**: 585–589.
2. McCarthy G et al. (1993) *Proc Natl Acad Sci USA* **90**: 4952–4956.

¹H magnetic resonance spectroscopy studies of cerebral metabolism in children

David G. Gadian* and Alan Connelly

Radiology and Physics Unit, Institute of Child Health, London, UK

This article summarizes some applications of ¹H magnetic resonance spectroscopy in the investigation of children with brain disease. Studies are described of children with inborn errors of metabolism, including lactic acidoses and mitochondrial disorders, ornithine carbamoyl transferase deficiency (a disorder of the urea cycle), and Canavan's disease (a disorder of *N*-acetylaspartate metabolism). Applications in epilepsy are also discussed.

Key words: magnetic resonance spectroscopy, brain, metabolism, metabolic disease, epilepsy.

INTRODUCTION

Over the last 4 years, we have been using ¹H magnetic resonance spectroscopy (MRS) to investigate cerebral metabolism in children with brain disease, and in this article we briefly summarize some of our main findings.

Our observations fall into two broad categories: (i) the accumulation of brain metabolites in children with inherited metabolic disease and (ii) spectral changes (more specifically a loss of signal from *N*-acetylaspartate) that are attributed to selective neuronal loss or damage. Examples are given from both of these categories to illustrate the scope and limitations of this noninvasive approach to the investigation of brain metabolism.

METHODS

All the clinical studies were carried out using a 1.5-T Siemens whole-body system, with a standard quadrature head coil. Most of the children were examined under sedation according to the protocol of the Hospital for Sick Children, Great Ormond Street, London, UK, as previously described [1]. Full diagnostic magnetic resonance imaging (MRI) was carried out together with the spectroscopy in each examination.

* Address for correspondence: Radiology and Physics Unit, Institute of Child Health, London, WC1N 1EH, UK.

Using the images as a guide, spectra were obtained from $2 \times 2 \times 2$-cm cubes centered on specific regions of interest, using a 90-180-180 spin-echo technique [2] with the three selective radio-frequency pulses applied in the presence of orthogonal gradients of 2 mT m^{-1}. Water suppression was achieved by preirradiation of the water resonance using a 90° Gaussian pulse with a 60-Hz bandwidth, followed by a spoiler gradient. TR was 1600 ms and TE was 135 ms. After global and local shimming and optimization of the water suppression pulse, data were collected in two to four blocks of 128 scans. The time-domain data were corrected for eddy-current-induced phase modulation using non-water-suppressed data as a reference [3]. Exponential multiplication corresponding to 1-Hz line broadening was carried out prior to Fourier transformation, and a cubic spline baseline correction was performed. In most examinations, spectra were obtained from two regions of interest.

RESULTS AND DISCUSSION

The dominant contributions to the spectra are normally from *N*-acetylaspartate (NAA), creatine + phosphocreatine (Cr), and choline-containing compounds (Cho). The relative intensities of these signals show both age dependence [4, 5] and regional dependence [5, 6], which must be taken into account when making comparisons.

Figure 1 shows a number of ¹H spectra obtained from children with brain disease. Figures 1A and 1B

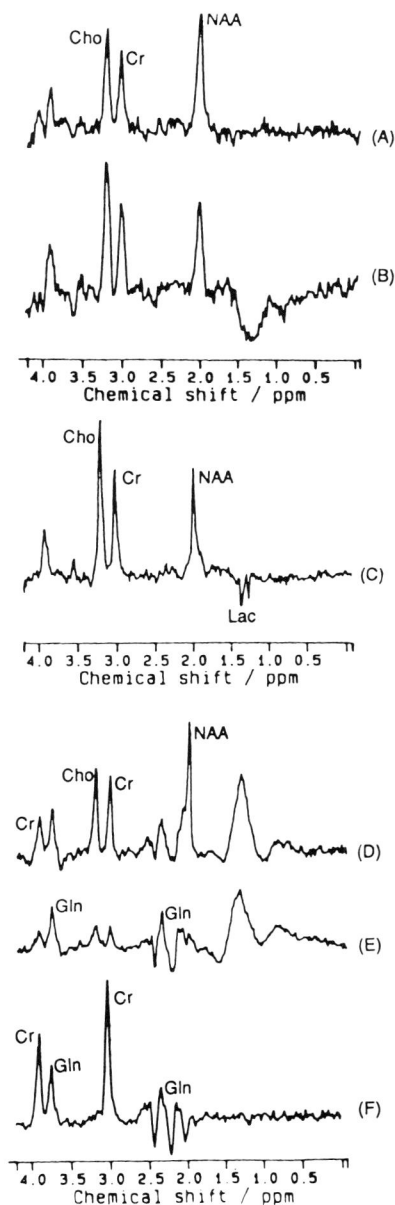

Fig. 1. (A) and (B): Spectra from the medial temporal regions of two age-matched children with epilepsy. In comparison with (A) and with the spectra of control subjects, (B) shows reduced NAA/Cho and NAA/Cr ratios. (C): Spectrum showing lactate (Lac) in occipital white matter, in a child aged 6 months with CSF lactate of 5.7 mmol L^{-1}. (D) and (E): Spectra of a child with OCT deficiency from an infarcted region (E) and from the contralateral hemisphere (D). On comparison with (F), it is clear that both spectra show signals that are characteristic of glutamine; (E) also shows very low NAA, Cr, and Cho signals, indicating a major loss of cellularity. (F): Spectrum of a solution containing 10 mM creatine and 40 mM glutamine, obtained with the same TE value (135 ms) as spectra (A)–(E).

show spectra from two patients with epilepsy, in one of which there are reduced NAA/Cho and NAA/Cr ratios, Fig. 1C shows a lactate signal in the spectrum of a patient with a lactic acidosis, and Fig. 1D-F shows two spectra from a child with ornithine carbomyl transferase deficiency, together with a spectrum from a solution containing creatine and glutamine. The roles of such spectra in the investigation of these children is discussed below.

Inherited metabolic diseases

Lactic acidosis and mitochondrial disorders

Congenital lactic acidoses form a large group of disorders that are commonly associated with profound neurological dysfunction. Difficulties are frequently encountered in establishing a precise diagnosis, and the mechanisms underlying brain damage are poorly understood. It has been shown that in several disorders of the brain, lactate can be seen by MRS at elevated concentrations [7–10]. We have performed 1H MRS on 24 patients under investigation for suspected metabolic disorder and have compared the MRS observations of brain lactate with measurements of cerebrospinal fluid (CSF) lactate [11].

Spectra were obtained from the basal ganglia in all 24 children, and from occipital white matter in 16 of the children. There was good concordance between the MRS and CSF investigations, in that all of the 9 children with CSF lactate concentrations of 2.5 mmol L^{-1} or less gave no detectable lactate signal on spectroscopy, whereas the 13 children with CSF lactates above 4 mmol L^{-1} all showed an inverted doublet signal characteristic of lactate (see Fig. 1C). This concordance serves to validate both types of measurement and suggests that 1H MRS may have a role in the investigation of those children who have neurological dysfunction in whom screening of blood or urine may not be adequate to establish a diagnosis.

Of further interest is the distribution of lactate in different areas of the brain. It is well recognized that the basal ganglia are particularly susceptible to damage in disorders of lactate metabolism, this being the hallmark of mitochondrial cytopathy and Leigh's disease. Eleven of 13 patients with CSF lactate concentrations above 4 mmol L^{-1} showed the peak in the basal ganglia, but lactate was also detected in the occipital white matter in all of the 8 examinations in which the spectra could be interpreted unambiguously. Regional variations in the lactate signal were observed in some cases. Further investigations of such variations, and of their relationship to focal brain damage, preferably using metabolic imaging methods [11], should help to explain the neurological patterns that are observed in these disorders.

Ornithine carbamoyl transferase deficiency

Ornithine carbamoyl transferase (OCT) deficiency is one of the five inherited disorders of the urea cycle. Affected individuals are prone to recurrent encephalopathy associated with hyperammonemia. The mechanism responsible for this encephalopathy remains uncertain. Possibilities include alterations in energy metabolism, neurotransmitter imbalance, astrocyte swelling, seizures, and changes in cerebral blood flow and intracranial pressure. Many of these phenomena could be secondary to the effects of glutamine, to which ammonia is converted, rather than directly to ammonia itself.

^{1}H MRS provides a noninvasive approach to the measurement of brain glutamine *in vivo*. However, because of the relatively complex magnetic response characteristics of the glutamine signals and because of spectral overlap with signals from other metabolites, the unambiguous detection of brain glutamine using clinical NMR systems poses difficulties. These difficulties were overcome by Kreis *et al.* [12], who, with the use of short echo times, reported the detection of brain glutamine in a series of patients with hepatic encephalopathy. In two children with OCT deficiency [13], we were also able to detect glutamine signals, even with relatively long (TE = 135 ms) echo times (see Fig. 1D and 1E). Confirmation of this assignment was obtained by comparison with the spectra of solutions acquired with the same pulsing conditions (Fig. 1F). In both children, glutamine was detected in two regions of the brain during episodes of acute hyperammonemic encephalopathy with focal neurological abnormalities. In one of the children, spectra obtained after treatment showed a marked decrease in these signals, indicating a return of brain glutamine toward normality.

In these studies we were able to obtain lower limits for the concentration of brain glutamine. The average of the four measurements in the two children was 13 mmol per kg wet weight, which is similar to the values of brain glutamine obtained in postmortem studies of patients who had died from hepatic failure, and four times the values given for normal human brain tissue (see Ref. 13 for a discussion). As this value of 13 mmol per kg wet weight is a lower limit, the actual concentrations within the brain are likely to be considerably higher, possibly by 50–100%, and could be even greater in the astrocytes, where the glutamine is synthesized. This could result in a rise in osmotic pressure, with consequent astrocytic swelling and, hence, cerebral edema and brain damage. These findings are, therefore, consistent with the hypothesis that intracerebral accumulation of glutamine contributes to the encephalopathy associated with hyperammone-

mia. Further work is required to establish why some areas of the brain are more affected than others, as MRI in these children clearly demonstrated.

Canavan's disease

Canavan's disease is an autosomal recessive disorder in which spongy degeneration of white matter is observed. Histologically, the affected white matter shows extensive vacuolation and demyelination. Recently, a deficiency of the enzyme aspartoacylase has been described in this disorder, and high levels of N-acetylaspartate (NAA) have been found in the urine and CSF of sufferers but not in patients with other leukodystrophies. We have described studies of two children with Canavan's disease [14]. MRI showed extensive high signal throughout the white matter, with little evidence of normal myelination. Spectra were acquired from regions centered on the basal ganglia and occipital white matter. Both regions showed very high signal intensity ratios of NAA/Cr and NAA/Cho, consistent with the known metabolic disorder in Canavan's disease. When taken together with the demyelination that is demonstrated by MRI in the same examination, they support the suggestion that the metabolic pathways involving NAA may play a role in the process of myelination. Such a role may be related to the finding that NAA has been found not only in neoronal cell cultures but also in a glial precursor cell, the O-2A progenitor [15].

N-Acetylaspartate and neuronal loss/damage

Much of the interest in ^{1}H MRS studies of the brain is currently focusing on the signal at 2.01 ppm. This signal arises from N-acetyl-containing compounds, the dominant contribution being from N-acetylaspartate (NAA). Although the function of NAA remains uncertain, it is believed to be located primarily within neurons, and, therefore, an unusually low NAA/Cr ratio is commonly interpreted in terms of selective neuronal loss or damage. However, some caution is required in interpreting NAA loss in young children, first because the ratio of NAA to the Cr and Cho signals increases with development, and second because, as mentioned earlier, it has recently been shown that NAA is present not only in neuronal cells but also in the glial cell precursor known as the O-2A progenitor [15]. Bearing in mind this cautionary note, a reduced NAA/Cr ratio has been observed in numerous disorders of the brain (see Ref 16), including stroke and tumors, multiple sclerosis, and epilepsy, and this is entirely consistent with the neuronal/axonal loss or damage that might be anticipated on clinical grounds. Below we describe some of our studies of patients with epilepsy, in which we use the NAA, Cr, and Cho signals to investigate the pathology associated with this disorder.

Temporal lobe epilepsy

The option of surgical treatment for patients with intractable temporal lobe epilepsy has become increasingly accepted in this disabling disorder. To offer definitive neurosurgical excision of epileptogenic tissue, the seizure focus must be determined with a high degree of accuracy. This frequently requires the implantation of intracerebral electrodes, which carries a significant risk of morbidity and can be particularly difficult to carry out and, indeed, to justify in children. We are using a combination of ¹H MRS, MRI, relaxation-time mapping, neuropsychology, EEG, and clinical assessment to identify noninvasively the underlying pathological basis of the seizure foci in temporal lobe epilepsy and to increase our understanding of the nature of such focal damage and its relationship to brain function. Here we consider the specific role of ¹H MRS in these investigations.

Spectra are obtained, as one part of integrated MRI/MRS examinations, from 2 × 2 × 2-cm cubes within the medial region of each temporal lobe. Many of the spectra from the patients with epilepsy show reduced NAA/Cho + Cr ratios in comparison with control subjects [17, 18; see Fig. 1A and 1B), and as discussed in Ref. 18, the metabolic abnormalities detected by MRS can aid lateralization of the seizure origin. Further information about the underlying cellular pathology is available from measurements of the absolute signal intensities. By multiplying the observed signal intensities by the 90° pulse voltage, it is possible to compensate for differences in radiofrequency coil loading [19] and thereby to compare signal intensities between different subjects. We have found that, in comparison with control subjects, the patients show not only a mean reduction in the NAA signal but also a mean increase in the Cr and Cho signals. The reduction in NAA is interpreted in terms of neuronal loss or damage. The explanation for the increase in the Cr and Cho signals remains unclear; but on the basis of our cell studies showing that the Cr and Cho concentrations (expressed relative to cellular protein content) were much higher in astrocyte and oligodendrocyte preparations than in cerebellar granule neurons [20], this increase may reflect reactive astrocytosis. Further studies are needed to establish whether this is, indeed, the basis of the increase in the Cr and Cho signals, but meanwhile it is apparent that the combination of *in vivo* and cellular studies provides a powerful approach to defining the cellular pathology associated with disorders of the brain.

Correlation of these MRS data with MRI, relaxation-time mapping, neuropsychology, EEG, and clinical assessment is currently in progress, and the initial analysis appears promising, both in terms of helping in the identification of the seizure focus [18] and also in investigating the pathological basis of functional deficits [21].

CONCLUSIONS

¹H MRS provides a noninvasive method of investigating brain metabolism in children with brain disease. Despite its limited spatial resolution, it is providing clinically useful information in children with inherited metabolic disease and with epilepsy. The technique can be incorporated into integrated MRI/MRS examinations and can provide new information about the biochemical and pathophysiological basis of neurological disorders.

REFERENCES

1. Shepherd JK, Hall-Craggs MA, Finn JP, Bingham RM (1990) Sedation in children scanned with high field magnetic resonance: the experience at the Hospital for Sick Children, Great Ormond Street. *Br J Radiol* **63**: 794–797.
2. Ordidge RJ, Bendall MR, Gordon RE, Connelly A (1985) Volume selection for *in vivo* spectroscopy. In: *Magnetic Resonance in Biology and Medicine* (Gorvind G, Khatrapal C, and Saran A, eds.) pp. 387–397. New Delhi: Tata-McGraw-Hill.
3. Klose U (1990). *In vivo* proton spectroscopy in presence of eddy currents. *Magn Reson Med* **14**: 26–30.
4. van der Knapp MS, van der Grond J, van Rijen PC, Faber JAJ, Valk J, Willemse K (1990). Age-dependent changes in localized proton and phosphorus spectroscopy of the brain. *Radiology* **176**: 509–515.
5. Connelly A, Austin SJ, Gadian DG (1991) Localised ¹H MRS in the paediatric brain: age and regional dependence. *Proc. 10th Ann Mtg Soc Magn Reson Med*, p. 379.
6. Frahm J, Bruhn H, Gyngell ML, Merboldt KD, Hanicke W, Sauter R (1989). Localized proton NMR spectroscopy in different regions of the human brain *in vivo*. Relaxation times and concentrations of cerebral metabolites. *Magn Reson Med* **11**: 47–63.
7. Bruhn H, Frahm J, Gyngell ML, Merboldt KD, Hanicke W, Sauter R (1989). Cerebral metabolism in man after acute stroke: new observations using localised proton NMR spectroscopy. *Magn Reson Med* **9**: 126–131.
8. Detre JA, Wang Z, Bogdan AR, Gusnard DA, Bay CA, Bingham PM, Zimmerman RA (1991). Regional variation in brain lactate in Leigh syndrome by localized ¹H magnetic resonance spectroscopy. *Ann Neurol* **29**: 218–221.

9. Grodd W, Krageloh-Mann I, Klose U, Sauter R (1991). Metabolic and destructive brain disorders in children: findings with localized proton MR spectroscopy. *Radiology* **181**: 173–181.

10. Luyten PR, Marien AJH, Heindel W, van Gerwen PHJ, Herholz K, den Hollander JA, Friedmann G, Heiss W-D (1990) Metabolic imaging of patients with intracranial tumors: H-1 MR spectroscopic imaging and PET. *Radiology* **176**: 791–799.

11. Cross JH, Gadian DG, Connelly A, Leonard JV (1993). Proton magnetic resonance spectroscopy in lactic acidosis and mitochondrial disorders. *J Inher Met Dis* **16**: 800–811.

12. Kreis R, Ross BD, Farrow NA, Ackerman Z (1992) Metabolic disorders of the brain in chronic hepatic encephalopathy detected with H-1 MR spectroscopy. *Radiology* **182**: 19–27.

13. Connelly A, Cross JH, Gadian DG, Hunter JV, Kirkham FJ, Leonard JV (1993). Magnetic resonance spectroscopy shows brain glutamine in ornithine carbamoyl transferase deficiency. *Pediatr Res* **33**: 77–81.

14. Austin SJ, Connelly A, Gadian DG, Benton JS, Brett EM (1991) Localised ^{1}H NMR spectroscopy in Canavan's disease: a report of two cases. *Magn Reson Med* **19**: 439–445.

15. Urenjak J, Williams SR, Gadian DG, Noble M (1992). Specific expression of *N*-acetyl-aspartate in neurons, oligodendrocyte-type 2 astrocyte (O-2A) progenitors and immature oligodendrocytes *in vitro*. *J Neurochem* **59**: 55–61.

16. Gadian DG, Shaw D, Moonen CTW, van Zijl P (1993) Advances in proton magnetic resonance spectroscopy of the brain: A report on a workshop held at the University of Oxford, December 1992. *Magn Reson Med* **30**: 1–3.

17. Gadian DG, Connelly A, Duncan JS, Cross JH, Kirkham FJ, Johnson CL, Vargha-Khadem F, Neville BGR, Jackson GD (1994) ^{1}H magnetic resonance spectroscopy in the investigation of intractable epilepsy. *Acta Neurol Scand (Suppl)* **152**, 116–121.

18. Connelly A, Jackson GD, Duncan JS, King MD, Gadian DG (1994). Magnetic resonance spectroscopy in temporal lobe epilepsy. *Neurology* **44**, 1411-1417

19. Hoult DI, Richards RE (1976) The signal-to-noise ratio of the nuclear magnetic resonance experiment. *J Magn Reson* **24**: 71–85.

20. Urenjak J, Williams SR, Gadian DG, Noble M (1993). Proton nuclear magnetic resonance spectroscopy unambiguously identifies different neural cell types. *J Neurosci* **13**: 981–989.

21. Gadian DG, Connelly A, Cross JH, Jackson GD, Isaacs EB, Vargha-Khadem F (1993) *Proc. 12th Ann Mtg Soc Magn Reson Med*, p. 430.

¹H spectroscopy in stroke

I. Marshall[1]* and R.J. Sellar[2]

Departments of [1]Medical Physics and [2]Clinical Neurosciences, University of Edinburgh, Edinburgh EH4 2XU, UK

We used proton spectroscopy to compare metabolite levels in infarcted brain tissue with the levels in corresponding normal white matter. In a preliminary study of six patients, the ratios (mean ± standard deviation) were 0.72 ± 0.25 ($p = 0.04$) for choline, 0.41 ± 0.24 ($p = 0.002$) for creatine, and 0.21 ± 0.22 ($p < 0.001$) for N-acetylaspartate.

Keywords: proton spectroscopy, stroke, ischaemia, infarct, brain metabolites.

INTRODUCTION

One of the potential clinical uses of proton (¹H) magnetic resonance spectroscopy (MRS) is in the study of cerebral ischemia resulting from stroke [1, 2]. ¹H MRS allows noninvasive measurement of several brain metabolites which reflect normal and pathological function. Spatial resolution is adequate to differentiate normal from pathological tissue, and examination times are clinically acceptable. We undertook a small preliminary study to investigate the feasibility of MRS examinations in stroke patients, who are often elderly and confused.

METHODS

Nine patients (mean age 62 ± 17 years) were studied within 2 weeks of onset of middle cerebral artery (MCA) territory ischemic stroke. MR imaging and proton spectroscopy were carried out in a 1.5-T Siemens Magnetom scanner using the standard head coil. T_2-weighted images were obtained in the transverse and coronal planes, and these images guided the selection of 8-ml volumes of interest (VOI) for spectroscopic examination. Volumes of interest were selected in the center of the infarct and in normal-appearing white matter for each subject. Spatially localized ¹H spectra were acquired from each VOI after local magnet shimming (to better than 0.15 ppm FWHM) on the water peak. The SE 135 point-resolved spectros-

* Address for correspondence: Department of Medical Physics, Western General Hospital, Edinburgh EH4 2XU, UK.

copy (PRESS) sequence [3] was used with TR = 1600 ms and TE = 135 ms. CHESS water suppression [4] was applied, and 256 acquisitions were collected. In addition, a water reference spectrum (16 acquisitions and no CHESS pulse) was collected from each VOI. The total examination time (imaging and spectroscopy) was approximately 1 h.

All data were analyzed on an IBM-compatible PC. Custom software was written to perform phase correction using the water reference [5, 6], 4-Hz Gaussian line broadening, removal of the residual water baseline, and spectral fitting. The water reference peak was used as a spectral "template" in the fitting procedure.

Ratios of metabolite levels in infarcts to the levels in the corresponding normal white matter were calculated, for each patient, for choline at 3.2 ppm, creatine at 3.0 ppm, and N-acetylaspartate (NAA) at 2.0 ppm.

RESULTS AND CONCLUSIONS

In all nine patients, satisfactory T_2-weighted images were obtained which clearly showed the infarcts as regions of high signal intensity. In six cases, we obtained satisfactory spectra from within the infarct and from normal white matter. In two further cases, the patients became uncomfortable and the examinations had to be terminated prematurely. In the remaining case, a bizarre spectrum was obtained from the infarct and was not analyzable.

Figure 1 shows the spectrum obtained from the infarcted region in one patient, and Fig. 2 shows the spectrum from the normal (contralateral) region. Choline, creatine, and NAA peaks are clearly visible in the normal spectrum but are much diminished in the

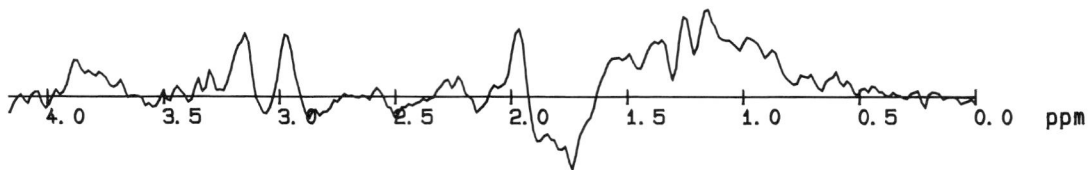

Fig. 1. ^{1}H magnetic resonance spectrum of an 8-ml volume of infarcted brain tissue in a stroke patient.

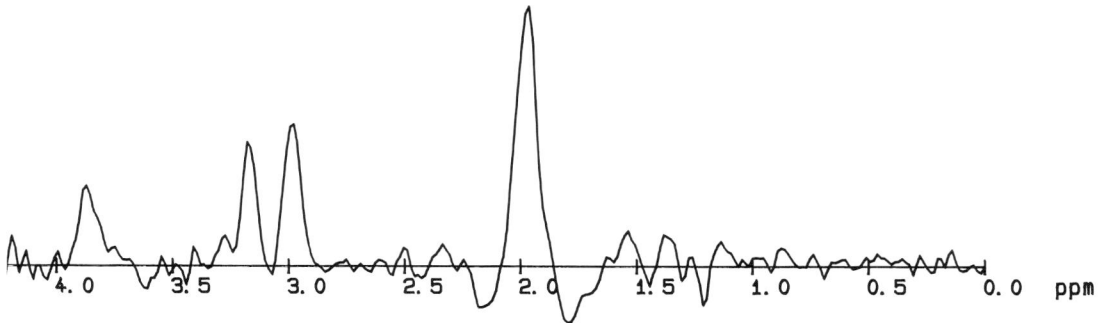

Fig. 2. Spectrum of corresponding normal white matter in the same patient.

infarct spectrum. Table 1 gives the mean ± standard deviation of the ratios of metabolite levels in the infarcts to the levels in the corresponding normal white matter for the six patients studied completely. We see from Table 1 that in infarcted tissue the levels of creatine and NAA are substantially lower than in normal tissue (41% and 21%, respectively), whereas there is a smaller decrease in choline, to 72% of its normal level. In calculating these ratios, we are implicitly assuming that the sensitivity of the head coil is the same over the two VOI regions. This assumption is probably valid because we expect its response to be laterally symmetric, and the normal tissue VOIs were located at the "mirror image" position of the infarcts. We believe that our ratios are clinically more useful than the NAA/choline and NAA/Creatine ratios sometimes quoted in the literature, because they separate out the pathological changes in each metabolite.

Although we did not set out to measure absolute metabolite levels in this study, retrospective calibration is possible using the (recorded) amplitude of either the water suppression pulse [7] or of the 90°

pulse [8] as a measure of coil loading, in conjunction with phantom studies using known concentrations of the metabolites. We found that the levels of choline, creatine, and NAA in normal white matter were 2.7 ± 1.0, 8.6 ± 2.7, and 15.6 ± 7.5 mM, respectively, for this patient group. These figures take no account of the partial volume effect of blood vessels and yet are somewhat greater than previously published literature values [7, 8].

Lactate was observed in four out of the six infarcts but was not sufficiently clear to be measurable. We believe this is partly due to lipid contamination of the spectra and partly due to our selection of patients. At 2 weeks poststroke, we would expect completely infarcted tissue to be producing no further lactate (although some groups have observed lactate even after several months [9]). In a more recent study, lactate was clearly observable (at approximately 10 mM concentration) in a patient measured within 2 days of onset of stroke.

REFERENCES

1. Felber SR et al. (1992) *Stroke* **23**: 1106–1110.
2. Gideon P et al. (1992) *Stroke* **23**: 1566–1572.
3. Bottomley PA (1987) *Ann New York Acad Sci* **508**: 333–348.
4. Frahm J et al. (1990) *J Magn Reson* **90**: 464–473.
5. Ordidge RJ, Cresshull ID (1986) *J Magn Reson Med* **3**: 151.
6. Klose U (1990) *Magn Reson Med* **14**: 26–30.
7. Danielsen ER, Henriksen O (1993) *SMRM Abstracts* 976.
8. Michaelis T et al. (1993) *Radiology* **187**: 219–227.
9. Graham GD et al. (1992) *Stroke* **23**: 333–340.

Table 1. Ratios of metabolite levels in infarcted tissue to levels in normal white matter ($n = 6$).

	Choline	Creatine	NAA
Mean	0.72	0.41	0.21
Standard deviation	0.25	0.24	0.22
p-Value	0.04	0.002	<0.001

¹H magnetic resonance spectroscopy of the brains of normal infants and after perinatal hypoxia–ischemia

Ernest B. Cady,[1]* Ann Lorek,[2] Juliet Penrice,[2] Richard Aldridge,[1] Marzena Wylezinska,[1] John S. Wyatt[2] and E. Osmund R. Reynolds[2]

Departments of [1]Medical Physics and Bioengineering, and [2]Paediatrics, University College London, London WC1E 6BT, UK

The aims of this study were to define proton (¹H) metabolite peak–area ratios in the brains of normal infants and to investigate abnormalities after perinatal hypoxia–ischemia. Point-resolved spectroscopy (PRESS) data were collected at 2.4 T with an echo time (TE) of 270 ms from 8-ml voxels located in the thalamus or occipito-parietal region. Fourteen normal and 9 asphyxiated infants were studied. The gestational plus postnatal ages (GPA) of these two groups were 31–41 (median 36) and 27–41 (37) weeks, respectively, and the asphyxiated infants were studied aged 0–10 (2) days. Peak–area ratios were determined in the normal infants for choline-containing compounds (Cho), creatine plus phosphocreatine (Cr), N-acetylaspartate (NAA) and lactate (Lac). Lactate was detected in all the normal infants and Lac/NAA was higher in the occipito-parietal region than in the thalamus ($p < 0.005$). Lac/NAA decreased with increasing GPA in both the thalamus ($p = 0.014$) and the occipito-parietal region ($p = 0.033$). In six of the nine asphyxiated infants, Lac/NAA was above 95% confidence intervals for either the thalamus and/or the occipito-parietal region. Of these six infants, two died and three were neurologically abnormal aged 2 months, indicating that elevated Lac/NAA after perinatal hypoxia–ischemia may convey a poor prognosis. Propan-1,2-diol (the phenobarbitone injection medium) was detected at ~1.1 ppm in three infants.

Keywords: ¹H-MRS, brain, birth asphyxia, lactate.

INTRODUCTION

¹H magnetic resonance spectroscopy (MRS) has potential both for the investigation of normal brain development and for monitoring changes in cerebral metabolism after hypoxia–ischemia. Data for ¹H metabolites in term infants and children have been published [1]. In that study, however, lactate was not detected. Others have suggested that lactate is commonly seen in premature infants [2]. The presence of lactate has also been noted after birth asphyxia [3]. Frequently, however, lactate has not been detected in infants with significant hypoxic–ischemic encephalopathy.

In this study, we aimed to establish normal ¹H metabolite peak–area ratios in healthy term and preterm infants, and as variation may exist between regions of the brain, we studied two separate areas.

We also investigated infants following perinatal hypoxia–ischemia.

METHODS

Point-resolved spectroscopy (PRESS) spectra (TE 270 ms; repetition time 2 s; 128 echoes) were collected on a

Table 1. Peak–area ratios in normal infants (mean ± standard deviation) at TE 270 ms.

	Thalamus ($n = 14$)	Occipito-parietal ($n = 8$)
NAA/Cho	0.75 (0.26)	0.67 (0.14)
Cr/Cho	0.49 (0.16)	0.45 (0.15)
NAA/Cr	1.58 (0.44)	1.60 (0.42)
Lac/NAA	0.23 (0.08)[a]	0.58 (0.30)[a]

[a]$p < 0.005$ for difference between thalamic and occipito-parietal voxels.

* Address for correspondence: Department of Medical Physics and Bioengineering, University College London, 11-20 Capper Street, London WC1E 6AU, UK.

Thalamus

Occipito-parietal

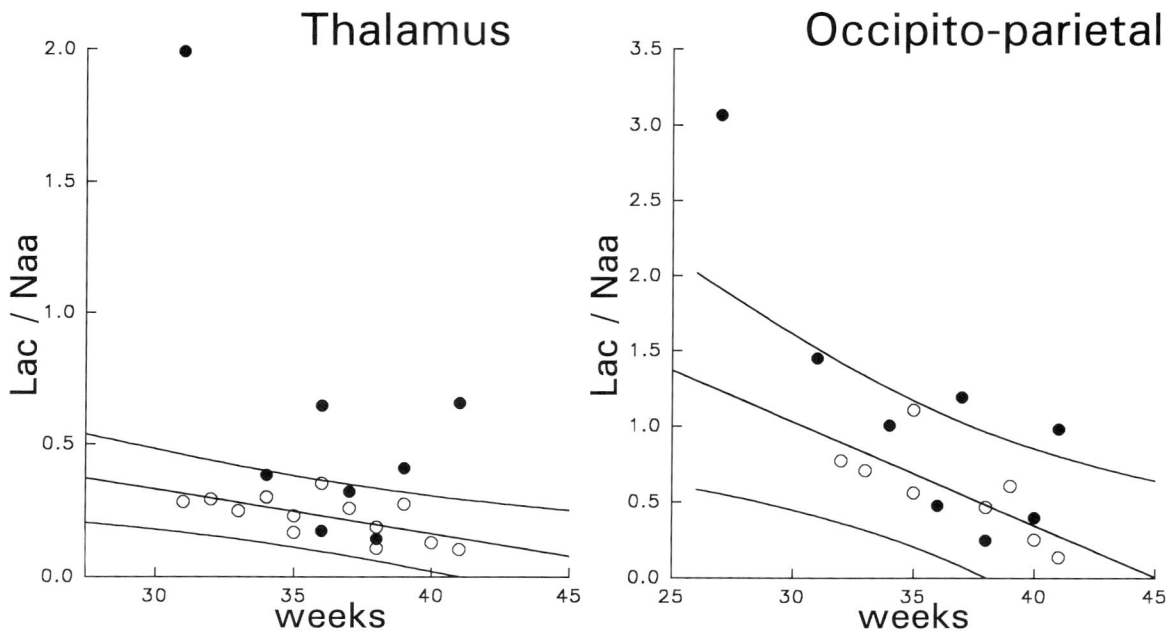

Fig. 1. Relation between Lac/NAA peak–area ratio at TE 270 ms in the thalamus and occipito-parietal region, and gestational plus postnatal age. ○ = normal infants, ● = maximum observed values for birth-asphyxiated infants. The regression line and 95% confidence limits for normal values are shown.

2.4-T (100-MHz) Bruker Biospec (actively shielded gradients, Helmholtz probe) from 8-ml voxels located in the thalamus or occipito-parietal region. Fourteen normal infants, born at 29–41 (median 33) weeks gestation were studied aged 1–46 (10) days at gestational plus postnatal age (GPA) of 31–41 (36) weeks. None of these control infants was small for gestational age and none had congenital anomalies. Nine asphyxiated infants born at 26–41 (37) weeks were studied on 18 occasions aged 0–10 (2) days. All had cord or first arterial base deficits less than -13 mmol L^{-1} as well as abnormal neurology. Two of these babies were treated with phenobarbitone at the time of study for seizures. In addition, an additional infant born at 39 weeks and treated with phenobarbitone and phenytoin for neonatal seizures, possibly secondary to a leukodystrophy, was studied on four occasions. Peak areas were determined by Lorentzian χ^2 minimization.

RESULTS

Peak–area ratios for the normal infants are given in Table 1. Lactate was detected in all the normal infants. Lactate/N-acetylaspartate (Lac/NAA) was higher in the occipito-parietal region than in the thalamus ($p < 0.005$; paired t-test). Lac/NAA decreased linearly with increasing gestational age in both the thalamus

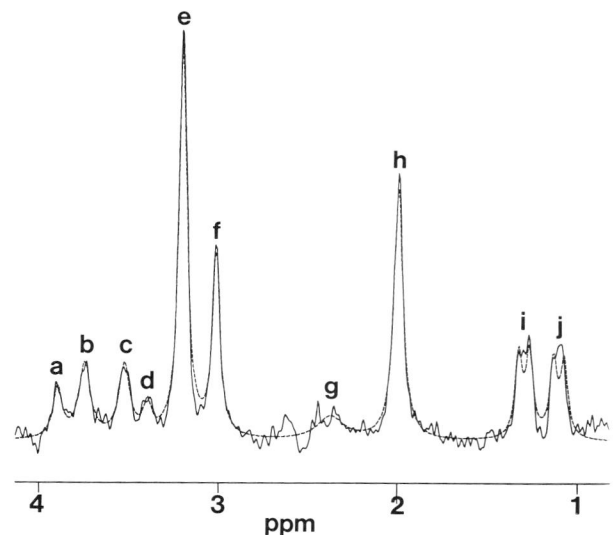

Fig. 2. A spectrum (solid line) from the thalamus of a birth-asphyxiated infant of 41 weeks gestation aged 2 h. Resonance identifications: (a) Cr; (b) glutamate/glutamine; (c) myoinositol/glycine; (d) scylloinositol/taurine; (e) choline-containing compounds; (f) creatine plus phosphocreatine; (g) glutamate/glutamine; (h) NAA; (i) Lac; (j) propan-1,2-diol. The dashed line is the Lorentzian fit to the spectrum.

($p < 0.02$, $m = -0.02$ per week, $c = 0.83$) and the occipito-parietal region ($p < 0.05$, $m = -0.07$ per week, $c = 3.07$) as shown in Fig. 1.

In six of the nine asphyxiated infants, Lac/NAA was above the 95% confidence limits for normal values in the thalamus and/or the occipito-parietal region. (See Fig. 1, which shows the maximum observed values.) Of these six infants, two died and three were neurologically abnormal at 2 months. All three infants with normal Lac/NAA had no detectable abnormalities aged 2 months.

The spectra from the three babies who were being treated with anticonvulsants showed a doublet at ~1.1 ppm attributed to propan-1,2-diol. This is the injection medium for both phenobarbitone and phenytoin. (See Fig. 2.)

CONCLUSIONS

In normal infants Lac/NAA was higher in the occipito-parietal region than in the thalamus, and it decreased with increasing GPA. Lac/NAA was raised following perinatal hypoxia–ischemia and may indicate a poor prognosis. In addition to raised lactate due to anerobic glycolysis, there may also have been a contribution from free fatty acids. The injection medium of commonly used anticonvulsants was seen resonating close to lactate. It is important to note this when interpreting spectra from babies both following hypoxia–ischemia and with suspected metabolic defects.

ACKNOWLEDGMENTS

The authors thank the Medical Research Council and the Wellcome Trust for financial assistance.

REFERENCES

1. Kreis R, Ernst T, Ross BD (1993) Development of the human brain: In vivo quantification of metabolite and water content with proton magnetic resonance spectroscopy. *Magn Reson Med* **30**: 424–437.
2. Leth H, Toft P, Pryds O, Lou H, Henriksen O (1994) Brain lactate increases with immaturity of healthy neonates. *Ped Res* **35**: 276.
3. Groenendaal F, Veenhoven RH, van der Grond J, Jansen GH, Witkamp TD, de Vries LS (1994) Cerebral lactate and N-acetylaspartate/choline ratios in asphyxiated full-term neonates demonstrated in vivo using proton magnetic resonance spectroscopy. *Ped Res* **35**: 148–151.

Proton MRS studies in Huntington's disease

M. Lowry,[1]* O. Quarrell,[2] L.W. Turnbull[1] and A. Horsman[1]

[1]*Yorkshire Cancer Research Campaign, and University of Hull Centre for Magnetic Resonance Investigations, Hull Royal Infirmary, Hull HU3 2JZ, UK*
[2]*Centre for Human Genetics, Sheffield, UK*

We studied six patients in the early stage of Huntington's disease, together with six unaffected normal subjects. Localized spectra were acquired from 4-ml voxels encompassing the combined putamen and caudate head using STEAM with TR = 1 s and TE = 40 ms. Metabolite concentrations were calculated using tissue water as an internal reference. Although MRI showed minor degenerative changes in the basal ganglia, we were unable to detect any differences in the neuronal marker, N-acetylaspartate, between the two groups (patient mean ± SD, 10.7 ± 2.1 µmol g wet wt^{-1}; controls 11.4 ± 1.3). Similarly, we were unable to detect differences in either choline or creatine. In contrast to other studies, we were unable to detect any increase in lactate content of the basal ganglia in these patients with early stage disease. We conclude that proton MR spectroscopy will not be a suitable technique to detect the very early changes in asymptomatic patients identified as having the mutation.

Keywords: proton MRS, N-acetylaspartate, Huntington's disease.

INTRODUCTION

Huntington's disease (HD) is a genetic disorder causing progressive neurodegeneration, characteristically in the basal ganglia. It is associated with an abnormal gene located on chromosome 4, but the molecular pathology of the disorder remains unknown. Because the disease causes neuronal loss through degeneration, it was anticipated that N-acetylaspartate (NAA) measurements might provide a diagnostic indication of presymptomatic HD in subjects at risk. Such an indication would be invaluable in cases where predictive testing by molecular genetic techniques is not possible. In reflecting the extent of neurodegeneration, results of MRS could possibly provide a better indication of likely time of onset of symptoms than other methods. Another expectation was that the neurotransmitter glutamate and its precursor glutamine could be detected in the basal ganglia.

* Address for correspondence: Centre for MRI, Hull Royal Infirmary, Anlaby Road, Hull HU3 2JZ, UK.

METHODS

Six male patients with HD aged between 32 and 49 years were studied. They had duration of disease between 2 and 11 years and their Shoulsan and Fahn disability scores [1] ranged between 5 and 13. The diagnosis of HD was confirmed in all six cases by the identification of the abnormal gene on chromosome 4 [2]. Six age-matched normal volunteers were also studied.

Images and spectra were acquired using an 1.5-T GE Signa Advantage with a standard 27-cm-diameter quadrature head coil. The basal ganglia were identified from T_2-weighted fast spin-echo images. Localized water-suppressed spectra (TR = 1 s, TE = 40 ms, NEX 1024) were acquired using STEAM from a 3–5-ml voxel encompassing the combined putamen and caudate head. Subsequently, a water reference spectrum was acquired at the same TE but with an extended TR (10 s) and only four averages. The reference provided the calibration for calculation of metabolite concentration [3]. Spectral processing included 3 Hz Gaussian apodization, zero-filling to 4096

Table 1. Metabolite concentrations determined in basal ganglia of HD patients and normal volunteers. Each value is the mean ± SD for six subjects.

	N-acetyl-aspartate	Creatine [μmol/g wet wt)$^{-1}$]	Choline
Normal volunteers	11.4 ± 1.3	10.0 ± 1.4	1.9 ± 0.3
HD patients	10.7 ± 2.1	8.7 ± 1.6	1.9 ± 0.4

data points, and Fourier transformation. Peak areas were obtained from the manually phased spectra by integration.

RESULTS

Axial T_2-weighted images of the HD patients demonstrated minor changes in signal intensity and anatomical organization of the basal ganglia. These changes may be associated with both HD specific events and generalized atrophy.

Spectra from the normal subjects and HD patients showed similar peak intensities for the three major metabolites (Fig. 1). Also detected were smaller peaks originating from amino acids and mobile lipids. In practice, however, although glutamate and glutamine peaks could be seen in the spectra from normal subjects and (less clearly) in those from patients, quantification of these peaks was not possible due to lack of resolution and the proximity of larger adjacent peaks. Contrary to recent reports for occipital white matter of HD patients [4], we were not able to detect lactate in any of the patients studied. The mean metabolite concentrations calculated from the spectra are shown in Table 1. There were no significant differences between patients and controls in concentrations of N-acetylaspartate, creatine, or choline.

DISCUSSION

The study of HD patients by proton MRS necessitates the consideration of several technical difficulties. HD eventually causes loss of those neurones in the basal ganglia controlling motor activity, leading to the characteristic chorea associated with later stages of the disease. Thus, only patients with early stage disease can be studied easily. Second, the basal ganglia are small, located close to the ventricles, and may contain significant quantities of iron. These factors can influence signal-to-noise ratio (S/N), homogeneity, and the quality of water suppression. In this study, we were

unable to acquire spectra of sufficiently high S/N from voxels containing only putamen or caudate.

NAA appears to be restricted to neurones in adult brain [5], yet we observed no decrease in this metabolite in HD patients, even though there is significant neuronal loss. It is possible that partial volume played a significant role in decreasing the sensitivity of the measurements, in that shrinkage of the basal ganglia would cause a concomitant increase in the contribution of other structures to the voxel. However, autopsy studies have shown that the primary effect of HD is on cell bodies, whereas axons remain intact [6]. It is possible that NAA is located predominantly in axons and, thus, would not decrease on loss of the cell body.

The lack of any significant differences between the spectra of basal ganglia in HD patients and controls is surprising particularly because a number of *in vitro* studies have demonstrated a functional impairment of mitochondria in HD [7] which might be expected to reveal itself in the proton spectrum. In support, previous proton MRS studies by Jenkins et al. have shown a significant elevation of lactate in both the occipital cortex and basal ganglia [4] of HD patients. There are, however, some important differences between these studies and our own. Jenkins et al. [4] acquired their spectra using an echo time of 272 ms, thus optimizing the detection of lactate. It is possible that, at the short TE used in our own studies, a resonance from lactate was masked by broad peaks from mobile lipid. They also used a much larger voxel, 14 ml, which may have included tissue from structures other than the basal ganglia.

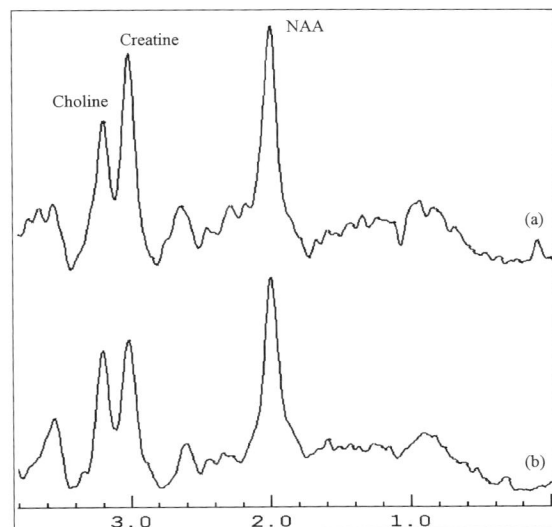

Fig. 1. Representative spectra of the basal ganglia acquired from (a) a normal volunteer and (b) an Huntington's disease patient.

It is concluded that MRS studies of HD patients are practicable, despite the requirement for them to remain still for some time, but that MRS is not a suitable technique to detect minor changes occurring during the early development of HD.

REFERENCES

1. Shoulson I, Fehn S (1979) Huntington's Disease: clinical care and evaluation. *Neurology* **29**: 1–3.
2. Warner JP, Barron LH, Brock DJH (1993) A new polymerase chain reaction (PCR) assay for the trinucleotide repeat that is unstable and expanded on Huntington's disease chromosomes. *Mol. Cell Probes* **7**: 235–239.
3. Barker PB, Soher BJ, Blackband SJ, Chatham JC, Mathews VP, Bryan RN (1993) Quantitation of proton NMR spectra of the human brain usingtissue water as an internal concentration reference. *NMR Biomed* **6**: 89–94.
4. Jenkins BG, Koroshetz WJ, Beal MF et al. (1993) Assessment of energy metabolism defects in Huntington's disease using ^{31}P and ^{1}H localized spectroscopy and functional MRI. Possible therapy with coenzyme Q10. *Proc Soc Mag Res Med* p. 134.
5. Urenjak J, Williams SR, Gadian DG et al. (1993) Proton nuclear magnetic resonance spectroscopy unambiguously identifies different neural cell types. *J Neurosci* **13**: 981–989.
6. Brownell A-L, Hamberg LM, Hantraye P et al. (1992) Combined assessment of blood volume, flow and glucose utilization in a primate model of Huntington's disease. *Proc Soc Mag Reson Med* p. 510.
7. Parker WD, Boyson SJ, Luder AS et al. (1990) Evidence for a defect in NADH: Ubiquinone oxidoreductase (complex I) in Huntington's disease. *Neurology* **40**: 1231–1234.

Quantitative proton MRS of brain tumors reveals increased choline T_2 in meningiomas

D.J. Manton, M. Lowry,[*] S.J. Blackband and A. Horsman

Yorkshire Cancer Research Campaign, and University of Hull Centre for Magnetic Resonance Investigations, Hull Royal Infirmary, Hull HU3 2JZ, UK

Quantitative proton spectroscopy was performed on 26 volunteers and 9 patients using STEAM. Voxels (8 ml) were localized within white matter or meningioma and water-suppressed spectra acquired with TR = 2 s at three echo times. Concentrations were calculated using individual relaxation parameter values with tissue water as an internal reference. Compared to white matter, meningiomas were characterized by an increased choline/creatine ratio, the absence of N-acetylasparate, and the presence of alanine. Further, the T_2 of choline and its concentration were both significantly greater in meningiomas than white matter ($p < 0.01$). Thus, the high choline/creatine ratio seen in meningioma spectra is the consequence of a greater concentration and a longer T_2. The longer T_2 may reflect differences in the relative proportions of choline-containing compounds. Our data demonstrate that individual measurements of relaxation parameters are important for long echo spectra and may reveal important metabolic information.

Keywords: proton MRS, quantitation, choline, T_2 relaxation, meningioma.

INTRODUCTION

Previous studies have demonstrated that spectra obtained from meningiomas differ from normal brain [1, 2]. The observed differences were obtained primarily from investigations using peak–area ratios, an approach which reduces the information available and may lead to misinterpretation of data. The differences could be the result of changes in metabolite concentration and/or differences in relaxation parameter values. Determination of these parameters would allow a more complete interpretation of the spectral differences to be made. In this study, we have used a recently described method [3] to determine the concentrations of the major metabolites in normal brain and meningiomas. The technique requires, in addition to signal amplitudes, estimates of both T_1 and T_2 for each metabolite. The results confirm that significant differences in glucose metabolism and membrane turnover exist in meningiomas.

* Address for correspondence: Centre for MRI, Hull Royal Infirmary, Anlaby Road, Hull HU3 2JZ, UK.

METHODS

Twenty-six normal volunteers and nine patients were investigated. The patients were examined prior to any surgical intervention and the diagnosis confirmed subsequently by histological examination of biopsy specimens. Images and spectra were acquired using an 1.5-T GE Signa Advantage with a standard 27-cm-diameter quadrature head coil. In all volunteers, an 8-cm^3 volume of interest (VOI) was selected in occipital white matter; in patients, the VOI was chosen to lie entirely within the boundaries of the lesion. Water-suppressed localized spectra were acquired using the Stimulated Echo Acquisition Mode STEAM sequence [4]. Spectra for T_2 determination were collected at echo times (TE) of 272, 136, and 30 ms (TR = 2 s). Each localized spectrum was followed by the acquisition of a water reference spectrum collected at the same TE but with an extended TR (10 s) and only four averages. Metabolite T_1 values for normal white matter were obtained from an additional series of studies in which six localized spectra were acquired with TRs of 0.8, 1.0, 1.2, 2.0, 5.0, and 10 s with a TE of 136 ms. Spectral processing included a B_0 correction, a convolution difference filter, 2 Hz Gaussian apodization, and zero

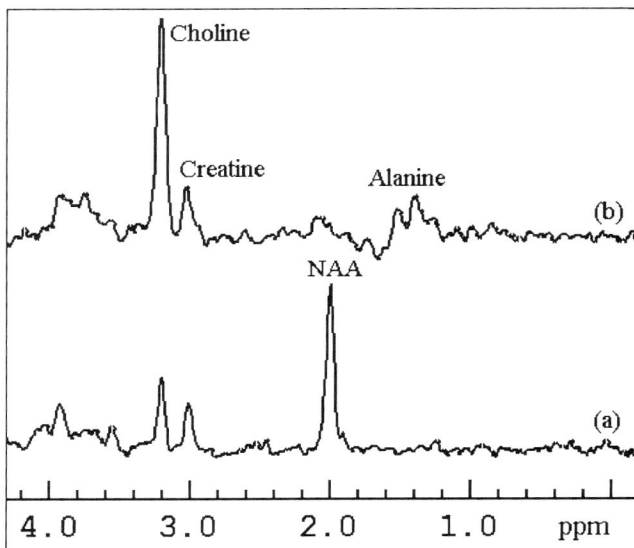

Fig. 1. Proton spectra of (a) normal white matter and (b) meningioma acquired from a 2 × 2 × 2-cm³ voxel using STEAM with TR = 2 s and TE = 272 ms.

filling before Fourier transformation. Peak areas were obtained by integration after manual phasing using a fixed width of ±0.09 ppm about the peak centers.

Relaxation parameters were estimated using an iterative nonlinear least squares algorithm, and the output used for the calculation of metabolite concentrations [3]. Tissue water was used as an internal concentration reference, with values calculated from published data [5, 6].

RESULTS

Representative spectra acquired from normal white matter and a meningioma are shown in Fig. 1. The major differences between spectra from the tumors and those from white matter are the almost complete absence of N-acetylasparate (NAA), a large increase in

the choline peak, and the appearance of a peak from the glycolytic end product, alanine. Lactate was detected in combination with alanine in three tumors.

Results of T_1 and T_2 calculations are presented in Table 1. Values of both parameters determined for white matter were similar to those reported elsewhere in the literature [3, 7]. We were able to obtain choline T_2 relaxation estimates for all the meningiomas; however, in most cases, it was impossible to determine values for either creatine or NAA due to the absence of these peaks from the spectra, particularly at the longer echo times. The only difference observed was for choline, where the T_2 value was 50% longer than for white matter. The metabolite concentrations determined using these parameters confirm the greater concentration of choline in meningiomas as suggested by the much larger peak in spectra of these tumors (Table 2). The concentrations of creatine and NAA are much lower than normal brain.

DISCUSSION

Although previous authors have shown spectra of meningiomas to be different from those of normal brain [1, 2], none have determined concentrations *in vivo* using tumor-specific relaxation times. For spectra acquired with short echo times, the use of T_2 values determined in normal tissue is a reasonable alternative because the influence of T_2 is minor under these conditions. However, acquisition of spectra at longer echo times may be necessary in these tumors to unequivocally determine the presence of alanine. Additionally, the relaxation times of tumor metabolites may provide useful information by themselves. Our results show that the differences between the spectra of normal brain and meningiomas are not solely due to differences in the concentrations of these metabolites. In meningiomas, both the T_2 and concentration of choline are greater than in normal brain;

Table 1. Relaxation parameters for normal brain and meningiomas.

Site	Parameter	n	Choline	Creatine [ms]	NAA [ms]	Water
White matter	T_1	6	1558 ± 244	1673 ± 258	1631 ± 197	966 ± 52
White matter	T_2	20	309 ± 84	195 ± 41	369 ± 124	100 ± 8
Meningioma	T_2	9	459 ± 146[a]	168 ± 44 (5)	N.D.[b]	107 ± 29

Note: T_2 and T_1 values were calculated for each subject from three to six spectra collected at a range of TE and TR values, respectively. Each value is the mean ± S.D. for the number of subjects indicated.
[a] $p \leq 0.01$ compared to white matter.
[b] N.D. = not detected.

Table 2. Metabolite concentrations in normal brain and meningiomas.

Site	n	Water (assumed)	Choline [μmol (g wet wt)$^{-1}$]	Creatine [μmol (g wet wt)$^{-1}$]	NAA
White matter	20	39200	2.0 ± 0.4	7.3 ± 1.1	11.4 ± 1.4
Meningioma	9	46337	3.3 ± 0.9[a]	3.7 ± 1.7 (5)[a]	N.D.[b]

Note: Concentrations were calculated for each subject using the mean T_1 value determined in white matter to correct for partial saturation. Each value is the mean ± S.D. for the number of subjects indicated.
[a] $p \leq 0.02$ compared to white matter.
[b] N.D. not detected.

consequently, the peak area at long echo times is considerably greater.

The mechanism of the observed difference in the T_2 of choline in meningiomas is unclear. However, variation in the relative concentrations of metabolites contributing to the peak would lead to differences in average T_2 if these compounds exhibited different relaxation rates. Phosphorylcholine and glycerophosphorylcholine, compounds involved in membrane lipid turnover, both contain the N-trimethylammonio functional group responsible for the peak at 3.21 ppm and may have different T_2 values. These two compounds also contribute to the phosphomonoester and phosphodiester peaks in ^{31}P spectra. Increases in the former peak in many tumors has been associated with changes in membrane metabolism [8]. Thus, the longer T_2 of the choline peak observed in meningiomas could be a consequence of the increase in membrane turnover associated with tumor growth.

An important characteristic of meningioma spectra is the presence of a peak from alanine, yet little is known regarding its production by these tumors. In other tissues, glutamine is a major precursor of alanine via the enzymes glutaminase and glutamate-pyruvate transaminase. The operation of the malate/aspartate shuttle in this pathway allows the mitochondrial reoxidation of glycolytically produced reducing equivalents. By producing alanine, meningiomas are able to obtain fourfold more ATP per molecule of glucose than if they produced lactate. Further the conversion of glutamine to alanine is also an ATP-producing process. The increased ATP synthesis obtained through alanine production and glutamine oxidation would enable meningiomas to maintain an intracellular envi-

ronment suitable for cell function and division and prevent the onset of necrosis.

In conclusion, we have measured metabolite concentrations in normal brain and in meningiomas using individually determined values for T_2 relaxation times. The measurements demonstrate that differences in T_2 relaxation can be an important factor in these calculations and may reveal new information concerning tumor cell metabolism.

REFERENCES

1. Gill SS, Thomas DGT, Van Bruggen N et al. (1990) Proton MR spectroscopy of intracranial tumours: In vivo and in vitro studies. *J Comput Assist Tomogr* **14:** 497–504.
2. Kugel HK, Heindel W, Ernestus RI et al. (1992) Human brain tumors: Spectral patterns detected with localized H-1 MR spectroscopy. *Radiology* **183:** 701–709.
3. Barker PB, Soher BJ, Blackband SJ et al. (1993) Quantitation of proton NMR spectra of the human brain using tissue water as an internal concentration reference. *NMR Biomed* **6:** 89–94.
4. Frahm J, Bruhn H, Gyngell ML et al. (1989) Localized high-resolution proton NMR spectroscopy using stimulated echoes: Initial applications to human brain *in vivo*. *Magn Reson Med* **9:** 79–93.
5. Lowry OH, Berger SJ, Chi MM-Y et al. (1977) Diversity of metabolic patterns in human brain tumors. I. High energy phosphate compounds and basic composition. *J Neurochem* **29:** 959–977.
7. Kreis R, Ernst T, Ross BD (1993) Absolute quantitation of water and metabolites in the human brain. II. Metabolite concentrations. *J Magn Reson B* **102:** 9–19.
8. de Certaines JD, Larsen VA, Podo F et al. (1993) *In vivo* 31P MRS of experimental tumours. *NMR Biomed* **6:** 345–365.

Whither human cardiac spectroscopy?

Paul A. Bottomley

G.E. Research and Development Center, Schenectady NY 12301, USA

Human cardiac magnetic resonance (MR) spectroscopy is presently comprised, almost exclusively, of phosphorus (^{31}P) studies. These provide access to supply-side energy metabolism in the anterior myocardium of patients with hypertrophy, with cardiomyopathies including heart failure, with heart transplants, and with ischemic disease and myocardial infarction. A link between reduced phosphocreatine (PCr) to adenosine triphosphate (ATP) ratios and heart failure has been identified which might assist diagnosis in the presence of other confounding factors. PCr/ATP is often reduced in transplanted hearts for reasons not understood, but the ratio is presently an unreliable predictor of significant histological rejection for many patients. Myocardial infarction may reduce overall metabolite levels. In reversible myocardial ischemia, ^{31}P exercise stress-testing can produce reversible PCr/ATP reductions, at least in anterior disease: these seem to be specific for ischemic disease and may be helpful, especially if new technologies such as phased detector arrays and Overhauser enhancement can provide access to more of the heart. Human cardiac spectroscopy with nuclei other than ^{31}P may potentially access citric acid cycle metabolites, oxymyoglobin and deoxymyoglobin, and creatine levels, which may also be altered in heart failure.

Keywords: to come.

INTRODUCTION

Energy metabolism has been the focus of human cardiac NMR spectroscopy [1]. The heart consumes more energy per unit tissue mass than any organ, and problems involving energy supply and demand are implicated in common disorders such as ischemic heart disease, myocardial infarction, and heart failure. Energy for muscular contraction, and many other processes besides, derives from adenosine triphosphate (ATP), which is broken into adenosine diphosphate and inorganic phosphate (P_i). ATP is maintained by the citric acid cycle which ultimately utilizes carbohydrates, glycogen, and fats as fuel sources, and, during short anaerobic periods, by the creatine kinase reaction

phosphocreatine (PCr) + ADP $\leftrightarrow$ ATP + creatine (Cr)

or from glycolysis, producing lactate.

Phosphorus (^{31}P) NMR spectroscopy permits direct measurements of the supply side of these energetic reactions: of naturally abundant ATP and PCr in the heart [2], and, albeit more difficult due to problems with overlapping 2,3-diphosphoglycerate resonances (DPG) from blood, of P_i when it is elevated and of intracellular pH, when the chemical shift of P_i can be measured. Carbon (^{13}C) NMR spectroscopy can see glycogen and fats, although the latter may be indistinguishable from metabolically relatively immobile stores [3], whereas proton (^{1}H) NMR could potentially provide measures of Cr and lactate, as well as the ubiquitous fat. Recent animal experiments also suggest a role for ^{1}H NMR in measuring myocardial oxygenation via oxymyoglobin and deoxymyoglobin resonances [4].

The myocardial concentrations of most of these metabolites is of the order of only micromoles per gram wet weight [5]. It is, therefore, a struggle to acquire their cardiac NMR spectra in tolerable human exams of about 1 h in contemporary whole-body magnets of 1.5–4 T, even with spatial resolution of about 10 ml [6] or more. The outstanding questions are: "What has been learned from patient studies so far?" "Is there a role for the technique in the clinic?" "What technical advances might be anticipated?" "What should be done next?" [1].

Address for correspondance: Department of Radiology, Johns Hopkins University, 600 North Wolfe Street, Baltimore, MD 21287-0843, U.S.A.

TECHNIQUES

Localization

All ^{31}P and ^{13}C *in vivo* human cardiac spectra to date have been acquired with surface detection coils located on the chest close to the anterior wall [2, 3] due to their superior signal-to-noise (S/N) performance relative to larger volume coils. In the limit where sample magnetic losses dominate the noise detected by the fully loaded coil (as suggested but not proven by a large decrease in coil Q when the coil is loaded with the chest), optimum sensitivity obtains when the coil diameter is approximately equal to the depth of the tissue of interest [7], which results in a coil of about 6–16 cm for the heart. Even so, the limited field of view offered by surface coils means that they must be carefully positioned using image guidance. A separate large NMR transmitter coil should be used to provide uniform excitation and avoid spatially dependent partial saturation [8]. Use of a prone versus a supine patient orientation, to decrease the coil-to-myocardium distance, and cardiac-synchronous acquisition are simple tricks which commonly afford significant sensitivity gains [8].

^{31}P spectra have been localized to the cardiac wall via DRESS (depth-resolved surface coil spectroscopy [2, 9]), ISIS (image selected *in vivo* spectroscopy [10]), 1D CSI (one-dimensional chemical shift imaging [8, 11]), the RFZ (rotating frame zeugmatography [12, 13]), and the 3D CSI (three-dimensional CSI [8, 14, 15]) techniques. DRESS and ISIS are single-volume-element (voxel) methods and are generally not optimal for studies in which the location of a metabolic abnormality is uncertain a priori, or for dynamic studies in which information is desired from multiple regions simultaneously [11]. 1D CSI, RFZ, and 3D CSI are all multiple-voxel techniques. 3D CSI provides full 3D resolution, but a large number of acquisitions, usually equal to at least the number of voxels in the final data set, are necessary, which may limit some studies, especially those in which transient changes are being monitored [11].

Distortion

Quantities representing PCr, ATP, etc., concentrations, and ratios are conventionally derived from integrals from the corresponding spectral resonances [16]. Myocardial values are almost invariably distorted by such factors as partial saturation and contamination from blood in the ventricles (^{31}P NMR) or pericardial fat (^{1}H, ^{13}C). Such distortion likely accounts for the published myocardial PCr/ATP values in normal subjects ranging from 0.9 ± 0.3 [14] to 2.1 ± 0.4 [17]. The 95% confidence intervals for the T_1 of myocardial PCr

is 4.4 ± 0.5 s compared to about 2.4 ± 0.6 s for ATP (γ or β) [18]. Hence, for repetition periods T_R gated at, say, once per cardiac cycle, the PCr/ATP ratio is reduced from its true value by a factor of between 1 and 2 depending on the precise T_R and excitation flip angle, α, employed [1, 19].

Fully relaxed, undistorted signals, S_0 can be derived from the T_1 values and α:

$$S_0 = \frac{S[1 - \cos \alpha \exp (-T_R/T_1)]}{[1 - \exp (-T_R/T_1)] \sin \alpha}$$

where S is the distorted signal and T_1 is generally assumed constant among study groups [19]. For myocardial PCr/ATP measurements by ^{31}P NMR, an alternative method of correcting the distortion is to directly measure the saturation factors for each subject from the ratios of short-T_R signals to fully relaxed ones. This can be accommodated in a few minutes using unlocalized, uniformly excited, surface coil spectra [11] if it is assumed that the ratio $T_1(PCr)/T_1(ATP)$ is similar in the chest and heart tissue that contribute to the unlocalized spectrum, which seems to be the case [18, 19]. Errors are minimized in both methods of correction by using small- or Ernst-angle excitation [1].

Blood contamination distorts myocardial PCr/ATP values in ^{31}P spectra because blood contains ATP but no PCr [20]. The distortion is corrected by quantifying the DPG resonances (at about 5.4 and 6.3 ppm relative to PCr) and subtracting about 15% of the result from the apparent ATP, because [ATP]/[DPG] ~ 0.3 [9, 21–23] and DPG has two phosphates. Blood corrections have a smaller effect on PCr/ATP values, increasing them about 13% on average [1].

Normal ^{31}P NMR parameters

When the above distortion factors are accounted for in human cardiac ^{31}P NMR spectroscopy, a mean normal myocardial PCr/ATP ratio of 1.83 ± 0.12 is obtained [1, 6, 20, 21, 24, 25]. This should be the best estimate of the ratio to date, as ATP and PCr are likely 100% NMR visible [26] and because PCr loss is probably inevitable in assays of surgical biopsy specimens [27]. Corrected measurements of the metabolite ratios can be translated into metabolite concentrations if measurements are done on a concentration standard and the tissue volume contributing to the heart spectrum is determined [15, 28]. Preliminary values of 11 ± 3 μmol g^{-1} for PCr and 7 ± 2 μmol g^{-1} wet weight for ATP agree [15, 28].

The forward flux of myocardial PCr through the creatine kinase reaction in the heart can be determined with spatially localized saturation transfer NMR experiments, wherein PCr is measured in the presence and absence of saturating irradiation applied to the γ-ATP resonance [29]. The forward rate is about 0.5 ± 0.2 s⁻¹ or 6 ± 3 μmol/(g wet wt. s), consistent with animal work [29].

Pi is often undetectable in the normal heart, even with decoupling [21], and may be partially NMR-invisible [26]. The presence of neighboring DPG resonances [30] also makes quantification difficult, with best estimates for P_i/PCr being 0.14 ± 0.06 [21], or at least <0.25 [30]. The intracellular pH, determined from the chemical shift of P_i, when detectable, is about 7.15 [21, 30].

New advances

Phased arrays of surface detection coils, as pioneered for conventional NMR imaging [7], can be adapted for cardiac spectroscopy [31]. The advantages are that they eliminate the need for careful patient positioning and they can provide a (quadrature) sensitivity improvement of up to about √2 relative to the best positioned single surface coil of the same diameter as

one of the phased-array component surface coils. A four-coil ³¹P cardiac phased array has been implemented on normal volunteers (Fig. 1) but not yet in a clinical setting [31].

A significant sensitivity improvement in cardiac ³¹P spectroscopy can also be realized from the proton nuclear Overhauser effect (nOe). This is about 60% for PCr (η ≈ 0.6) and 30–60% for ATP (η ≈ 0.3–0.6) [32, 33]. Care is needed to avoid excessive RF power deposition when applying the requisite ¹H irradiation. Differences in nOe for PCr and ATP may distort the observed PCr/ATP ratio, necessitating additional corrections for comparative studies [32]. A net potential sensitivity improvement of about 2.3-fold is, thus, anticipated from implementation of both phased-array coil technology and nOe.

Finally, signal loss and data scatter resulting from misset or nonoptimum flip angles can be avoided, and the time required for setting up pulses in patient studies eliminated altogether through use of adiabatic

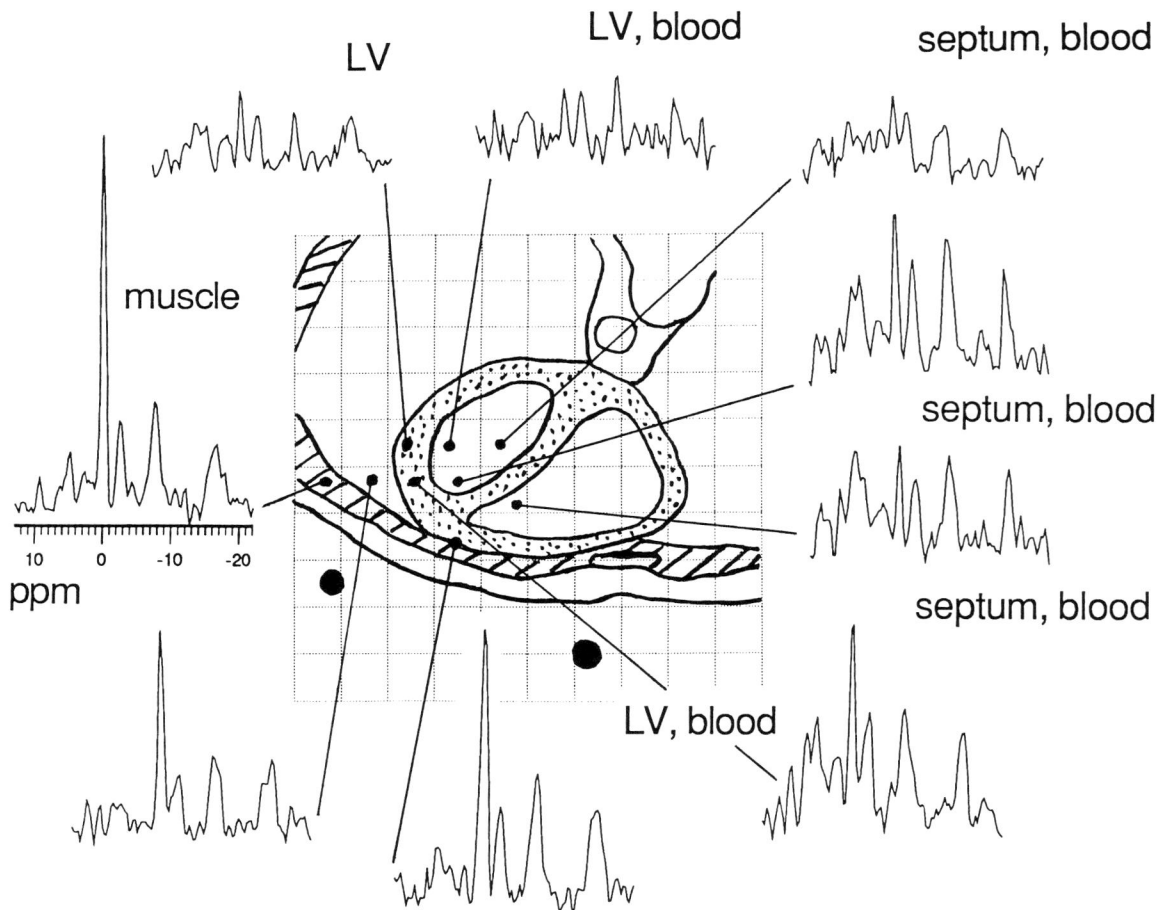

Fig. 1. ³¹P NMR spectra acquired with a ³¹P cardiac phased array of four 6.5-cm-diameter surface detector coils. For a CSI study, the four data sets must be first reconstructed and phased prior to combination into a single set with improved S/N. (Reproduced from Ref. 31 with permission.)

low-angle pulses with the flip angle chosen to minimize signal loss over the range of uncertainties of the T_1's of the moieties of interest [18].

PATIENT STUDIES

Cardiac NMR spectroscopy studies of patients have thus far been limited to ^{31}P.

Cardiomyopathy

Despite human surgical biopsy studies [27, 34] and ^{31}P NMR studies of animal cardiomyopathic models of cardiomyopathy showing reduced high-energy phosphates, *in vivo* ^{31}P NMR studies of patients are mixed [1]. Myocardial PCr/ATP ratios were reported as lower in cardiomyopathy due to muscular dystrophy, beriberi, and amyloidosis [17], in hypertrophic cardiomyopathy (HCM) [9, 17, 21], and in heart failure patients

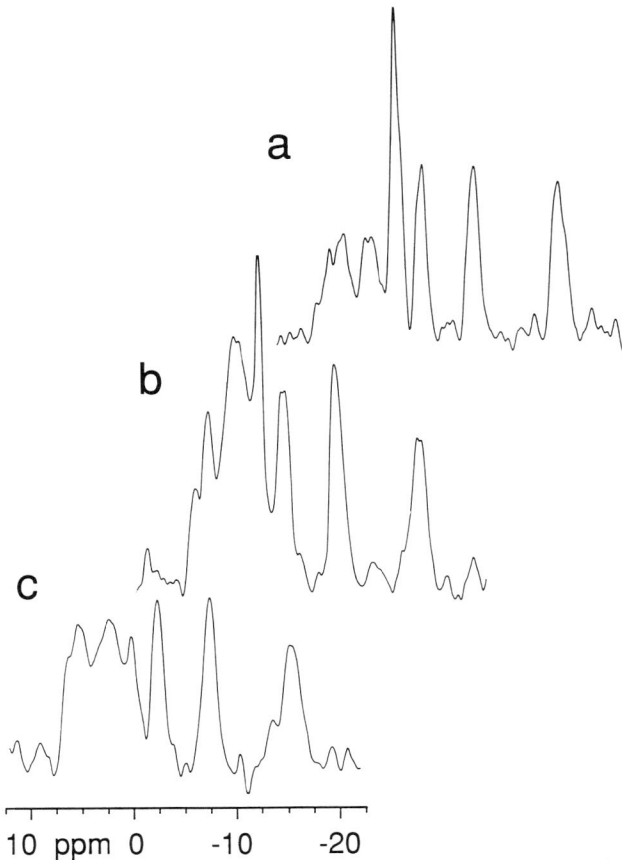

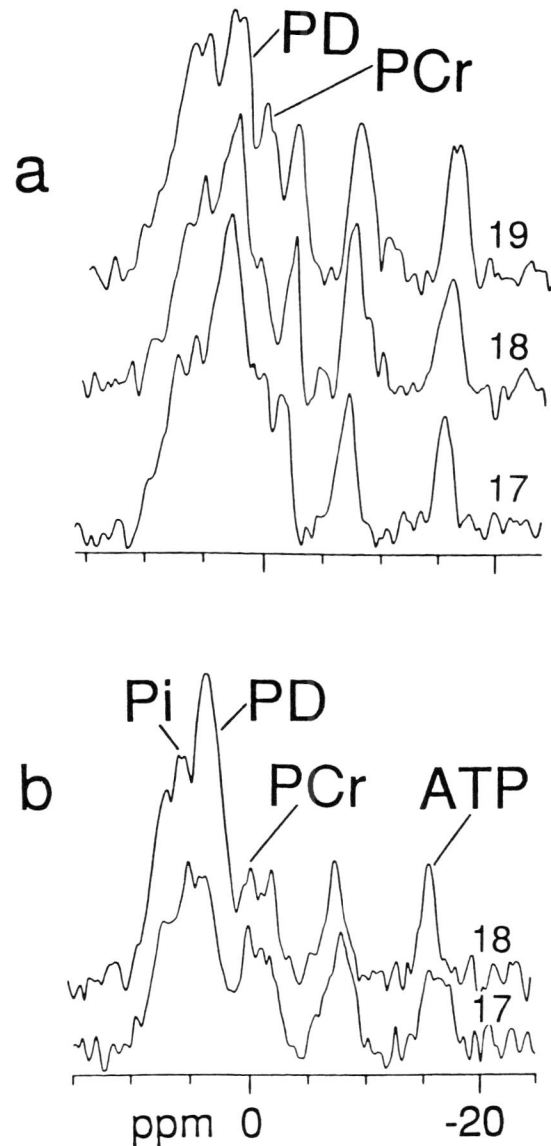

Fig. 2. Cardiac ^{31}P NMR spectra from the anterior left ventricular wall of (a) a normal volunteer, (b) a patient with DCM and coronary artery disease, and (c) a patient with DCM not due to ichemic disease. The PCr/ATP ratio is lower in the patients. (Reproduced from Ref. 20 with permission.)

Fig. 3. Adjacent cardiac ^{31}P NMR spectra from 1-cm-thick sections through the anterior left ventricular wall of two patients with moderate rejection with histological evidence of myocyte necrosis. The PCr/ATP ratio is reduced to 0.9 ± 0.04 in (a) and 0.9 ± 0.3 in (b), compared with a normal range of 1.93 ± 0.21. Phosphodiester resonances (PD) are also elevated. (Reproduced from Ref. 24 with permission.)

with left ventricular hypertrophy (LVH) [13] and dilated cardiomyopathy (DCM) (Fig. 2) [20, 25]. Other studies report no significant PCr/ATP changes in LVH [14, 17] or DCM [14, 17, 21, 35, 36]. Myocardial PCr/ATP ratios correlated neither with ejection fractions nor fractional shortening [20, 25, 35] nor etiology [20]. However, PCr/ATP changes were linked to advanced heart failure in two studies: (1) PCr/ATP was

Table 1. Anterior myocardial PCr/ATP ratios in normal volunteers and patients with anterior ischemic disease, nonischemic heart disease, and with fixed thallium radionuclide defects indicative of myocardial infarction (MI).

Phase	Controls	Ischemia	Non-CAD	MI	Ref.
Rest	1.72 ± 0.15	1.45 ± 0.31	1.59 ± 0.31		11
Exercise	1.74 ± 0.17	0.91 ± 0.24[a]	1.55 ± 0.24		11
Recovery	1.77 ± 0.16	1.27 ± 0.38	1.54 ± 0.28		11
Change	1%	−37%	−3%		
Rest	1.80 ± 0.28	1.56 ± 0.19		1.18 ± 0.28	45
Exercise	1.84 ± 0.24	0.94 ± 0.27[a]		1.12 ± 0.24	45
Change	1%	−40%		−5%	

[a]$P < 0.001$ versus rest.

lower in valve disease patients undergoing treatment for heart failure but not in patients not requiring therapy [13] and (2) declining PCr/ATP ratios correlated with the severity of failure indexed by the New York Heart Association (NYHA) clinical classification scheme [25].

Two factors likely account for much of the variability in findings. First, it seems that the range and severity of heart failure present in the study groups was a critical factor, as evidenced by the observations that PCr/ATP was not altered in mild failure [13, 25] and that statistical changes in PCr/ATP are masked when patients are not grouped according to the severity of symptoms of failure [18]. The other factor is statistical sensitivity [20], as evidenced by the lower mean myocardial PCr/ATP ratios in virtually all studies [1]. Of the causes, it is possible that the lower energy reserve suggested by the reduced myocardial PCr/ATP in the more advanced stages of heart failure, is related to contractile dysfunction [37, 38]. A remaining question, though, is why ^{31}P metabolic changes are not seen earlier, even prior to the onset of failure, and, in light of some HCM studies showing reduced PCr/ATP in the absence of severe failure [21], whether other factors may be involved.

^{31}P NMR might be useful for identifying heart failure in the presence of confounding factors including age [13] and lung disease or for the management of valve patients to minimize permanent damage to the heart [39], but much work would be needed to define the conditions under which benefit might result.

Heart transplants

The idea that ^{31}P NMR might have a role in the management of transplant patients stems from animal studies showing PCr/P$_i$ or PCr/ATP reductions in acute rejection [40–42]. The standard method for diagnosis of rejection requiring augmented immuno-suppressive therapy in transplant patients is histological evidence of myocyte necrosis in endomyocardial biopsies obtained from regular cardiac catheterization. Conference abstracts, from 1988 on, have generally confirmed that PCr/ATP or PCr/P$_i$ are reduced in transplanted human hearts (Fig. 3) [1]. However, ^{31}P NMR does not appear to be a reliable predictor of significant histological rejection, in the clinical sense, as agreement between NMR and histology may be realized in only about 60%–70% of cases [24].

Nevertheless, the cause of the metabolic changes are not easily linked to other heart disease [24], and the clinical problem of relating the metabolic indices to the histology illustrates the fundamental difficulty that dead cells seen histologically would have no PCr or ATP that could influence the PCr/ATP ratio seen by ^{31}P NMR. P$_i$ might index necrosis better if difficulties in its quantification were ameliorated [1]. If the PCr/ATP changes mark a rejection phase preceding cell death, studies involving a more frequent NMR/biopsy schedule of NMR exams and biopsies would need to be explored to establish the correlation. The cause and effect of the reduced myocardial energy reserve in these patients is an outstanding problem.

Coronary artery disease

In human myocardial infarction, PCr/ATP ratios are commonly unaltered [25, 30, 43]. Animal studies show ATP and PCr depletion in the initial hours of ischemic injury [44], so the observed PCr/ATP ratio in human infarction must reflect surrounding metabolically normal, though possibly jeopardized, myocardium. However, the overall PCr and ATP levels would be expected to be lower in proportion to the infarction size [1]. This is supported by the observed correlation between the ^{31}P NMR ATP level and estimates of the size of perfusion deficits derived from radionuclide images [43].

In patients with ischemic heart disease involving severe coronary stenosis, the resting myocardial PCr/ATP in the affected region is nearly normal [11, 25]. However, reversible decreases can be elicited by stress-testing of the patient in the magnet, for example, using isometric hand-grip exercise (Table 1) [11]. A continuous exercise at 30% of the maximum force increases the heart-rate blood-pressure product by about 30% and can induce some vasoconstriction when significant stenosis is present. In patients with $\geq 70\%$ stenoses of the main anterior vessels, a 37% decrease in anterior wall PCr/ATP was observed during exercise, whereas the same protocol produced no change in patients with nonischemic disease and in normal controls [11]. Similar results have been reported at conferences [45]. The lack of stress-induced changes seen in normal controls [11, 46] and in patients with nonischemic disease [11], cardiomyopathy [36], and with fixed perfusion deficits on radionuclide imaging [45] suggest that the stress-induced PCr/ATP reductions may be specific to ischemic disease.

A clinical ^{31}P NMR stress test would be enhanced by extension of the technology to the inferior and posterior walls, which the technical advances alluded to above may help address. Studies comparing the sensitivity and cost efficacy of the procedure relative to existing modalities would be needed.

OTHER NUCLEI

Because the isotopic abundance of ^{13}C is only 1.1%, natural abundance ^{13}C NMR of energy-rich metabolites like glucose and glutamate are unrealistic in an hour-long human study. Fatty acid resonances, much from pericardial fat, dominate the localized natural abundance ^{13}C human heart spectrum: Glycogen may be visible with ^{1}H decoupling and nOe [3]. Access to glycolytic and citric acid cycle intermediaries generally requires infusion of ^{13}C-labeled substrates such as glucose, which, animal studies suggest, may be highly sensitive to conditions involving low blood flow [47]. This provides the impetus for improving ^{1}H/^{13}C detection methods to enable better sensitivity for human studies [48].

Fat resonances also dominate human ^{1}H cardiac spectra [49] and fall in a spectral region neighboring on many metabolites of interest, including lactate and glutamate. Total creatine should be accessible however, and is expected to be lower in heart failure and cardiomyopathy [34, 38]. At chemical shifts far from water and fat, resonances of oxymyoglobin and deoxymyoglobin have been seen in rat heart ^{1}H spectra and correlated with tissue oxygen content [4], offering

another means of addressing ischemia. These approaches have a way to go in technology and protocol development before patient studies can be contemplated.

ACKNOWLEDGMENTS

I thank RG Weiss, M. Conway, B. Rajagopalan, and G.K. Radda for many helpful discussions.

REFERENCES

1. Bottomley PA (1994) MR spectroscopy of the human heart: the status and the challenges. *Radiology* **191:** 593–612.
2. Bottomley PA (1985) Noninvasive study of high-energy phosphate metabolism in human heart by depth-resolved ^{31}P NMR spectroscopy. *Science* **229:** 769–772.
3. Bottomley PA, Hardy CJ, Roemer PB, Mueller OM (1989) Proton-decoupled, Overhauser-enhanced, spatially localized carbon-13 spectroscopy in humans. *Magn Reson Med* **12:** 348–363.
4. Kreutzer U, Wang DS, Jue T (1992) Observing the ^{1}H NMR signal of the myoglobin Val-E11 in myocardium: an index of cellular oxygenation. *Proc Natl Acad Sci USA* **89:** 4731–4733.
5. Bottomley PA (1989) Human in vivo NMR spectroscopy in diagnostic medicine: clinical tool or research probe? *Radiology* **170:** 1–15.
6. Menon RS, Hendrich K, Hu X, Ugurbil K (1992) ^{31}P NMR spectroscopy of the human heart at 4 T: detection of substantially uncontaminated cardiac spectra and differentiation of subepicardium and subendocardium. *Magn Reson Med* **26:** 368–376.
7. Roemer PB, Edelstein WA, Hayes CE, Souza SP, Mueller OM (1990) The NMR phased array. *Magn Reson Med* **16:** 192–225.
8. Bottomley PA, Hardy CJ (1990) Strategies and protocols for clinical ^{31}P research in the heart and brain. *Phil Trans Roy Soc Lond A* **333:** 531–544.
9. Sakuma H, Takeda K, Tagami T, Nakagawa T, Okamoto S, Konishi T, Nakano T (1993) ^{31}P MR spectroscopy in hypertrophic cardiomyopathy: comparison with Tl-201 myocardial perfusion imaging. *Am Heart J* **125:** 1323–1328.
10. Schaefer S, Gober J, Valenza M, Karczmar GS, Matson GB, Camacho SA, Botvinick EH, Massie B, Weiner MW (1988) Nuclear magnetic resonance imaging-guided phosphorus-31 spectroscopy of the human heart. *J Am Coll Cardiol* **12:** 1449–1455.
11. Weiss RG, Bottomley PA, Hardy CJ, Gerstenblith G (1990) Regional myocardial metabolism of high-energy phosphates during isometric exercise in patients with coronary artery disease. *N Engl J Med* **323:** 1593–1600.
12. Blackledge MJ, Rajagopalan B, Oberhaensli RD, Bolas NM, Styles P, Radda GK (1987) Quantitative studies of

human cardiac metabolism by P-31 rotating frame NMR. *Proc Natl Acad Sci USA* **84**: 4283–4287.

13. Conway MA, Allis J, Ouwerkerk R, Niioka T, Rajago-palan B, Radda GK (1991) Detection of low phosphocre-atine to ATP ratio in failing hypertrophied human myocardium by ^{31}P magnetic resonance spectroscopy. *Lancet* **338**: 973–976.

14. Schaefer S, Gober JR, Schwartz GG, Twieg DB, Weiner MW, Massie B (1990) In vivo phosphorus-31 spectro-scopic imaging in patients with global myocardial dis-ease. *Am J Cardiol* **65**: 1154–1161.

15. Bottomley PA, Hardy CJ, Roemer PB (1990) Phosphate metabolite imaging and concentration measurements in human heart by nuclear magnetic resonance. *Magn Reson Med* **14**: 425–434.

16. Bottomley PA (1991) The trouble with spectroscopy papers. *Radiology* **181**: 344–350.

17. Masuda Y, Tateno Y, Ikehira H, Hashimoto T, Shishido F, Sekiya M, Imazeki Y, Imai H, Watanabe S, Inagaki Y (1992) High-energy phosphate metabolism of the myo-cardium in normal subjects and patients with various cardiomyopathies—the study using ECG gated MR spec-troscopy with a localization technique. *Jpn Circ J* **56**: 620–626.

18. Bottomley PA, Ouwerkerk R (1994) Optimum flip-angles for exciting NMR with uncertain T_1 values. *Magn Reson Med* **32**: 137–141.

19. Bottomley PA, Hardy CJ, Weiss RG (1991) Correcting human heart ^{31}P NMR spectra for partial saturation. Evidence that saturation factors for PCr/ATP are homo-geneous in normal and disease states. *J Magn Reson* **95**: 341–355.

20. Hardy CJ, Weiss RG, Bottomley PA, Gerstenblith G (1991) Altered myocardial high-energy phosphate me-tabolites in patients with dilated cardiomyopathy. *Am Heart J* **122**: 795–801.

21. de Roos A, Doornbos J, Luyten PR, Oosterwaal LJMP, van der Wall EE, den Hollander JA (1992) Cardiac metabolism in patients with dilated and hypertrophic cardiomyopathy: assessment with proton-decoupled P-31 MR spectroscopy. *J Magn Reson Imaging* **2**: 711–719.

22. Minakami S, Suzuki C, Saito T, Yoshikawa H (1965) Studies on erythrocyte glycolysis. I. Determination of the glycolytic intermediates in human erythrocytes. *J Biochem* **58**: 543–550.

23. Beutler E (1983) The erythrocyte. In *Hematology,* 3rd ed (Williams WJ, Beutler E, Erslev AJ and Lichtman MA, eds) pp. 283–284. New York: McGraw-Hill.

24. Bottomley PA, Weiss RG, Hardy CJ, Baumgartner WA (1991) Myocardial high-energy phosphate metabolism and allograft rejection in patients with heart transplants. *Radiology* **181**: 67–75.

25. Neubauer S, Krahe T, Schindler R, Horn M, Hillenbrand H, Entzeroth C, Mader H, Kromer EP, Riegger GAJ, Lackner K, Ertl G (1992) ^{31}P magnetic resonance spectros-copy in dilated cardiomyopathy and coronary artery disease. *Circulation* **86**: 1810–1818.

26. Humphrey SM, Garlick PB (1991) NMR-visible ATP and

Pi in normoxic and reperfused rat hearts: a quantitative study. *Am J Physiol* **260**: H6–H12.

27. Swain JL, Sabina RL, Peyton RB, Jones RN, Wechsler AS, Holmes EW (1982) Derangements in myocardial purine and pyrimidine nucleotide metabolism in patients with coronary artery disease and left ventricular hypertro-phy. *Proc Natl Acad Sci USA* **79**: 655–659.

28. Okada M, Mitsunami K, Yabe T, Kinoshita M, Morikawa S, Inubushi T (1992) Quantitative measurements of phosphorus metabolites in normal and diseased human hearts by ^{31}P NMR spectroscopy (abstract). *Proceedings Society for Magnetic Resonance in Medicine* **2**: 2305.

29. Bottomley PA, Hardy CJ (1992) Mapping creatine kinase reaction rates in human brain and heart with 4 tesla saturation transfer ^{31}P NMR. *J Magn Reson* **99**: 443–448.

30. Bottomley, PA, Herfkens RJ, Smith LS, Bashore TM (1987) Altered phosphate metabolism in myocardial infarction: P-31 MR spectroscopy. *Radiology* **165**: 703–707.

31. Hardy CJ, Bottomley PA, Rohling KW, Roemer PB (1992) An NMR phased array for human cardiac ^{31}P spectros-copy. *Magn Reson Med* **28**: 54–64.

32. Bottomley PA, Hardy CJ (1992) Proton Overhauser enhancements in human cardiac phosphorus NMR spec-troscopy at 1.5 T. *Magn Reson Med* **24**: 384–390.

33. Kolem H, Sauter R, Friedrich M, Schneider M, Wicklow K (1993) Nuclear Overhauser enhancement and proton decoupling in phosphorus chemical shift imaging of the human heart. In *Cardiovascular Applications of Magnetic Resonance* (Pohost GM, ed) pp. 417–426. Mt Kisco NY: Futura.

34. Ingwall JS, Kramer MF, Fifer MA, Lorell BH, Shemin R, Grossman W, Allen PD (1985) The creatine kinase system in normal and diseased human myocardium. *N Engl J Med* **313**: 1050–1054.

35. Auffermann W, Chew WM, Wolfe CL, Tavares NJ, Parmley WW, Semelka RC, Donnelly T, Chatterjee K, Higgins CB (1991) Normal and diffusely abnormal myo-cardium in humans: functional and metabolic character-ization with P-31 MR spectroscopy and cine MR imag-ing. *Radiology* **179**: 253–259.

36. Schaefer S, Schwartz GG, Steinman SK, Meyerhoff DJ, Massie BM, Weiner MW (1992) Metabolic response of the human heart to inotropic stimulation: in vivo phospho-rus-31 studies of normal and cardiomyopathic myocar-dium. *Magn Reson Med* **25**: 260–272.

37. Krause SM (1988) Metabolism in the failing heart. *Heart Failure* 267–273.

38. Ingwall JS (1993) Is cardiac failure a consequence of decreased energy reserve? *Circulation* **87**(Suppl VII): VII-58–VII-62.

39. Editorial (1991) When to operate in aortic valve disease. *Lancet* **338**: 981.

40. Canby RC, Evanochko WT, Barrett LV, Kirklin JK, McGiffen DC, Sakai TT, Brown ME, Foster RE, Reeves RC, Pohost GM (1987) Monitoring the bioenergetics of cardiac allograft rejection using in vivo P-31 nuclear magnetic resonance spectroscopy. *J Am Coll Cardiol* **9**: 1067–1074.

41. Haug CE, Shapiro JL, Chan L, Weil R (1987) P-31 nuclear magnetic resonance spectroscopic evaluation of heterotopic cardiac allograft rejection in the rat. *Transplantation* **44:** 175–178.

42. Fraser CD, Chacko VP, Jacobus WE, Soulen RL, Hutchins GM, Reitz BA, Baumgartner WA (1988) Metabolic changes preceding functional and morphological indices of rejection in heterotopic cardiac allografts. *Transplantation* **46:** 346–351.

43. Mitsunami K, Okada M, Inoue T, Hachisuka M, Kinoshita M, Inubishi T (1992) In vivo ^{31}P nuclear magnetic resonance spectroscopy in patients with old myocardial infarction. *Jpn Circ J* **56:** 614–619.

44. Jennings RB, Reimer KA (1981) Lethal myocardial ischemic injury. *Am J Pathol* **102:** 241–255.

45. Yabe T, Mitsunami K, Okada M, Morikawa S, Inubushi T, Kinoshita M (1993) Detection of myocardial ischemia by ^{31}P-magnetic resonance spectroscopy during hand-grip exercise. *Circulation* **89:** 1709–1716.

46. Conway MA, Bristow JD, Blackledge MJ, Rajagopalan B, Radda GK (1991) Cardiac metabolism during exercise in healthy volunteers measured by ^{31}P magnetic resonance spectroscopy. *Br Heart J* **65:** 25–30.

47. Weiss RG, Chacko VP, Glickson JD, Gerstenblith G (1989) Comparative ^{13}C and ^{31}P NMR assessment of altered metabolism during graded reductions in coronary flow in intact rat hearts. *Proc Natl Acad Sci USA* **86:** 6426–6430.

48. van Zijl PCM, Barker PB, Soher BJ, Gillen J, Bottomley PA, Duyn J, Moonen CTW, Weiss RG (1993) Proton spectroscopic imaging of ^{13}C-labelled compounds on a 1.5 Tesla standard clinical imager (abstract). *Proceedings Society of Magnetic Resonance in Medicine* **1:** 373.

49. den Hollander JA, Evanochko WT, Pohost GM (1992) Observation of cardiac lipids by localized ^{1}H magnetic resonance spectroscopic imaging. In: *Book of Abstracts: Society of Magnetic Resonance in Medicine 1992, Works in Progress.* p. 849. Berkeley, CA: Society of Magnetic Resonance in Medicine.

Ions, transport, and energetics in normal and diseased skeletal muscle

George K. Radda

MRC Biochemical & Clinical Magnetic Resonance Unit, John Radcliffe Hospital, Oxford OX3 9DU, UK

Magnetic resonance spectroscopy (MRS) has highlighted the relationship between intracellular ionic homeostasis and the control of muscle energetics. In skeletal muscle, the oxidative rate of ATP synthesis is largely controlled by ADP, the concentration of which is determined by the creatine kinase equilibrium that includes the concentration of H^+. At the onset of aerobic dynamic exercise, ATP is maintained largely by glycolysis, producing lactic acid and PCr breakdown. Vasodilation follows and ATP synthesis becomes predominantly oxidative. During recovery, PCr resynthesis gives a measure of mitochondrial function, and pH recovery reflects the $Na^+:H^+$ antiport activity. Dynamic ^{31}P MRS measurements can be used to derive quantitative information about the processes (fluxes and concentrations) described above. In diseased muscle (e.g., mitochondrial myopathy, dystrophy, hypertension) specific changes are observed in some of the control functions, ionic fluxes, or mitochondrial oxidative rates.

Keywords: oxidative metabolism; glycolysis; creatine kinase; ATP.

INTRODUCTION

Metabolic control in skeletal muscle accommodates a wide dynamic range of energy demand from at rest, through during exercise to in recovery. During exercise, both the anaerobic and aerobic pathways are activated, whereas in recovery, aerobic adenosine triphosphate (ATP) production is dominant. In skeletal muscle, phosphorus-containing metabolites are the most important regulators of the synthesis of ATP by the mitochondrion. There remains disagreement about the precise mechanism of the control of oxidative phosphorylation *in vivo* [1]. Several mechanisms may be involved, including control by orthophosphate (P_i), adenosine diphosphate (ADP), phosphorylation potential, and substrate availability. It is unlikely that a single mechanism regulates ATP production under all conditions.

We, and others, have used phosphorus (^{31}P) magnetic resonance spectroscopy (MRS) of skeletal muscle in humans and in animals to analyze the concentrations of ATP, ADP, phosphocreatine (PCr), P_i, and H^+,

at rest, during exercise at different workloads, and in recovery from exercise (for a review, see Ref. 2). The measurements provided a basis not only for investigating normal healthy muscle but for the study of a whole variety of muscle diseases [3]. In recent years we have shown how we can go beyond qualitative inferences of estimating rates of glycogenolytic ATP synthesis, aerobic ATP synthesis, and proton efflux, and to study their relationships to the concentrations of their putative regulators. The quantitative treatments we have developed can now be routinely applied to derive *in vivo* flux parameters in healthy and diseased muscle, thereby giving us valuable information about the nature and mechanism of specific disease processes. The investigations can be considered under three main categories, and in each of these groups particular disease phenomena can be readily recognized. The three categories are energetics in the resting muscle, recovery from exercise which represents an entirely aerobic oxidative process in normal conditions, and metabolic changes and energetics during exercise where several processes contribute. In the last grouping, the relative contributions of different pathways is dependent on muscle mass, time of exercise, and nature of exercise. This last category provides the most complex set of results but in many ways, provided that analysis can be carried out quanti-

Address for correspondence: MRC Biochemical & Clinical Magnetic Resonance Unit, John Radcliffe Hospital, Oxford OX3 9DU, UK.

tatively, it gives a wealth of new information about disease.

SKELETAL MUSCLE ENERGETICS AT REST

The relative and absolute concentrations of PCr, ATP, P_i, and of intracellular pH at rest are relatively invariant in normal individuals and across muscle groups. In general, the pH is close to 7.03 and the phosphorylation potential is

phosphorylation potential = $([ATP]/[ADP])[P_i]$
$$= .24 \times 10^6 \, M^{-1}$$

Not a great deal is known about what regulates total phosphate concentrations in the muscle, and for that matter, total creatine, but these two concentrations will determine both the concentration of ADP through the creatine kinase equilibrium and the phosphorylation potential. There are a number of diseases where, even at rest, specific changes occur. For example, in mitochondrial myopathies, the phosphorylation potential is the best descriminator of abnormality, being lower than that of the normal range [4]. In the majority of cases, PCr/ATP and [ADP] are also abnormal, and there is a significant increased mean of P_i/ATP although this is not a good descriminator in most patients. Intracellular pH, though mildly elevated, is not significantly different from controls in this disease.

In contrast, in Duchenne and Becker muscular dystrophy and in manifesting carriers of the disease, the most significant and earliest observable change in skeletal muscle is an elevation in intracellular pH [4]. The most likely explanation of this increase in pH, shown on the basis of studies of the mouse equivalent of the human disease, the MDX mouse, is that there is increased intracellular sodium, possibly following from an increase in cellular calcium concentrations [5]. Thus, at rest, all the ion regulatory mechanisms are reset to a new steady-state level. The observations would also explain why the rate of proton clearance after exercise is decreased, as at high intracellular sodium the proton sodium exchange rates would be slowed down.

Intracellular P_i does depend on the plasma phosphate concentration, and this has been studied in a group of patients in renal failure. There is a linear relationship in plasma P_i and cellular P_i. The slope of the relationship of extracellular over intracellular is about 3.5, showing that intracellular P_i concentrations are more tightly controlled than the extracellular levels. Although intracellular P_i does vary, it is interesting that the phosphorylation potential that accompanies this change remains constant in this group of patients.

PCR RESYNTHESIS DURING RECOVERY IS A MEASURE OF OXIDATIVE PHOSPHORYLATION

The analysis of the dependence of mitochondrial oxidation rate on phosphorus–metabolite concentrations in muscle is complicated by the near-equilibrium process catalyzed by creatine kinase, which ensures that PCr, ADP, and intracellular pH are related by the expression (6)

[ADP]/[ATP]
$$= \{([\text{total creatine}]/[PCr]) - 1 \, (1/K_m)\} \times 10^{pH}$$

In addition, during exercise and recovery, $[PCr + P_i]$ is approximately constant. These constraints impose correlations on metabolite concentrations; For example, if pH is constant, then $[P_i]/[PCr]$ is proportional to [ADP], the free energy of ATP hydrolysis is proportional to [PCr], and the contributions of [ADP], [PCr], [creatine], $[P_i]$, and phosphorylation potential to the overall mitochondrial driving function cannot be distinguished [1]. This is the reason why it has not been possible to reconcile the model based on hyperbolic ADP control with those based on linear driving function. If the pH is allowed to vary, the additional degree of freedom should enable the dependence on ADP and on PCr concentrations to be dissociated. We have shown that, under such conditions in human muscle, the recovery kinetics of ADP and of PCr show that mitochondrial ATP synthesis has a hyperbolic dependence on [ADP] but remains approximately linear with respect to $[P_i]$, [PCr], and the free energy of ATP hydrolysis [6]. The first of these is consistent with the kinetic control of the adenine–nucleotide translocase by [ADP] [2]. This can explain all the other correlations, although other regulators cannot be excluded. The K_m for ADP control is 30 μmol (1 of cell water)$^{-1}$ and the apparent maximal rate for mitochondrial ATP synthesis (Q_{max}) is approximately 40 mmol per 1 of cell water per minute [2].

Based on the observations above, we developed a model that substantially reproduces the metabolic response in recovery of a wide range of PCr and of pH values and that can be used to assess quantitatively the changes that are observed in diseased muscle [7].

The main postulates of the model are as follows:

1. ATP production is controlled only by [ADP], according to a hyperbolic function with a K_m and a Q_{max} [2].
2. ATP production during recovery is used to supply a resting demand and to resynthesize PCr.
3. The creatine kinase reaction is at equilibrium.

4. The synthesis of PCr produces protons, which is dependent on the pH [8].
5. The proton efflux is proportional to the cellular acidification [8].
6. The cell has a constant buffering capacity.

The model is run by entering the initial conditions of [PCr] and of pH, calculating [ADP] and, hence, the ATP production over a short time interval, determining the associated proton load and efflux, and thus arriving at new values for the next time increment.

The calculated recovery curves reproduce the main features of the observed ^{31}P MRS studies of normal muscle, namely, (1) PCr recovery is slowed when the pH is low; (2) pH recovery shows an initial acidification when the proton load from PCr resynthesis exceeds the proton extrusion; (3) ADP recovery is rapid and is not much changed by the metabolic state at the end of exercise.

We have used the hyperbolic relationship between the cytosolic [ADP] and the rate of PCr resynthesis after exercise to estimate the apparent maximum rate of mitochondrial ATP synthesis (Q_{max}) in several diseases in which mitochondrial oxidation may be impaired, either as a result of reduced mitochondrial numbers, intrinsic mitochondrial defect, or impaired supply of substrate or oxygen [9]. We have demonstrated how muscle responds by increasing the rate of anaerobic ATP synthesis and/or by allowing [ADP] to rise, so as to increase the mitochondrial drive. This requires an appropriate balance between lactic acid production (which tends to lower [ADP], by lowering pH) and proton efflux (which has the opposite effect). We have identified four patterns of results. In Group A, apparent Q_{max} is reduced and [ADP] is appropriately increased. In mitochondrial myopathy this is because upregulation of proton efflux reduces the pH change in exercise despite increased lactic acid production. Other conditions that show similar behavior in muscle energetics include patients with peripheral vascular disease and uremic patients on dialysis. In Group B, apparent Q_{max} is reduced, but there is no compensatory rise in [ADP], probably because anaerobic ATP synthesis during exercise is increased without a compensatory increase in proton efflux. Patients with cyanotic heart disease, cardiac failure, and myelodisplastic anemia show this kind of muscle response. In Group C, [ADP] is increased during exercise, but apparent Q_{max} is normal, suggesting either an abnormal increase in proton efflux or a decrease in anaerobic glycogenolysis during exercise. In some diseases, e.g., hypertension, the former explanation is more likely where it has been shown in animal studies that not only the amiloride-sensitive sodium proton anti-

port activity is increased but other ionic fluxes such as the ATP-driven sodium potassium exchange are also upregulated. Patients with myotonic dystrophy and carriers of Duchenne dystrophy also appear in this category. In Group D, we put conditions such as respiratory failure and iron deficiency, where, despite impaired oxygen supply, both apparent Q_{max} and end-exercise [ADP] are normal. The factors that determine whether, during exercise, glycolysis or increased ADP-enhancing oxidative metabolism are the primary mechanisms for maintaining the concentration of ADP are not clearly understood. In the next section I shall discuss some of the basic principles and regulatory mechanisms during exercise.

BIOENERGETIC CHANGES IN SKELETAL MUSCLE DURING EXERCISE

We can dissect the various contributions to ATP synthesis during exercise by comparing the changes observed under ischaemic and aerobic conditions at the same muscle performance. We have carried out such a study on the *flexor digitorum superficialis* in four adult males during dynamic ischaemic and aerobic exercise at three different work rates and during recovery from aerobic exercise. During exercise, changes in pH and PCr were larger at higher power, but in aerobic exercise neither end-exercise [ADP] nor the initial postexercise PCr resynthesis rate altered with power. In ischemic exercise we estimated total ATP resynthesis from the rates of PCr depletion and glycogenolysis inferred using an analysis of proton buffering. The estimate of total ATP turnover remained constant with time and was shown to be proportional to work rate. As PCr decreased, the relative contribution from glycogenolysis to ATP synthesis increased in parallel so as to maintain the total ATP synthesis rate. Comparison of the calculated ATP turnover in ischemic and aerobic exercise suggested that oxidative ATP synthesis was small during the first minute of aerobic exercise and increased with a half-time of around 0.5–1 min. This suggests that oxidative ATP synthesis is negligible during the first half-minute of aerobic exercise at mechanical power output levels of 0.5, 0.67, and 1 W. Using the values of proton efflux derived from studying pH recovery after exercise, we Acould estimate ATP synthesis by glycogenolysis during aerobic exercise from the measured pH changes. We showed that glycolytic ATP synthesis is approximately linearly dependent on P_i concentration throughout ischemic exercise and during the first 1–2 min of aerobic exercise. This relationship with P_i may be of regulatory significance, as P_i is a substrate for glycogen phosphorylase and an activator of phosphofructokinase.

We used near-infrared spectroscopy to measure hemoglobin desaturation during aerobic and ischemic exercise at 0.5 W. The results showed that hemoglobin desaturation was higher at the end of the first minute of aerobic exercise (in fact as high as during ischemic exercise) than at the end of exercise. This mirrors the calculated rate of oxidative ATP synthesis. A possible explanation is a delayed increase in blood flow so that oxidative ATP synthesis is limited first by the rate of arterial oxygen supply and then, at later stages, by the cytosolic ADP concentration when oxygen supply is adequate. There are, however, other possible explanations (see Ref. 10).

This type of analysis during exercise has been used to evaluate quantitatively the glycogenolytic response in a variety of conditions where oxygen delivery is limited. These include respiratory failure, anemia, and patients where the hemoglobin oxygen dissociation curve is modified either as a result of genetic condition or by drugs such as BW 12C79, which is an agent that left-shifts the oxygen dissociation curve of hemoglobin [11]. Recently, we have also investigated the effect of an agent called Bryostatin, a modulator of protein kinase C, which is being used in Phase I cancer trials. This agent was known to have a quite severe side effect in producing myalgia; a detailed study on a group of patients has shown that this is a result of the vasoconstrictory effect of Bryostatin in skeletal muscle producing severe oxygen deficiency.

CONCLUSION

The essential problem in the quantitative study of bioenergetics and bioenergetic abnormalities is to infer rates of oxidative and glycogenolytic ATP turnover and proton efflux from measurements of pH and metabolite concentrations. In steady-state exercise, the oxidative ATP synthesis rate can only be measured by oxygen consumption or ^{31}P MR saturation transfer or taken as being proportional to the mechanical work. In non-steady-state exercise or recovery from exercise, absolute rates of ATP synthesis and proton efflux are obtainable from ^{31}P MRS measurements. For many of these calculations we need to know the cytosolic buffering capacity. Knowledge of metabolic control relationships (e.g., between aerobic ATP synthesis and [ADP]) also allows estimation of oxidative capacity from steady-state or kinetic measurements. Quantitative bioenergetic interpretation of skeletal muscle ^{31}P magnetic resonance spectroscopy will become more reliable and informative as our knowledge of these processes improves.

ACKNOWLEDGEMENT

This summary is based on the work of many colleagues given in the reference list. The work was supported by the Medical Research Council and the British Heart Foundatin.

REFERENCES

1. Radda GK, Kemp GJ, Styles P, Taylor DJ (1993) Control of oxidative phosphorylation in muscle. *Biochem Soc Trans* **21**: 762–764.
2. Kemp GJ, Radda GK (1994) Quantitative interpretation of bioenergetic data from ^{31}P and ^1H magnetic resonance spectroscopic studies of skeletal muscle: an analytical review. *Magn Reson Quart* **10**: 43–63.
3. Radda GK, Taylor DJ (1992) The study of bioenergetics *in vivo* using nuclear magnetic resonance. In *Molecular Mechanism of Bioenergetics* (Ernster L, ed), pp. 463–481. New York: Elsevier.
4. Kemp GJ, Taylor DJ, Dunn JF, Frostick SP, Radda GK (1993) Cellular energetics in dystrophic muscle. *J Neurol Sci* **116**: 201–206.
5. Dunn JF, Tracey I, Radda GK (1992) A ^{31}P NMR study of muscle exercise metabolism in mdx mice: evidence for abnormal pH regulation. *J Neurol Sci* **113**: 108–113.
6. Kemp GJ, Taylor DJ, Radda GK (1993) Control of phosphocreatine resynthesis during recovery from exercise in human skeletal muscle. *NMR Biomed* **6**: 66–72.
7. Styles P, Kemp GJ, Radda GK (1992) A model for metabolic control which reproduces the main features of recovery which are observed by ^{31}P MRS. *Proceedings of the 11th Annual Meeting, Society for Magnetic Resonance Medicine*, p. 2702.
8. Kemp GJ, Taylor DJ, Styles P, Radda GK (1993) The production, buffering and efflux of protons in human skeletal muscle during exercise and recovery. *NMR Biomed* **6**: 73–83.
9. Kemp GJ, Taylor DJ, Thompson CH, Hands LJ, Rajagopalan B, Styles P, Radda GK (1993) Quantitative analysis by ^{31}P magnetic resonance spectroscopy of abnormal mitochondrial oxidation in skeletal muscle during recovery from exercise. *NMR Biomed* **6**: 302–310.
10. Kemp GJ, Thompson CH, Barnes PRJ, Radda GK (1994) Comparisons of ATP turnover in human muscle during ischaemic and aerobic exercise using ^{31}P magnetic resonance spectroscopy. *Magn Reson Med* **31**: 248–258.
11. Philip PA, Thompson CH, Carmichael J, Rea D, Mitchell K, Taylor DJ, Stuart NSA, Dennis I, Rajagopalan B, Ganesan T, Radda GK, Harris AL (1993) A Phase I study of the left-shifting agent BW12C79 plus mitomycin C and the effect on the skeletal muscle metabolism using ^{31}P Magnetic Resonance Spectroscopy. *Cancer Res* **53**: 5649–5653.

Reduced purine catabolite production in the postischemic rat heart: a ^{31}P NMR assessment of cytosolic metabolites

Ryszard T. Smolenski, Magdi H. Yacoub and Anne-Marie L. Seymour*

Magnetic Resonance Spectroscopy Group, Department of Cardiothoracic Surgery, National Heart and Lung Institute at Harefield Hospital, Harefield, Middlesex UB9 6JH, UK

Ischemia can cause release of adenosine and purine catabolites from the heart, through the breakdown of ATP. If repeated periods of ischemia are induced, the efflux of purines is markedly reduced, although it is not clear if this is beneficial for the long-term survival of the heart. We have investigated changes in high-energy phosphates and purine release in the isolated perfused rat heart using ^{31}P NMR spectroscopy and high-performance liquid chromatography. Hearts were subjected to one of the following protocols: Group A—1 min of total global ischemia (TGI) after 40 min, 60 min, and 85 min of perfusion (a total of 3 × 1 min ischemia); Group B—1 min of TGI after 40 min of perfusion, 10 min of TGI after 50 min of perfusion, and a final 1 min of TGI after 85 min of perfusion. The profile of high-energy phosphate metabolites, P_i accumulation and purine release was similar for each 1-min period of TGI in Group A, whereas phosphocreatine content was increased and ATP content reduced by an extended period of TGI in Group B, leading to a less severe acidosis and purine efflux in the final 1 min of TGI at 85 min of perfusion. In conclusion, the reduced purine release observed in Group B may be related to the preischemic ATP pool size and accessibility and the increased myocardial energy reserve in the form of phosphocreatine.

Keywords: ^{31}P-NMR, ischemia, energy metabolism, purine release.

INTRODUCTION

Myocardial ischemia causes an imbalance between energy production and energy utilization, resulting in the breakdown of ATP to its purine constituents. These components can then be released into the coronary circulation and, hence, are lost from the myocardial cell.

The efflux of purines may be considered either beneficial or detrimental to the long-term survival of the heart. One important component of purine release is adenosine, which can exert a number of protective effects on the heart [1], including coronary vasodilation, inhibition of catecholamine actions, platelet aggregation, and leukocyte infiltration. On the other hand, release of purines from the myocardium results in a substantial depletion of the intracellular adenine nucleotide pool, thus rendering the heart more vulnerable to reperfusion injury [2].

Previous studies have shown that repeated periods of ischemia can markedly reduce the efflux of purines [3]. In contrast, short episodes of ischemia followed by reperfusion have been shown to increase myocardial tolerance to a subsequent more prolonged period of ischemia—described as "preconditioning" [4]. However, the mechanisms underlying these observations are unresolved.

In this study, we have investigated the relationship between myocardial intracellular high-energy phosphates and purine efflux following repeated brief periods of ischemia and the effects on functional recovery of the heart.

MATERIALS AND METHODS

Hearts from male Wistar rats were perfused in the Langendorff mode with a modified Krebs–Henseleit buffer (containing 118 mM NaCl, 24 mM NaHCO$_3$, 4.8 mM KCl, 1.2 mM KH$_2$PO$_4$, 1.2 mM MgSO$_4$, 1.25 mM

---

* Address for correspondence: M.R.S. Group, Dept. of Cardiothoracic Surgery, Heart Science Centre, N.H.L.I. at Harefield Hospital, Harefield, Middlesex UB9 6JH, UK.

$CaCl_2$, and 11 mM glucose) under a constant pressure of 100 cm H_2O. Left ventricular function was monitored via a fluid-filled balloon inserted into the left ventricle, and coronary flow was measured by timed collection of perfusate.

^{31}P-NMR spectra were acquired in 1-min time blocks using a 9.4-T superconducting magnet with a 7-cm bore (phosphorus frequency = 162 MHz) interfaced with a Bruker AMX spectrometer. Partially saturated spectra were recorded using a 90° pulse and 0.9-s interpulse delay to assess relative changes in myocardial high-energy phosphate content. Samples of coronary effluent were collected immediately before each period of ischemia and for 3 min during reperfusion and subsequently analyzed for purine content using reverse-phase high-performance liquid chromatography (HPLC) [5].

Hearts were perfused for 90 min total and were exposed to one of the following protocols: Group A was subjected to 1 min of total global ischemia (TGI) after 40 min, 60 min, and 85 min of perfusion (a total of 3 × 1 min ischemia). Group B was subjected to 1 min of TGI after 40 min of perfusion, 10 min of TGI after 50 min of perfusion, and a final 1 min of TGI after 85 min of perfusion. Data are presented as percentage changes based on the average of control measurements taken after 30 min normoxic perfusion. The mean and S.E. of six hearts for Group A and nine hearts for Group B are presented.

RESULTS

In Group A, the extent of purine efflux was similar following each of the 1-min periods of TGI (Table 1 and Fig. 1, upper panel). In Group B, following 10 min of TGI, the production of purines was markedly decreased during the final 1 min of TGI at 85 min of perfusion (Table 1 and Fig. 1, lower panel), consistent with previous reports [3].

There was no alteration in the profile of high-energy phosphate depletion and inorganic phosphate (P_i) accumulation during each 1 min of TGI in Group A as shown in the ^{31}P-NMR spectra (Fig. 1, upper panel) and Table 1. In contrast, following 10 min of TGI, hearts in Group B showed an elevated phosphocreatine (PCr) level (146% of control) but a markedly decreased ATP content at 85 min of perfusion (Table 1). In consequence, the increased PCr content available reduced the extent of acidosis that occurred in the final 1 min of TGI (pH 6.97 ± 0.01 and Table 1). In both groups, the changes in cytosolic P_i mirrored inversely those of PCr. Myocardial function (assessed by left ventricular developed pressure) was maintained at

Table 1. Percentage changes in cytosolic energy metabolites and inorganic phosphate and purine release in hearts exposed to repeated periods of ischemia.

	PCr	ATP	P_i	pH	Purine Release
Group A (n = 6)					
40 min perfusion	100 ± 14	100 ± 11	100 ± 5	7.04	100
1 min TGI at 40 min	52 ± 28	99 ± 10	176 ± 18	6.91	511
60 min perfusion	111 ± 10	101 ± 12	101 ± 13	7.04	51
1 min TGI at 60 min	39 ± 19	96 ± 6	173 ± 12	6.90	506
85 min perfusion	107 ± 9	100 ± 8	88 ± 8	7.03	48
1 min TGI at 85 min	53 ± 12	94 ± 12	180 ± 11	6.90	467
Group B (n = 9)					
40 min perfusion	100 ± 11	100 ± 7	100 ± 5	7.04	100
1 min TGI at 40 min	59 ± 18	101 ± 7	203 ± 15	6.93	448
85 min perfusion	146 ± 11	78 ± 8	102 ± 13	7.03	122
1 min TGI at 85 min	77 ± 18	68 ± 11	211 ± 10	6.97	163

100% throughout the protocol in Group A and recovered to 100% following 10 min of TGI in Group B.

CONCLUSIONS

This study demonstrates that myocardial production of purines and the degree of acidosis during a brief 1-min period of ischemia are markedly reduced following an extended period of TGI (10 min). However, it is not clear if these effects are detrimental to the survival of the heart, as no significant difference in functional recovery is observed between Groups A and B.

The decreased purine release may be explained by a number of different mechanisms. First, 5′-nucleotidase and AMP deaminase, key enzymes in adenine nucleotide catabolism, may be inhibited by ischemia. Changes in the intracellular milieu both during and after ischemia may affect the activities of these important regulatory enzymes, thus reducing the extent of nucleotide breakdown. Second, the remaining intracellular adenine nucleotide pool may not be accessible to the enzymes involved in catabolism. Two major com-

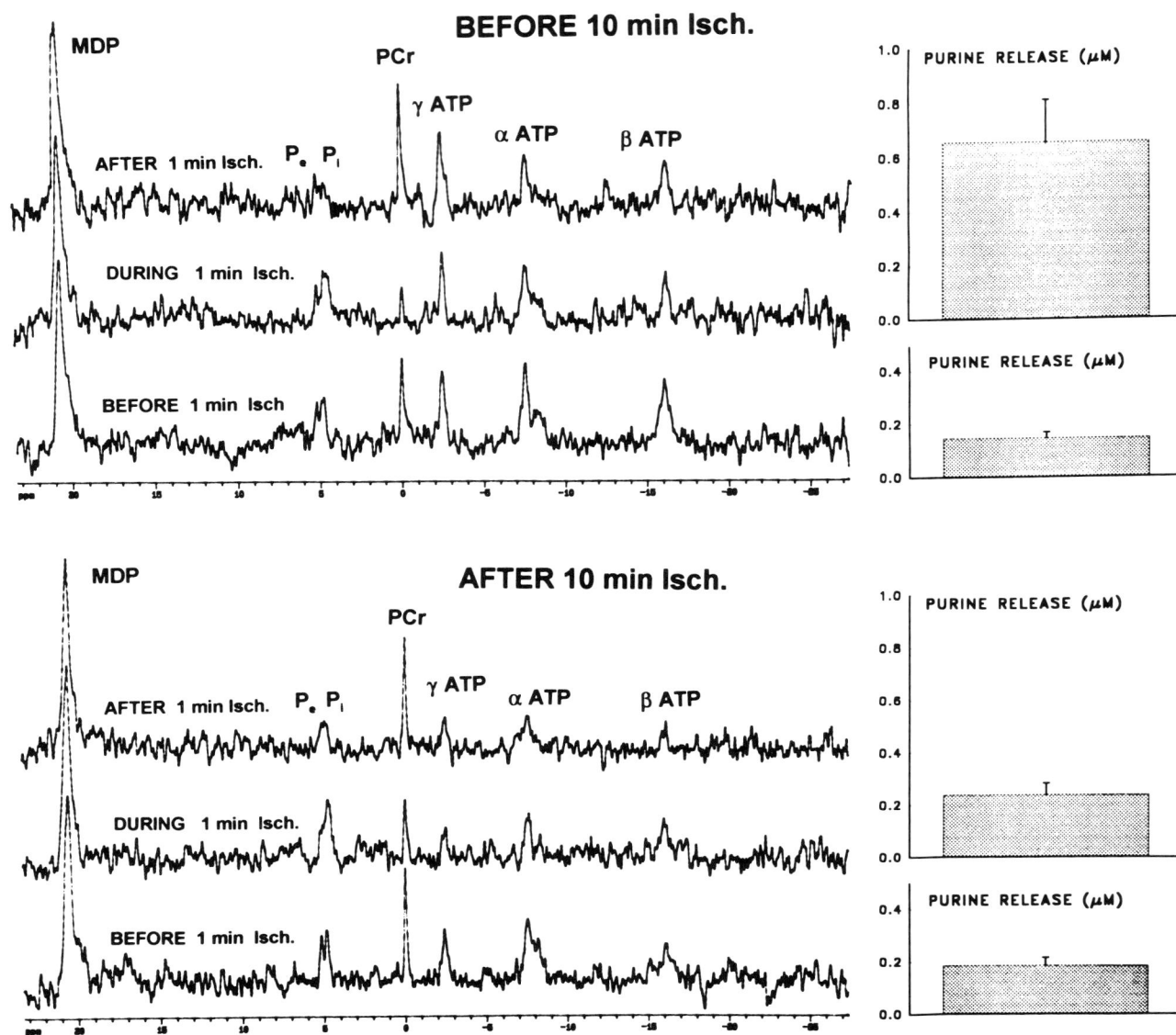

Fig. 1. ^{31}P-NMR spectra of an isolated perfused rat heart and myocardial purine release prior to, during, and following 1 min of TGI after 40 min of perfusion (upper panels) or after 85 min of perfusion (lower panels). Details are included in the Methods section.

partments of adenine nucleotides exist inside the cell, the cytosolic pool, and the mitochondrial pool. There is some evidence to suggest that the cytosolic compartment is depleted more rapidly than the mitochondrial one. This is not surprising in that the enzymes of nucleotide catabolism are situated within the cytosol. Thus, the cytosolic compartment will be depleted to a greater extent than the mitochondrial pool, contributing to the reduced adenine nucleotide content observed (Table 1, Group B) and the decreased purine efflux. Third, the rate of energy utilization may be depressed following repeated bouts of ischemia. However, there is less evidence to support this latter view,

as no significant differences in left-ventricular-developed pressure or heart rate were observed between Groups A and B.

The extended period of TGI (10 min) causes an overshoot in the recovery of PCr. This may reflect the reestablishment of intracellular metabolic equilibrium and has a beneficial effect in enhancing the myocardial energy reserve. The protective effect can be observed in the final 1 min of TGI, where the decline in intracellular pH is essentially buffered by the augmented PCr utilization through the creatine kinase reaction.

In summary, these results show that myocardial

energy metabolism and purine efflux are modified by repeated periods of ischemia. Such changes may alter the susceptibility of the heart to ischemic damage. Use of a blood-perfused preparation may help to clarify these issues.

ACKNOWLEDGMENT

We thank the British Heart Foundation for financial support.

REFERENCES

1. Nees S, Herzog V, Becker BF, Bock M, Des Rosiers Ch, Gerlach E (1985) The coronary endothelium: a highly active metabolic barrier for adenosine. *Basic Res Cardiol* **80:** 515–529.
2. Bailey IA, Seymour A-ML, Radda GK (1981) A 31P-NMR study of the effects of reflow on the ischemic heart. *Biochim Biophys Acta* **637:** 1–7.
3. Smolenski RT, Simmonds HA, Garlick PB, Venn GE, Chambers DJ (1993) Depressed adenosine and total purine catabolite production in the post-ischemic rat heart. *Cardioscience* **4:** 235–240.
4. Reimer KA, Jennings RB (1992) Preconditioning. In *Myocardial Protection: The Pathophysiology of Reperfusion and Reperfusion Injury* (Yellon DM, Jennings RB, eds.) pp. 165–183. New York: Raven Press.
5. Smolenski RT, Lachno DR, Ledingham SJM, Yacoub MH (1991) Determination of sixteen nucleotides, nucleosides and bases using high performance liquid chromatography and its application to the study of purine metabolism in hearts for transplantation. *J Chromatogr* **527:** 414–420.

Mechanisms of ^{31}P relaxation in phosphorus metabolites

E. R. Andrew* and R. Gaspar

Departments of Physics and Radiology, University of Florida, Gainesville, FL 32611, USA

Measurements have been made of the longitudinal relaxation time T_1 of ^{31}P for the individual resonances of the metabolites AMP, ADP, ATP, P_i, and PCr (phosphocreatine) in H_2O and D_2O solutions from 5 to 60°C at various concentrations and at frequencies of 40 MHz (2.3 T) and 120 MHz (7 T). The contributions of dipolar, chemical shift anisotropy, and spin-rotation mechanisms have been separated, and activation parameters of the underlying molecular reorientations have been determined.

Keywords: phosphorus metabolites, ^{31}P relaxation, relaxation mechanisms, chemical shift anisotropy, spin rotation.

INTRODUCTION

High-resolution ^{31}P-NMR spectra of metabolites obtained *in vivo* from humans, animals, and cells provide valuable information concerning the biochemistry of living systems in normal and diseased states. For quantitation, saturation transfer, NOE, and studies of molecular mobility and exchange, relaxation knowledge is very important, but few systematic measurements have been made and no analysis of mechanisms. As a first step, we have measured T_1 for the five principal metabolites in pure aqueous solutions from 5 to 60°C and at frequencies of 40 MHz and 120 MHz.

The principal mechanisms to be considered are as follows:

1. Dipolar, both intramolecular and intermolecular, always present
2. Chemical shift anisotropy (CSA), present for nuclei in less than tetrahedral symmetry
3. Spin rotation (SR), likely to be significant for smaller molecules
4. Paramagnetic, from dissolved oxygen and other paramagnetic species
5. Scalar, when couplings are modulated by exchange or a fast relaxing partner

In the fast motion regime, the dipolar and CSA relaxation rates are proportional to the molecular correlation time τ_c, but the SR rate is inversely proportional to τ_c. Consequently, measurement of T_1 over a temperature range enables dipolar and CSA contributions to be discriminated from SR. As dipolar and SR relaxation contributions are independent of magnetic field strength B_0, whereas CSA is proportional to B_0^2, measurements in two field strengths enable the CSA contribution to be separated. Use of H_2O and D_2O solvents varies the dipolar contribution in a known way and assists in separating dipolar and SR contributions. The concentration dependence of T_1 enables a discrimination to be made between intramolecular and intermolecular dipolar contributions. Relaxation due to paramagnetic contributions was minimized by careful sample preparation [1, 2]. Scalar relaxation could be estimated from the known ^{31}P and ^{1}H T_1 values and was found to be negligible.

RESULTS AND CONCLUSIONS

The measured temperature dependence of T_1 for the five metabolites is shown in Figs. 1–5 as activation plots, $\log T_1$ against $1/T$. If τ_c follows an Arrhenius activation law, a pure dipolar or CSA mechanism yields a straight line with a negative slope, whereas a pure SR mechanism yields a straight line with a positive slope. It is clear from the figures that for AMP, ADP, ATP, and phosphocreatine (PCr), there is no significant SR contribution for these metabolites.

For P_i, T_1 showed no field dependence, indicating an absence of CSA contribution, which is not surpris-

---

* Address for correspondence: Department of Physics, 215 Williamson Hall, University of Florida, Gainesville, FL 32611, USA.

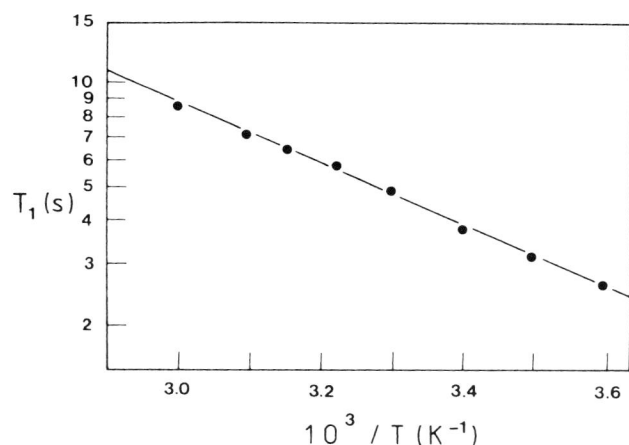

Fig. 1. AMP in H_2O.

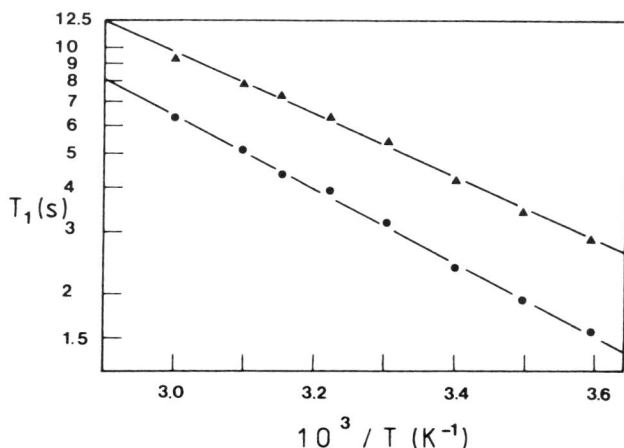

Fig. 3. ATP in H_2O. Circles = P_α; triangles = P_β; squares = P_γ.

ing for this tetrahedrally symmetric ion. The activation plots in Fig. 4 are nonlinear and indicate a significant SR contribution. A computer fit of the experimental points to theory gives a 27% SR contribution in H_2O and 57% in D_2O. From the SR contribution, the SR coupling constant was found to be 1.81×10^{-41} kg m^2 s^{-1}, very similar to values obtained experimentally for six other small phosphorus molecules [3] which range from 1.48×10^{-41} to 1.87×10^{-41} kg m^2 s^{-1}, thus lending support for the relaxation model used. The computer fit of the theoretical lines to the experimental points in Fig. 4 yields activation energies E_A of 12.1 kJ mole^{-1} in H_2O and 11.1 kJ mole^{-1} in D_2O. Accuracies of E_A are $\pm 7\%$.

The straight-line plots in Figs. 1, 2, 3, and 5 yield the following activation energies for the molecular reorientations which generate the relaxation: for ATP, values of E_A are 19.6, 19.2, and 17.7 kJ mole^{-1} for P_α, P_β, and P_γ, respectively; for ADP, values of E_A are 20.0 and 17.1 kJ mole^{-1} for P_α and P_β respectively; for AMP, the value

of E_A is 17.1 kJ mole^{-1}. It is seen that the outermost groups are somewhat less hindered. For PCr, the values of E_A are 15.4 kJ mole^{-1} in H_2O and 14.6 kJ mole^{-1} for D_2O. The slightly smaller value of E_A in D_2O, which we also noted for P_i above, although barely outside experimental error, may, thus, represent a small but real difference in the two solvents for both metabolites.

The field dependence of T_1 at 37°C showed that in AMP, the CSA contribution was 51% and 11% at 120 and 40 MHz, respectively; in ADP, it was 53% and 11% for P_α, and 25% and 4% for P_β; in ATP, it was 59% and 14% for P_α, 68% and 19% for P_β, and 34% and 5% for P_γ. The CSA contribution is, thus, significantly smaller for the end groups either because the shielding anisotropy of the end groups is less, or because τ_c is less due to the less restricted motion we noted earlier.

T_1 was found to be independent of concentration in the range 0.01–0.1 M, implying that the dipolar relax-

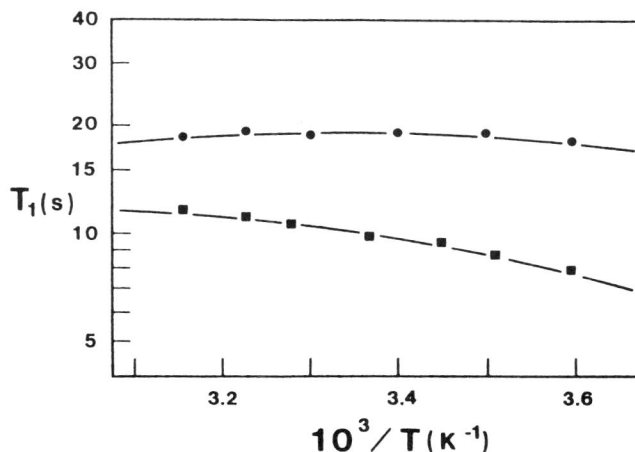

Fig. 2. ADP in H_2O. Circles = P_α; triangles = P_β.

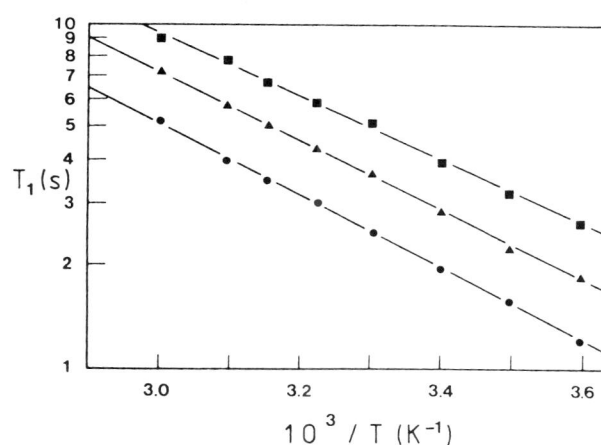

Fig. 4. P_i in H_2O (squares) and in D_2O (circles).

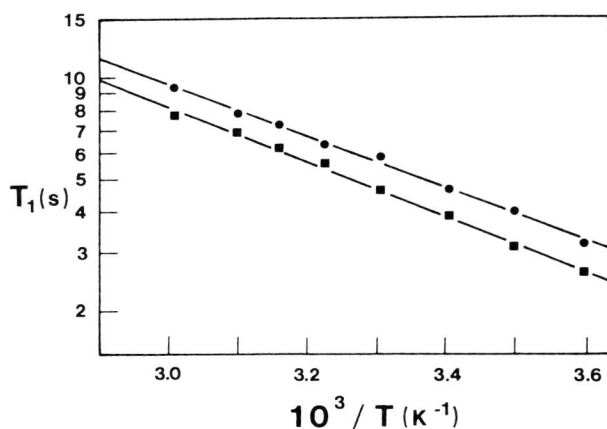

Fig. 5. PCr in H_2O (squares) and in D_2O (circles).

ation contributions were predominantly intramolecular.

Finally, we should note that values of T_1 reported *in vivo* are shorter than the values reported here for pure aqueous solutions by typically a factor of order 2. In cells and tissues, relaxation pathways are supplied by the small concentration of paramagnetic ions and by dissolved oxygen and from the presence of large molecules and organelles to which the metabolite

molecules become attached for variable residence times.

ACKNOWLEDGMENTS

The authors are grateful to Professor W. S. Brey for assistance with measurements at 40 MHz. They gratefully acknowledge support from Johnson and Johnson, from NIH grants 1 P41 RR02278 and CA42283, and from the Hungarian Academy of Sciences.

REFERENCES

1. Andrew ER, Gaspar R (1988) Proton magnetic relaxation of adenosine monophosphate in solution. *Chem Phys Lett* **146**: 184–188.
2. Andrew ER, Gaspar R (1988) Proton magnetic relaxation of adenosine diphosphate and adenosine triphosphate in solution. *Chem Phys Lett* **147**: 551–556.
3. Gillen KT (1972) Comparison of ^{31}P spin-rotation interaction constants derived from chemical shift data and from NMR relaxation and viscosity data. *J Chem Phys* **56**: 1573–1581.

In vivo ^{13}C chemical shift imaging of the human liver

E. Thiaudière,[1]* M. Biran, C. Delalande,[1] B. Bouligand[2] and P. Canioni[1]

[1]Unité de Résonance Magnétique des Systèmes Biologiques, C.N.R.S. UMR 9991,
Université de Bordeaux II, F-33076 Bordeaux, France
[2]Siemens S.A., F-93527 St-Denis, France

Chemical shift imaging (CSI) was applied to measure natural abundance proton-decoupled ^{13}C-NMR spectra of the human liver. Large surface coils were designed for ^{13}C spectra acquisition (16-cm-diameter circular coil) as well as for proton imaging and decoupling (21 × 20-cm butterfly coil). Such sizes allowed deep observations of the abdomen. A space matrix of 8 × 4 voxels (4 × 8 cm each) was defined using 32 phase-encoding steps. Magnetic field gradients were adjusted on multicompartment phantoms to limit contamination between voxels. Spectral maps containing {[1]H}-^{13}C spectra of liver from healthy volunteers with an acceptable signal-to-noise ratio were recorded within 20 min. Liver spectra exhibited well-defined resonances corresponding to fatty acyl chains, carbonyl groups, and sugars. The (C-1)-glycogen resonance was also detected under such conditions. Such a technique would be of interest in the development of metabolic investigations on the human liver *in vivo*.

Keywords: *in vivo* spectroscopic imaging, human liver, ^{13}C-NMR.

INTRODUCTION

In vivo chemical shift imaging (CSI) [1, 2] is expected to be widely used to obtain NMR spectral data from different parts of an organ within a single experiment. Proton and ^{31}P-CSI from the human brain is already documented [3, 4]; the technique is being developed for other organs such as the liver [5, 6]. Very little data are available concerning proton-decoupled natural abundance ^{13}C-CSI due to the very low sensitivity of the nucleus. Moreover, the liver is known to be heterogenous from a magnetic point of view, which does not make it easy to get relevant localized spectral information. However, *in vivo* nonlocalized {[1]H}-^{13}C spectra from the abdominal region of humans were successfully obtained and were used to assess glycogen metabolism [7, 8].

In this article, we describe the achievement of large surface coils for ^{1}H- and ^{13}C-NMR and the feasibility of performing {[1]H}-^{13}C-CSI experiments at 2 T on human liver within a limited amount of time.

---

* Address for correspondence: Unité de Résonance Magnétique des Systèmes Biologiques, C.N.R.S. UMR 9991, Université de Bordeaux II, 146 rue Léo Saignat, F-33076 Bordeaux, France.

MATERIALS AND METHODS

Experiments were carried out on a Siemens Magnetom 63 SP equipped with a superconducting magnet operating at 2 T. For ^{1}H imaging and decoupling, a 21 × 20-cm butterfly coil [9] was designed and tuned at 84.4 MHz. [13]C spectra were obtained using a 16-cm-diameter circular coil tuned at 21.2 MHz. Both coils were operating in the transmit/receive mode. Healthy volunteers were placed in the prone position and proton images were recorded for liver localization with a classical fast low-angle shot (FLASH) sequence [TE = 135 ms, field of view (FOV) = 320 mm, slice thickness = 10 mm]. For 2D-CSI experiments, 32 phase-encoding steps made it possible to define a matrix of 8 × 4 voxels in the transverse mode. Natural abundance {[1]H}-^{13}C spectra were recorded via a slice-selective (8-cm thickness) ^{13}C excitation pulse (225° flip angle at the center of the ^{13}C coil). Proton decoupling was achieved using a WALTZ 16 sequence [10] for 66 ms. The repetition time was 1–1.5 s and the radiofrequency (RF) deposition was determined to be less than 2 W kg^{-1}. Typically, 32 free-induction decay (FID) of 2048 points were recorded within 20 min and a line broadening of 50 Hz was applied before Fourier transformation.

RESULTS

{¹H}-¹³C 2D-CSI experiments were first carried out on multicompartment phantoms containing ethanol, methanol, and sunflower oil in order to check the spectral contamination between voxels. It was found to be less than 10% by adjusting the phase-encoding gradients (data not shown).

We tried then to obtain spectral maps of 64 voxels measuring 4×4 cm on humans. It followed that an acceptable S/N for 20 min acquisition time was only found in voxels located close to the ¹³C coil, that is, for abdominal muscles. As a consequence, we halved the number of phase-encoding steps in the horizontal axis, resulting in an increase of $\sqrt{8}$ of the S/N. Figure 1 shows a typical spectral map showing voxels well

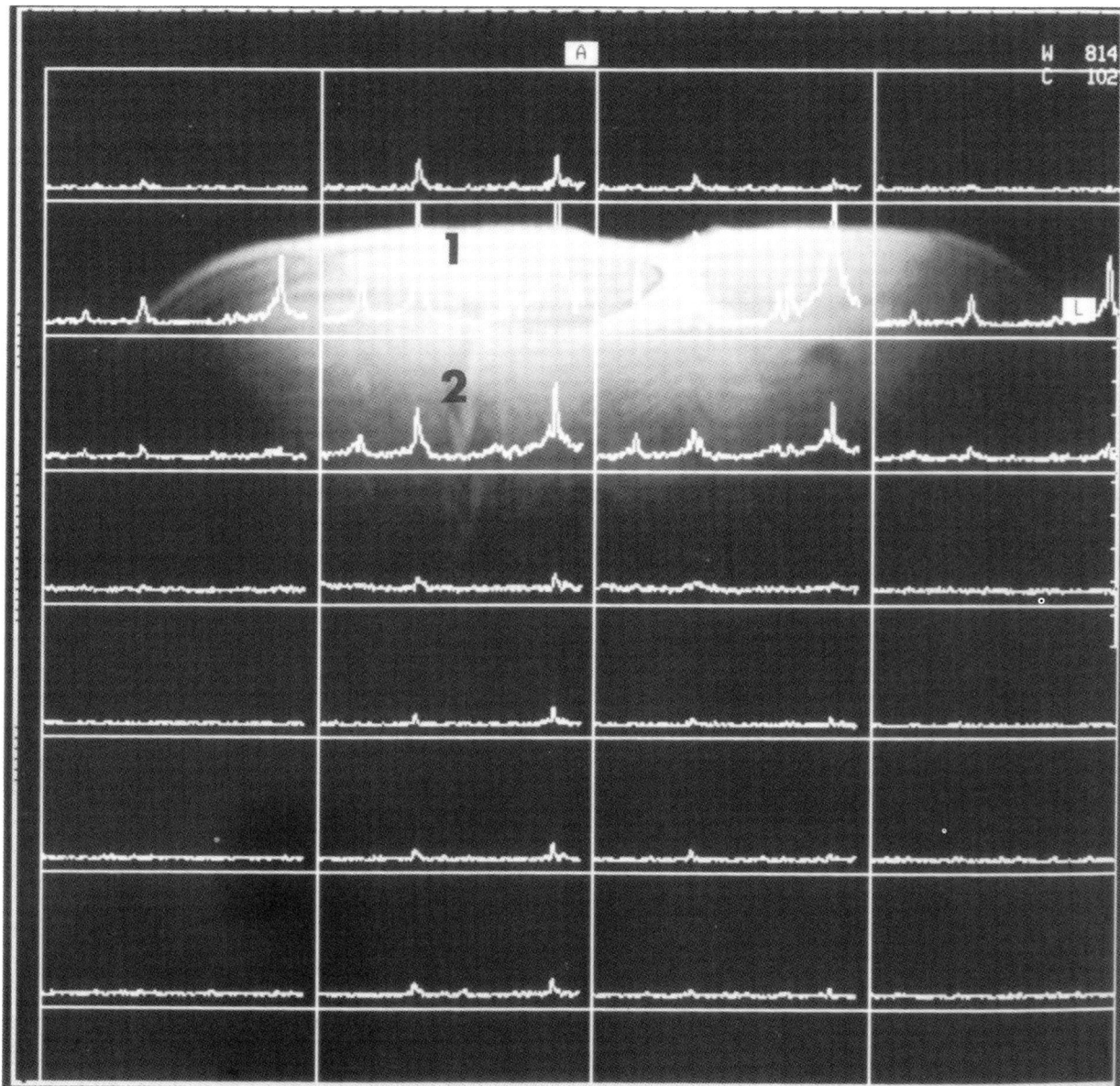

Fig. 1. {¹H}-¹³C spectral map of a healthy volunteer obtained from a 2D-CSI experiment. Overlaid is a proton image acquired in the transverse mode. The abdominal muscles can be distinguished in the upper part, whereas the liver appears in dark. ¹H-decoupled ¹³C-NMR spectra are represented in their respective 4×8 cm voxel. The spectral width is 200 ppm (4200 Hz) and the signal scale is the same for every spectrum. Spectra from voxels 1 (muscle + adipose tissue) and 2 (liver alone) are depicted in Fig. 2.

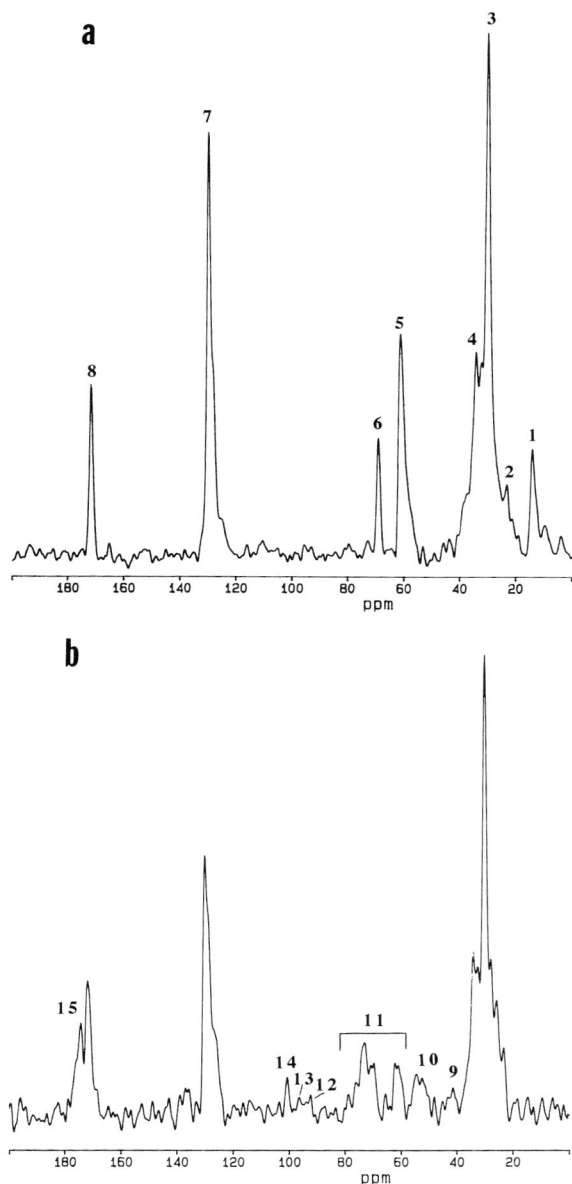

Fig. 2. {^{1}H}-^{13}C spectra from the spectral map of Fig. 1. (a) Spectrum from voxel 1. Assignment of resonances: 1, *CH$_3$–CH$_2$–CH$_2$, fatty acyl chain; 2, CH$_3$–*CH$_2$–CH$_2$, fatty acyl chain; 3, (CH$_2$)$_n$; 4, CH$_2$–*CH$_2$–CO, fatty acyl chain; 5, C-1, C-3, glycerol (ester); 6, C-2, glycerol (ester); 7, CH=*CH–CH$_2$–*CH=CH, fatty acyl chain; 8, CH$_2$–CH$_2$–*CO, fatty acyl chain. (b) Spectrum from voxel 2. Assignment of resonances: 9, *CH$_2$–NH$_2$, ethanolamine; 10, (*CH$_3$)$_3$–N, choline + creatine + carnitine; 11, glycerol (ester) and carbohydrates (C-2, C-3, C-4, C-5, C-6, glucose, and glycogen); 12, C-1 α-glucose; 13, C-1 β-glucose; 14, C-1 glycogen; 15, CO–OR, proteins, phospholipids. Assignments were given according to Refs. 7 and 13.

localized in the human liver. {^{1}H}-^{13}C spectra corresponding to voxels 1 (muscle + liver) and 2 (liver only) are depicted in Fig. 2. The S/N of the liver spectrum was significantly lower than that of the muscle spectrum. This emphasized the difficulty of obtaining spectroscopic data from the deep abdomen even with large surface coils. In voxel 2, fatty acyl chains, carbonyl groups, glucose, and related carbohydrates resonances were well resolved. It was also possible to detect the natural abundance C-1 glycogen resonance.

CONCLUSIONS

Single-voxel localized spectroscopy could be achieved on the liver, but it is less informative than multivoxel spectroscopic imaging. In the present work, it was shown that acquiring several {^{1}H}-^{13}C spectra from different parts of the abdomen was possible, provided that coils bearing a quality factor >150 are used. It has to be noted that our spectra were recorded within a reasonably short amount of time with rather low-RF deposition. From this point of view, NMR spectroscopic imaging is a very mild investigational technique. In order to further study some feature of liver metabolism, the S/N of spectrum 2 in Fig. 2 must be improved. This could be done with a better decoupling between coils: even though the butterfly geometry of the proton coil is useful for limiting the mutual inductance with the circular ^{13}C coil, this compromise might not be the best one. Work is in progress to find alternatives to this problem. Furthermore, the use of ^{13}C-enriched substrates such as ^{13}C-1 glucose [11, 12] would bring significant improvement for the detection of weak resonances and would allow a marked reduction of the voxel size. The latter point could permit investigations of topical lesions within the organ.

REFERENCES

1. Brown TR, Kincaid BM, Ugurbil K (1982) NMR chemical shift imaging in three dimensions. *Proc Natl Acad Sci USA* **79**: 3523–3526.
2. Maudsley AA, Hilal SK, Perman WH, Simon HE (1983) Spatially resolved high resolution spectroscopy by "four dimensional" NMR, *J Magn Reson* **51**: 147–152.
3. Xue M, Galvez N, Ng TC, Majors AW, Rudick R, Modic M (1992) Evaluation of the ^{1}H spectroscopy of sclerosing vasculopathy using chemical shift imaging. *SMRM Abstracts* **1**: 646.
4. Srinivasan R, Arias-Mandoza F, Murphy-Boesch J, Stoyanova R, Willard T, Negendank W, Brown T (1992) Proton

decoupled ^{31}P CSI of human brain in a rampable magnet at 2.0 Tesla. *SMRM Abstracts* **1**: 1901.

5. Buchthal SD, Thoma WJ, Taylor JS, Nelson SJ, Brown TR (1989) *In vivo* T_1-values of phosphorus metabolites in human liver and muscle determined at 1.5 T by chemical shift imaging. *NMR Biomed* **2**: 298–304.

6. Cox IJ, Menon DK, Sargentoni J, Bryant DJ, Collins AG, Coutts GA, Iles RA, Bell JD, Benjamin IS, Gilbey S, Hodgson HJF, Morgan MY (1992) Phosphorus-31 magnetic resonance spectroscopy of the human liver using spectroscopic imaging techniques. *J Hepatol* **14**: 265–275.

7. Beckmann N, Seelig J, Wick H (1990) Analysis of glycogen storage disease by *in vivo* ^{13}C NMR: Comparison of normal volunteers with a patient. *Magn Reson Med* **16**: 150–160.

8. Jue T, Rothman DL, Tavitian BA, Shulman RG (1989) Natural abundance ^{13}C study of glycogen repletion in human liver and muscle. *Proc Natl Acad Sci USA* **86**: 1439–1442.

9. Heerschap A, Luyten PR, van der Heyden JI, Oosterwaal LJMP, den Hollander JA (1989) Broadband proton-decoupled natural abundance ^{13}C NMR spectroscopy of humans at 1.5 T. *NMR Biomed* **2**: 124–132.

10. Shaka AJ, Keeler J, Frenkiel T, Freeman R (1983) An improved sequence for broadband decoupling: WALTZ-16. *J Magn Reson* **52**: 335–338.

11. Beckmann N, Turkalj I, Seelig J, Keller U (1991) ^{13}C NMR for the assessment of human brain glucose metabolism *in vivo*. *Biochemistry* **30**: 6362–6366.

12. Gruetter R, Novotny EJ, Boulware SD, Rothman DL, Mason GF, Shulman GI, Shulman RG, Tamborlane WV (1992) Direct measurement of brain glucose concentrations in human by ^{13}C NMR spectroscopy. *Proc Natl Acad Sci USA* **89**: 1109–1112.

13. Canioni P, Alger JR, Shulman RG (1983) Natural abundance carbon-13 magnetic resonance spectroscopy of liver and adipose tissue of the living rat. *Biochemistry* **22**: 4974–4980.

Glycogen resynthesis in liver and muscle after exercise: measurement of the rate of resynthesis by ^{13}C magnetic resonance spectroscopy

K.T. Moriarty,[1] D.G.O. McIntyre,[2] K. Bingham,[2] R. Coxon,[2] P.M. Glover,[2]
P.L. Greenhaff,[1] I.A. Macdonald,[1]* H.S. Bachelard[2] and P.G. Morris[2]

[1]*Department of Physiology and Pharmacology, Queen's Medical Centre, University of Nottingham,*
[2]*Magnetic Resonance Centre, University of Nottingham, Nottingham NG7 2RD, UK*

We have used natural abundance ^{13}C magnetic resonance spectroscopy (MRS) to measure glycogen content of muscle and liver before and after heavy exercise, and after consumption of different carbohydrate-based drinks. After an overnight fast, five healthy men (mean ± SEM age 23 ± 1 years) exercised to exhaustion at 75% of VO_{2max} on two occasions (mean work rate 165 ± 8 W for 78 ± 14 min) and then, in a single blind random order, consumed either of two drinks containing the same carbohydrate load (177 g). Spectra were recorded over Vastus Lateralis muscle and the liver before and after exercise, and hourly for 5 h after the carbohydrate load. In muscle, glycogen content after exercise was 37% and 31% of basal (preexercise) concentration before consuming the drinks. After carbohydrate loading, glycogen concentration had increased significantly ($p < 0.05$) to 70% and 64% of basal concentration respectively after 5 h. Hepatic glycogen concentration did not change significantly throughout. The study demonstrates the feasibility of sequential MRS measurement of muscle and liver glycogen before and after exercise and after carbohydrate loading.

Keywords: Magnetic resonance spectroscopy, glycogen, liver, muscle.

INTRODUCTION

Until recently, tissue biopsy with direct biochemical measurement has been the only method of assessing metabolite concentrations in human skeletal muscle [1–3]. Inevitably, this may be unpleasant, painful, and dangerous for subjects and operators alike, and the biopsy technique itself may also introduce artifactual changes which could affect the metabolic profile of any subsequent biopsy. Repeated liver biopsies are not acceptable because of the significant risks associated and there is limited information as to what happens to hepatic glycogen with heavy exercise.

In 1983, Sillerud and Shulman showed that glycogen gives a well-resolved ^{13}C-MRS (magnetic resonance spectroscopy) spectrum [4], which allowed liver and muscle glycogen concentrations to be measured

in man [5–7]. Natural abundance ^{13}C-MRS measurement of human muscle glycogen has been shown to detect small sequential changes in muscle glycogen related to low-intensity exercise [8] and has been validated by direct biochemical assay of needle biopsy samples [9].

The aim of this study was to use ^{13}C magnetic resonance spectroscopy to measure the glycogen content of muscle and liver before and after heavy exercise undertaken to deplete muscle glycogen stores, and then after loading two different carbohydrate drinks.

MATERIALS AND METHODS

Five healthy men, mean (±SEM) age 23 (±1) years, attended the Magnetic Resonance Centre on the university campus on two separate occasions. After refraining from exercise, smoking, and drinking any caffeine-containing drinks or alcohol for 24 h before each study, subjects had spectroscopy of liver and

---

Address for correspondence: IA MacDonald Department of Physiology and Pharmacology, Queen's Medical Centre, Nottingham, NG7 2UH, UK.

muscle performed at rest after an overnight fast. Subjects then exercised to voluntary exhaustion at 75% of maximal O_2 uptake (VO_{2max}). This had been measured for each subject on two previous occasions. The workload was 165 (± 8) W for 78 (± 14) min. After the exercise period, spectra were recorded from muscle and liver again, and then after consumption of two different carbohydrate-based drinks (drink A was a mixture of glucose polymers and drink B was sucrose). The total carbohydrate content of each was 177 g (900 ml), consumed over 5 min. Liver spectra were recorded after 30 min and then hourly; muscle spectra were recorded after 60 min and then hourly. A typical set of seven spectra from muscle is shown in Fig. 1.

Natural abundance ^{13}C-MR spectra were recorded using a magnetic resonance system constructed at the University of Nottingham, operating inside the room-temperature bore of a 3-T whole-body superconducting magnet (Oxford Magnet Technology). For the liver, a circular surface coil of radius 6 cm was con-

structed from a single turn of 6-mm-diameter copper pipe. This was mounted on a plastic spacer and taped to the skin of the volunteer. For the muscle measurements, an elliptical surface coil of major axis 12 cm and minor axis 7 cm was constructed from the same copper pipe and attached to a thermoplastic cast moulded to fit the thigh of each subject. The coil was positioned over Vastus Lateralis. ^{13}C-NMR spectra were recorded at 32 MHz without proton decoupling. Blocks of 30 000 free-induction decays (FIDs), each excited by a single square radio-frequency pulse of 130 μs duration were averaged. The pulse length corresponded to a flip angle of approximately 180° at the coil center. The block acquisition time was 16 min.

Data processing was performed using NMRI software (New Methods Research Inc.). The time-domain data set size was 512 points, and all FIDs were zero-filled to 2048 points. A Lorentz–Gauss filter with Lorentzian narrowing of 35 Hz and Gaussian broadening of 70 Hz was applied, followed by a trapezoidal weighting function prior to Fourier transformation. The zero- and first-order phases were set manually. A ninth-order polynomial correction and baseline deconvolution was applied to produce a near linear baseline. Chemical shifts were calibrated relative to a sodium acetate standard, labeled in the C-1 position and positioned at the center of both coils, which generates a reference peak at 182.3 ppm. Glycogen peak areas were measured by integration and expressed as a percentage of the lipid peak; the limits of integration were chosen after averaging all spectral data for a single subject to maximize signal to noise. All data were analyzed by three-factor analysis of variance (ANOVA) with repeated measures (BMDP Statistical Software, Los Angeles, CA, USA). Where significant, post hoc testing was performed using paired *t*-tests, with Bonferroni's correction for multiple comparisons.

RESULTS

Muscle

The individual preexercise and postexercise values ($n = 5$) for each subject, each of whom attended twice, are shown Fig. 2. Each symbol refers to a single subject. Muscle glycogen fell significantly ($p < 0.001$) from 0.77% of the lipid resonance preexercise to 0.26% postexercise, which is approximately one-third of the preexercise value. After consumption of the two drinks, muscle glycogen rose significantly ($p < 0.01$) to approximately double the postexercise value after 5 h. There were no differences between the two visits at any time point (Fig. 3).

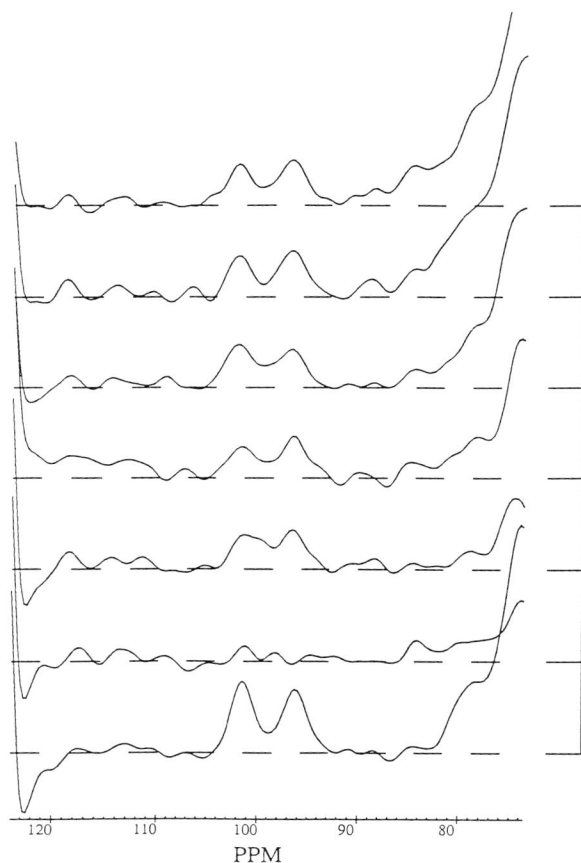

Fig. 1. A typical set of spectra derived from muscle. The lowest spectrum is that recorded preexercise, and the one above it postexercise. The other spectra show resynthesis, with the final spectrum at the top recorded 5 h after carbohydrate loading.

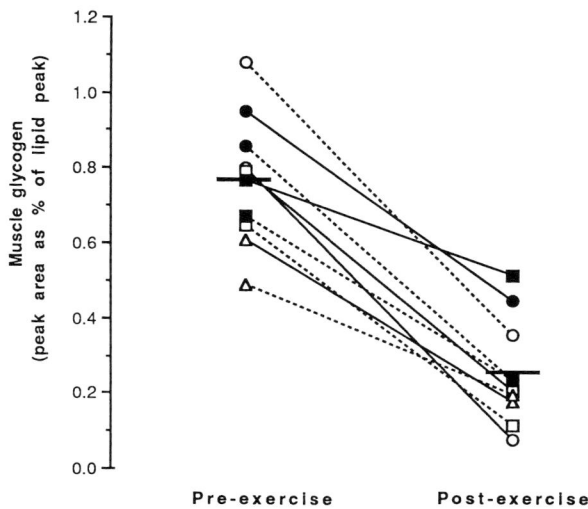

Fig. 2. Muscle glycogen content before and after exercise to exhaustion. Each subject is represented by a unique symbol. The values before drink A are linked by a solid line, those before drink B by a dashed line. The mean values before and after exercise are shown by the horizontal bars. There was a highly significant fall in muscle glycogen after exercise ($p < 0.01$).

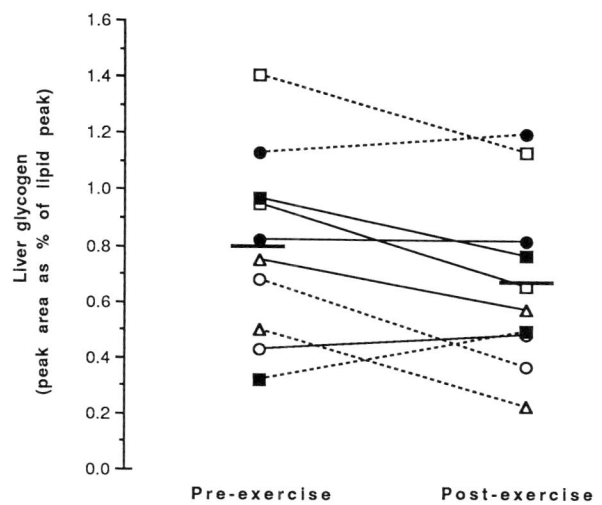

Fig. 4. Liver glycogen content before and after exercise to exhaustion. Each subject is represented by a unique symbol. The values before drink A are linked by a solid line, those before drink B by a dashed line. The mean values before and after exercise are shown by the horizontal bars. Note the considerable intersubject and intrasubject variation and that there was no significant change with exercise.

Liver

The individual preexercise and postexercise values for each subject ($n = 5$), each of whom attended twice, are shown in Fig. 4; the symbols are the same as those shown in Fig. 2 for each subject. Liver glycogen fell from 0.80% of the lipid resonance preexercise to 0.68% postexercise; the difference did not reach significance. After consumption of the two drinks (Fig. 5), although

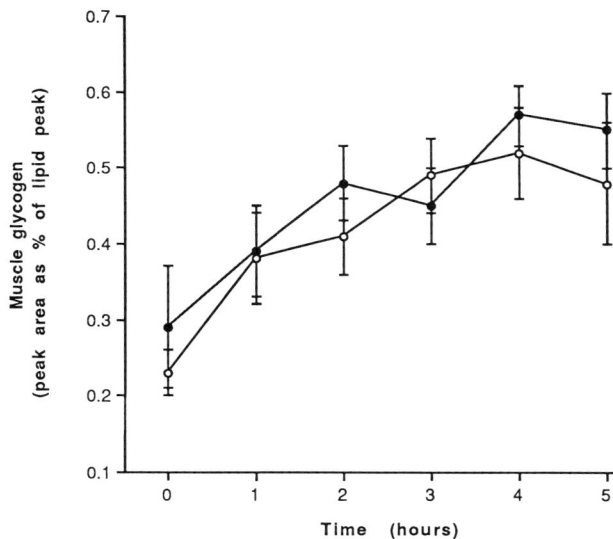

Fig. 3. Muscle glycogen content in the postexercise recovery period. Immediately after the measurements were made at time 0, a drink containing 177 g carbohydrate was consumed. (● denotes values after drink A, ○ after drink B.) There were similar rates of increase in muscle glycogen content after the two drinks, with no significant difference between them.

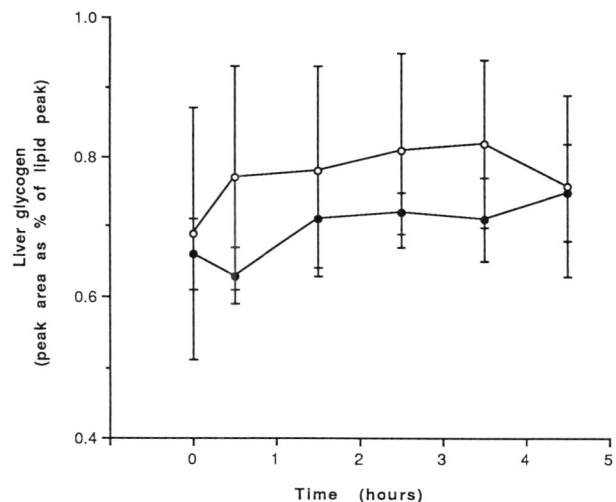

Fig. 5. Liver glycogen content in the postexercise recovery period. Immediately after the measurements were made at time 0, a drink containing 177 g carbohydrate was consumed. (● denotes values after drink A, ○ after drink B.) There was no significant change in liver glycogen content over this period, although there was a trend for the values to be higher after drink B ($p = 0.06$.)

there was an apparent rise in liver glycogen with one of the carbohydrate-based drinks, this fell short of significance ($p = 0.06$).

CONCLUSIONS

This study shows that measurement of muscle and liver glycogen content can be estimated in the same study by recording interleaved spectra from the two sites. The study also demonstrates that two different aspects of glycogen metabolism, depletion and repletion, can be combined in the same study. The results reaffirm the power of natural abundance ^{13}C-MRS for the study of human glycogen metabolism. The technique used was well within current safety guidelines for irradiation. More significantly, the results obtained in this study by MRS replace the equivalent number of muscle and liver biopsies, 70 of each, with consequent avoidance of significant morbidity.

Significant changes in muscle glycogen were demonstrated with a small subject number, suggesting that variance due to the technique is small, as the variance between subjects is comparable with results obtained by biopsy [9]. Variance in liver glycogen between subjects was much higher in our study, probably due to a combination of intrasubject variation in positioning of the coil, and intersubject and intrasubject differences in glycogen content due to diet and fasting prior to the study [10]. Such error is likely to be systematic; because the mean postexercise liver glycogen content between visits was comparable, the trend toward a significant difference between visits merits further investigation, as it is likely to be due to the intervention, that is, differences in the composition of the two carbohydrate-based drinks.

ACKNOWLEDGMENTS

The magnetic resonance system was constructed in the M.R. Centre at the University of Nottingham with funding from the British Technology Group. The study was funded by SmithKline Beecham Consumer Healthcare.

REFERENCES

1. Hultman E (1967) Muscle glycogen in man determined in needle biopsy specimens: method and normal values. *Scand J Clin Lab Invest* **19**: 209–217.
2. Maehlum S (1978) Muscle glycogen synthesis after a glucose infusion during post exercise recovery in diabetic and non-diabetic subjects. *Scand J Clin Lab Invest* **38**: 349–354.
3. Dietrichson P, Coakley J, Smith PEM, Griffiths RD, Helliwell TR, Edwards RHT (1987) Conchotome and needle percutaneous biopsy of skeletal muscle. *J Neurol Neurosurg* **50**: 1461–1467.
4. Sillerud LO, Shulman RG (1983) Structure and metabolism of mammalian liver glycogen monitored by carbon-13 nuclear magnetic resonance. *Biochemistry* **22**: 1087–1094.
5. Avison MJ, Rothman DL, Nadel E, Shulman RG (1988) Detection of human muscle glycogen by natural abundance ^{13}C NMR. *Proc Natl Acad Sci (USA)* **85**: 1634–1636.
6. Jue T, Rothman DL, Tavitian BA, Shulman RG (1989). Natural abundance ^{13}C NMR study of glycogen repletion in human liver and muscle. *Proc Natl Acad Sci (USA)* **86**: 1439–1442.
7. Price TP, Rothman DL, Avison MJ, Buonamico P, Shulman RG (1991) ^{13}C-NMR measurements of muscle glycogen during low intensity exercise. *J Appl Physiol* **70**: 1836–1844.
8. Shulman GI, Rothman DL, Jue T, Stein P, DeFronzo RA, Shulman RG (1990) Quantitation of muscle glycogen synthesis in normal subjects and subjects with non-insulin-dependent diabetes by ^{13}C nuclear magnetic resonance spectroscopy. *New Engl J Med* **322**: 223–228.
9. Taylor R, Price TB, Rothman DL, Shulman RG, Shulman GI (1992). Validation of ^{13}C NMR measurement of human skeletal muscle glycogen by direct biochemical assay of needle biopsy samples. *Magn Res Med* **27**: 13–20.
10. Hultman E, Nilsson LH (1975). Factors influencing carbohydrate metabolism in man. *Nutr Metab* **18** (Suppl 1): 45–64.

MRS studies of cancer

J.R. Griffiths,* R.J. Maxwell,[1] S.L. Howells, F.A. Howe,[1] S.P. Robinson,[1]
M. Stubbs,[1] C.L. McCoy,[1] L.M. Rodrigues,[1] C.L. Parkins[2] and D.J. Chaplin[2]

[1]CRC Biomedical Magnetic Resonance Research Group, St. George's Hospital Medical School,
London, SW17 ORE, UK [2]CRC Gray Laboratory, Mount Vernon Hospital,
Northwood, Middlesex HA6 2RN, UK

Cancer was an obvious disease to study by magnetic resonance spectroscopy (MRS); it produces large lesions that give clearly abnormal spectra, all treatment methods leave much to be desired, and radiotherapy, in particular, is limited by tissue hypoxia, a process that can be investigated by MRS. ^{31}P MRS has shown that tumor cells are not acidic, as had been thought; instead, the pH gradient across the tumor cell membrane is the reverse of that in a normal cell. This change in hydrogen-ion gradient is accompanied by changes in gradients of many other ions.

Tumor oxygenation can be monitored in animal tumor models using the techniques employed for functional magnetic resonance imaging (MRI) of the brain. Large changes in signal are observed when drugs that reduce tumor blood flow are administered.

^{1}H NMR spectra of acid extracts of tumor or normal tissue biopsies contain sufficient information to permit classification (and thus, perhaps, diagnosis) if computer-based pattern recognition techniques are employed. Surprisingly, the same technique gives quite good classification of ^{31}P spectra taken *in vivo*.

Can MRS be *applied* in cancer therapy? Studies on tumor ion balance will help in the design of anticancer drugs and other therapies. Tumor blood flow studies using MRI could be applied to individual patients to predict the usefulness of radiotherapy and to assist in radiotherapy planning. Pattern recognition methods could automate the screening of biopsies and could also assist in interpretation of human spectra taken *in vivo*.

Keywords: Magnetic resonance spectroscopy, tumors, ion balance, functional MRI, blood flow, pattern recognition.

INTRODUCTION

The use of magnetic resonance spectroscopy (MRS) to study cancer *in vivo* was a relatively late development compared with heart, muscle, and other body tissues, although in retrospect it was an obvious choice. Cancer is a common disease, and tumors contain abnormal concentrations of some metabolites. Many are several centimeters in diameter before they are detected, and a reasonable number are found in locations in which they can give adequate MRS signals with current techniques. Furthermore, there is an

*Address for correspondence: CRC Biomedical Magnetic Resonance Research Group, St. George's Hospital Medical School, London SW17 ORE, UK.

urgent need to improve the efficacy of cancer therapy. Nonsurgical anticancer therapies such as radiotherapy, chemotherapy, and endocrine therapy are all of limited use against the major solid tumors. The same is true of the newer therapies, including hyperthermia, photodynamic therapy, immunotherapy, and those based on biological response modifiers (e.g., tumor necrosis factor or interferon). Using noninvasive measurements of tumor chemistry, we should be able to improve our understanding of these therapies and, perhaps, to monitor and thus optimize the treatment of individual patients. So far, however, the major successes of MRS in cancer have been concerned with research. As with many other diseases, we have learned much about the physiology and biochemistry of cancer from MRS, but we have not yet been able to apply it routinely in the clinic.

TUMOR pH

The chemical shift of the P_i peaks in the first ^{31}P spectra of tumors *in vivo* showed that their intracellular pH was not acidic, as had been thought for many years, but neutral or slightly basic [1, 2]. The acidic tumor pH values that had previously been obtained with micro-electrodes were mainly due to the extracellular fluid, which contains a high concentration of hydrogen ions extruded from the cells. The corollary of this observation was not immediately understood, however. This was that the pH gradient across the tumor cell membrane was reversed: Tumor cells are more alkaline than their surroundings, whereas normal cells are usually more acidic than the pH 7.4 extracellular fluid in which they are bathed [3]. Because this fundamental gradient is reversed, there are changes in the distribution of many other ionic species.

Studies on this topic have recently been facilitated by the introduction of 3-aminopropylphosphonate (3-APP), a pH indicator for the extracellular fluid [4]. Using this, we have been able to measure simultaneously both the intracellular and extracellular pH of tumors. The administration of 3-APP I.P. does not detectably alter intracellular pH (pH_i) (as measured from the chemical shift of the P_i peak) or other metabolic indices, and the extracellular pH (pH_e) detected correlates with calculations based on an assumed equilibrium of the protonated and unprotonated species of lactate across the cell membrane [5, 6].

ELIMINATING THE CHEMICAL SHIFT ARTIFACT BY DIVA

A major technical problem with single-voxel localization methods such as Image Selective in Vivo Spectroscopy (ISIS) is that frequency is used to encode both chemical shift and spatial position. Because of this, each peak in the spectrum comes from a slightly different voxel; this is a serious nuisance if (as in the case of pH determinations) the chemical shift between two peaks (Δ) is what is being measured. The separation is given by

$$\text{Displacement (mm)} = \Delta \text{ (ppm)}$$
$$\times B_0 \text{ (T)/Gradient (mT m}^{-1})$$

This effect is relatively trivial for peaks separated by a small chemical shift, such as P_i and α-NTP. (α-NTP is used as a chemical shift standard in these experiments.) However, the chemical shift difference between 3-APP and α-NTP, 31 ppm, is so great that the displacement becomes

$$\text{Displacement} = 31 \times 4.7/75 = 2 \text{ mm}$$

This is sufficient to reduce the volume overlap of the two voxels, 1 cm³, to an unacceptable 44%. Magnetic field inhomogeneities could result in the signal of the chemical shift standard being measured at a different magnetic field to that at which the pH_e probe is measured. We have devised a simple way to minimise this problem for a pair of peaks, by performing, in effect, two separate ISIS experiments with the offset frequency centered on each peak in turn. We term it Double ISIS Volume Acquisition, or DIVA. The spectra in a study on pH_i are centered on the offset frequencies of α-NTP and 3-APP so each peak is measured from the same voxel. The DIVA method, in combination with a quantitation technique such as Variable Projection [VARPRO], can also be used to measure ratios of peak areas.

ION DISTRIBUTION ACROSS THE CANCER CELL MEMBRANE

We have been studying the distribution of ions across the cancer cell membrane *in vivo* and have found many unexpected abnormalities. Tumor cells have an elevated Na^+ and decreased K^+, increased P_i, Ca^{2+}, and lactate⁻, and decreased HCO_3^- and Mg^{2+}; the ratio ATP:ADP $\times$ P_i is also decreased [5]. The most likely explanation of these changes is that the lactic acid produced by the enhanced glycolytic metabolism of tumor cells is rapidly exported as lactate⁻ and H^+ (to maintain electrical neutrality) and the H^+ is slow to clear from the tumor extracellular space, perhaps because of poor tumor blood flow. The reversal of the normal H^+ gradient results in changes in many other linked ionic equilibria.

TUMOR BLOOD FLOW AND OXYGENATION

There has been much interest in the study of tumor blood flow and oxygenation because radiotherapy is ineffective in hypoxic cells. We have used the D_2O wash-in method [7] to measure tumor blood flow in transplanted and primary rodent tumors. The results can be displayed as volume-averaged spectra or as images; the latter give important information about the heterogeneous distribution of blood supply in the tumor. It is also possible to calculate absolute flow rates if the arterial input function is known; we find it best to obtain this from the signal of the blood in the heart.

We have experimented with hypotensive drugs to reduce tumor blood flow [8, 9], but we found that these effects were largely confined to transplantable tumors: Most primary tumors (induced by chemicals or radiation) were resistant [10]. There have also been reports that naturally occurring murine tumors fail to respond to hypotensives [11]. This may be because the action of such drugs is thought to be due to dilation of the host blood vessels, whereas tumor blood vessels, lacking receptors for the drug, fail to respond. The combination of a fall in blood pressure and redirection of flow to host tissues results in tumor hypoperfusion and hypoxia. Primary tumors grow relatively slowly and may have time to develop blood vessels that are able to respond to hypotensives. Quick-growing transplants, however, develop blood vessels that do not respond to hypotensives, so such tumors are vulnerable [10, 11]. Slower-growing transplants seem to behave more like primaries [12].

Lately, we have been developing a noninvasive method for measuring changes in tumor blood flow and oxygenation [13]. This is based on the functional MRI (F-MRI) technique that has been used so successfully in the brain to delineate changes during mental activity. The same methodology, a pulse sequence that is very sensitive to the T_2^* phenomena induced by the paramagnetic red cells in the blood, can be used to delineate changes in subcutaneous rodent tumors caused by agents that affect the tumor vasculature. Our original experiments utilized the hypotensive agent calcitonin gene-related peptide, which reduces blood flow transiently in the GH3 prolactinoma and causes a fall in the cellular energy status as measured by ^{31}P MRS [9]. In tumors that show a transient ^{31}P change, there is a marked change in the ^{1}H MRI image detected by a gradient echo-pulse sequence [13]. It is unclear, at present, whether this is due to changes in blood oxygen level dependence (BOLD) or blood volume or blood flow, but the effect is marked and reproducible in the GH3 tumor, although not in the RIF-1 fibrosarcoma [14]. We have found that excellent registration can be maintained between images, so it is possible to detect the marked heterogeneity in vascular response that would be expected from the chaotic architecture and blood supply in transplanted rodent tumors.

F-MRI has the great advantage that tissues are imaged with the sensitivity of the ^{1}H nucleus and that the signal is derived from the tissue water, which is several orders of magnitude higher in concentration than any metabolite. In general, the introduction of "physiological MRI" techniques that obtain images of dynamic processes has been an important development in recent years. Because their sensitivity is so much higher than that of MRS, it is possible to trade it off for more rapid scan times or detailed spatial images.

PATTERN RECOGNITION

MR spectra, even when taken *in vivo*, contain enormous amounts of information rarely considered by conventional interpretation techniques. We have been developing automated statistical methods for data analysis, based on the entire spectrum rather than selected peaks. Our approach has been described in detail by Howells et al. [15, 16]; briefly, it consists of digitizing the spectra by taking the highest peak in each of (typically) 200 windows, taking the principal components (PCs) of the resulting database, selecting those that give most of the information (typically about 10–15), and subjecting these PC scores to cluster analysis. The chosen PCs for the database are then used to train an artificial neural network (a computer program based on a putative model for the interaction of neurones) to learn how to classify the spectra. Data from spectra not used in the training stage are then processed by the network, using the learned parameters, to test the classification scheme that has been developed.

Our original studies were on 1D ^{1}H NMR spectra of perchloric acid extracts of three normal rat tissues and five rat tumors [15, 16]. Recently, we have expanded the database of tumors used in this study to 200 spectra. The same methods [16] were applied and the results of a neural network analysis are shown in Table 1. The neural network was tested on the "leave-one-out" principle, in which it "learns" from 199 of the 200 samples and classifies the remaining 1. The accuracy of the classification is remarkable: 96% of the samples were classified correctly, a further 2.5% were classified correctly but not to the arbitrary degree of certainty that we required (these were termed "partly correct"), 3% could not be classified, and only 0.5%—one sample—was incorrectly classified. The success of the method with this artificial problem is promising and has prompted us to undertake tests on more realistic data sets of human biopsies.

Another extension of this method would be to study spectra taken noninvasively, *in vivo*. At present, most studies outside the brain are performed by ^{31}P MRS, and the spectra generated are not encouraging. They contain few peaks, some of them poorly resolved, line shapes are irregular, the signal-to-noise ratio is much lower than can be obtained *in vitro*, and the metabolite

Table 1. Classification of a 200 sample data set of ^1H spectra from normal rat tissues and rat tumors by the neural network. Sample preparation, NMR, and pattern recognition were as in Ref. 16. The network "learned" from 199 of the samples and then attempted to classify the remaining 1.

Class	Correct	Partly correct	Unclas- sified	Wrong
Fibrosarcoma	15	1	0	0
Pituitary Tumor	8	1	1	0
Walker carcinosarcoma	7	1	0	0
Morris hepatoma H7777	10	0	2	1
Morris hepatoma 9618A	11	1	0	0
Spleen	42	0	0	0
Kidney	49	1	2	0
Liver	46	0	1	0
% of total	94.0	2.5	3.0	0.5

signals are superimposed on a broad and variable hump due to membrane and macromolecular phosphates. Nevertheless, we have had some success with the same general approach as was used for the ^1H pattern recognition [15]. A database of 58 ISIS spectra from brain ($n = 7$), muscle ($n = 6$), liver ($n = 6$), pituitary tumors ($n = 9$), Morris hepatomas 9618A ($n = 8$), MNU-induced mammary tumors ($n = 14$) (all in rats), and RIF-1 fibrosarcomas ($n = 8$) in mice was studied. In this case, PC analysis did not improve the final classification, so it was omitted. The neural network, using the "leave-one-out" principle, classified 62% correctly, with a further 19% partially correct (i.e., correct but not with the required degree of certainty): 12% unclassified and 7% wrong [17]. Not surprisingly, this was not as good as with the biopsy dataset, but the results were still surprisingly good. Again, we have been encouraged to proceed to a trial of tumor spectra from patients, to see whether it is possible to predict the response of tumors to therapy.

CONCLUSIONS

How far will the techniques described in this article be applicable in cancer therapy? Our studies on tumor pH_i, pH_e, and the associated shifts of ion balance across the cell membrane may help in the design of anticancer drugs and in the interpretation of the action of other therapeutic modalities such as hyperthermia. Tumor oxygenation is thought to be of central importance in radiotherapy, one of the major present-day therapeutic modalities. Studies using F-MRI techniques, if they are as successful in patients as in animals, could easily be applied to individual patients. Thus, the response of different parts of a tumor to radiotherapy might be predictable; resistant areas might be given higher doses during radiotherapy planning (or vice versa) or chemotherapy might be preferred in some cases. F-MRI has much higher resolution than MRS techniques and could be applied to much smaller malignant deposits.

The role of pattern recognition methods could be widespread. They could provide automated and objective analysis of spectra obtained from biopsies in screening programs (e.g., cervical tissues) or they may be able to help classify some histological specimens whose degree of malignancy cannot easily be established by pathologists. In general, it is not difficult to diagnose most tumors by conventional means, so the main use of high-resolution NMR of biopsies could be in establishing the grade or degree of malignancy. Extensive studies on realistic databases will be required to test these ideas. MRS spectra obtained noninvasively seem to indicate the response of tumors to therapy before tumor regression is observable [18]; pattern recognition methods may refine these tests and make them objective. In general, it should be easy to incorporate a pattern recognition algorithm into a conventional MRS examination because the powerful computer workstations used to control spectrometers are able to perform the necessary computations. Testing a spectrum against a preprogrammed neural network, for instance, takes only a few seconds on a SUN-10.

REFERENCES

1. Griffiths JR, Stevens AN, Iles RA, Gordon RA, Shaw D (1981) ^{31}P NMR investigation of solid tumours in the living rat. *Biosci Rep* **1:** 177–182.
2. Griffiths JR, Cady E, Edwards RHT, McCready VR, and Wiltshaw E (1983) ^{13}P NMR studies of a human tumour *in situ. Lancet* 1 1436–1437.
3. Griffiths JR (1991) Are cancer cells acidic? *Br J Cancer* **64:** 425–427.
4. Gillies RJ, Lui Z, Bhujwalla Z (1994) ^{31}P NMR measurement of extracellular pH of tumours and tumour cells *in vitro* using 3-aminopropylphosphonate. *Am J Physiol Cell* **267:** C195–C203.
5. Stubbs M, Rodrigues L, Howe FA, Wang J, Jeong K-S, Veech RL, Griffiths JR (1994) The metabolic consequences of a reversed pH gradient in rat tumours. *Cancer Res* **54:** 4011–4016.

6. Stubbs M, Bhujwalla ZM, Tozer GM, Rodrigues LM, Maxwell RJ, Morgan R, Howe FA, Griffiths JR (1992) An assessment of ^{31}P MRS as a method of measuring pH in rat tumours. *NMR Biomed* **5:** 351–359.

7. Mattiello J, and Evelhoch JL (1991) Relative volume-average murine tumor blood flow measurement via deuterium nuclear magnetic resonance spectroscopy. *Magn Reson Med* **18:** 320–334.

8. Tozer GM, Maxwell RJ, Griffiths JR, Pham P (1990) Modification of the ^{31}P magnetic resonance spectra of a rat tumour using vasodilators and its relationship to hypertension. *Br J Cancer* **39:** 857–863.

9. Burney IA, Maxwell RJ, Griffiths JR, Field SB (1991) The potential for prazosin and calcitonin gene-related (CGRP) in causing hypoxia in tumours. *Br J Cancer* **64:** 683–688.

10. Field SB, Needham S, Burney IA, Maxwell RJ, Coggle JE, Griffiths JR (1991) Differences in vascular response between primary and transplanted tumours. *Br J Cancer* **63:** 723–726.

11. Wood PJ, Stratford IJ, Sansom JM, Cattanach BM, Quinney RM, Adams GE (1992) The response of spontaneous and transplantable murine tumors to vasoactive agents measured by ^{31}P magnetic resonance spectroscopy. *Int J Radiat Oncol Biol Phys* **22:** 473–476.

12. Robinson SP, van den Boogaart A, Hamilton E, Waterton JC, Griffiths JR (1994) Differences in vascular response between early and late generation transplanted tumours Proceedings 2nd Meeting, Society of Magnetic Resonance, p 1336, 1994.

13. Howe FA, Robinson SP, Griffiths JR (1993) Monitoring changes in oxygenation and blood perfusion of a subcutaneous tumour by functional MRI *Proceedings 12th Annual Meeting. Society for Magnetic Resonance in Medicine,* p. 1002.

14. Griffiths JR, Howe FA, Robinson SP (1994) Changes in tumour perfusion and oxygenation monitored by physiological MRI. *Br J Cancer* **69:** 53.

15. Howells SL, Maxwell RJ, Griffiths JR (1992) Classification of tumour 1H spectra by pattern recognition. *NMR Biomed* **5:** 59–64.

16. Howells SL, Maxwell RJ, Griffiths JR (1992) An investigation of tumor ^{1}H nuclear magnetic resonance spectra by the application of chemometric techniques. *Magn Reson Med* **28:** 214–236.

17. Howells SL, Maxwell RJ, Howe FA, Peet AC, Stubbs M, Rodrigues LM, Robinson SP, Baluch S, Griffiths JR (1993) Pattern recognition of ^{31}P magnetic resonance spectra obtained *in vivo. NMR Biomed* **6:** 237–241.

18. Negendank W (1992) Studies of human tumors of MRS: a review. *NMR Biomed* **5:** 303–324.

^{13}C-MRS studies on cerebral metabolism

Herman Bachelard,* Ronnitte Badar-Goffer, Oded Ben-Yoseph, Peter Morris,
Andrew Taylor and Nicola Thatcher

MR Centre, Department of Physics, University of Nottingham, Nottingham NG7 2RD, UK

^{13}C from labeled glucose is normally incorporated rapidly into cerebral glutamate with little detectable glutamine or citrate. In contrast, glutamine and citrate only show significant labeling from ^{13}C acetate, which reflects metabolism in glial cells. When brain slices are depolarized with 40 mM KCl (which mirrors some of the conditions of epilepsy) the ^{13}C enrichment of glutamine and citrate from glucose is accelerated in contrast to that of glutamate, which is not. This clearly indicates that depolarizing conditions stimulate glial rather than neuronal consumption of glucose.

In tissues subjected to hypoxia, there is greatly increased labeling of glycerol 3-phosphate, which was confirmed by its increased presence in ^{31}P-MR (magnetic resonance) spectra. Analysis of the labeling of lactate, alanine, and glycerol 3-phosphate demonstrated that the ability of the brain to maintain normal function in hypoxia is limited by the capacity of the key enzyme, lactate dehydrogenase. This has implications in the clinical assessment and management of stroke. These results also have implications in the interpretation of activation studies, where increased lactate could be due either to depolarization or hypoxia, or both.

The spectra observed in studies on metabolism of U-[^{13}C] glutamate in cerebral preparations revealed clear signals from glutamine and lactate released to the media. The isotopomer patterns of the lactate showed that it must have arisen from the exogenous glutamate, because if it were due to naturally abundant ^{13}C in the lactate, only singlets would have appeared. Comparison of the isotopomer patterns and the percentage ^{13}C enrichments of the glutamine and lactate showed that there is higher incorporation of ^{13}C from exogenous glutamate into lactate than into glutamine. The enrichment of the lactate indicated that very little was derived from glucose and suggests that the glutamate is converted to lactate in the glia for use by the neurones.

Keywords:

INTRODUCTION

Cerebral metabolism is studied in guinea pig cortical slices by following incorporation of ^{13}C from labeled precursors (1-[^{13}C] glucose or 2-[^{13}C] acetate) into selected metabolites. The percentage ^{13}C enrichment of individual C atoms in the metabolites is calculated from resonances in ^{13}C-MR spectra, corrected for naturally abundant ^{13}C, and their tissue concentrations. Due to the inherent relative insensitivity of ^{13}C-MRS, the analyses are performed on tissue extracts.

Normally, glutamine and citrate are considerably more enriched when acetate rather than glucose is used as a precursor. Because acetate is taken up exclusively by glial cells, labeling patterns can be used to distinguish between neuronal and glial metabolisms [1]. The technique has been applied to studies on the effects of depolarization [2], an excitatory condition relevant to the consequences occurring in epilepsy, and hypoxia [3] which is of interest in the metabolic effects of asphyxiation and stroke.

The relationship between neuronal and glial metabolism has also been explored by following the incorporation of ^{13}C from labeled glutamate into glutamate and lactate, where isotopomer patterns and percentage ^{13}C enrichments revealed considerably more incorporation into lactate than into glutamine.

---

* Address for correspondence: MR Centre, Department of Physics, University of Nottingham, University Park, Nottingham NG7 2RD, UK.

METHODS

Guinea pig cortical slices (0.35 mm thick) were prepared and incubated in media containing (mM) NaCl, 124; KCl, 5; KH_2PO_4, 1.2; $MgSO_4$, 1.2; $CaCl_2$, 2.4; $NaHCO_3$, 26; and glucose, 10, gassed with $O_2:CO_2$ (95:5) at 37°C for 30 min to allow for reestablishment of their optimal metabolic state and then transferred to the same media containing the appropriate ^{13}C-labeled precursor. After various time periods, neutralized perchloric acid extracts were prepared. ^{13}C-MR spectra were acquired on Bruker AMX 500 or AM 400 spectrometers using 90° radiofrequency pulses and an interpulse interval of 4 s in a 10-mm ^{13}C probe head. Spectra were broad-band decoupled at 10 W, only during acquisition in order to avoid differential nuclear Overhauser effects and to minimize sample heating. Blocks of 4000 scans were summed and multiplied by an exponential function giving a line broadening of 4 Hz. Chemical shifts are given relative to an internal dioxan standard set at 67.4 ppm [3]. Absolute ^{13}C enrichments were calculated on the basis of quantitation of the resonances in the spectra compared with the dioxan standard and direct measurement of the total pool size of the metabolite from amino acid analyses and enzymatic determinations [1].

The total amount of ^{13}C in a particular resonance is given by

$$[^{13}C]_{m(total)} = \frac{[^{13}C]_D (area)(SF)}{(area)_D (SF)_D} \quad (1)$$

where area is the measured area beneath the ^{13}C resonance, SF is the saturation factor of the resonating species, m is the metabolite, and D is the dioxan standard. From this, the absolute percentage ^{13}C enrichment is calculated as

$$\% \text{ enrichment} = \frac{([^{13}C]_{m(total)} - [^{13}C]_{m(n.a.)}) \times 100}{[m]} \quad (2)$$

where $[^{13}C]_{m(total)}$ is the total amount of ^{13}C [Eq. (1)], $[^{13}C]_{m(n.a.)}$ is the naturally abundant ^{13}C in the metabolite, and $[m]$ is pool size of the metabolite from chemical or enzymatic analysis.

RESULTS AND DISCUSSION

Depolarization

The effects of depolarization using high (40 mM) K$^+$ are known to include stimulated rates of intermediary metabolism, decreased levels of phosphocreatine, and increased release of calcium and neurotransmitters [4, 5]. Comparison of the spectrum observed from depo-

larized tissue after labeling with 1-[^{13}C] glucose with that of control (Fig. 1) shows the increased labeling of lactate, glutamine, γ-aminobutyrate (GABA), and citrate, with no change in glutamate resonances. This strongly suggests that utilization of glucose in glial cells rather than in neurones had increased [2], in line with earlier evidence for greater sensitivity of glial cells to depolarization [5]. The isotopomers of the glutamate and glutamine resonances in Fig. 1 also provide quantitative information on sequential rates of flux through the tricarboxylic acid cycle, and the increased rate of lactate enrichment can be derived from observation of the protons attached to the $^{13}CH_3$ group using ^1H-NMR spectroscopy [6].

Hypoxia

The brain is known to be the most vulnerable part of the body to deprivation of glucose and/or oxygen, with large increases in lactate and decreases in energy intermediates, with eventual cell death [5]. ^1H- and ^{31}P-MR spectroscopy has been regularly applied to monitoring these parameters and correlated them with blood flow thresholds in the hypoxic or ischaemic cerebral cortex *in vivo*, and whereas these studies have proved largely confirmatory, they have been very important in demonstrating the feasibility of investigating the metabolic consequences of such insults *in vivo* and in the human brain. These changes in key cerebral metabolites are now being monitored in stroke patients (see Ref. 6 for a review).

The general decrease in oxidative metabolism with the concomitant increase in glycolysis known to occur in hypoxia can be more fully characterized using ^{13}C-NMR spectroscopy. In mild hypoxia, the spectra confirmed the expected decreases in tricarboxylic acid cycle intermediates and associated amino acids, and increases in lactate and alanine. However, in severe hypoxia (Fig. 2) the labeling of alanine increased further, whereas that of lactate did not, suggesting that in severe hypoxia the ability of lactate dehydrogenase to maintain normal levels of NADH had been overcome and that the accumulating pyruvate had been diverted by transamination to alanine [Eq. (3)]. A new resonance occurred in severe but not in mild hypoxia in the region where trioses might be expected and was confirmed as glycerol 3-phosphate by ^{31}P-MR spectroscopy and direct enzymatic analysis [3]. The metabolite pool concentrations are summarized in Table 1. As glycerol 3-phosphate could also arise from a buildup of NADH from the reaction involving a glycolytic intermediate [dihydroxyacetone phosphate, DHAP, Eq. (4)], these increases in alanine and glycerol 3-phosphate provide new possibilities of monitoring cytoplasmic NADH/NAD$^+$ ratios noninvasively in se-

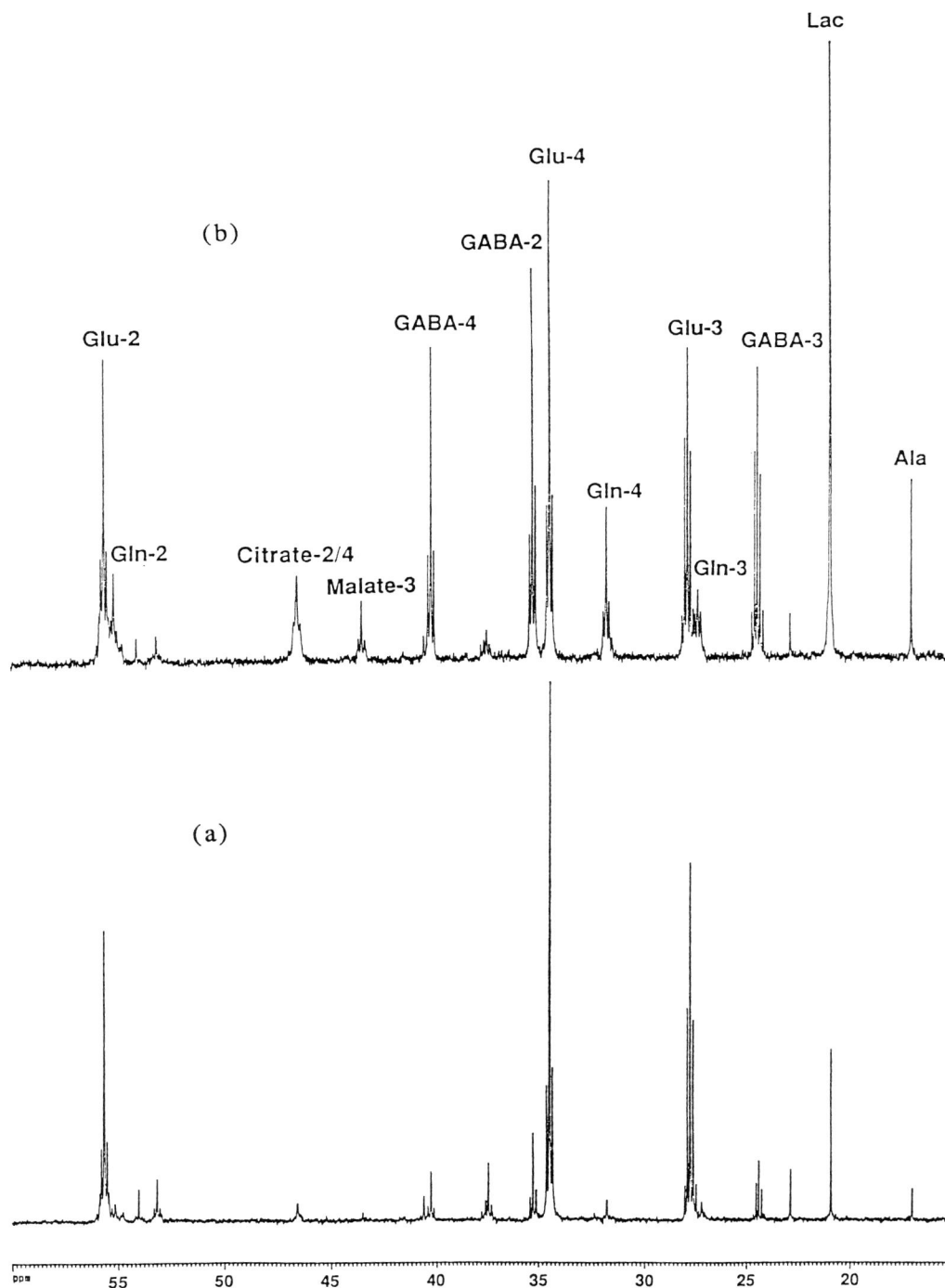

Fig. 1. ^{13}C-MR spectra of depolarized cerebral tissue [6]. Extracts were prepared after incubation in media containing 5 mM 1-[^{13}C] glucose to near steady-state ^{13}C enrichment, which took 4 h under control and 3 h under depolarization conditions. (a) Control, (b) depolarization with 40 mM K$^+$. (Reproduced with permission from *Journal of Neurochemistry*.)

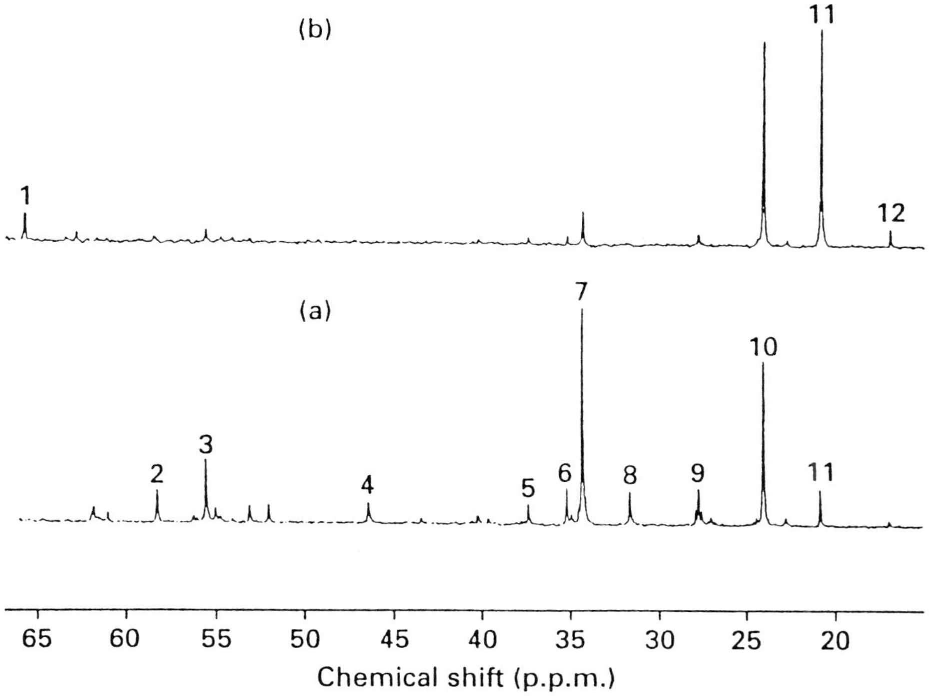

Fig. 2. ^{13}C-MR spectra of cerebral tissues exposed to severe hypoxia [3]. Extracts were prepared from tissues incubated in media containing 1-[^{13}C] glucose and 2-[^{13}C] acetate for 45 min. (a) Control, (b) severe hypoxia. (Reproduced with permission from *Biochemistry Journal.*)

vere hypoxia *in vivo.*

$$Glycerol\ 3\text{-}P$$
$$Alanine$$
$$Lactate + NAD^+ \longleftrightarrow Pyruvate + NADH + H^+ \qquad (3)$$
$$Acetyl\ CoA$$

$$NADH + H^+ + DHAP \longleftrightarrow NAD^+ + Glycerol\ 3\text{-}P \qquad (4)$$

Glial production of lactate and glutamine

Glutamate is known to be taken up preferentially into glial cells where it is converted to glutamine, which is

Table 1. Changes in metabolite concentrations in cerebral tissues exposed to mild and severe hypoxia [3]. Values, from enzymatic estimations, are for NADH are nmol/100 mg protein [9] and for the other metabolites, μmol per 100 mg protein.

Condition	NADH	Lactate	Alanine	Glyc.3-P	Glyc.3-P[a]
Control	43	1.5	0.15	0.03	U.D.[b]
Mild	55	2.8[c]	0.2	0.07	U.D.
Severe	89[c]	2.9[c]	0.5[c]	0.76[c]	0.77

[a]Glycerol 3-phosphate was also calculated from ^{31}P-NMR spectra.
[b]U.D. Undetectable in spectra. [c]Different from control values at $P < 0.01$.

then transferred to neurones. Neuronal neurotransmitter pools of glutamate and also of GABA are thought to be derived from this glutamine. Spectra obtained from tissues incubated with U-[^{13}C] glutamate revealed clear signals from glutamine and lactate released to the media. The isotopomers of the lactate (Fig. 3) show doublets in both C-3 and C-2 positions, confirming that the lactate must have arisen from the exogenous glutamate, because if it were due to naturally abundant ^{13}C in the lactate, only singlets would have appeared. The isotopomer patterns (which reveal the sequence of labeling of the different C atoms within the molecules) of the glutamine and lactate were qualitatively similar to those observed in cultured astrocytes by Sonnewald et al. [7] but were quantitatively different, suggesting higher rates of turnover in the intact tissue. The doublet of the glutamine C-3 of Fig. 3 (i.e., ^{13}C-3 with an adjacent ^{13}C on C-2 or C-4), which indicates the relative amount of incorporation of ^{12}C from the endogenous pool of glutamate and from the unlabeled glucose of the medium (Fig. 3), accounted for 30% of the total label; i.e., some 70% was derived from the exogenously applied ^{13}C-glutamate. The percentage ^{13}C enrichments (from the dioxan standard) of the glutamine released to the medium were C-3, 15.2%; C-2, 12.8%; and C-4, 9.7%. The percentage ^{13}C enrichment for the

a b

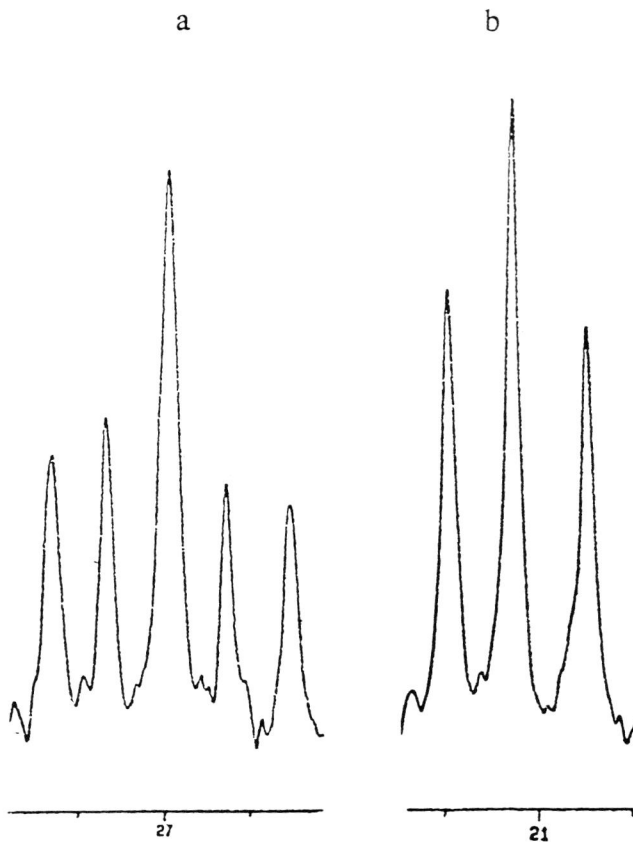

Fig. 3. ^{13}C-MR spectra of glutamine C-3 (a) and lactate C-3 (b) isolated from the incubation medium of cerebral tissues after exposure to 0.2 mM U-[^{13}C] glutamate for 3 h.

C-3 of lactate was over 80%. These results clearly show considerably more incorporation of ^{13}C from glutamate into lactate than into glutamine and suggest that the lactate is being produced almost entirely from the exogenous glutamate than the endogenous glucose. It can be tentatively concluded that this lactate is being produced by the glia for consumption by neurones, as has been indicated from studies on cultured astrocytes [7].

Comments on functional activation studies

The lactate observed to increase in ^{1}H-MR spectra in activation studies of visual stimulation in the human brain has been attributed to anaerobic glycolysis [8], with implied lack of oxygen. On activation of neurones, Na$^+$ moves into the cells and K$^+$ out, where it is taken up by neighboring glial cells. ATP is consumed via the Na$^+$, K$^+$-dependent ATPase, and both glycoly-

sis and metabolism through the tricarboxylic acid cycle are stimulated, essentially in the glial cells which are known to be more sensitive to depolarization [5]. Under such conditions, the increased oxygen consumption is likely to be small relative to the amount available, and the increase in lactate could be attributed to increased aerobic glycolysis. The above results on depolarization could, therefore, serve to indicate that the activation produced by photic stimulation is more likely to be due to depolarization rather than to oxygen deprivation, which may have important implications for future interpretation of the results of activation studies.

REFERENCES

1. Badar-Goffer RS, Bachelard HS, Morris PG (1990) Cerebral metabolism of acetate and glucose studied by ^{13}C-NMR spectroscopy: a technique for investigating metabolic compartmentation in the brain. *Biochem J* **266**: 133–139.
2. Badar-Goffer RG, Ben-Yoseph O, Bachelard HS, Morris PG (1992) Neuronal–glial metabolism under depolarizing conditions—a ^{13}C-n.m.r. study. *Biochem J* **282**: 225–230.
3. Ben-Yoseph O, Badar-Goffer RS, Morris PG, Bachelard HS (1993) Glycerol 3-phosphate and lactate as indicators of the cerebral cytoplasmic redox state in severe and mild hypoxia respectively: a ^{13}C- and ^{31}P-NMR study. *Biochem J* **291**: 915–919.
4. Bachelard HS, Badar-Goffer RS, Brooks KJ, Dolin SJ, Morris PG (1988) Measurement of free intracellular calcium in the brain by ^{19}F–nuclear magnetic resonance spectroscopy. *J Neurochem* **51**: 1311–1313.
5. McIlwain H, Bachelard HS (1985) *Biochemistry and the Central Nervous System,* 5th ed. Edinburgh: Churchill-Livingstone.
6. Bachelard HS, Badar-Goffer RS (1993) NMR spectroscopy in neurochemistry. *J Neurochem* **61**: 412–429.
7. Sonnewald U, Westergaard N, Petersen SB, Unsgard G, Schousboe A (1993) Metabolism of [U-^{13}C] glutamate in astrocytes studied by ^{13}C NMR spectroscopy: incorporation of more label into lactate than into glutamine demonstrates the importance of the tricarboxylic acid cycle. *J Neurochem* **61**: 1179–1182.
8. Prichard J, Rothman D, Novotny E, Petroff O, Avison M, Howseman A, Hanstock C, Shulman R (1989) Photic stimulation raises lactate in human visual cortex [Abstract]. *Proceedings of the 8th Annual Meeting, Society of Magnetic Resonance in Medicine.* p. 1071.
9. Garafola O, Cox DWG, Bachelard HS (1988) Brain levels of NADH and NAD$^+$ under hypoxic and hypoglycaemic conditions in vitro. *J Neurochem* **51**: 172–176.

MRS studies on calcium and zinc in metabolizing cerebral slices exposed to glutamate and NMDA

Nicola Thatcher,[1] Ronnitte Badar-Goffer,[2] Herman Bachelard[1]* and Peter Morris[1]

[1]Magnetic Resonance Centre, University of Nottingham, Nottingham NG7 2RD, UK
[2]Department of Organic Chemistry, Weizmann Institute of Science, Rehovot, Israel

The ^{19}F-NMR calcium indicator 5FBAPTA has been used to measure changes in free intracellular calcium, $[Ca^{2+}]_i$, in superfused guinea pig cerebral cortical slices. Increases in $[Ca^{2+}]_i$ have been observed with depolarization and the combined insult of hypoxia and hypoglycemia. These increases in $[Ca^{2+}]_i$ can be explained by the excitotoxic hypothesis which proposes a central role for the neurotransmitter glutamate and the NMDA receptor in cell death. We, therefore, investigated the effects of glutamate and NMDA directly on $[Ca^{2+}]_i$ in cerebral cortical slices with ^{31}P-NMR to monitor the energy state. In the presence of glutamate ($\pm$Mg) a new resonance was observed in the ^{19}F spectra and was attributed to the Zn–5FBAPTA complex. The zinc peak appears with or just following an increase in $[Ca^{2+}]_i$ and with a drop in PCr. Similar results were obtained on exposing the tissues to NMDA. Zinc has been reported to be enriched in various parts of the brain and have a multiplicity of possible roles. This is the first time zinc has been shown in actively metabolizing tissue. The observation that the zinc resonance does not appear with depolarization or hypoxia and hypoglycemia suggests that the mechanisms of damage in these latter insults are not solely attributable to the release of excitotoxins.

Keywords: MR spectroscopy, ^{19}F-MR spectroscopy, calcium, zinc, glutamate, NMDA.

INTRODUCTION

The events leading to cell death in ischemia have been explained by the excitotoxic hypothesis which proposes a central role for the excessive release of the neurotransmitter glutamate, a rise in free intracellular calcium ($[Ca^{2+}]_i$) via the N-methyl-D-aspartate (NMDA) receptor, and the triggering of a cascade of damaging chemical events [1]. In our previous studies, we have used the ^{19}F-MRS (magnetic resonance spectroscopy) indicator, 5,5'-F_2-1,2-bis (o-aminophenoxy) ethane-N,N,N',N'-tetraacetic acid (5FBAPTA), to measure changes in $[Ca^{2+}]_i$ in actively metabolizing guinea pig cerebral cortical slices and obtained ^{31}P-NMR spectra to monitor changes in the energy state. Increases in $[Ca^{2+}]_i$ were observed with combined hypoxia and hypoglycemia (studied as the two major components

of ischaemia) and also with depolarization [2]. To better understand these results in terms of the excitotoxic hypothesis we decided to investigate the effects of glutamate and NMDA directly on $[Ca^{2+}]_i$ and the energy state using the MRS techniques previously reported [2].

MATERIALS AND METHODS

Treatment of tissues

Tissue slices from the guinea pig cerebral cortex were prepared as previously described [2], transferred to the superfusion apparatus and placed within the NMR magnet. After control ^{19}F and ^{31}P spectra had been acquired, the superfusion medium was replaced with media containing glutamate (1 or 0.5 mM) or the racemic mixture of NMDA (NMDLA, 200 μM) in the presence and absence of magnesium. Further NMR spectra were then acquired. NMR data were obtained using an AMX-500 Bruker narrow-bore spectrometer operating at 202.46 MHz for ^{31}P and 470.51 MHz for

* Address for correspondence: Magnetic Resonance Centre, Department of Physics, University of Nottingham, University Park, Nottingham NG7 2RD, UK.

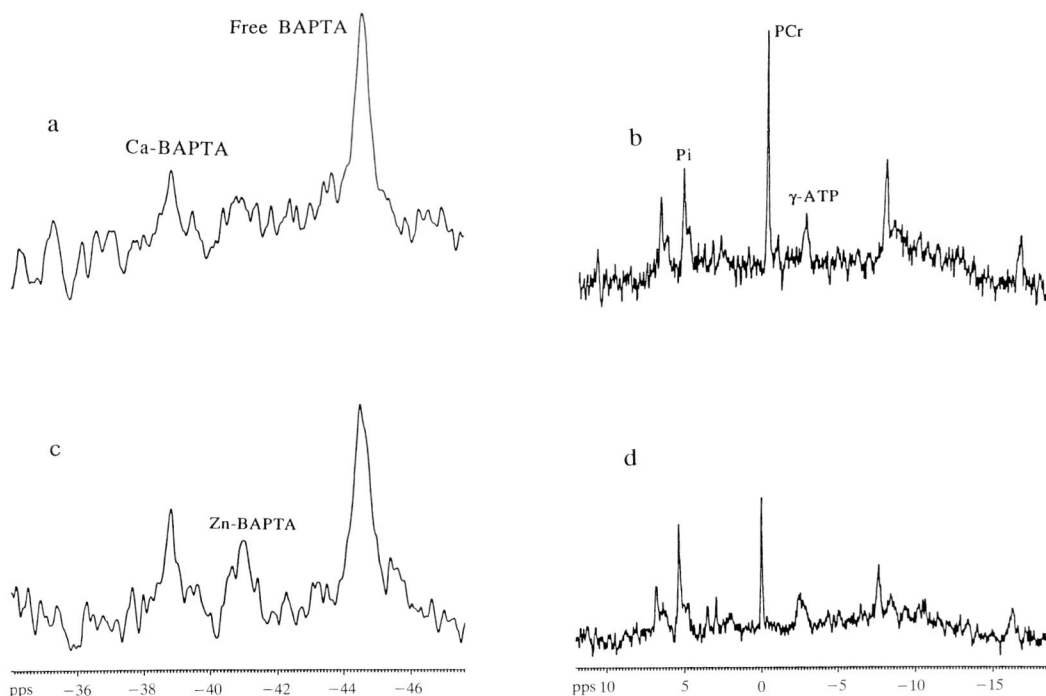

Fig. 1. ^{19}F (a, c) and ^{31}P (b, d) spectra of guinea pig cerebral cortical slices showing changes with 0.5 mM glutamate, + Mg^{2+}, in [Ca^{2+}]$_i$, [Zn^{2+}]$_i$ (c) and PCr (d) from control (a and b).

^{19}F. Values for [Ca^{2+}]$_i$ were calculated from the ratios of the measured areas of bound and free resonances for 5FBAPTA in the ^{19}F spectrum multiplied by the dissociation constant for Ca–5FBAPTA (600 nM).

RESULTS

Glutamate (1 or 0.5 mM)

On exposure of cerebral slices to 0.5 mM glutamate + Mg^{2+}, ^{19}F spectra showed an increase in [Ca^{2+}]$_i$ and a new resonance appeared with a chemical shift specific to the zinc–5FBAPTA complex. PCr decreased to 42% of control (Fig. 1). Almost identical results were obtained with 0.5 mM glutamate in the absence of Mg^{2+} or with 1 mM glutamate ± Mg^{2+} (Table 1). Exposure of the tissue slices to 200 μM NMDLA caused similar but slower increases in [Ca^{2+}]$_i$, with zinc appearing in most but not all experiments. PCr decreased to 39% of control (Table 1). Previous studies on depolarization (40 mM [K$^+$]$_e$) or with combined hypoxia and hypoglycemia were repeated, and although [Ca^{2+}]$_i$ increased (Table 1), no zinc was observed.

TPEN [N,N,N',N'-tetrakis(2-pyridylmethyl)ethylenediamine] is a chelator of divalent cations with a very high affinity for zinc and much lower affinities for calcium and magnesium. TPEN (50 μM) had no effect on control ^{19}F and ^{31}P spectra, but on exposure of the tissues to 1 mM glutamate in the presence of TPEN, no zinc was detected although calcium increased as previously.

Table 1. Effects of excitotoxic amino acids on Ca^{2+} and Zn^{2+}.

Condition	Mg	(n)	Control	Ca^{2+} [nM]	% Control	PCr^a
Glu (0.5 mM)	–	(2)	215	380	177^b	
Glu (0.5 mM)	+	(2)	178	302	170^b	42%
Glu (1 mM)	–	(4)	191 ± 64	345 ± 38	181^b	
Glu (1 mM)	+	(4)	149 ± 22	360 ± 65	242^b	35%
NMDLA (0.2 mM)	–	(1)	187	294	157	
NMDLA (0.2 mM)^c	+	(3)	152 ± 75	257 ± 10	169^b	39%
Depolarization^d	+	(1)	185	352	190	35%

^{a}PCr as percentage of control; no significant changes in PCr/ATP.
$^b P < 0.05$. Note: Zinc appeared in all conditions except ^{c}where zinc showed in two of three experiments and ^{d}where no zinc appeared.

CONCLUSIONS

We feel confident that the new resonance that appears in the study can be attributed to zinc due to its specific chemical shift and the use of TPEN, and we believe this is the first time zinc has been shown in actively metabolizing cortical tissue. This MRS technique has the advantage over fluorescence methods in its ability to distinguish between Ca^{2+} and Zn^{2+}. The $[Zn^{2+}]_i$ was calculated, from the ratio of the zinc–5FBAPTA resonance to the total 5FBAPTA resonances in the ^{19}F spectrum (assuming an intracellular concentration of 5FBAPTA of 100 µM), to range between 10 and 20 µM [3].

Zinc has been reported to be enriched in the hippocampus, cerebellum, and pineal gland with a high enrichment within synaptic vesicles [4]. Release of zinc to the medium, in a calcium-dependent manner, by superfused hippocampal slices with electrical stimulation and depolarization has also been reported [5, 6], as has a movement of zinc from nerve endings to cell bodies after kainate-induced seizures and ischemia [7]. A speculative role of zinc released from nerve endings has been to act postsynaptically as a neuromodulator of the effects of both glutamate and GABA and has been shown to attenuate NMDA-induced toxicity. Zinc can be compared to calcium in the multiplicity of its possible roles in the brain. The zinc observed in this study is intracellular because this is the location of the 5FBAPTA. Its appearance on exposure to glutamate and NMDA suggests that it is being released from a 5FBAPTA-inaccessible to a 5FBAPTA-accessible site, for example, from a protein-bound form [3].

It is important to note that a zinc resonance was not observed when cortical slices were exposed to depolarization or the combined insult of hypoxia and hypoglycemia, although increases in $[Ca^{2+}]_i$ were observed. This contradicts the idea that the appearance of zinc is a consequence of elevated $[Ca^{2+}]_i$ and also suggests that the mechanisms of cell damage under such conditions cannot be explained solely by the current excitotoxic hypothesis.

These studies were supported by the Medical Research Council.

REFERENCES

1. Olney JW (1983) Excitotoxins; an overview In *Excitotoxins* (Fuxe K, Roberts P, Schwarts R, eds) pp. 82–96. London: MacMillan.
2. Badar-Goffer, RS, Thatcher NM, Morris PG, Bachelard HS (1993) Neither severe hypoxia nor hypoglycaemia alone causes any significant increase in $[Ca^{2+}]_i$—only a combination of the two insults has this effect. A ^{31}P- and ^{19}F-NMR study. *J Neurochem* **61**: 2207–2214.
3. Badar-Goffer R, Morris P, Thatcher N, Bachelard H (1994) Excitotoxic amino acids cause appearance of MRS-observable zinc in superfused cortical slices. *J Neurochem* **62**: 2488–2491.
4. Perez-Clausell J, Danscher G (1985) Intravesicular localization of zinc in rat telencephalic boutons. A histochemical study. *Brain Res* **337**: 91–98.
5. Howell GA, Welch MG, Frederickson CJ (1984) Stimulation-induced uptake and release of zinc in hippocampal slices. *Nature* **308**: 736–738.
6. Assaf SY, Chung S-H (1984) Release of endogenous Zn^{2+} from brain tissue during activity. *Nature* **308**: 734–736.
7. Tonder N, Johansen FF, Frederickson CJ, Zimmer J, Diemer JH (1990) Possible role of zinc in the selective degeneration of dentate hilar neurons after cerebral Possible role of zinc in the selective degeneration of denate hilar neurons after cerebral ischemia in the adult rat. *Neurosci Lett* **109**: 247–252.

Severity of delayed ("secondary") cerebral energy failure after acute hypoxia–ischemia is related to the time integral of acute ATP depletion

Ernest B. Cady,[2]* Ann Lorek,[1] Yakito Takei,[1] John S. Wyatt,[1] Juliet M. Penrice,[1] A. David Edwards,[1] Donald Peebles,[1] Marzena Wylezinska,[2] Huw Owen-Reece,[1] Vincent Kirkbride,[1] Christopher E. Cooper,[1] Richard F. Aldridge,[2] Simon C. Roth,[1] Guy Brown,[3] David T. Delpy[2] and E. Osmund R. Reynolds[1]

Departments of [1]Paediatrics, [2]Medical Physics and Bio-Engineering, and [3]Biochemistry and Molecular Biology, University College London, London WC1E 6JA, UK

The aim of this study was to reproduce the delayed ("secondary") cerebral energy failure previously described in birth-asphyxiated newborn infants and to investigate relationships between primary insult severity and the extent of the delayed energy failure. Phosphorus (^{31}P) magnetic resonance spectroscopy (MRS) at 7 T was used to study the brains of 12 newborn piglets during an acute, reversible, cerebral hypoxic–ischemic episode which continued until nucleotide triphosphates (NTP) were depleted. After reperfusion and reoxygenation, spectroscopy was continued for 48 h. High-energy metabolite concentrations returned to near normal levels after the insult, but later they fell as delayed energy failure developed. The time integral of NTP depletion in the primary insult correlated strongly with the minimum [phosphocreatine (PCr)]/[inorganic orthophosphate (P_i)] observed 24–48 h after the insult. (Linear regression analysis gave slope $-8.04\ h^{-1}$; ordinate intercept = 1.23; $r = 0.92$; $P < 0.0001$.) This model is currently being used to investigate the therapeutic potential of various cerebroprotective strategies including hypothermia.

Keywords: ^{31}P-MRS, brain, birth asphyxia, cerebroprotection.

INTRODUCTION

^{31}P-MRS (magnetic resonance spectroscopy) of the brains of severely birth-asphyxiated human infants often gives normal results on the first day of life, but later changes indicate the development of cerebral energy failure. ([Phosphocreatine (PCr)]/inorganic orthophosphate (P_i)] and eventually [nucleotide triphosphates (NTP)] fall, but there is no intracellular acidosis. These changes convey a very unfavourable prognosis [1]). The aim of this study was to reproduce this delayed ("secondary") energy failure in the newborn piglet following severe acute cerebral hypoxia–

ischemia and to investigate possible relationships between primary insult severity and outcome.

METHODS

Twelve newborn Large-white piglets less than 24 h old were anesthetized (inhaled isoflurane and nitrous oxide) and subjected to reversible, bilateral, common-carotid occlusion and hypoxemia (mean PaO_2 3.1 (SD 0.6) kPa) for up to 1.5 h by which time NTP had fallen by 30% as quantified by the ratio [NTP]/[EPP], where EPP is the exchangeable phosphate pool P_i + PCr + ($\gamma + \alpha + \beta$)-NTP. This was followed by reperfusion and normal oxygenation. Vital physiological signs were monitored and kept within normal ranges throughout the 48 h. An additional six piglets were studied as sham-operated controls.

^{31}P spectra were collected before and during the

---

* Address for correspondence: Department of Medical Physics and Bio-Engineering, University College London, 11–20 Capper Street, London WC1E 6JA, UK.

insult and for the following 48 h using a 7-T Bruker Biospec and a 25-mm-diameter surface coil on the intact scalp. A DANTE [2] pulse-acquire sequence was used with a 180° coil-center flip angle and a 10-s repetition time. Data were analyzed using Lorentzian χ^2 minimization in the frequency domain [3] and intracellular pH (pH$_i$) was estimated from the P$_i$ chemical shift (δ_{P_i}) using the Henderson–Hasselbalch relationship: $pH_i = 6.77 + \log[(\delta_{P_i} - 3.29)/(5.68 - \delta_{P_i})]$ [4].

RESULTS

During the insult, cerebral [PCr]/[P$_i$] fell from 1.40 (0.29) to 0.01 (0.02; $P < 0.001$; unpaired t-test), and [NTP]/[EPP] decreased from 0.19 (0.02) to 0.06 (0.04; $P < 0.001$). Following reperfusion and reoxygenation, these ratios rose to 1.43 (0.29) after 4.0 (2.2) h and 0.19 (0.02) after 5.3 (2.7) h, respectively. As delayed energy failure developed, [PCr]/[P$_i$] again fell to 0.62 (0.61; $P < .01$) 24 h after the insult and 0.49 (0.37; $P < 0.001$) at 48 h (see Fig. 1) in spite of normal values for PaO$_2$, mean arterial blood pressure, and blood glucose. [NTP]/[EPP] fell to 0.15 (0.03; $P < .01$) at 48 h. pH$_i$ remained unchanged. Linear regression analysis (see Fig. 2) showed that the time integral of [NTP]/[EPP] depletion during the primary insult and recovery was related to the minimum [PCr]/[P$_i$] observed between

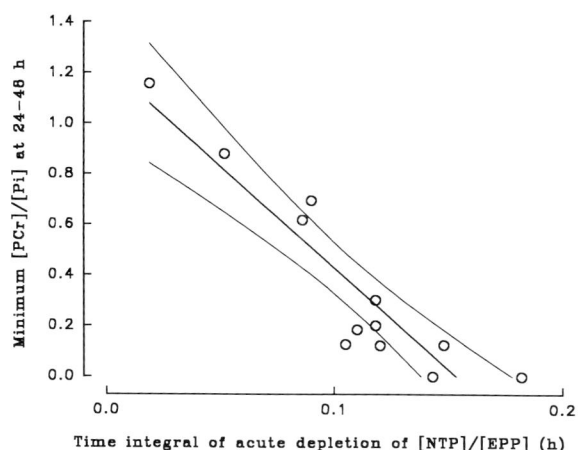

Fig. 1. A ^{31}P spectrum (solid line) of the brain of a newborn piglet 47 h after the primary insult, showing greatly elevated P$_i$ and reduced PCr but with a pH$_i$ (7.05) near normal. Three hundred and ninety-two transients were averaged. Resonance identifications: a—phosphoethanol-amine; b—phosphocholine; c—P$_i$; d—glycerolphosphory-lethanolamine; e—glycerolphosphorylcholine; f—PCr; g, h, and k—γ-, α-, and β-NTP, respectively; i—nicotinamide dinucleotides; j—uridine diphosphosugars. The dashed line is the Lorentzian fit to the spectrum via χ^2 minimization.

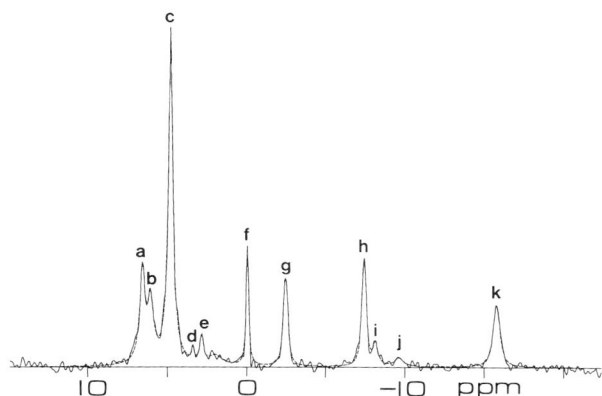

Fig. 2. The relationship between primary insult severity and extent of delayed energy failure.

24 and 48 h after the insult. (Linear regression analysis gave slope -8.04 h^{-1}; ordinate intercept = 1.23; $r = 0.92$; $P < 0.0001$). In the control piglets, no changes in cerebral metabolites occurred throughout the 48 h for which they were studied.

DISCUSSION AND CONCLUSIONS

These studies indicate that the metabolic events detected by ^{31}P-MRS in the brains of birth-asphyxiated human infants can be reproduced in the newborn piglet. The severity of the acute episode of energy failure, quantified by the time integral of [NTP]/[EPP] depletion, was related to that of the subsequent delayed energy failure using the minimum [PCr]/[P$_i$] at 24–48 h as an index. This relationship appears to indicate that the amount of irreversible tissue damage depends on both the primary failure of energy generation and its duration. This model is proving useful for the investigation both of mechanisms of delayed energy failure and of clinically feasible cerebroprotective strategies such as hypothermia.

ACKNOWLEDGMENTS

The authors thank the Medical Research Council, the Royal Society, the Wellcome Trust, and the Wolfson Foundation for financial assistance.

REFERENCES

1. Azzopardi D, Wyatt JS, Cady EB, Delpy DT, Baudin J, Stewart AL, Hope PL, Hamilton PA, Reynolds EOR (1989)

Prognosis of newborn infants with hypoxic/ischemic brain injury assessed by phosphorus magnetic resonance spectroscopy. *Pediatr Res* **25:** 445–451.

2. Morris GA, Freeman R (1978) Selective excitation in Fourier transform magnetic resonance. *J Magn Reson* **29:** 433–462.

3. Cady EB (1991) A reappraisal of the absolute concentra-

tions of phosphorylated metabolites in the human neonatal cerebral cortex obtained by fitting Lorentzian curves to the ^{31}P NMR spectrum. *J Magn Res* **91:** 637–643.

4. Petroff OAC, Prichard JW, Behar KL, Alger JR, den Hollander JA, Shulman RG (1985) Cerebral intracellular pH by ^{31}P nuclear magnetic resonance spectroscopy. *Neurology* **35:** 781–788.

Large increases in ^{1}H metabolite T_2's after cerebral hypoxia–ischemia correlate with ATP depletion

Ernest B. Cady,[1]* Ann Lorek,[2] Juliet Penrice,[2] A. David Edwards,[2] Guy Brown,[3]
Huw Owen-Reece,[2] Vincent Kirkbride,[2] Christopher E. Cooper,[2]
John S. Wyatt[2] and E. Osmund R. Reynolds[2]

*Departments of [1]Medical Physics and Bio-Engineering, [2]Paediatrics, and [3]Biochemistry and Molecular Biology,
University College London, Gower Street, London WC1E 6BT, UK*

In vivo proton (^{1}H) magnetic resonance spectroscopy (MRS) can measure cerebral metabolite concentrations and nuclear relaxation times. Function of the sodium (Na^+)/potassium (K^+) pump in cell membranes depends on adequate adenosine triphosphate (ATP) levels: intracellular Na^+ is normally extruded in exchange for extracellular K^+. Low ATP will cause pump dysfunction and loss of K^+ accompanied by influx of Na^+ and water. Raised intracellular water may increase molecular mobility and this might be detectable as increased apparent transverse relaxation times (T_2's). ^{1}H-MRS of the brains of newborn piglets during acute hypoxia–ischemia revealed enigmatic increases in the peak area of creatine + phosphocreatine (Cr) relative to those of choline-containing compounds (Cho) and *N*-acetylaspartate (NAA). Interleaved ^{1}H and phosphorus (^{31}P) MRS showed that the T_2's of both Cr and lactate (Lac) increased during acute hypoxia–ischemia and these changes correlated with reductions in nucleotide triphosphate (NTP; largely ATP). Within 50 h of metabolic recovery from the primary insult, as delayed energy failure developed, the T_2's of Cho, Cr, NAA, and Lac increased greatly. These T_2 changes also correlated with NTP depletion. These observations demonstrate important relationships between T_2's and function of the ATP-dependent Na^+/K^+ pump.

Keywords: ^{1}H-MRS, ^{31}P-MRS, proton metabolite T$_2$'s, ATP, brain.

INTRODUCTION

In healthy brain, the metabolites with the strongest ^{1}H-MRS (magnetic resonance spectroscopy) signals are due to Cho (choline), Cr (creatine & phosphocreatine) and NAA (*N*-acetylasparate). Lactate (Lac) is often detectable during and following hypoxia–ischemia. Although ^{1}H metabolite T_2's (transverse relaxation times) have been measured in many studies, no clear dependence on energy metabolism has been ascertained and the relevance of altered T_2's in pathological conditions remains unclear.

Using interleaved ^{1}H- and ^{31}P-MRS, we have investigated the aftermath of acute reversible cerebral hypoxi-a–

ischemia that caused severe energy failure (very low [phosphocreatine (PCr)]/[inorganic phosphate (P_i)] ratio; falling [NTP] (nucleotide triphosphate mainly ATP [1]); and profound intracellular acidosis) in the newborn piglet [2]. Following resuscitation, PCr and NTP were replenished, but, in spite of maintained systemic physiological homeostasis, observations during the next 50 h demonstrated the slow development of delayed energy failure similar to our findings in birth-asphyxiated infants [3]. At the end of the acute insult, the amplitude of the Cr resonance (at ~3.0 ppm) was increased relative to both Cho (at ~3.2 ppm) and NAA (at ~2.0 ppm), as shown in Fig. 1. Although ^{31}P-MRS indicated that [PCr] had fallen, [total Cr] should not have increased. The high Cr signal may have been caused by a raised T_2 associated with increased cytosolic water following failure of the Na^+/K^+ pump due to low [ATP] [4]. To investigate this observation, cerebral metabolite T_2's in six newborn piglets were

* Address for correspondence: Department of Medical Physics and Bioengineering, University College London, 11–20 Capper Street, London WC1E 6AU, UK.

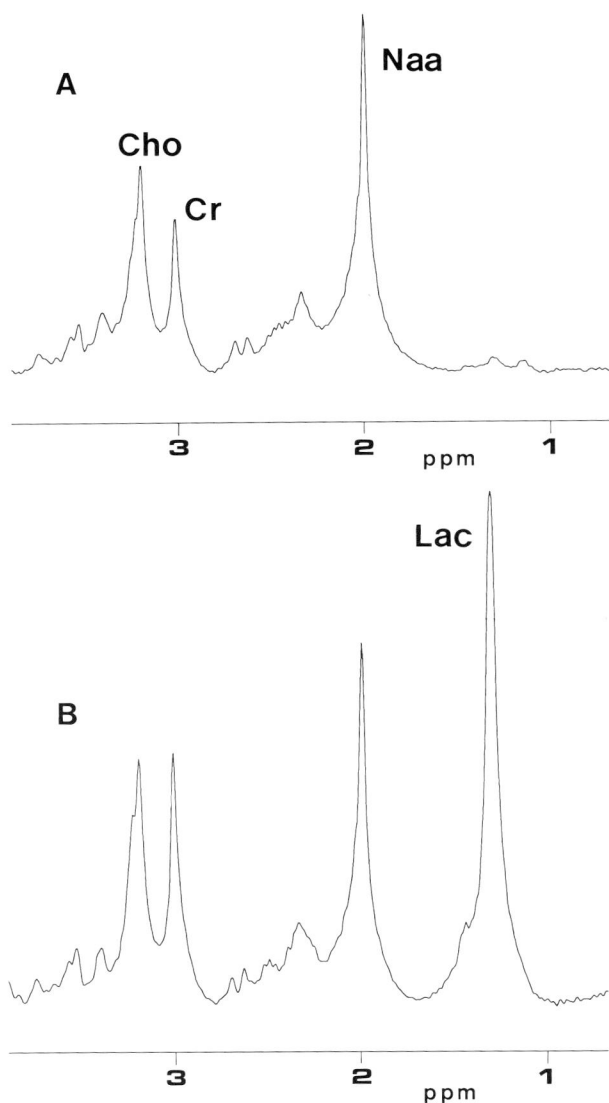

Fig. 1. ^1H spectra from piglet brain before (A) and after 35 min of hypoxia–ischemia (B). At the end of the insult, raised Cr T_2 was suggested by the relatively high Cr peak amplitude.

related to NTP levels before, during, and after acute hypoxia–ischemia.

METHODS

Anesthesia was induced (5% inhaled isoflurane) and maintained (1% isoflurane, 70% nitrous oxide, and morphine sulphate infusion at 0.2–0.7 mg kg^{-1} h^{-1}) and each piglet (Large-white; <24 h old) was then subjected to reversible, bilateral common carotid occlusion and hypoxaemia (PaO$_2$ ~ 3.5 kPa) for approxi-

mately 1 h followed by reperfusion and normal oxygenation. Physiological variables were monitored and kept within normal ranges.

Spectra were collected using a 7-T Bruker Biospec (^{31}P, 121 MHz; ^{1}H, 300 MHz) and a 25-mm-diameter surface coil on the intact scalp. A $1\bar{1}$-$2\bar{2}$ water-suppression spin-echo sequence [5] optimized for NAA at ~ 2 ppm was used for ^{1}H spectroscopy. For the spectra in Fig. 1, acquisition conditions were as follows: echo time (TE) 270 ms; repetition time (TR) 5 s; EXORCYCLE phase-cycling [6]; and 64 echoes averaged. So that T_2's could be estimated with minimal effects due to concentration changes, during the acute insult ^{1}H data were collected as in Fig. 1 but in clusters of five spectra with TE 540, 270, 132, 270, and 540 ms and a 1-s TR. The TE 540 ms and TE 270 ms collections were analysed in pairs and T_2's were calculated assuming monoexponential decay [7]. After recovery from the insult, data were collected as in Fig. 1 with TE 132, 270, and 540 ms. For ^{31}P, a DANTE [8] (500, 10-μs pulses/200-μs TR; for suppression of bone/phospholipid signal) pulse-acquire sequence was used (180° coil-center flip angle; 10-s TR). Peak areas were measured by fitting Lorentzians to the spectra using χ^2 minimization with prior knowledge [9]. The NTP level was quantified as the fraction [NTP]/[EPP], where EPP is the exchangeable phosphate pool P$_i$ + PCr + ($\gamma + \alpha + \beta$)–NTP.

RESULTS

Before the acute insult, T_2's were as follows: Cho 255 ± 50 ms (mean ± SD); Cr 160 ± 23 ms; and NAA 215 ± 34 ms (Lac T_2 was not measured due to low preinsult concentration); NTP/EPP was 0.21 ± 0.01. At the end of the acute insult, NTP/EPP had fallen to 0.05 ± 0.05 ($P < 0.0005$; paired t-test) and Cr T_2 had risen to 263 ± 51 ms ($P < 0.0002$) at which time Lac T_2 was 223 ± 17 ms. No change was seen in the T_2's of either Cho or NAA during the acute insult. Linear regression analyses showed significant correlations of T_2's with NTP/EPP depletion for both Cr and Lac ($P < 0.001$). Approximately 1 h after resuscitation, NTP/EPP had risen to 0.15 ± 0.03 ($P < 0.02$) and the T_2's of Cr and Lac were 226 ± 88 ms and 206 ± 58 ms, respectively. Over the next 50 h, NTP/EPP fell again as delayed energy failure developed and the T_2's of Cho, Cr (see Fig. 2), NAA, and Lac showed large increases that also correlated linearly with NTP/EPP depletion ($P < 0.02$, <0.001, <0.001, and <0.001, respectively). No correla-

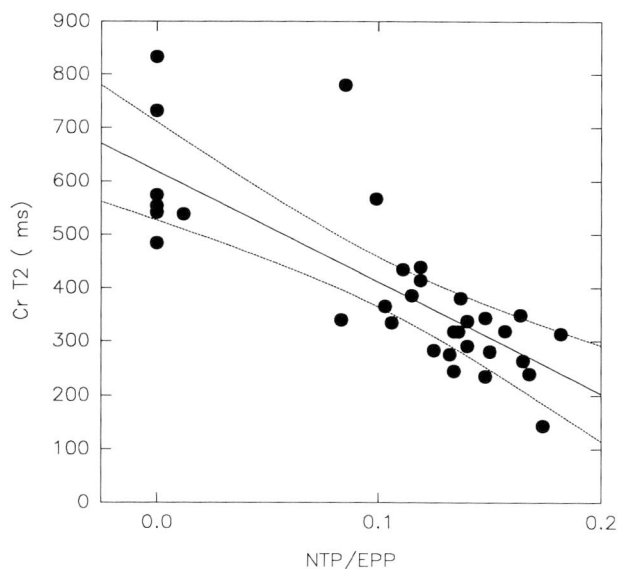

Fig. 2. Cr T_2 and NTP/EPP during the development of delayed energy failure in three piglets from 1 to 49 h after an acute hypoxic–ischemic cerebral insult. The linear regression (solid, middle curve) and the 99% confidence limits (dashed, top and bottom curves) are indicated.

tions were found between metabolite T_2's and PCr/EPP, insult duration, or intracellular pH.

DISCUSSION AND CONCLUSIONS

The dependences of cerebral metabolite T_2's on NTP deficit were likely to have been caused by increased cytosolic water due to Na^+/K^+ pump failure [4]. Greater molecular mobility may result from increased intracellular water and, if molecules become more mobile, according to theory T_2 should increase [10]. Relationships between water T_2 and concentration have been investigated in several systems. For example, in agarose–gel studies [11], it was found that T_2 increased approximately linearly with water content.

It was surprising that neither NAA nor Cho T_2 increased during acute hypoxia–ischemia and also surprising that during delayed energy failure, T_2's were much higher for a given NTP/EPP than during the primary insult. Deoxyhemoglobin is paramagnetic and high levels of this during acute hypoxia might reduce metabolite T_2's [12] thereby countering, to an as yet uncertain extent, increases due to raised cytosolic water.

During delayed energy failure, the dynamic range of T_2 was greater than the changes in signal-intensity ratio recently reported in diffusion-weighted MR imag-

ing studies [13]. Further investigations, utilizing improved T_2 measurements and other methods for monitoring both cellular edema and deoxyhemoglobin levels are necessary to elucidate the causal mechanisms of the T_2 increases. The results presented here suggest that T_2 measurements may have great potential for monitoring cerebral edema.

ACKNOWLEDGMENTS

The authors thank D. Peebles, S. Roth, and Y. Takei for help with earlier experiments, R.F. Aldridge for technical assistance, and The Medical Research Council, The Royal Society, The Wellcome Trust, and The Wolfson Foundation for financial assistance.

REFERENCES

1. Chapman AG, Westerberg E, Siesjo BK (1981) The metabolism of purine and pyrimidine nucleotides in rat cortex during insulin-induced hypoglycemia and recovery. *J Neurochem* **36**: 179–189.
2. Lorek A, Takei Y, Cady EB, Wyatt JS, Penrice J, Edwards AD, Peebles D, Wyleznska M, Owen-Reece H, Kirkbride V, Cooper CE, Aldridge RF, Roth SC, Brown G, Delpy DT, Reynolds EOR (1994) Delayed ("secondary") cerebral energy failure following acute hypoxia-ischaemia in the newborn piglet: continuous 48-hour studies by phosphorus magnetic resonance spectroscopy. *Pediatr. Res.* (in press).
3. Azzopardi D, Wyatt JS, Cady EB, Delpy DT, Baudin J, Stewart AL, Hope PL, Hamilton PA, Reynolds EOR (1989) Prognosis of newborn infants with hypoxiia-ischemia brain injury assessed by phosphorus magnetic resonance spectroscopy. *Pediatr Res* **25**: 445–451.
4. Flynn CJ, Farooqui AA, Horrocks LA (1989) Ischemia and hypoxia. In *Basic Neurochemistry: Molecular, Cellular, and Medical Aspects* (Siegel GJ, Agranoff B, Albers RW, Molinoff P, eds) p. 783. New York: Raven Press.
5. Hore PJ (1983) Solvent suppression in Fourier transform magnetic resonance. *J Magn Reson* **55**: 283–300.
6. Bodenhausen G, Freeman R, Turner DL (1977) Suppression of artifacts in two-dimensional J spectroscopy. *J Magn Reson* **27**: 511–514.
7. Williams SR, Proctor E, Allen K, Gadian DG, Crockard HA (1988) Quantitative estimation of lactate in brain by ¹H NMR. *Magn Reson Med* **7**: 425–431.
8. Morris GA, Freeman R (1978) Selective excitation in Fourier transform magnetic resonance. *J Magn Reson* **29**: 433–462.
9. Cady EB (1991) A reappraisal of the absolute concentrations of phosphorylated metabolites in the human neonatal cerebral cortex obtained by fitting Lorentzian curves to the ³¹P NMR spectrum. *J Magn Reson* **91**: 637–643.

10. Slichter CP (1990) *Principles of Magnetic Resonance* 3rd ed. pp. 212–214. Berlin: Springer-Verlag.

11. Ablett S, Lillford PJ, Baghdadi SMA, Derbyshire W (1978) Nuclear magnetic resonance investigations of polysaccharide films, sols, and gels. *J Coll Interf Sci* **67**: 355–376.

12. Gasparovic C, Matwiyoff NA (1992) The magnetic properties and water dynamics of the red blood cell: A study by proton NMR lineshape analysis. *Magn Reson Med* **26**: 274–299.

13. Busza AL, Allen KL, King MD, van Bruggen N, Williams SR, Gadian DG (1992) Diffusion-weighted imaging studies of cerebral ischaemia in gerbils: Potential relevance to energy failure. *Stroke* **23**: 1602–1612.

Magnetic resonance spectroscopy data analysis: time or frequency domain?

Aad van den Boogaart,[1]* Mika Ala-Korpela,[2] Franklyn A. Howe,[1]
Loreta M. Rodrigues,[1] Marion Stubbs[1] and John R. Griffiths[1]

[1]*St. George's Hospital Medical School, London, UK*
[2]*University of Oulu, Oulu, Finland*

Comparisons of time and frequency domain methods are presented for *in vitro* [1]H and *in vivo* [31]P magnetic resonance spectroscopy (MRS) data. Many distortions in the MR spectrum, introduced by applying the Fourier transform to a nonideal free-induction decay (FID), can be handled more elegantly in the time domain, where operations are carried out directly on the measured signal. It was found that if the measured signal is well conditioned—high signal-to-noise ratio (S/N), no truncation, no baseline problems—then both time and frequency domain methods give the same results within the error limits. However, distortions in the measured signal make analysis by time domain methods preferable over frequency domain methods. In all applications, the use of prior knowledge appeared to play an important role.

Keywords: quantitation, ^{1}H and ^{31}P MRS, water removal, prior knowledge, signal-to-noise ratio, VARPRO.

INTRODUCTION

Quantitative analysis of magnetic resonance spectroscopy (MRS) data can be conducted either in the time or frequency domain. Time domain methods avoid any preprocessing of the measured data, carrying out operations on the measured signal, whereas frequency domain methods process the Fourier transform (FT) spectrum of the original signal. Distortions of the FT spectrum due to imperfections in the measured time domain signal cause problems for frequency domain analysis methods. Receiver-distorted initial data points and truncation of the free-induction decay (FID) distort the spectrum, which then needs deconvolution for repair. Also, quickly decaying signals from immobile components give a broad, rolling baseline in the FT spectrum, demanding baseline approximation by a straight line (for small spectral intervals) or a polynomial. These "frequency domain problems" can be elegantly handled using time domain analysis. If the measured signal is free from the mentioned problems, the use of a frequency domain method may become more attractive, especially with respect to current computer requirements. Whatever the choice of method, the FT spectrum is an invaluable tool for interpreting the data and quantitation results.

For *in vitro* ^{1}H-MRS data of ultracentrifuged lipoprotein fractions from human blood plasma, the rapid time domain method HLSVD was used to remove the large residual water signal [1, 2], after which the nonlinear least-squares fitting algorithms VARPRO [3] (time domain) and FITPLA[c] [4] (frequency domain) were compared. For *in vivo* ^{31}P-MRS data of rat tumors, VARPRO was compared to linear least-squares Lorentzian fitting (FITSPEC, Varian NMR Instruments) and simple peak integration in the spectrum at both high and low S/N.

MATERIALS AND METHODS

In vitro ^{1}H-MRS

[1]H-MR spectra of ultracentrifuged lipoprotein fractions from a normolipidemic volunteer were recorded

* Address for correspondence: CRC Biomedical Magnetic Resonance Research Group, St. George's Hospital Medical School, Division of Biochemistry, Cranmer Terrace, London SW17 0RE, UK.

at 310 K on a Jeol JNM–GX400 FT NMR spectrometer (operating at 399.6 MHz). Water suppression was done using a standard binomial 1–$\bar{1}$ pulse sequence. Two hundred fifty-six FIDs (32 768 data points) were accumulated using a 28–30-μs 45° pulse and a pulse repetition time of 6.6 s.

In vivo ³¹P-MRS

³¹P spectra were obtained on a 4.7-T, 33-cm-bore SISCO instrument from a cubic voxel (typically 1 cm³) within the tumor, using the ISIS localization technique. Adiabatic inversion and excitation pulses were used with a 10-s repetition time. The ISIS FIDs represented 400 transients (4096 data points) which were collected as 5 blocks of 80.

RESULTS

In vitro ¹H-MRS

The HLSVD method enabled rapid removal of the residual water resonance from the spectrum, without affecting the peaks of interest, even though these were superimposed on the massive wings of the water peak. No equivalent method is available in the frequency domain. Comparative VARPRO and FITPLA^c analyses conducted on the heavily overlapping peaks in the methylene and methyl region of the spectrum showed good agreement in peak areas and linewidths for all constituents of overlapping resonances to within the error limits. Results for a low-density lipoprotein

(LDL) fraction spectrum are shown in Fig. 1. It should be mentioned that FITPLA^c has a good way of obtaining the best available starting values for the nonlinear least-squares algorithm. The results of this "scan" were also used as starting values for the VARPRO run. Extensive results of this study can be found in Ref. 5.

In vivo ³¹P-MRS

VARPRO, FITSPEC, and Integration agreed well with each other when analyzing FIDs consisting of 400 acquired transients (see Fig. 2a). The performance of the three MRS data analysis techniques at lower S/N was assessed by analyzing the individual blocks of 80 transients, which reduced the S/N of these spectra by a factor of $\sqrt{5}$ compared to the 400—transient spectra (see Fig. 2b). For Integration and FITSPEC, the means of the peak areas estimated from the low-S/N spectra deviated substantially from the results obtained from the averaged spectra. VARPRO, using prior knowledge of the metabolites, hardly showed any degradation in performance at low S/N. When analyzing the low-S/N blocks, no use was made of findings from the high-S/N analysis for that particular signal.

DISCUSSION

In the *in vitro* ¹H-MRS study, both the time and frequency domain methods resolved the severe peak

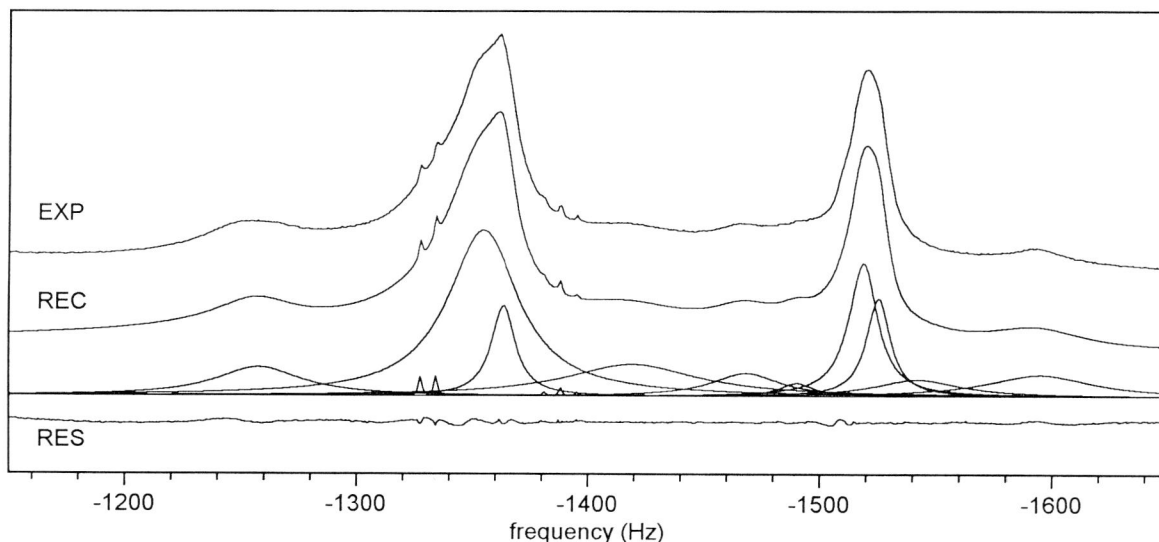

Fig. 1. The methylene and methyl region of an LDL ¹H-MR spectrum; spectrum after water removal (EXP), reconstructed spectrum (REC), individual Lorentzians, and residual (RES). FITPLA^c results are shown; however, VARPRO gave near identical results.

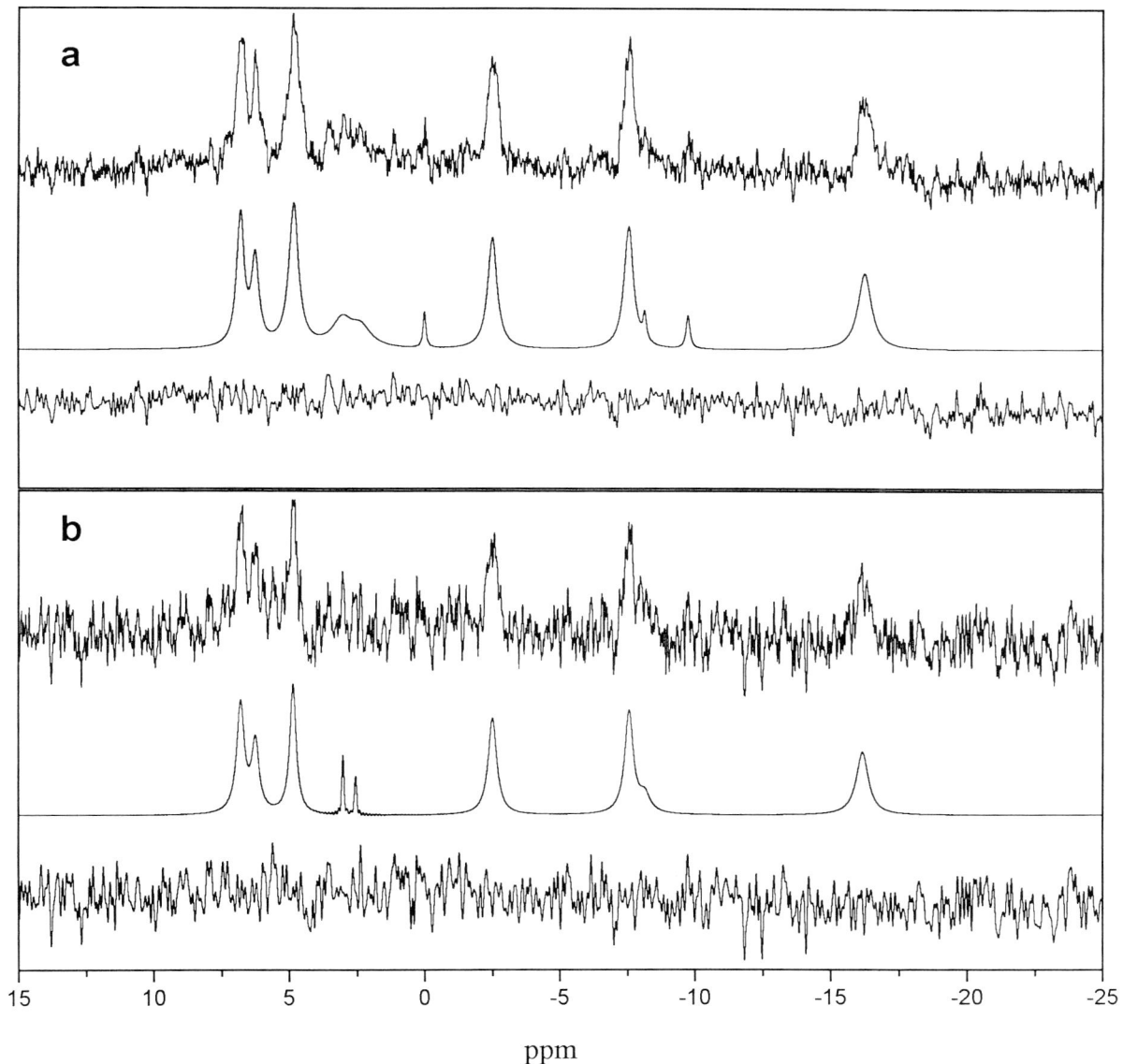

Fig. 2. VARPRO time domain fitting results of *in vivo* ^{31}P-MRS data of high (a) and low S/N (b). VARPRO results did not suffer from the drop in S/N FITSPEC and Integration performed well at high S/N but failed at low S/N.

overlap. FITPLA[c] and VARPRO performed equally well, as there were no other distortions: Residual water was removed, S/N was high, and there were many data points and no missing initial data points. In the *in vivo* ^{31}P-MRS study with shorter data lengths, the S/N and distorted initial data points formed a limiting factor for the frequency domain methods, whereas VARPRO still produced reliable results. Distortions in the measured MRS signal make time domain methods preferable to frequency domain methods. Current studies show the same findings for short-TE *in vivo* ^{1}H-MRS data from the human brain.

ACKNOWLEDGMENTS

This work was supported by the Cancer Research Campaign, UK; grant number SP1971/0402. The ^{1}H-MRS project was also supported by the Academy of Finland and the British Council.

REFERENCES

1. Pijnappel WWF, van den Boogaart A, de Beer R, van Ormondt D (1992) *J Magn Reson* **97**: 122.
2. van den Boogaart A, van Ormondt D, Pijnappel WWF, de

Beer R, Ala-Korpela M (1994) In *Mathematics in Signal Processing III* (McWhirter JG, ed) p. 175. Oxford: Clarendon Press.

3. van der Veen JWC, de Beer R, Luyten PR, van Ormondt D (1988) *Magn Reson Med* **6:** 92.

4. Hiltunen Y, Ala-Korpela M, Jokisaari J, Eskelinen S, Kiviniitty K, Savolainen M, Kesäniemi YA (1991) *Magn Reson Med* **21:** 222.

5. van den Boogaart A, Ala-Korpela M, Jokisaari J, Griffiths JR (1994) *Magn Reson Med* **31:** 347.

Quantitative proton MRS assessment of citrate heterogeneity in normal prostate

M. Lowry, D.J. Manton, L.W. Turnbull, S.J. Blackband and A. Horsman

Yorkshire Cancer Research Campaign and University of Hull Centre for Magnetic Resonance Investigations, Hull Royal Infirmary, Hull HU3 2JZ, UK

Water-suppressed proton spectra of the two major anatomical regions of the normal prostate were acquired with a commercial phased-array multicoil. The spectra demonstrated excellent signal-to-noise ratio and spectral resolution allowing identification of peaks from choline, creatine, and amino acids, as well as a major peak from citrate. Quantification of the citrate peak using tissue water as an internal concentration reference revealed a marked variability among different volunteers. In each case, citrate was consistently twofold to threefold greater in the peripheral zone than in the central gland. The results demonstrate heterogeneity of citrate within the prostate and suggest significant differences in the cytology and hormonal control of citrate synthesis among individuals.

Keywords: proton MRS, quantitation, citrate, prostate, heterogeneity.

INTRODUCTION

The current inability of magnetic resonance imaging (MRI) to differentiate among various pathologies of the prostate [1] has stimulated the application of magnetic resonance spectroscopy (MRS) to this problem. Human prostatic epithelial cells synthesize and secrete large quantities of citrate [2] which is easily detectable in the proton spectrum [3–5]. Biochemical studies *in vitro* have demonstrated that the citrate content of prostatic adenocarcinoma (ACP) is decreased, whereas that of benign prostatic hypertrophy (BPH) is increased compared to normal tissue [6]. These pathologies also differ in their principal sites of presentation, with ACP appearing primarily in the peripheral zone and BPH in the central gland [7]. Correct clinical interpretation of proton MRS data therefore requires a knowledge of the anatomical distribution of citrate. This study demonstrates considerable regional heterogeneity in citrate concentration of the normal prostate which could have a significant impact on the application of proton MRS to the diagnosis of prostatic lesions.

Address for correspondence: Centre for MRI, Hull Royal Infirmary, Anlaby Road, Hull HU3 2JZ, UK

METHODS

Five healthy volunteers aged between 25 and 52 years were studied using a GE 1.5-T Signa. Images and spectra were acquired using a commercial pelvic phased-array multicoil (GE Medical Systems, Milwaukee, WI) for signal reception. Spectroscopic voxels were identified from axial T_2-weighted, fast spin-echo images obtained with TR/TE of 2500/168 ms. The stimulated echo acquisition mode (STREAM) sequence with outer volume suppression was used to acquire two separate localized spectra from 3–5 ml voxels positioned in the central gland and peripheral zone. Each spectrum was followed by the acquisition of water reference spectra at four different echo times with a TR of 10 s and four averages.

The acquired free-induction decays (FIDs) were apodized using a 4-Hz Gaussian filter and zero-filled to 2K complex points before Fourier transformation. Citrate and water peak areas were obtained from manually phased spectra by fitting a single Lorentzian to each peak. The method of Barker et al. [8] was used to calculate concentrations from these peak areas assuming that T_1 of citrate and tissue water content were 1.2 s and 44 mmol g^{-1}, respectively. The value of 184 ms used for the T_2 of citrate was taken from the work of Heerschap et al. [3]. The irregular shape of the

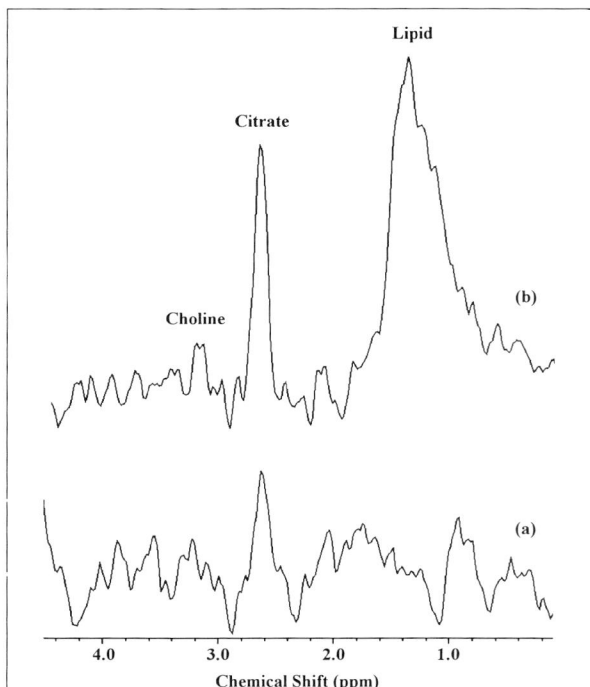

Fig. 1. Proton spectra acquired from (a) central gland and (b) peripheral zone of the prostate gland of a normal young male. Each spectrum is the sum of 512 averages collected using STEAM with TR = 1 s and TE = 50 ms.

peripheral zone precluded the acquisition of spectra from this tissue without contamination from the central gland. Tissue volumes estimated from the axial localizer images were therefore used to correct peripheral zone peak areas for the variable proportion of included central gland.

RESULTS

Figure 1 shows representative proton spectra acquired from central gland and from peripheral zone of the prostate. In all spectra, a major peak at 2.6 ppm arising from the coupled methylene protons of citrate was visible. In some spectra, particularly those of the peripheral zone, contributions from choline-containing compounds, and mobile lipids were observed at 3.2 and 1.4 ppm, respectively.

The T_2 of water used to calculate citrate concentrations was obtained from the unsuppressed reference spectra acquired separately from the two regions. The mean value obtained for the peripheral zone, 145 ± 33 ms (mean ± S.D.), was significantly greater than that for central gland, 88 ± 15 ms. Citrate concentrations calculated for the two regions showed considerable interindividual heterogeneity. For the peripheral zone,

values ranged from 28 to 102 μmol g^{-1} fresh weight and for the central gland from 12 to 58 μmol g^{-1} fresh weight (Fig. 2). In all five volunteers, however, the peripheral zone consistently demonstrated a greater concentration than the central gland (61 ± 30 vs. 34 ± 20 μmol g^{-1} fresh weight; mean ± S.D., $P < 0.05$ by paired t-test).

DISCUSSION

The use of a phased-array receiver coil to acquire high-quality spectra of the prostate has several advantages over the use of an endorectal coil. Apart from the increase in comfort for the patient, the body coil provides homogenous excitation over the whole of the pelvic region, whereas the phased-array provides homogenous signal reception at distances beyond those attainable with an endorectal coil. This coil combination has enabled the accurate quatification of citrate within the two major regions of the prostate. The use of a 17-cm Helmholtz coil by Schick et al. [5] represents a similar approach. However, they did not aquire reference spectra and were, thus, unable to quantify citrate.

The concentrations reported here are of the same magnitude as those measured in prostatic fluid and semen [9]. Further, our value of 34 μmol g^{-1} fresh

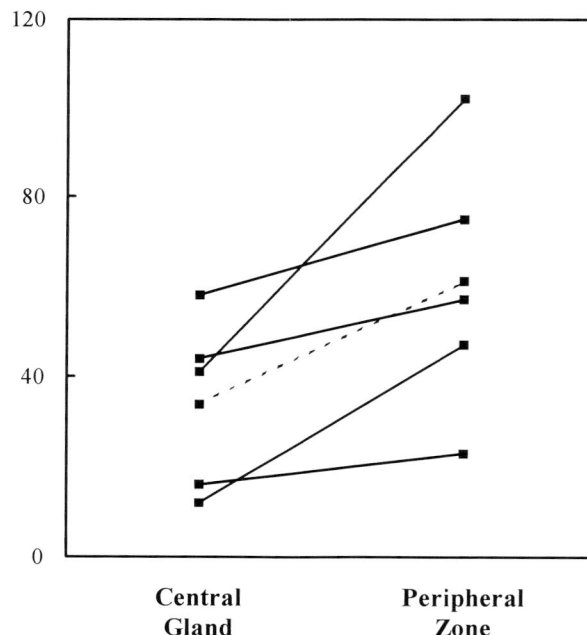

Fig. 2. Variation in citrate concentration within normal prostate gland. Citrate concentration was determined from spectra acquired separately from both the central gland and peripheral zone of each volunteer (—). The mean citrate concentration for each region is also plotted (- - -).

weight for the normal central gland is consistent with that of 53 μmol g^{-1} fresh weight reported by Heerschap et al. [3] for BPH tissue *in situ*. The calculation of citrate concentrations requires values for citrate T_1, citrate T_2, and tissue water content. For our calculations, we have assumed that these three parameters are identical in the two regions. This may not be valid for the relaxation parameters, particularly because the T_2 of water differs significantly between the two regions (see the preceding section). Nevertheless, citrate T_2 would need to be reduced from 184 ms to 60 ms in order to produce a central gland citrate concentration equal to that of the peripheral zone. Similarly, the T_1 of citrate would need to increase twofold. For water content, the assumption of equality is not unreasonable, as proton density-weighted images show no signal intensity difference between the peripheral zone and central gland.

Costello and Franklin [2] originally proposed that citrate concentrations might differ between the peripheral zone and central gland. Numerous *in vitro* studies and embryological observations in rats and monkeys suggested that the peripheral zone was responsible for the bulk of hormonally mediated citrate production. Although the central gland in man may be functionally different and responsible for some citrate production, our observation of considerable quantities of citrate in this region may be explained by the presence of citrate-rich fluid in the ejaculatory ducts. Within the peripheral zone, citrate is synthesized predominantly by epithelial cells. Stromal cells show little capacity for citrate synthesis and do not contribute to its accumulation. Thus, the variation in citrate concentration of this zone between individuals could be produced by a variation in the relative proportions of epithelial and stromal cells. Consistent with this suggestion, Schiebler et al. [10] recently demonstrated with perchloric acid extracted radical prostatectomy specimens that some cases of BPH cannot be distinguished from ACP by high-resolution ^{1}H spectroscopy. Histological examination of these cases showed only small areas of glandular tissue with extensive stromal hyperplasia. Further variation in peripheral zone citrate concentration could arise through the hormonal action of testosterone and prolactin [11]. Both act to increase the transcription of the gene for mitochondrial aspartate aminotransferase, a key enzyme in citrate synthesis. Thus, variations in the serum concentration of these hormones could modulate the concentration of citrate within the prostate by changing its rate of synthesis.

This study clearly demonstrates both the regional and interindividual variation in citrate concentration of the prostate. The results question the clinical utility of unlocalized tissue sampling at transurethral resection and suggest that citrate concentration should be measured *in vivo* and directly compared with whole mounted prostate specimens.

ACKNOWLEDGMENTS

We are grateful to the Yorkshire Cancer Research Campaign and the Jeremy Drake Foundation for funds to support this work.

REFERENCES

1. Ling D, Lee JKT, Heiken JP, Balfe DM, Glazer HS, McClennan GL (1986) Prostatic carcinoma and benign prostatic hyperplasia: Inability of MR imaging to distinguish between the two diseases. *Radiology* **158**: 103–107.
2. Costello LC, Franklin RB (1991) Concepts of citrate production and secretion by prostate 1. Metabolic Relationships. *Prostate* **18**: 25–46.
3. Heerschap A, de Jager G, de Koster A, Barentz J, de la Rosette J, Debruyne F, Ruijs J (1993) 1H MRS of prostate pathology. *Proc Soc Magn Reson Med* p. 213.
4. Thomas MA, Narayan P, Kurhanewicz J, Jajodia P, Weiner MW (1990) 1H MR Spectroscopy of normal and malignant human prostates in vivo. *J Magn Reson* **87**: 610–619.
5. Schick F, Bongers H, Kurz S, Jung WI, Pfeffer M, Lutz O (1993) Localized proton MR spectroscopy of citrate in vitro and of the human prostate in vivo at 1.5 T. *Magn Reson Med* **29**: 38–43.
6. Costello LC, Littleton GK, Franklin RB (1978) Regulation of citrate-related metabolism in normal and neoplastic prostate *in* "Endocrine Control in Neoplasia." Eds. Sharma RK, Criss WE. pp. 303–314. Raven Press. New York.
7. McNeal J, Redwine E, Freiha M, Stamey TA (1988) Zonal distribution of prostatic carcinoma: correlation with histological pattern and direction of spread. *Am J Surg* **12**: 897–906.
8. Barker PB, Soher BJ, Blackband SJ, Chatham JC, Mathews VP, Bryan RN (1993) Quantitation of proton NMR spectra of the human brain using tissue water as an internal concentration reference. *NMR Biomed* **6**: 89–94.
9. Dondero F, Sciarra F, Isidori A (1972) Evaluation of relationship between plasma testosterone and human seminal citic acid. *Fert Steril* **23**: 168–171.
10. Schiebler M, Miyamoto K, Gabel S, White M, Luyten P, Mohler J (1991) In vitro high resolution proton spectroscopy of the human prostate: benign prostatic hypertrophy and adenocarcinoma. *Proc Soc Magn Reson Med* p. 322.
11. Costello LC, Franklin RB (1991) Concepts of citrate production and secretion by prostate: 2. Hormonal relationships in normal and neoplastic prostate. *Prostate* **19**: 181–205.

ABSTRACTS OF INVITED PAPERS

P03

The interdependence of functional MRI and MRS in the human brain

R.G. SHULMAN, A.M. BLAMIRE, W. CHEN,
E.J. NOVOTNY and D.L. ROTHMAN
Yale University, New Haven, Connecticut, USA

During brain activity there are numerous indications that energy consumption increases. However, the quantitative extent of this increase is not known. The question has been raised directly by PET measurements [1] of stimulation of the visual cortex by a flashing light pattern. These results showed $\sim 50\%$ increase in CMRglc, whereas $CMRO_2$ only increased by $\sim 5\%$. We have recently introduced two NMR methods which measure these two parameters and are using them to measure the effects of visual stimulation. The values of $CMRO_2$ are measured by infusing 1-^{13}C glucose and determining the turnover rate of the glutamate–glutamine pool. Our values [2] of this rate in the visual cortex agree with the $CMRO_2$ values determined by ^{15}O PET measurements [1].

We have developed a method of measuring changes in CMRglc and measured $\sim 22\%$ changes averaged over 12 cm^3 of the visual cortex during stimulation [3].

In order to avoid partial volume effects, it is necessary to obtain signals from several cubic centimeters of the brain and to be focused accurately on the stimulated regions. Sensitivity on our 2.1-T system is now sufficient to obtain ^{1}H-NMR spectra of the glucose and glutamate changes from ~ 6 cc of the cortex. Functional echo-planar MRI has been used to locate the activated regions [3] from which spectra are now being obtained.

Cognitive functional MRI studies on word generation and working memory tasks suggest that similar spectroscopic measurements can be made on regions.

1. Fox PT et al. (1988) *Science* **241**: 462.
2. Rothman DL et al. (1992) Proc. Natl. Acad. Sci. **89**: 9603.
3. Chen W et al. (1993) Proc. Natl. Acad. Sci. **90**: 9896.

P09

Localized NMR spectroscopy, neurometabolism, and the functioning human brain

J. FRAHM
Biomedizinische NMR Forschungs GmbH, 37018 Göttingen, Germany

Localized magnetic resonance spectroscopy (MRS) and advanced magnetic resonance imaging (MRI) techniques have opened new insights into the functioning human brain. Thus, access to cerebral anatomy and pathology has been complemented by a regional analysis of cellular metabolism as well as by a visualization of neural activity via physiologic alterations such as task-related changes in cerebral blood oxygenation.

The purpose of this presentation is to illustrate spectroscopic aspects of brain function and dysfunction in man as well as to relate MRS approaches to recent studies using functional neuroimaging. In general, biomedical applications of neurometabolism using localized proton and phosphorus MRS of the central nervous system require a transformation of spectral findings into absolute substrate concentrations.

Current questions address issues such as the uptake and distribution of substrates, metabolic correlates of brain function, and studies of disease states of the brain ranging from ischemia, neoplasms, and inherited metabolites disorders to psychiatric diseases. Examples will emphasize neurometabolic diseases in children.

POSTERS

PI01

In vivo T_2 measurements with a CPMG–OSIRIS sequence.

P. POULET, F. GIRARD,* I.J. NAMER and
J. CHAMBRON
*Institut de Physique Biologique, URA CNRS 1173, Faculté
de Médecine, 4, rue Kirschleger, 67085 Strasbourg Cedex,
France.*

T_2 measurements performed with imaging experiments are often complicated by diffusion processes and spin–spin interactions during long interpulse delays in the presence of encoding magnetic field gradients.

The CPMG–OSIRIS sequence presented uses a OSIRIS (ISIS + out of slice presaturation) localization scheme followed by a train of refocusing pulses which allows the acquisition of numerous echoes with a short, easy to select, interpulse delay. The transverse magnetization decay can be analyzed in a precise way, and a multiparametric approach can be considered.

The sequence was written and experiments were performed on a Bruker MSL200 with a wide-bore vertical magnet. Validations were made on test objects, for proton, on gels and $CuSO_4$ solutions, and for fluorine 19 on suspensions of a blood substitute, perfluorooctylbromide PFOB.[1] The tranverse and longitudinal relaxation rates of the fluorine nuclei of PFOB are linearly related to the partial oxygen pressure PO_2 of the suspension.

The sequence has then been applied to T_2 measurements on animal models. For proton experiments, 27-μl volumes were localized in rat brain areas mainly composed of white matter. Control and edemateous areas were studied.

Localized measurements of ^{19}F T_2 were performed on rat brains and tongues after injection of PFOB. The volume used was 125 μl. The T_2 obtained on the different peaks allows the calculation of the PO_2 of the investigated area. Typical experiments were performed in 35 s and have an accuracy of 10 mm Hg.

The results obtained will be presented, as well as the advantages and limitations of the described methodology.

---

* *Present address: FORENAP, MR Unit, 68250 Rouffach, France.*
[1]* *Gift from Pr. J. Riess, Université de Nice, France.*

PI02

T_1 maps using U-STEAM

A. VÄTH and P.M. JAKOB
*Unité INSERM 318, Groupe d'Application de la RMN à la
Neurobiologie, Hôpital Albert Michallon, BP 217x 38043
Grenoble Cedex, France*

Introduction: Recently, we have developed a fast imaging technique called U-STEAM that is very similar to high-speed STEAM [1] but has no need for fast switching gradient systems. This technique allows to accurately measure T_1 relaxation times in reasonable experimental times.

Methods: The U-STEAM technique 90°–TE/2–90°–TM–(α-TE/2-STE)$_n$ generates a train of n differently phase-encoded stimulated echoes STE. The initial slice selective 90° pulse and the 90° hard pulse in combination with the gradients prepare a pool of longitudinal magnetization in the slice of interest that is attenuated by T_1 during a relaxation delay TM. The STE are acquired by applying nonselective α pulses in the presence of the read gradient. Phase encoding can be either done by incrementing the gradient stepwise or by using a conventional phase-encoding scheme. A TR of 2 ms and a 64 × 128 data matrix were used, yielding a one shot image in 130 ms.

For T_1 mapping a series of 16 one-shot U-STEAM images with increasing relaxation delays TM has been acquired in less than 3 min.

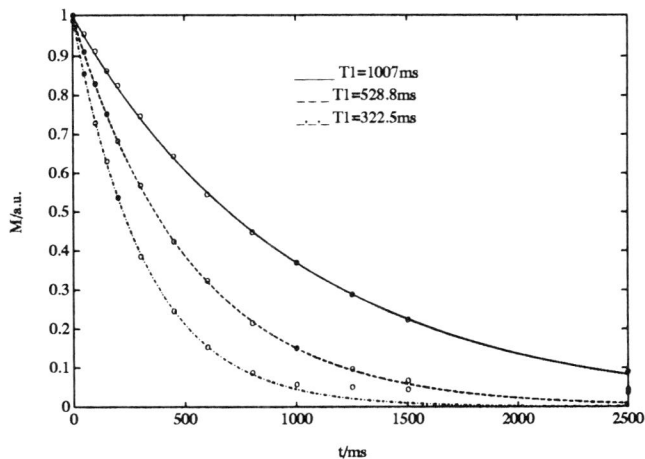

Results and discussion: Multicompartment phantom studies indicate that U-STEAM allows fast and accurate T_1 measurements (see graphic). Additional experiments are necessary to confirm the ability of U-STEAM in biological systems.

Acknowledgments: This work was supported by a grants of the DAAD/HSPII and the European Community BIOMED I program

1. Frahm J, Merboldt KD, Hänicke W, Haase A (1985) "Stimulated Echo Imaging" *J Magn Reson* **64**: 81–93.

PI03

Fitting of amplitude magnetization transfer curves
D. GOUNOT, Y. MAUSS, B. DUMITRESCO and J. CHAMBRON
Institut de Physique Biologique, Faculté de Médecine, Strasbourg, France

Aim: Magnetization transfer experiments highlight the relations existing between the two main components of a biological tissue: water (A) and macromolecules (B). Our experiment consists in irradiating the tissue with a RF field of frequency offset f and effective magnetic field $\mathbf{B}_1$ (expressed in μT) during a time τ. After this irradiation, the amplitude of the NMR signal is measured by a 90° impulsion. The measurements give the amplitude magnetization transfer curves (AMT). Our aim was to fit a whole set of AMTs acquired systematically with f and $\mathbf{B}_1$ variables using the two-compartment model and Bloch equations.

Material and methods: Experiments were performed on agarose gels (0.5, 1, 1.5, and 2%) doped with a solution of $MnCl_2$ 0.0001 M on freshly excised bovine cerebral tissues (white and gray matter, medula). The device is a Bruker CXP 100 spectrometer operating at 19.973 MHz. The irradiation was performed in a range of $\pm$ 130 kHz, with seven values of irradiation power (from $\mathbf{B}_1 = 2.5\ \mu$T to 170 μT), during a time τ long enough to reach equilibrium. All the data obtained for a substance were fitted together using a dedicated program based on the Bloch–McDonnell solutions of the magnetization equations at equilibrium. The whole set of equations was taken in account (six equations). As we considered a bicompartimental model, six parameters are sufficient to characterize the model: $R_{1A}, R_{2A}, R_{1B}, R_{2B}$ (R being the relaxation rate), R_{AB} is the rate of exchange from A to B, and $F = M_{B0}/M_{A0}$, the relative proportion of protons in the two compartments. The aim of the program was to determine all the sets of these six parameters which fit the AMTs.

Results and discussion: A direct determination of the six parameters by a nonlinear regression method fails because the parameters are found to be mathematically dependent. So it is necessary to reduce the set of independent variables. The best way is to introduce some relaxation rates obtained independently. The parameter set can then be reduced to four or five independent variables. Concerning agarose gels, satisfactory parameters sets were found. Concerning the tissues, we did not found satisfactory parameter sets. An additional compartment seems necessary in order to improve the fit.

PI04

Predominance of signals from extracerebral veins in functional MRI of motor activity in the human brain
C. DELON-MARTIN, V. BELLE, R. MASSARELLI, J. DECETY, J.F. LE BAS, M. DÉCORPS, A.L. BENABID, and C. SEGEBARTH
INSERM U.318 (GARN), CHU, BP217X, F38043 Grenoble, France

A vast majority of the functional MRI (fMRI) studies published so far have applied the gradient-echo MR techniques on clinical 1.5-T MR systems. Usually, these studies exhibit a limited spatial resolution, due either to instrumental limitations (as in the case of echo-planar acquisition), or to constraints of temporal resolution. Hence, it has been difficult to assign precisely the origin of the gradient-echo fMRI signals.

In the present 1.5-T study, the gradient-echo fMRI response to different finger-tapping paradigms has been investigated over a 3D volume. The results show that this response is due predominantly to veins located on the surface of the cortex.

The demonstration of the predominance of extracerebral vascular signals in fMRI of motor activity is based on a novel approach. A large set of contiguous 2D fMRI images is thus acquired, and MIP images derived from this set are compared with MR angiograms obtained from the volume covered by the fMRI images. The advantages of this approach are twofold. First, the full 3D fMRI response is obtained in experimental conditions which match those applied in the usual 2D fMR (gradient-echo techniques). Second, the vascular predominance in the fMRI response can be demonstrated conveniently by superposing the fMRI MIPs and MR angiograms.

These results constitute a first example of functional angiography in the human brain. They have been confirmed by means of alternative functional MR angiography methods, based on phase-contrast MR images acquired during rest and during performance of a motor task [1].

1. Belle V, Delon-Martin C, Massarelli R, et al. Functional MR angiography of the human brain. Abstract at this symposium.

PI05

The development of targeted MRI systems at Exeter

W. VENNART, S. PITTARD, M.E. FRY, R.E. ELLIS, G. SHERMAN, J. GASSON, J. FOSTER, I.R. SUMMERS and A. HOWSEMAN

Department of Physics, University of Exeter, Exeter EX4 4QL, UK

There is a need in MRI to understand more fully how different tissue states determine the signals obtained if some attempt to quantify disease is to be realized. We have developed targeted MRI systems capable of relatively high-resolution imaging to study joints in arthritis and distal tissues for assessment of peripheral vascular disease in diabetes. This research has led to some novel hardware developments and the ability to explore fundamental changes in MR signals from diseased tissues hitherto not possible. For specific applications, we have designed special radio-frequency coils, e.g. a U-shaped birdcage for the metacarpophalangeal joints of the hand and a split coil (with a ladder network driver) for the knee. Along with standard birdcage design for studying the distal interpalangeal joints, these developments have enabled the normal joint to be investigated *in vivo* at high resolution and changes in joint tissues elucidated as arthritis progresses. All the systems are based on small horizontal-bored superconducting magnets with actively screened gradient sets (Magnex Scientific Ltd) to provide optimum access; the operating consoles (Surrey Medical Imaging Systems Ltd) are based on a modular design utilizing IBM-compatible personal computers. This poster will describe some of the more exciting technical developments and give an outline of the systems developed and their particular niche applications.

PI06

A low-cost current driver circuit for pulsed gradient NMR experiments

J.S. THORNTON, M.A. BROWNE and P.A. PAYNE

Department of Instrumentation and Analytical Science, University of Manchester Institute of Science and Technology, Manchester, UK

Introduction: A low-cost gradient current driver has been designed and implemented, forming part of a distributed intelligence NMR imaging system developed in our laboratory. The circuit was required to generate the precise, stable, bipolar current waveforms required in MR imaging experiments and pulsed gradient diffusion coefficient measurements. Gradient waveform voltages were generated by an intelligent controller based around a BBC microcomputer, the pulse timing being determined by trigger signals from the system pulse programmer.

Methods: The circuitry to be described consisted of two sections, namely, a precision, voltage-controlled current sink combined with a current steering arrangement, allowing the magnitude and direction of the current produced by a 0–20 A unipolar commercial laboratory power supply to be accurately controlled.

The current sink was a conventional arrangement consisting of an op-amp in a noninverting configuration driving a power MOSFET transistor, the output current being sensed by a precision, water-cooled, "4-wire," 100W resistor. Closed-loop feedback compensation components were selected empirically to optimize the current pulse rise times and pulse stability.

The current steering section consisted of an "H-bridge" array of four power MOSFETs configured as voltage-controlled switches, effectively allowing the polarity of the current applied to the gradient coil to be reversed under digital control.

Results: The accuracy of the output current immediately subsequent to a switching point exceeded 0.05%. For a nominal value of 10 A DC, the temporal stability of the output current was $0.6\% \text{ h}^{-1}$. Following a switching point, the output rose smoothly to the final value within 0.3 ms for all current levels, no significant overshoot or ringing being observed (load inductance $\approx 22 \ \mu H$, resistance $\approx 0.5 \ \Omega$).

Conclusion: A simple, economical gradient current driver circuit has been developed which is capable of the high performance required for modern pulsed gradient NMR experiments.

PI07

A versatile digital gradient controller for NMR imaging experiments

J.S. THORNTON, M.A. BROWNE and P.A. PAYNE

Department of Instrumentation and Analytical Science, University of Manchester Institute of Science and Technology, Manchester UK

Introduction: An intelligent gradient control unit based around a proprietary microcomputer has been designed and constructed as a part of a low-cost MR imaging system developed in our laboratory.

Methods: The gradient controller to be described was required to generate output voltage signals proportional to preprogrammed gradient values at times accurately synchronized with trigger pulses from the system pulse controller. A BBC Master microcomputer was employed, the required sequence of gradient values being calculated and stored in memory prior to the start of an experiment. The new gradient value for each channel was transferred to an external register in advance of each switching point, the contents of this buffer then being clocked to the digital-to-analog converter (DAC) upon receipt of a "next gradient" trigger pulse. An interrupt was then generated, causing the next gradient values to be transferred to the external registers.

A separate 12-bit DAC (AD667JN) was employed for each of the three output channels, each being interfaced to the BBC machine's 1-MHz expansion bus via a 6522 Versatile Interface Adapter chip. These memory-mapped devices provided a convenient method of data transfer between the 8-bit data bus of the BBC machine and the 12-bit DACs and were also required to handle the necessary interrupt functions.

The DACs were configured to provide unipolar output voltages in the range 0–10 V. A single TTL logic signal was used to control the polarity of the output produced by home-built current driver circuits.

Software was developed (using BBC BASIC and 6502 assembly language as appropriate) to provide data transfer and interrupt service routines and also to generate the sequence of gradient values required to execute 2DFT and Filtered Back Projection MR imaging sequences.

Results: The system described has been successfully employed in a number of MR imaging experiments.

Conclusion: A useful, versatile gradient controller system has been developed at modest cost.

PI08

Software pulse sequence generator based on DSP96000 for NMR tomography and spectroscopy
K. BARTUŠEK and Z. DOKOUPIL
Institute of Scientific Instruments,† ASCR Královopolská 147, 61264 Brno, Czech Republic

The development of magnetic resonance imaging (MRI) techniques puts increasingly higher demands on the time coordination of the operation of spectrometer circuits and on the automation of the MRI experiment. Especially, generation of several different AM rf selective pulses in one sequence and generation of gradient pulses of defined shapes are concerned.

The properties of generators of pulse sequences (GPS) which control the tomograph performance are limited, above all, by their hardware, and their application versatility is limited by their software. Therefore, a software GPS has been tested which has a markedly simpler hardware, increases its reliability, and decreases its price. The program loop determines the length of time intervals, no timer is necessary, and the generator has better flexibility.

The basic part of the GPS hardware is the 32-bit DSP96000/40-MHz digital signal processor from Motorola, complemented with a 96-bit output register and a 64-kword program memory. GSP has a time resolution of 50 ns, shortest timing event of 180 ns, and eight mutually nested hard loops. The pulse sequence and control signals are defined by the DSP program which is transferred from the host computer (PC 486) via the series line and started. Four 12-bit GSP signals are used for the generation of modulation signals for selective radiofrequency pulses and gradients in one pulse sequence.

The software GPS with DSP is part of the control system, and owing to its properties, it meets the present demands of NMR tomography and spectroscopy.

PI09

Improved selective pulses for the MR spin-echo experiment
A. AL-BESHR, C. OESTERLE, D. McINTYRE,*
and P. MORRIS
M.R. Centre, University of Nottingham, Nottingham, UK
*Division of Biochemistry, Department of Cellular and Molecular Science, St. George's Hospital, Medical School, London, UK

Spin-echo experiments are still widely used in MRI. Usually, the $\pi/2$ and π selective pulses are curtailed sinc functions. Sometimes, the $\pi/2$ sinc pulse is "optimized," but little effort is usually expended in optimizing the refocusing π pulse; generally, a pulse that is simply twice the amplitude of the $\pi/2$ pulse is used. Because the spin system is nonlinear, this can lead to substantial signal loss, particularly if multiple spin echoes are generated.

We have used the SPINCALC scheme [Ngo JT, Morris PG (1985) *Magn Reson Med* 5: 217], an optimisation method that operates in a switched stationary reference frame, to design refocusing pulses with a performance substantially improved over that of the standard sinc pulse. Because the SPINCALC method effectively linearizes the Bloch equation, acceptable results are achieved in just a few iterations. The benefits are twofold: better refocusing, hence higher signal to noise ratio, and sharper slice selection.

Rather than optimize the $\pi/2$ and π selective pulses separately, it is also possible to optimize the spin-echo sequence as a whole. In principle, imperfections in one pulse can be compensated by changes in the excitation profile of the second. Various approaches to this are possible using the SPINCALC algorithm.

PI10

Symmetrical shielded head gradient coil

T. SKÓRKA and A. JASINSKI

H. Niewodniczański Institute of Nuclear Physics, 31-342 Kraków, Poland

Functional MRI requires high-speed gradient coils capable of generating large gradients. A local head gradient coil should meet conflicting requirements: be short and easy to fit over patient's head, have no mechanical torque, generate linear gradient in largest possible volume, and have small inductance, small field outside, and efficiency. A number of solutions to this problem has been presented [1].

In this paper, a discrete winding approach was used based on calculating field from the Biot–Savart law of current elements, optimizing the positions of wires to produce the desired field in ROI using the conjugate gradient descent method. The error function E is defined as [2]

$$E = \sum_{i=1}^{N} (B_{zi} - B_{zi}(X))^2$$

where N = number of target points having field B_{zi} and $B_{zi}(X)$ = calculated field values for a given configuration of wires. The target points are defined inside and outside of the coil. Optimization is carried out for fixed geometry and number of turns of wire for gradient and screen coils by changing positions of wires. It is computation-intensive, requiring large

number of iterations to produce reasonable coil layout. The starting wire configuration used in this design was a four-quadrant spiral for the gradient and screen coils having unequal number of turns.

A screened head gradient coil having an inside diameter of 300 mm, outside diameter of 600 mm, efficiency of 0.2 (mT/m) · A, gradient linearity of 5% over a sphere of 200 mm was designed. Field profiles and calculation details will be presented.

1. Turner R (1993) *Magn Reson Imaging* 11: 903.
2. Wong EC, Jesmianowicz A, Hyde JS (1991) *Magn Reson Med* 21: 39.

PI11

Measurement of Gradient Magnetic Field for NMR Tomography

K. BARTUŠEK and B. JÍLEK

Institute of Scientific Instruments, ASCR Královopolská 147, 61264 Brno, Czech Republic

We present a technique for measuring the time dependence of magnetic fields due to eddy currents (EC) produced by time-dependent magnetic field gradients.

The described NMR method is based on the measurement of an instantaneous frequency of the FID signal, recorded immediately after switching off the gradient pulse. This technique makes use of a large-volume sample (diameter 15 mm) and 90° selective RF excitation pulses and free-induction decay (FID) (or a spin or gradient echo) to measure the out-of-phase component of the FID (echo), which is proportional to $\gamma \Delta B$, i.e., the amount the signal is off resonance. The time of measurement was 300 ms. The data were processed in several steps. The first was the determination of the instantaneous phase of the complex FID signal. The second step was the derivation of the phase and adaptive moving average filtration of the instantaneous frequency, because the phase noise is nonlinearly proportional to the S/N ratio drop of the FID amplitude. The third step was the implementation the Nelder–Mead simplex algorithm for nonlinear fitting and for determination of the preemphasis constants.

The measurement was carried out using a homebuilt 200-MHz spectrometer with a probe allowing microthomography (max. diameter 20 mm). Preemphasis constants for the same magnet system measured by different methods are confronted, and the preemphasis compensation of our magnet by the gradient system with the digital signal processor DSP96000 will be made. The measuring technique is sensitive and easy to implement and interpret.

PI12

Elimination from NMR spectra of baseline distortions caused by the response of audiofilters
Z. STARČUK, K. BARTUŠEK, B. JÍLEK, and Z. STARČUK, JR.
Institute of Scientific Instruments, ASCR Královopolská 147, 61264 Brno, Czech Republic

Flat baselines are often a perequisite for the successful analysis of 2D NMR spectra, especially NOE spectra, and it is important to be able to cope with various baseline artifacts such as baseline roll, t_1 ridges, and t_1 noise. There are several mechanisms, as a rule closely interrelated, which participate in the baseline distortion. The analysis of the problem showed that in most cases it is much easier to prevent the creation of the baseline distortions than to eliminate them from the spectra.

One of the sources of baseline distortions belonging to the class of so-called "first-points problems" is the transient response of the low-pass audiofrequency filters to the abrupt appearance of the NMR signal.

Hoult et al. have analyzed these phenomena for a four-pole Butterworth filter and, to solve the transient response problem, suggested synchronizing properly the data sampling with the filter response [1]. Quite recently, an improved Hoult's technique has been presented by Froystein [2].

In this contribution, we describe an approach to the elimination of the distortion caused by the transient response in case audiofilters (analog or digital) with symetric impulse response are employed. The basic demand of this approach is to locate the in-phase point (the point in which all magnetization vectors have the same phase) into the middle of the symmetric transient response. Then the samples ahead of the midpoint are added to the samples occurring in symmetrical positions behind the midpoint of the transient response. The obtained FID signal provides a spectrum free of distortions caused by filter ringing.

A somewhat different technique based on the processing of the whole NMR signal has been developed by Halámek et al. [3].

1. Hoult DI et al. (1983) *J Magn Reson* **51**: 110.
2. Froystein NA (1993) *J Magn Reson Series A* **103**: 332.
3. Halámek J, Vondra V, Kasal M, *J Magn Reson* (submitted for publication).

PI13

An approach to the solution of the first data-point problem in indirectly detected dimensions in *m*D NMR experiments
Z. STARČUK, K. BARTUŠEK and Z. STARČUK, JR.
Institute of Scientific Instruments, ASCR Královopolská 147, 61264 Brno, Czech Republic

Because of finite widths of 90° pulses flanking the evolution periods, the data acquisition in indirectly detected dimensions in multidimensional NMR experiments often start at finite durations. These "sampling delays" necessitates the use of a linearly frequency-dependent phase correction, which introduces baseline distortions.

Several strategies for overcoming this problem have been proposed. Frenkiel et al. [1] obtained good baselines by using a sequential acquisition scheme with the receiver phase adjusted to give sine modulation in indirectly detected dimensions. Bax et al. [2] and Archer et al. [3] have showed that one avoids the problem of baseline distortion when acquiring the data with a sampling delay of one-half the dwell time or one dwell time in case complex or real acquisition scheme is employed. Finally, Lippens and Hallenge [4] and Frøystein [5] cure baseline and phase problems in *m*D NMR experiments by inserting a refocusing 180° pulse in between the excitation end deexcitation 90° pulses flanking the evolution period.

In this contribution, we describe an approach to the solution of the first data-point problem in the indirectly detected dimensions of *m*D NMR experiments, which is based on the use of a "reverse rotation pulse" $[90°(-x)]^1 = 360° (+x) 270°(-x) - \Delta t$, developed by Freeman et al. [6], for excitation and its in-time inverted, counterpart Δt-$270°(-x)360°(+x)$ for deexcitation in evolution periods of *m*D NMR spectroscopic schemes.

1. Frenkiel T, Bauer C, Carr MD, Birdsall B, Feeney J (1990) *J Magn Reson* **90**: 420.
2. Bax A, Ikura M, Kay LE, Zhu G (1991) *J Magn Reson* **91**: 174.
3. Archer SJ, Boldisseri DM, Torchia DA (1992) *J Magn Reson* **97**: 602.
4. Lippens G, Hallenga K (1990) *J Magn Reson* **88**: 619.
5. Frøystein NA (1993) *J Magn Res Series A* **103**: 332.
6. Freeman R, Friedrich J, Xi-Li W (1988) *J Magn Reson* **79**: 561.

PI14

Image reconstruction from EPR spectra

C.M. SMITH and A.D. STEVENS
*Department of Radiology, Leicester Royal Infirmary,
Leicester LE1 5WW, UK*

This paper shows images which have been reconstructed from EPR spectra obtained from our continuous-wave, 250-MHz, (radio-frequency) EPR spectrometer.

An automatic technique that rotates the nonhorizontal baselines which are caused by stray magnetic effects onto the horizontal axis is explained. This treats each spectrum consistently.

Our results using the convoluted back-projection method show the effect that the deconvolution cutoff frequency has on the image reconstructions (both 2D and 3D).

A slower, indirect, iterative method, which does a nonlinear minimization, is shown to give a very smooth reconstructed image when the method of maximum entropy is used to determine the value of the final residual sum of squares. This method is more flexible than the convoluted back-projection method and overcomes the problem of numerical instability encounted in deconvolution.

Images from phantom samples *in vitro* are discussed. These show that as few as 16 spectra, which have been accumulated quickly and therefore contain much noise, can still be processed to give a good image. Artifacts due to a small number of projections in the convoluted back-projection method which may be removed by a threshold are not present in the maximum entropy reconstruction. Animal *in vivo* images will be included if available.

PI15

Acquisition of simultaneous blood and tissue contrast agent intensity/time curves and quantification to give brain tumour permeability

N.J. TAYLOR, R.A. FOX*, S.F. TANNER
and M.O. LEACH
*C.R.C. Clinical Magnetic Resonance Research Group,
Institute of Cancer Research and Royal Marsden Hospital,
Downs Road, Sutton, Surrey SM2 5PT, UK *Royal Perth
Hospital, Perth 6000, Western Australia*

We have developed an interleaved spin-echo projection and gradient-echo sequence to allow rapid simultaneous monitoring of both the blood input function and image intensities of regions of interest (ROI) within the brain. It provides improved quantification compared with our previous sequence [1], has good spatial and temporal resolution, and can be applied in various body regions.

1D projections are interleaved with the Fourier lines of an image, giving a temporal resolution of 120 ms for the projections. Image time resolution is 34 s for a full 256^2 data set, and 17 s for half-Fourier. The projections are gradient moment refocused, with saturation pulses being used prior to the projection to reduce signal due to inflow effects and ensure that the final signal is proportional to the Gd-DTPA concentration. The full sequence produces 256 projections and 1 image per acquisition, with 15–30 acquisitions per investigation.

The projection intensities corresponding to blood vessels must be corrected by subtracting the contribution arising from overlaying tissue. For brain work, the internal carotid arteries are the most suitable vessels. Blood signal intensities in the projections are corrected for geometrical factors by normalizing to the signal from the blood in the sagittal sinus, obtained with an identical imaging sequence.

All data must be adjusted to compensate for the effects of B_1 inhomogeneity and for tissue-dependent proton densities. Comparing the corrected data with two reference samples placed by the head provides T_1 values which can then be converted to Gd-DTPA concentrations. The software then deconvolves the measured blood curve from the tissue curve. The final curve is then fitted to an adaptation of an existing model [2] for the blood-brain barrier permeability to give values for its rate constants.

Normal volunteers were imaged without Gd-DTPA in the head coil of our 1.5-T clinical MR scanner to test the sequence and method. These measurements were followed by preliminary clinical studies, which indicate the viability of the method, giving clear concentration/time curves which can be successfully fitted to the model.

1. Taylor NJ et al. (1993) *Magn Reson Med* **30**: 744–750.
2. Tofts, Kermode (1991) *Magn Reson Med* **17**: 357–367.

PC01

MRI criteria for spinal cord surgical decompression

S.S. RABINOVICH, G.P. STRELTSOVA
and M.U. SIZIKOV
*Research Institute of Traumatology, International
Tomography Center, Novosibirsk, Russia*

Treatment effectiveness of traumatically caused spinal

cord (SC) compression can be prognosed by MRI. We conducted retrospective study of decompressive surgery on 42 patients with spine and spinal cord injuries (SSCI). Neurological deficit was appraised in the Frankel scale. MRI was conducted in 30 days after the trauma for 6 patients, in 6–8 months after the trauma for 17 patients, and in some years after the trauma for 11 patients. Eight patients in the residual period of SSCI underwent bypass surgery after MRI. Received MRI scans have been appraised using the following criteria: status of spine itself (discs and centrums); spine and SC relations; and SC and liquor space status. Compression degree by the Takahashy method was appraised: 0–10%, as small; 11–39%; as middle; 40% and over, as considerable. SC safety and injuried place structural changes have been studied too. All patients underwent bypass surgery, either ventral or dorsal stabilization of the injuried spinal segment with SC decompression simultaneously. If SC compression is small (up to 10%), a good clinical result of SC decompression was observed even in the residual period of trauma cases. In 16 patients with middle degree of SC compression, surgery brings nonsignificant improvement. Our results correlate with the data of Silberstein et al. (1992) in acute SSCI. Top valuable MRI is in case of SC contusion process, always preceded with the phenomena of SC tissue ischemia. MRI allows us to trace the dynamics of the ischemic square development. MRI control is of special importance in surgery of ischemia by means of omentum transplantation for SC revascularization. Thus, MRI is the valuable method for studying of relations between SC and spine. SC compression degree, calculated by MRI, under conditions of SC surviving can be a prognostical criterium. The same applies for surgery in the concrete case. It must be admitted that SC compression detected by MRI coupled with its atrophia is a bad prognostic symptom.

PC02

Exercise-related changes in aortic flow measured by spiral echo-planar phase-shift velocity mapping
R.H. MOHIADDIN, P.D. GATEHOUSE
and D.N. FIRMIN
Royal Brompton Hospital, London, UK

Conventional cardiovascular magnetic resonance is limited by its inability to acquire reliable images during dynamic exercise. Although different forms of stress are available, dynamic exercise is preferable, as it simulates the stress experienced by the patient in

everyday life. We used spiral echo-planar velocity mapping to measure exercise-related changes of aortic flow in 10 healthy volunteers. Flow in the descending thoracic aorta was measured at rest and immediately following dynamic exercise using a 0.5-T machine with a surface receiving coil and ECG triggering. Supine dynamic exercise was performed using a pedaling system designed and built by the authors. Resting spiral velocity mapping was acquired in a transverse plane transecting the descending thoracic aorta. The subjects were asked to perform maximum exercise, then to stop and hold their breath during a single heart-beat acquisition time. Eight cine frames with a temporal resolution of 50 ms were acquired through systole. Each image was acquired in 40 ms during a spiral trajectory of k-space starting at the center 8 ms after the RF excitation. Flow was computed from aortic mean velocity and cross-sectional area. The field of view was 30 cm, slice thickness was 10 mm, and reconstructed images were 64^2. Reproducibility of the technique was established by repeating the flow measurement in four consecutive heart beats. At rest, the heart rate (mean $\pm$ SD), mean aortic flow, peak aortic flow, and the time to peak flow were 68.0 ± 6.0 beats min^{-1}, 40.7 ± 7.5 ml beat^{-1}, 107.0 ± 20.0 ml s^{-1} and 175.0 ± 25.0 ms, respectively. These parameters were similar in the four consecutive resting heart beats. Following exercise, the heart rate and mean and peak aortic flows were significantly increased, measuring 101.0 ± 12.0 beats min^{-1}, 56.7 ± 10.7 ml min^{-1}, and 157.9 ± 29.3 ml s^{-1}, respectively, whereas the time to peak flow (115.0 ± 32.0 ms) was significantly reduced. We have demonstrated the feasibility of using spiral echo-planar velocity mapping to measure aortic flow at rest and have demonstrated the expected changes in aortic flow following dynamic exercise. The clinical application of this method will depend on the availability of equipments and the refinement of the technique.

PC03

Obstetric echo-planar imaging
V. ADAMS, P. GOWLAND, P. HARVEY,
A. FREEMAN, J. HYKIN, P. BAKER, I. JOHNSON,
B. WORTHINGTON and P. MANSFIELD
Magnetic Resonance Centre, University of Nottingham, Nottingham, NG7 2RD, UK

Thirty-two singleton pregnancies were scanned using echo-planar magnetic resonance imaging (EPI). All pregnancies were suffering complications, 11 of which

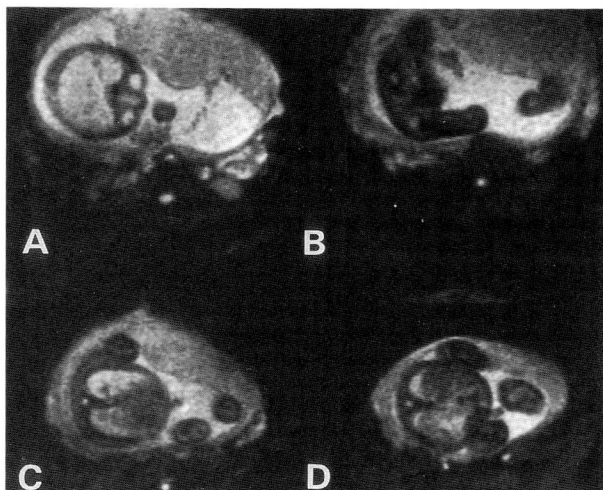

Transectional snapshot image through a fetus *in utero* at 36 weeks' gestation. (A) Section through brain and orbits; (B) section through shoulders; (C) section through lungs; (D) section through bowel.

were found at birth to be growth retarded. Gestational age ranged from 23 weeks to term. Problems caused by fetal motion are overcome by EPI, enabling acquisition of a full set of images through the uterus in 10 s, each image taking only 100 ms.

Volumes of fetal organs, placenta, amniotic fluid, and the entire uterus were measured and growth profiles formed. Measurements and observations were compared with ultrasound results and fetal outcome.

The first T_1 maps of a few selected pregnancies have been obtained in order to investigate the possibility of providing information about perfusion and structural development in the fetus and placenta.

We are grateful to Action Research for initial funding of the obstetric work and to MRC for support of the EPI program.

1. Mansfield P, Stehling M, Ordidge et al. (1990) *Br J Radiol* **63:** 833–841.

PC04

MRI of interstitial laser photocoagulation in breast cancer
M. CLEMENCE, S.A. HARRIES, Z. AMIN,
W.M.W. GEDROYC* and S.G. BOWN
National Medical Laser Centre, London, UK
St. Mary's Hospital, London, UK

There is increasing interest in the technique of interstitial laser photocoagulation (ILP) for percutaneous tumor destruction. The technique is being studied for application to the treatment of early breast cancer where it could potentially replace lumpectomy. Clearly, ILP would have no clinical application unless some form of imaging technique were available that could accurately predict the extent of the laser damage. MRI is emerging as an ideal method for both monitor and follow-up.

Forty-two patients have had ILP before surgery. Initially, ultrasound was used to monitor the therapy but was unsatisfactory. Five patients have undergone pre-ILP and 24-h post-ILP MRI evaluation to investigate the potential of this imaging technique. MRI was performed using a gradient-echo sequence with fat suppression on a GE Signa 1.5-T system and the GE breast coil, both with and without a Gd-DTPA contrast agent. Subsequent surgery made the lesion available for comparison between imaging and histology.

The results demonstrate that with a contrast agent good correlation can be obtained between the imaging and histological specimen. MRI shows considerable promise as an accurate predictor of the extent of laser-induced necrosis and is currently undergoing further evaluation.

PC05

Spinal complications of ankylosing spondylitis—MR assessment
J.S. DAWSON, K.J. FAIRBAIRN, J.K. WEBB,
K. LLOYD JONES and B.J. PRESTON
University Hospital, Nottingham, UK

The precise role of MR in the assessment of ankylosing spondylitis has not been defined. We present the MR findings in patients presenting with the spinal complications of ankylosing spondylitis. In a 2-year study period (1991–1993), there were 14 patients (11 M, 3 F) with a mean age of 48.7 years (range 27–63 years). Most patients had long-standing and advanced disease. Sagittal and axial MR images of the spine (T_1 and T_2 weighted) were obtained using either a surface coil or a body coil. The spinal complications of ankylosing spondylitis had either a traumatic or a nontraumatic etiology. Traumatic complications included fracture, extradural hematoma, cord contusion, posttraumatic syrinx, and pseudoarthrosis. Nontraumatic complications featured deformity, disco-vertebral inflammatory lesions, atlanto-axial subluxation, cauda equina syndrome, and accelerated disc degeneration/osteoarthritic change adjacent to fused spinal segments ("last joint" syndrome). Recognition of the spinal complications associated with ankylosing spondylitis is important. MR appears to be uniquely suited to this task and can evaluate all the relevant anatomical structures (vertebrae, spinal ligaments, intervertebral discs, vertebral joints, thecal sac, extradural space, and spinal cord) in a noninvasive manner.

PS01

Accuracy of time-domain data analysis in ^{31}P-MRS—tissue-like phantom studies

M. WYLEZINSKA and E.B. CADY
Department of Medical Physics and Bioengineering, University College London Medical School, London, UK

For clinical application, reliable estimates of metabolites absolute concentration are required. These values may depend on data processing techniques, particularly if the S/N is low.

The purpose of this work was to investigate the performance of three time-domain data analysis methods applied for absolute concentrations quantification, using a tissue substitute phantom.

Methods: The phantom used, was a $10 \times 10 \times 10$-cm^3 Perspex cube, filled with tissue substitute material with known metabolite concentrations [1] mimicking ^{31}P spectrum obtained from normal neonatal brain.

All spectra were collected on a 2.4 T Bruker Biospec, using 9 cm surface coil and single pulse-acquire sequence (TR 30s). For absolute quantification, load—matched standard phantom, calibration protocol [2] was applied. Each of FID signal was analyzed using three techniques: LPSVD, HSVD, VARPRO.

Results and conclusions: PCr concentrations in mM [mean (propagated CR errors)] obtained for different data analysis methods were:

Noise	LPSVD	HSVD	VARPRO	True [PCr] = 1.56
20%	1.42 (0.25)	1.44 (0.16)	1.60 (0.36)	
50%	1.21 (0.39)	1.13 (0.49)	1.50 (0.35)	
90%	1.08 (1.05)	1.84 (1.33)	1.62 (0.73)	

Noise standard deviation was given as a percentage of PCr amplitude. It can be seen that VARPRO gave most accurate values. LPSVD tended to give too low concentrations, while HSVD gave too high values at low S/N.

We also found that number of points truncated had an effect on quantification results.

Acknowledgment: We are grateful to R. de Beer for supplying the VARPRO software.

1. Wylezinska MM, Cady EB (1992) Proc. SMRM 11th Annual Meeting, p. 4268.
2. Buchli R et al. (1992) Proc. SMRM 11th Annual Meeting, p. 1903.

PS02

Alterations in glucose transport during development and regression of cardiac hypertrophy

N.S. BHUTTA, J.F. UNITT* and A-ML SEYMOUR
*M.R.S. Group, N.H.L.I. at Harefield Hospital, *Department of Biochemistry, Fisons Pharmaceuticals, Loughborough, UK Harefield, UK*

Cardiac hypertrophy (HT) is the adaptive response of the heart to chronic overload and is characterized by an increased capacity for glycolysis. We have investigated the rate of glucose uptake and phosphorylation (GUP) and energy status in HT, regression from HT (R), and control (C) rat hearts using ^{31}P-NMR. The model used was the hyperthyroid rat, induced by daily administration of thyroxine (T4) [35 µg/100g BW] over 7 days. Regression of HT was produced by discontinuing T4 administration for a further week. Hearts were perfused in the isovolumic Langendorff mode, initially with 5 mM glucose as substrate and subsequently with 5 mM glucose + 1 mM 2-deoxyglucose (2-DOG). The initial rate of GUP [µmol min^{-1} (g wet wt)$^{-1}$] was measured by following the accumulation of 2-DOG-6-P in the ^{31}P spectrum.

	C ($n = 6$)	HT ($n = 3$)	R ($n = 5$)
Hwt : T1	0.46	0.54	0.50
*PCr	5.39	4.72	6.35
*P$_i$	1.44	2.08	1.40
GUP	0.06	0.23	0.16

*µmol (g wet wt.)$^{-1}$

Results are given as the mean from n experiments (Hwt : T1, heart weight : tibia length). These results suggest that in the hyperthyroid model of HT, glucose uptake is increased and, following regression, returns to control, as do the changes in high-energy phosphates. Thus, the metabolic adaptations accompanying HT are reversible upon regression of HT.

PS03

^{13}C-NMR spectroscopic measurements of oxidative flux in the denervated canine myocardium

S.B. CLARKE*, A.J. DRAKE-HOLLAND, M.H. YACOUB, M.I.M. NOBLE* and A-ML SEYMOUR
M.R.S. Group, N.H.L.I. at Harefield Hospital, Harefield, UK
*AUCVM, *Department of Medicine, Charing Cross* and Westminster Medical School, Westminster, UK

The chronically denervated dog heart (DN) has a higher oxygen consumption for the same amount of external work than control (C). This observation suggests that oxidative metabolism in the DN myocardium may be altered. We have determined the oxidative flux through the tricarboxylic acid (TCA) cycle using [13]C-2 acetate as a substrate analogue of fatty acids and ^{13}C-NMR in DN and C hearts. The *in vivo* characteristics of acetate uptake by the myocardium were measured separately and found to parallel those of lactate. Dogs were denervated by the method of surgical regional neuroablation at least 3 weeks prior to experimentation. Two grams of [13]C-2 acetate were administered intravenously over a period of 20 min to DN or C dogs. Subsequently, a sample of heart tissue was removed and rapidly frozen. Tissue extracts were analyzed using proton-decoupled ^{13}C-NMR. The incorporation of the ^{13}C label into the C-4 and C-2 positions of glutamate was measured and the ratio of ^{13}C-labeled C-2/C-4 used as an index of oxidative flux. DN ratio = 0.61 ($n = 2$) and C ratio = 2.18 ($n = 2$). These data suggest that the metabolism of the DN myocardium differs from that of C and that oxidation of acetate (and fatty acids) via the TCA cycle may be reduced in the DN myocardium.

PS04

Quantitation of the effects of an aldose reductase inhibitor in peripheral nerve using ^{13}C-NMR

S.A. BREEN, C.M. SENNITT, D.J. MIRRLEES, F. CAREY and J.C. WATERTON
Zeneca Pharmaceuticals, Alderley Park, Macclesfield, Cheshire SK10 4TG, UK.

In diabetes, an increased flux through the sorbitol pathway via activation of aldose reductase by hyperglycemia is associated with detrimental effects in the lens, nerve, and other tissues. Aldose reductase (ALR) catalyzes the conversion of glucose or galactose to sorbitol or dulcitol. ALR is active in human nerve, and sorbitol accumulation has been verified in this tissue. Treatment with aldose reductase inhibitors (ARIs) could therefore, potentially, diminish the detrimental side effects of diabetes. ^{13}C-NMR spectroscopy has previously been used to measure ARI flux in lens [1, 2]. We now report studies in peripheral nerve.

Quantitation of enzyme flux in isolated peripheral rat nerve was achieved using 1-^{13}C galactose as substrate, measuring the rate of production of 1-^{13}C dulcitol. NMR spectra were recorded on a Brüker AM400 spectrometer incorporating a 10-mm broadband probe, using both internal extracellular and external standards (respectively polyvinylpyrrolidone and silicone).

The sulphonylnitromethane ARI, 3,5-dimethyl-4-((nitromethyl)sulphonyl)-benzenamine proved to be an effective inhibitor of ALR flux at a concentration of 100 μM. The mean net forward flux was 4.1 ± 2.3 nmol (ml nerve water)$^{-1}$ min^{-1}. In the presence of the inhibitor, flux was reduced significantly ($P < 0.001$) to 14% of control. Because dulcitol is symmetrical, an estimate of the backward flux, to 6-^{13}C galactose, is also possible. Under our conditions, this was negligible.

1. Earl D, Mirrlees D, Pickford R, Slater AM, Sheard B (1978) 8th International Congress on Magnetic Resonance in Biological Systems.
2. Williams WF, Odom JD (1986) *Science* **233**: 223.

PS05

Manipulation of the physiology of murine tumors monitored by *in vivo* ^{31}P-MRS

P.J. WOOD, J.M. SANSOM, J.C.M. BREMNER, I.J. STRATFORD and G.E. ADAMS
MRC Radiobiology Unit, Chilton, Didcot, Oxon OX11 ORD, **UK**

One novel approach to improvement of anticancer therapies is the manipulation of tumor oxygenation by vasoactive agents. Increased tumor hypoxia may improve the efficiency of bioreductive cytotoxic agents, which require a hypoxic environment for activity. Conversely, increased tumor oxygenation may improve sensitivity to X-rays.

The metabolic response of experimental murine tumors KHT, RIF-1, and SCCVII to vasoactive agents was monitored by *in vivo* ^{31}P MRS. A 4.7-T, 30-cm horizontal bore magnet was used for these studies, with a 7-mm surface coil placed over the tumor on the mouse back. Mice were anesthetized for experiments using Hypnorm/Hypnovel, or unanesthetized but restrained in jigs. Spectra were analyzed using a baseline and Lorentzian curve-fitting program, and data were expressed as the ratio of the inorganic phosphate peak area to the sum of all peak areas or P_i/total.

Increased tumor hypoxia was observed as a reduction in ATP; thus, P_i total was increased and was brought about by agents such as the vasodilator hydralazine at 5 mg kg^{-1} I.V. and the nitric oxide synthase inhibitor, nitro-L-arginine at 10 mg kg^{-1} I.V. The increases in hypoxia were sufficient to enhance the cytotoxicity of bioreductive drugs such as RB 6145.

Increased tumor oxygenation was observed as a reduction in P_i/total and was brought about by agents such as the calcium antagonist flunarizine at 5 mg kg^{-1} I.P. and the nitric oxide donor SIN-1 at 2 mg kg^{-1} I.V. These agents also increase tumor sensitivity to X-rays.

Clearly, *in vivo* ^{31}P-MRS is a useful technique for determining the metabolic responses of tumors to physiological manipulation, with the aim of evaluating agents as potential adjuncts to conventional anticancer therapies.

PS06

Use of ^{31}P-MRS and ^{2}H uptake studies to assess novel photosensitisers used in photodynamic therapy of murine tumors

J.K. BRADLEY, J.C.M. BREMNER, I.J. STRATFORD,
S. BROWN,* S. WOOD* and G.E. ADAMS
MRC Radiobiology Unit, Oxon OX11 0RD,
Department of Biochemistry and Molecular Biology, Leeds University, Leeds LS2 9JT, UK

Photodynamic therapy (PDT) consists of the systemic administration of a photosensitiser followed by localized irradiation of the tumor with monochromatic light from an optical fiber. The cytotoxic effects of this treatment are both by direct cell killing and indirectly following severe damage to the tumor vasculature.

Using a fiber-optic setup in the magnet, we have made measurements of phosphorus metabolism before, during, and up to 24 h after irradiation for a number of novel phthalocyanine photosensitizers. These have been compared with aluminium disulphonated phthalocyanine and photofrin. ^{31}P-MRS of the tumor has shown that the rate and duration of the increase in P_i and concomitant decrease in ATP are highly dependent on the photosensitizer used and its physical location in the tumor at the time of irradiation.

We have also evaluated the ^{2}H tracer uptake technique for measuring tumor blood flow (TBF) and found it compares well with results obtained from other tracer techniques [1]. In these experiments, TBF readings are made before, immediately after, and 1 and 24 h postirradiation. We have observed very rapid decreases in TBF which can remain low for 24 h. We have seen that the extent of decrease in TBF varies between photosensitizers used and correlates well with the changes seen in phosphorus metabolism.

^{31}P-MRS and ^{2}H-MRS are proving very useful for comparing the action of different photosensitizers.

1. Bradley JK et al. (in press). *Nuclear Magn Reson Biomed.*

PS07

[Ca^{2+}]$_i$ and the energy state during cerebral metabolic insults

N.M. THATCHER, R.S. BADAR GOFFER,
P.G. MORRIS and H.S. BACHELARD
M.R. Centre, University of Nottingham, Nottingham NG7 2RD, UK

In order to investigate the mixed biochemical insult of ischemia, we have followed the effects of mild hypoglycemia and moderate hypoxia on free intracellular calcium [Ca^{2+}]$_i$ (using the ^{19}F-NMR calcium indicator 5FBAPTA) and the energy state (by ^{31}P-NMR) in superfused guinea pig cerebral cortical slices.

With the single insults of hypoxia or hypoglycemia, [Ca^{2+}]$_i$ did not increase above control values (there was an initial decrease in hypoxia), and decreases in PCr which reversed on return to control conditions were observed. The combined insult was introduced either sequentially, following the single insult of hypoxia or hypoglycemia, or directly after control spectra had been acquired. When preceded by the single insult, an increase in [Ca^{2+}]$_i$ to 100% above control was observed with a large decrease in PCr and ATP and only slight recovery. When the tissues were subjected to the immediate combined insult, the increase in [Ca^{2+}]$_i$ was much higher, to 350% above control, with PCr reduced, and again with only a slight recovery.

That [Ca^{2+}]$_i$ did not increase with hypoxia or hypoglycemia was contrary to current excitotoxic hypotheses which propose a role for increases in [Ca^{2+}]$_i$ in cell death resulting from these insults. An increase in [Ca^{2+}]$_i$ was only observed with the combined insult which was much more severe when introduced immediately than when preceded by the single insult. This indicates some sort of adaption of the cerebral tissue slices to the single insult, rendering them less vulnerable to the combined insult.

PS08

Changes in ^{31}P spectrum of serum of patients with myeloma multiplex during chemotherapy

M. KULISZKIEWICZ-JANUS* and S. BACZYŃSKI**
*Department of Haematology, Medical University, Wroolaw, Poland
**Institute of Chemistry, University of Wroolaw, Poland

^{31}P spectra were performed in 21 healthy volunteers and 20 patients with multiple myeloma on the beginning of the disease and were repeated up to five times during therapy. Studies were carried out on AMX 300 Brüker spectroscope. Spectra were obtained using an interpulse delay of 40 s. As a reference compound, 85% ortophosporus acid was applied. All spectra consisted of an inorganic phosphate (P_i) peak (considered as a rise pattern) and two peaks from phospholipids (PL): phosphatidylcholine (PC) and phosphatidylethanolamine (PE) with sphingomyelin (SM).

Prior to therapy, all ^{31}P spectra showed strongly reduced peak areas at intensities from phospholipids. During therapy resulting in remission resonance from PL progressively increased, resembling the shape received from a healthy sera. Long-term follow-up ^{31}P-MRS studies showed a good correlation between evaluation of MRS parameters and response of the disease to the therapy.

By acquiring ^{31}P spectra it is possible to characterize phospholipid metabolism of cancers. Our results showed significant correlations between area and intensities of two peaks of PL and of HDL concentrations (correlation coefficient 0.44, 0.42, 0.58, respectively; P-level <0.001). Moreover, we found a statistically significant decline of concentration of HDL in serum of patients with multiple myeloma, which statistically increased in the response patient. In patients not responding to the therapy, HDL concentration did not change significantly.

PS09

Observation of amino acid labeling in the human brain by localized ^{13}C-NMR

R. GRUETTER, G.F. MASON, D.L. ROTHMAN,
E.J. NOVOTNY, S.D. BOULWARE, G.I. SHULMAN,
J.W. PRICHARD and R.G. SHULMAN
Yale University, New Haven, Connecticut, USA

Cerebral metabolism of [1-^{13}C] D-glucose was studied with localized ^{13}C-NMR spectroscopy during intravenous infusion of enriched glucose in four healthy subjects aged 18–22 years.

The use of a three-dimensional localization resulted in the complete elimination of triacylglycerol resonances, which originated in scalp and subcutaneous fat. The sensitivity and spectral resolution were sufficient to allow a 4-min time-resolved observation of label incorporation into the resolved C3 and C4 resonances of glutamate and C4 resonance of glutamine, as well as C3 of aspartate with lower time resolution. C4 glutamate labeled rapidly reaching close to maximum labeling at 60 min, yielding a Krebs cycle rate of 0. mM min^{-1}. The label flow into C3 glutamate clearly lagged behind that of C4 glutamate and peaked at a similar value at 110–140 min, consistent with a 50-fold faster α-ketoglutarate–glutamate exchange rate compared to the Krebs cycle rate.

A slight but significant lag of glutamine C4 behind glutamate C4 consistent with rapid glutamine synthesis in the human brain above 0.5 mM min^{-1}.

Doublets due to homonuclear ^{13}C–^{13}C coupling between the C3 and C4 peaks of the glutamate molecule were observed *in vivo*. Isotopomer analysis yielded a ^{13}C isotopic fraction at C4 glutamate of 27 $\pm$ 2%, which was 4.5% less than half of the enrichment of plasma glucose ($P < 0.05$).

Quantification of glutamate C4 was performed by comparison with an external standard giving 2.4 $\pm$ 0.1 mM. Combined with the isotopomer analysis, a minimum estimate for the total brain glutamate concentration of 9.1 mM was calculated. Similarly, minimum total brain concentration was estimated for glutamine at 4.3 mM, for GABA at 1.2 mM, and for aspartate at 1.0 mM. These values are consistent with quantification of respective total brain concentrations by other methods. The agreement suggests that chemically inert pools are small, and almost all of the carbon is derived from plasma glucose in healthy human brain.

Index*

*Italic page numbers indicate illustrations.